Health Care for Older Adults

Health Care for Older Adults

Editors

**Francisco José Tarazona Santabalbina
Sebastià Josep Santaeugènia Gonzàlez
José Augusto García Navarro
José Viña**

MDPI • Basel • Beijing • Wuhan • Barcelona • Belgrade • Manchester • Tokyo • Cluj • Tianjin

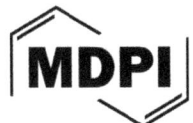

Editors
Francisco José Tarazona Santabalbina
Hospital Universitario de la Ribera
Spain

Sebastià Josep Santaeugènia Gonzàlez
Generalitat de Catalunya
Spain

José Augusto García Navarro Spanish
Society of Geriatrics and Gerontology
Spain

José Viña
University of Valencia
Spain

Editorial Office
MDPI
St. Alban-Anlage 66
4052 Basel, Switzerland

This is a reprint of articles from the Special Issue published online in the open access journal *International Journal of Environmental Research and Public Health* (ISSN 1660-4601) (available at: https://www.mdpi.com/journal/ijerph/special_issues/_health_care_for_older_adults).

For citation purposes, cite each article independently as indicated on the article page online and as indicated below:

LastName, A.A.; LastName, B.B.; LastName, C.C. Article Title. *Journal Name* **Year**, *Volume Number*, Page Range.

ISBN 978-3-0365-1823-7 (Hbk)
ISBN 978-3-0365-1824-4 (PDF)

© 2021 by the authors. Articles in this book are Open Access and distributed under the Creative Commons Attribution (CC BY) license, which allows users to download, copy and build upon published articles, as long as the author and publisher are properly credited, which ensures maximum dissemination and a wider impact of our publications.

The book as a whole is distributed by MDPI under the terms and conditions of the Creative Commons license CC BY-NC-ND.

Contents

About the Editors ix

Francisco José Tarazona-Santabalbina, Sebastià Josep Santaeugènia Gonzàlez, José Augusto García Navarro and Jose Viña
Healthcare for Older Adults, Where Are We Moving towards?
Reprinted from: *Int. J. Environ. Res. Public Health* **2021**, *18*, 6219, doi:10.3390/ijerph18126219 . . . 1

Ho-Jin Shin, Sung-Hyeon Kim, Suk-Chan Hahm and Hwi-Young Cho
Thermotherapy Plus Neck Stabilization Exercise for Chronic Nonspecific Neck Pain in Elderly: A Single-Blinded Randomized Controlled Trial
Reprinted from: *Int. J. Environ. Res. Public Health* **2020**, *17*, 5572, doi:10.3390/ijerph17155572 . . . 5

Chien-Ying Lee, Yih-Dih Cheng, Wei-Yuan Cheng, Tung-Han Tsai and Kuang-Hua Huang
The Prevalence of Anticholinergic Drugs and Correlation with Pneumonia in Elderly Patients: A Population-Based Study in Taiwan
Reprinted from: *Int. J. Environ. Res. Public Health* **2020**, *17*, 6260, doi:10.3390/ijerph17176260 . . . 17

Charmaine Childs, Jennifer Elliott, Khaled Khatab, Susan Hampshaw, Sally Fowler-Davis, Jon R. Willmott and Ali Ali
Thermal Sensation in Older People with and without Dementia Living in Residential Care: New Assessment Approaches to Thermal Comfort Using Infrared Thermography
Reprinted from: *Int. J. Environ. Res. Public Health* **2020**, *17*, 6932, doi:10.3390/ijerph17186932 . . . 31

Laura M. Pérez, Carmina Castellano-Tejedor, Matteo Cesari, Luis Soto-Bagaria, Joan Ars, Fabricio Zambom-Ferraresi, Sonia Baró, Francisco Díaz-Gallego, Jordi Vilaró, María B. Enfedaque, Paula Espí-Valbé and Marco Inzitari
Depressive Symptoms, Fatigue and Social Relationships Influenced Physical Activity in Frail Older Community-Dwellers during the Spanish Lockdown due to the COVID-19 Pandemic
Reprinted from: *Int. J. Environ. Res. Public Health* **2021**, *18*, 808, doi:10.3390/ijerph18020808 . . . 53

Hana Ko and SuJung Jung
Association of Social Frailty with Physical Health, Cognitive Function, Psychological Health, and Life Satisfaction in Community-Dwelling Older Koreans
Reprinted from: *Int. J. Environ. Res. Public Health* **2021**, *18*, 818, doi:10.3390/ijerph18020818 . . . 67

Boyuan Chen and Sohee Shi
Bibliometric Analysis on Research Trend of Accidental Falls in Older Adults by Using Citespace—Focused on Web of Science Core Collection (2010–2020)
Reprinted from: *Int. J. Environ. Res. Public Health* **2021**, *18*, 1663, doi:10.3390/ijerph18041663 . . . 77

José Luis García-Giménez, Salvador Mena-Molla, Francisco José Tarazona-Santabalbina, Jose Viña, Mari Carmen Gomez-Cabrera and Federico V. Pallardó
Implementing Precision Medicine in Human Frailty through Epigenetic Biomarkers
Reprinted from: *Int. J. Environ. Res. Public Health* **2021**, *18*, 1883, doi:10.3390/ijerph18041883 . . . 95

Francisco José Tarazona-Santabalbina, Cristina Ojeda-Thies, Jesús Figueroa Rodríguez, Concepción Cassinello-Ogea and José Ramón Caeiro
Orthogeriatric Management: Improvements in Outcomes during Hospital Admission Due to Hip Fracture
Reprinted from: *Int. J. Environ. Res. Public Health* **2021**, *18*, 3049, doi:10.3390/ijerph18063049 . . . 113

Cristina González de Villaumbrosia, Pilar Sáez López, Isaac Martín de Diego,
Carmen Lancho Martín, Marina Cuesta Santa Teresa, Teresa Alarcón, Cristina Ojeda Thies,
Rocío Queipo Matas, Juan Ignacio González-Montalvo and
on behalf of the Participants in the Spanish National Hip Fracture Registry
Predictive Model of Gait Recovery at One Month after Hip Fracture from a National Cohort of 25,607 Patients: The Hip Fracture Prognosis (HF-Prognosis) Tool
Reprinted from: *Int. J. Environ. Res. Public Health* **2021**, *18*, 3809, doi:10.3390/ijerph18073809 . . . **143**

Anna Torné, Emma Puigoriol, Edurne Zabaleta-del-Olmo, Juan-José Zamora-Sánchez,
Sebastià Santaeugènia and Jordi Amblàs-Novellas
Reliability, Validity, and Feasibility of the Frail-VIG Index
Reprinted from: *Int. J. Environ. Res. Public Health* **2021**, *18*, 5187, doi:10.3390/ijerph18105187 . . . **161**

Laura Coll-Planas, Dolors Rodríguez-Arjona, Mariona Pons-Vigués, Fredrica Nyqvist,
Teresa Puig and Rosa Monteserín
"Not Alone in Loneliness": A Qualitative Evaluation of a Program Promoting Social Capital among Lonely Older People in Primary Health Care
Reprinted from: *Int. J. Environ. Res. Public Health* **2021**, *18*, 5580, doi:10.3390/ijerph18115580 . . **175**

Nicolás M. González-Senac, Jennifer Mayordomo-Cava, Angela Macías-Valle,
Paula Aldama-Marín, Sara Majuelos González, María Luisa Cruz Arnés, Luis M. Jiménez-Gómez,
María T. Vidán-Astiz and José Antonio Serra-Rexach
Colorectal Cancer in Elderly Patients with Surgical Indication: State of the Art, Current Management, Role of Frailty and Benefits of a Geriatric Liaison
Reprinted from: *Int. J. Environ. Res. Public Health* **2021**, *18*, 6072, doi:10.3390/ijerph18116072 . . . **195**

Keisuke Fujii, Yuya Fujii, Yuta Kubo, Korin Tateoka, Jue Liu, Koki Nagata,
Shuichi Wakayama and Tomohiro Okura
Association between Occupational Dysfunction and Social Isolation in Japanese Older Adults:
A Cross-Sectional Study
Reprinted from: *Int. J. Environ. Res. Public Health* **2021**, *18*, 6648, doi:10.3390/ijerph18126648 . . . **217**

Kyosuke Oki, Yoichiro Ogino, Yuriko Takamoto, Mikio Imai, Yoko Takemura,
Yasunori Ayukawa and Kiyoshi Koyano
The Significance of Posterior Occlusal Support of Teeth and Removable Prostheses in Oral Functions and Standing Motion
Reprinted from: *Int. J. Environ. Res. Public Health* **2021**, *18*, 6776, doi:10.3390/ijerph18136776 . . . **227**

Nath Adulkasem, Phichayut Phinyo, Jiraporn Khorana, Dumnoensun Pruksakorn and
Theerachai Apivatthakakul
Prognostic Factors of 1-Year Postoperative Functional Outcomes of Older Patients with Intertrochanteric Fractures in Thailand: A Retrospective Cohort Study
Reprinted from: *Int. J. Environ. Res. Public Health* **2021**, *18*, 6896, doi:10.3390/ijerph18136896 . . . **239**

Valentina Buda, Andreea Prelipcean, Carmen Cristescu, Alexandru Roja,
Olivia Dalleur, Minodora Andor, Corina Danciu, Adriana Ledeti,
Cristina Adriana Dehelean and Octavian Cretu
Prescription Habits Related to Chronic Pathologies of Elderly People in Primary Care in the Western Part of Romania: Current Practices, International Recommendations, and Future Perspectives Regarding the Overuse and Misuse of Medicines
Reprinted from: *Int. J. Environ. Res. Public Health* **2021**, *18*, 7043, doi:10.3390/ijerph18137043 . . . **253**

Honoria Ocagli, Daniele Bottigliengo, Giulia Lorenzoni, Danila Azzolina, Aslihan S. Acar, Silvia Sorgato, Lucia Stivanello, Mario Degan and Dario Gregori
A Machine Learning Approach for Investigating Delirium as a Multifactorial Syndrome
Reprinted from: *Int. J. Environ. Res. Public Health* **2021**, *18*, 7105, doi:10.3390/ijerph18137105 . . . **273**

About the Editors

Francisco José Tarazona Santabalbina, MD, PhD. Specialist in Geriatric Medicine, he is associate professor Catholic University of Valencia. Member of Executive board of Spanish Society of Geriatrics and Gerontology (SEGG), he is Finance Director European Geriatric Medicine Society (EUGMS) too. He has published more than 50 papers on geriatrics in indexed journals.

Sebastià Josep Santaeugènia Gonzàlez, MD, PhD, MHA. Specialist in Internal Medicine. Member of the Central Catalonia Chronicity Research Group (C3RG), Centre for Health and Social Care Research (CESS), Universitat de Vic–University of Vic-Central University of Catalonia (UVIC-UCC). He has published more than 40 papers on geriatric and palliative care indexed journals.

José Augusto García Navarro, MD, PhD. Specialist in Geriatric Medicine. He is President of the Spanish Society of Geriatrics and Gerontology (SEGG) and General Director of the Health and Social Consortium of Catalonia.

José Viña was born in Valencia, Spain. After pursuing his studies in Medicine at the University of Valencia, and doing research work under Prof Hans Krebs in Oxford, he obtained his PhD in 1976. He taught Physiology at Extremadura University and then returned to Valencia and took up his present position as full Professor of Physiology at the University of Valencia. Here Prof. Viña combines his teaching duties with research work, the latter in two main lines, ageing and exercise. José Viña leads a successful research group named FRESHAGE working on different aspects of ageing, including healthy ageing, exercise, and Alzheimer's disease.

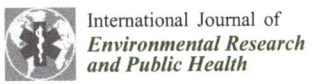

Editorial

Healthcare for Older Adults, Where Are We Moving towards?

Francisco José Tarazona-Santabalbina [1,2,*], Sebastià Josep Santaeugènia Gonzàlez [3,4], José Augusto García Navarro [5,6] and Jose Viña [2,7]

1. Departmanet of Geriatric Medicine, Hospital Universitario de la Ribera, Carretera de Corbera km 1, 46600 Alzira, Spain
2. Centro de Investigación Biomédica en Red Fragilidad y Envejecimiento Saludable (CIBERFES), 28029 Madrid, Spain; jose.vina@uv.es
3. Chronic Care Program, Health Department, Generalitat de Catalunya, 08002 Barcelona, Spain; sebastia.santaeugenia@gencat.cat
4. Central Catalonia Chronicity Research Group (C3RG), Centre for Health and Social Care Research (CESS), Universitat de Vic–University of Vic-Central University of Catalonia (UVIC-UCC), C. Miquel Martí i Pol, 1, 08500 Vic, Spain
5. Consorci de Salut i Social de Catalunya, 08022 Barcelona, Spain; jagarcia@segg.es
6. Spanish Society of Geriatrics and Gerontology, 28006 Madrid, Spain
7. Freshage Research Group, Department of Physiology, Faculty of Medicine, Institute of Health Research-INCLIVA, University of Valencia, 46010 Valencia, Spain
* Correspondence: Tarazona_frasan@gva.es

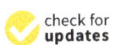

Citation: Tarazona-Santabalbina, F.J.; Santaeugènia Gonzàlez, S.J.; García Navarro, J.A.; Viña, J. *Healthcare for Older Adults, Where We Moving towards?*. IJERPH **2021**, *18*, 6219. https://doi.org/10.3390/ijerph18126219

Received: 2 June 2021
Accepted: 3 June 2021
Published: 8 June 2021

Publisher's Note: MDPI stays neutral with regard to jurisdictional claims in published maps and institutional affiliations.

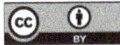

Copyright: © 2021 by the authors. Licensee MDPI, Basel, Switzerland. This article is an open access article distributed under the terms and conditions of the Creative Commons Attribution (CC BY) license (https://creativecommons.org/licenses/by/4.0/).

Since the end of World War II, science has not stopped progressing. Health and social advances have increased human longevity as never before [1]. We live longer, partially due to an increase in our knowledge of the physiological processes of successful aging, but also due to the pathophysiological processes of unhealthy aging. Among the least favorable aging trajectories, a syndrome that stands out from the gerontological and geriatric perspective is frailty. Since Linda Fried described the physiological cycle of this geriatric syndrome in 2001 [2], the presence of frailty in the elderly has been associated with a loss of functionality, hospital admissions, disability, mortality and institutionalization in nursing homes. In fact, it is a more robust predictor of adverse events than some variables that are still used abnormally in clinical inertia, such as chronological age [3]. This ageism remains in force in clinical practice, as has been possible to verify with the COVID-19 pandemic [4] that has devastated the planet. As it has been published, the elderly found it difficult to access the necessary clinical resources due to a simple matter of age.

Our Special Issue deals with the following issue: how to improve healthcare for our elders. One of the reviews included could not be more revealing in this regard, detailing the epigenetic factors linked to successful trajectories of aging [5]. Our life expectancy depends mainly on environmental factors, but we should not forget how the environment modifies our genetic expression through epigenetic mechanisms. Identifying the molecular and cellular epigenetic mechanisms can contribute to the early detection of changes or deficits associated with the different aging trajectories, including those that lead to frailty. The era of biomarkers has arrived. The biological clock shows the states of robustness and frailty in adults. With this information, clinicians can predict adverse events and improve decision-making processes.

Frailty, as should be remembered, is associated with multiple geriatric syndromes, including polypharmacy and pharmacological iatrogenesis. The periodic review of the pharmacological history of the elderly should be part of usual clinical routine. In this context, evaluating and reducing the anticholinergic load of prescribed medications has a positive effect on the cognitive status of our older adults and also reduces the incidence of some adverse events, such as respiratory infections [6]. Likewise, the analysis of frailty allows access to key prognostic information, in both community-dwelling and hospitalized older adults [7]. Similarly, advances in geriatric knowledge allow us to predict walking recovery after hip fracture surgery [8]. Thus, variables such as age and the estimation of anesthetic risk (due to its link with the prevalence of comorbidity), independence in walking prior to the fracture, the presence of cognitive impairment and pressure ulcers (both geriatric syndromes), the delay in surgery and early mobilization (two of the great challenges of clinical management), and the destination at discharge strongly influence gait recovery. Falls is another important geriatric syndrome and is linked to hip fracture incidence. Even if undervalued by the clinical practice, falling has important social and health implications, among which are the non-negligible associated costs. Falls are considered normal in the elderly by a great number of clinicians; this ageist principle is gradually being broken as indicated by the significant number of articles published between 2010 and 2020 on the matter [9]. These published studies should highlight the implication of geriatric factors in falling, such as sarcopenia, cognitive status, frailty, depression and fear of falling. The prevention of falls in older adults continues to be a great public health challenge. Accustomed to associating frailty with functional and clinical factors, clinicians often forget the social conditioning factors and constructs, such as social frailty [10]. Social frailty is associated with a worse clinical, nutritional, psycho-affective, cognitive situation, and with lower life satisfaction. In fact, physical activity is linked with social and psychological factors, such as the presence of depressive symptoms [11], the perception of fatigue, loneliness and social isolation. In this Special Issue, two studies pay attention to clinical application of thermal points. In older adults with dementia and verbal fluency impairments, thermal sensation could be useful to communicate with patients [12]. Moreover, thermotherapy could be effective in pain control [13].

Finally, interdisciplinary teams develop an important role in complex processes management, such as elective colorectal cancer surgery [14]. Holistic approaches, with a correct continuity of care, prolongs the benefits of enhanced recovery after surgery (ERAS) protocols, in the nutritional state and in hemoglobin blood levels, reducing transfusion rates.

This Special Issue offers different manuscripts to readers trying to improve life satisfaction, quality of life and life expectancy in older adults in different scenarios. It is up to us to achieve these goals. We are sure that these interesting papers will contribute to improve the clinical practice. Enjoy these articles.

Funding: This research received no external funding.

Institutional Review Board Statement: Not applicable.

Informed Consent Statement: Not applicable.

Data Availability Statement: Not applicable.

Conflicts of Interest: The authors declare no conflict of interest.

References

1. Vaupel, J.W.; Villavicencio, F.; Bergeron-Boucher, M.P. Demographic perspectives on the rise of longevity. *Proc. Natl. Acad. Sci. USA* **2021**, *118*, e2019536118. [CrossRef] [PubMed]
2. Fried, L.P.; Tangen, C.M.; Walston, J.; Newman, A.B.; Hirsch, C.; Gottdiener, J.; Seeman, T.; Tracy, R.; Kop, W.J.; Burke, G.; et al. Frailty in older adults: Evidence for a phenotype. *J. Gerontol. A Biol. Sci. Med. Sci.* **2001**, *56*, M146–M156. [CrossRef] [PubMed]
3. Romero-Ortuno, R.; Forsyth, D.R.; Wilson, K.J.; Cameron, E.; Wallis, S.; Biram, R.; Keevil, V. The Association of Geriatric Syndromes with Hospital Outcomes. *J. Hosp. Med.* **2017**, *12*, 83–89. [CrossRef] [PubMed]
4. Cesari, M.; Proietti, M. COVID-19 in Italy: Ageism and Decision Making in a Pandemic. *J. Am. Med. Dir. Assoc.* **2020**, *21*, 576–577. [CrossRef] [PubMed]
5. García-Giménez, J.L.; Mena-Molla, S.; Tarazona-Santabalbina, F.J.; Viña, J.; Gomez-Cabrera, M.C.; Pallardó, F.V. Implementing Precision Medicine in Human Frailty through Epigenetic Biomarkers. *Int. J. Environ. Res. Public Health* **2021**, *18*, 1883. [CrossRef] [PubMed]
6. Lee, C.Y.; Cheng, Y.D.; Cheng, W.Y.; Tsai, T.H.; Huang, K.H. The Prevalence of Anticholinergic Drugs and Correlation with Pneumonia in Elderly Patients: A Population-Based Study in Taiwan. *Int. J. Environ. Res. Public Health* **2020**, *17*, 6260. [CrossRef] [PubMed]
7. Torné, A.; Puigoriol, E.; Zabaleta-del-Olmo, E.; Zamora-Sánchez, J.-J.; Santaeugènia, S.; Amblàs-Novellas, J. Reliability, Validity, and Feasibility of the Frail-VIG Index. *Int. J. Environ. Res. Public Health* **2021**, *18*, 5187. [CrossRef] [PubMed]

8. De Villaumbrosia, C.G.; Sáez López, P.; de Diego, I.M.; Lancho Martín, C.; Cuesta Santa Teresa, M.; Alarcón, T.; Ojeda Thies, C.; Queipo Matas, R.; González-Montalvo, J.I. Predictive Model of Gait Recovery at One Month after Hip Fracture from a National Cohort of 25,607 Patients: The Hip Fracture Prognosis (HFPrognosis) Tool. *Int. J. Environ. Res. Public Health* **2021**, *18*, 3809. [CrossRef] [PubMed]
9. Chen, B.; Shin, S. Bibliometric Analysis on Research Trend of Accidental Falls in Older Adults by Using Citespace—Focused on Web of Science Core Collection (2010–2020). *Int. J. Environ. Res. Public Health* **2021**, *18*, 1663. [CrossRef] [PubMed]
10. Ko, H.; Jung, S. Association of Social Frailty with Physical Health, Cognitive Function, Psychological Health, and Life Satisfaction in Community-Dwelling Older Koreans. *Int. J. Environ. Res. Public Health* **2021**, *18*, 818. [CrossRef] [PubMed]
11. Pérez, L.M.; Castellano-Tejedor, C.; Cesari, M.; Soto-Bagaria, L.; Ars, J.; Zambom-Ferraresi, F.; Baró, S.; Díaz-Gallego, F.; Vilaró, J.; Enfedaque, M.B.; et al. Depressive Symptoms, Fatigue and Social Relationships Influenced Physical Activity in Frail Older Community-Dwellers during the Spanish Lockdown due to the COVID-19 Pandemic. *Int. J. Environ. Res. Public Health* **2021**, *18*, 808. [CrossRef] [PubMed]
12. Childs, C.; Elliott, J.; Khatab, K.; Hampshaw, S.; Fowler-Davis, S.; Willmott, J.R.; Ali, A. Thermal Sensation in Older People with and without Dementia Living in Residential Care: New Assessment Approaches to Thermal Comfort Using Infrared Thermography. *Int. J. Environ. Res. Public Health* **2020**, *17*, 6932. [CrossRef] [PubMed]
13. Shin, H.J.; Kim, S.H.; Hahm, S.C.; Cho, H.Y. Thermotherapy Plus Neck Stabilization Exercise for Chronic Nonspecific Neck Pain in Elderly: A Single-Blinded Randomized Controlled Trial. *Int. J. Environ. Res. Public Health* **2020**, *17*, 5572. [CrossRef] [PubMed]
14. González-Senac, N.M.; Mayordomo-Cava, J.; Macías-Valle, A.; Aldama-Marín, P.; González, S.M.; Arnés, M.L.C.; Jiménez-Gómez, L.M.; Vidán-Astiz, M.T.; Serra-Rexach, J.A. Colorectal Cancer in Elderly Patients with Surgical Indication: State of the Art, Current Management, Role of Frailty and Benefits of a Geriatric Liaison. *Int. J. Environ. Res. Public Health* **2021**, *18*, 6072. [CrossRef]

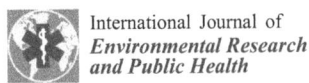

Article

Thermotherapy Plus Neck Stabilization Exercise for Chronic Nonspecific Neck Pain in Elderly: A Single-Blinded Randomized Controlled Trial

Ho-Jin Shin [1,†], Sung-Hyeon Kim [1,†], Suk-Chan Hahm [2,*] and Hwi-Young Cho [1,3,*]

1. Department of Health Science, Gachon University Graduate School, Incheon 21936, Korea; sports0911@hanmail.net (H.-J.S.); 315201@hanmail.net (S.-H.K.)
2. Graduate School of Integrative Medicine, CHA University, Seongnam 13488, Korea
3. Department of Physical Therapy, Gachon University, Incheon 21936, Korea
* Correspondence: schahm@cha.ac.kr (S.-C.H.); hwiyoung@gachon.ac.kr (H.-Y.C.); Tel.: +82-31-881-7101 (S.-C.H.); +82-32-820-4560 (H.-Y.C.)
† These two authors contributed equally to this work as co-first authors.

Received: 26 June 2020; Accepted: 29 July 2020; Published: 1 August 2020

Abstract: Neck pain is a serious problem for public health. This study aimed to compare the effects of thermotherapy plus neck stabilization exercise versus neck stabilization exercise alone on pain, neck disability, muscle properties, and alignment of the neck and shoulder in the elderly with chronic nonspecific neck pain. This study is a single-blinded randomized controlled trial. Thirty-five individuals with chronic nonspecific neck pain were randomly allocated to intervention ($n = 18$) or control ($n = 17$) groups. The intervention group received thermotherapy with a salt-pack for 30 min and performed a neck stabilization exercise for 40 min twice a day for 5 days (10 sessions). The control group performed a neck stabilization exercise at the same time points. Pain intensity, pain pressure threshold (PPT), neck disability index, muscle properties, and alignment of the neck and shoulder were evaluated before and after the intervention. Significant time and group interactions were observed for pain at rest ($p < 0.001$) and during movement ($p < 0.001$), and for PPT at the upper-trapezius ($p < 0.001$), levator-scapula ($p = 0.003$), and splenius-capitis ($p = 0.001$). The disability caused by neck pain also significantly changed between groups over time ($p = 0.005$). In comparison with the control group, the intervention group showed significant improvements in muscle properties for the upper-trapezius (tone, $p = 0.021$; stiffness, $p = 0.017$), levator-scapula (stiffness, $p = 0.025$; elasticity, $p = 0.035$), and splenius-capitis (stiffness, $p = 0.012$), and alignment of the neck ($p = 0.016$) and shoulder ($p < 0.001$) over time. These results recommend the clinical use of salt pack thermotherapy in addition to neck stabilization exercise as a complementary intervention for chronic nonspecific neck pain control.

Keywords: neck stabilization exercise; nonspecific neck pain; salt pack; thermotherapy

1. Introduction

Neck pain is a common health problem with a lifetime prevalence of 14.2% to 71% in the adult population and is considered a major problem for public health [1]. In particular, Korean women of middle and older age have a prevalence of 20.8% [2]. The common presentation of neck pain is nonspecific neck pain, defined as simple neck pain without a specific underlying disease causing the pain, which results from postural and mechanical causes [3,4]. Appropriate management of nonspecific neck pain is essential because chronic neck pain results in increased muscle tone, restricted cervical range of motion, functional impairments of activities of daily living, and decreased quality of life [4].

Nonspecific neck pain can be treated with a variety of interventions, such as medication, manual therapy, heat, and exercise [3–6]. In particular, exercise is an evidence-based practice to not only relieve pain in individuals with nonspecific neck pain, but also to improve muscle strength, motor function, and quality of life [7]. The efficacy of cervical-scapulothoracic stabilization exercise and neck stabilization exercise for the management of neck pain have been reported in previous studies [8–10].

Thermotherapy has been used to reduce chronic musculoskeletal pain and has been reported as a complementary intervention [11–19]. Since the application of thermotherapy to the skin increases the temperature and blood flow to the muscle and decreases muscle fatigue [14–16], it may be associated with an increase in muscle flexibility [17]. These effects of thermotherapy can also decrease muscle spasms [13]. Considering these findings, the application of thermotherapy followed by exercise during the rehabilitation process may strengthen the stability of neck muscles; thus, thermotherapy combined with neck stabilization exercise may be more effective than exercise alone for relieving nonspecific neck pain.

A hot pack is one of the most common methods of thermotherapy, and various heat transfer substances, such as silicate gel, polymer gel, and water, were used in the hot pack [20–23]. Salt can be an option for a heat transfer substance in hot packs. Considering that thermotherapy using salt have analgesic and anti-inflammatory effects [24,25], hot packs using salt can be used for management of musculoskeletal pain. However, no clinical trial has been specifically conducted to investigate the feasibility of salt packs in patients with nonspecific neck pain, and the efficacy of thermotherapy combined with neck stabilization exercise for nonspecific neck pain has not been investigated. Thus, the aim of this study was to investigate the efficacy of a combination of a salt pack with neck stabilization exercise on pain, pain pressure threshold (PPT), neck disability, and alignment in individuals with chronic nonspecific neck pain. To this end, we compared the effects of thermotherapy using a salt pack plus neck stabilization exercise versus a neck stabilization exercise alone for symptomatic relief from chronic nonspecific neck pain.

2. Methods

2.1. Study Design

This study was designed as a single-blinded, randomized controlled trial. The experimental protocol was approved by the Gachon University Institutional Review Board (1044396-201903-HR-040-01). The study was performed in accordance with the protocol, and all participants provided written informed consent prior to their enrollment in the study.

2.2. Participants and Sample Size

For this study, we enrolled elders (>60 years) with chronic nonspecific neck pain that had lasted longer than 6 months (visual analogue scale (VAS) > 3/10), who had not undertaken regular physical activity in the past year. Chronic nonspecific neck pain was defined as neck pain provoked by neck postures, movements, or pressure for at least 3 months without a known pathology (neurological, trauma-induced, etc.) as the cause of the complaints [26]. The exclusion criteria were neck pain associated with inflammatory, hormonal, and neurological disorders or structural deformity in the upper extremities; neck pain related to previous surgery; positive radicular signs consistent with nerve root compression; severe referred pain; severe psychological disorder; or pregnancy. In addition, participants were excluded if they were under anti-inflammatory, analgesic, anticoagulant, muscle relaxant, or antidepressant medication use 1 week before the study commenced [26].

The sample size was calculated using the computer software G-power (Heinrich-Heine-University Düsseldorf, version 3.1.9.4, Düsseldorf, Germany) In the present study, the effect size was set to 0.25 (medium effect size) [27], and the alpha level was 0.05. On the basis of these values, 34 participants (17 participants per group) were needed to achieve 80% power using a 2-sided test. Thus, with a 10% dropout rate, a total of 38 participants were required.

2.3. Experimental Procedures and Interventions

All participants were randomly assigned to treatment or control groups using a stratified randomization method [28]. Participants were stratified by age (60–69/70–79) and baseline VAS at rest (3–5/6–8) and randomization was performed within each stratum by using permuted block randomization (block size 4). The group allocation was concealed to the outcome assessor by blinding the group assignment, and primary and secondary variables were assessed before and after the intervention. Pre-test were performed on the morning (9 a.m. to 10 a.m.) before the first intervention, and post-tests were performed in the morning (9 a.m. to 10 a.m.) on the next day after the intervention. All assessments were conducted in a random order to exclude potential fatigue and order effects due to measurement order.

The intervention group performed neck stabilization exercise and thermotherapy using a salt pack, and the control group performed only neck stabilization exercises at Saesum Resort in Taean-gun. The neck stabilization exercise was applied by slightly modifying the exercise intervention performed in the previous study [10]. It consisted of a warm-up (5 min), main exercise (30 min), and cool-down (5 min), and was performed in both the intervention and control groups. The warm-up and cool-down consisted of neck and upper extremity stretching, and the main exercise was as follows: (1) Deep neck flexor isometric exercise in supine position; (2) Multi-directional isometric exercise (cervical flexion, extension, rotation, side bending) in a sitting position; (3) Upper extremity movement exercise; (4) Resistive exercise with Thera-band. The neck stabilization exercise was performed according to the therapist's instruction.

After the neck stabilization exercise, the intervention group performed additional thermotherapy using a salt pack. For thermotherapy, bay salt was used in packs. The salt was collected at Taean-gun, Chungcheongnam-do, Republic of Korea in April 2019 and then packed in cotton cloth. The far infrared radiation (FIR) emissivity of bay salt used in this study was 0.900 µm and the FIR emission power was 3.89×10^2 W/m^2·µm (Table A1 in Appendix A). The salt packs were kept in a warming cabinet (LH-1043G, Lassele Co., Ltd., Ansan, Korea) set at 60 °C until the start of the intervention. The participant was in a prone position. A salt pack set at 55 °C was applied to the neck and shoulder [29]; even after 30 min of application, it was maintained at about 40–50 °C. All interventions were conducted twice a day for 5 days, neck stabilization exercise was performed for 40 min and additional thermotherapy using salt pack was performed for 30 min.

2.4. Outcome Measures

2.4.1. Primary Variables

The visual analogue scale (VAS) [30] was used to assess pain intensity at rest and during movement. VAS at rest (resting pain) was defined as an unpleasant feeling or pain without movement, and VAS during movement (movement-induced pain) was defined as unpleasant feelings or pain incurred by neck movement (flexion, extension, lateral flexion, rotation) [31]. Patients marked their pain intensity at rest and during movement on a VAS table.

To assess the PPT of the neck, the PPT assessment method described in a previous study was used with a distal algometer (Somedic AB, Farsta, Sweden) containing a 1-cm^2 probe [11,32,33]. The pressure head of the algometer was applied to the upper trapezius, levator scapula, and splenius capitis of the neck and shoulder area, as in a previous study [34]. The assessor gradually increased the application pressure in 10-kPa/s increments until the participants expressed a pain response, such as a pain-induced vocalization and a gesture related to pain (hand grasp or eye blink) [32]. The measurement was repeated twice, and the measurement interval was 30 s. The mean threshold was calculated for the left- and right-side points.

The neck disability index (NDI) was used to assess functional disability due to neck pain; this assessment consists of 10 items describing the impact of pain on different daily living activities [33]. Each item is rated on a six-point Likert scale (range 0–5), with 0 indicating no limitation due to pain and 5 indicating that an activity is impossible to perform. The total score ranges from 0 to 50, with a higher score indicating a higher level of disability. The NDI is the most widely used tool for assessing functional outcomes in patients with neck pain and is recommended for evaluation of the effectiveness of neck pain treatment.

2.4.2. Secondary Variables

A handheld myotonometer (Myoton AS, Tallinn, Estonia) with excellent intra and inter-tester reliability (ICC = 0.97) was used to measure the mechanical properties of muscle (muscle tone, stiffness, and elasticity) [35]. The skeletal muscle assessments were performed at the same region where PPT was measured. Each time, the probe (3 mm diameter) of equipment was placed perpendicular to the skin's surface and five repeated measurements were obtained. The myofascial tissue oscillations were evoked with 5 brief (15 ms) mechanical impulses at 0.4 N force and frequency of 1 Hz. The mean threshold was calculated for the left- and right-side points. Muscle tone is a value expressing muscle tone in a passive or resting state without voluntary contraction. Muscle stiffness is a value representing the resistance of tissue to external mechanical impulse. Muscle elasticity is a value expressing the ability to recover to the initial shape after the disappearance of the external force of deformation.

Changes in cervical and shoulder alignments were assessed using the cervical angle and shoulder angle, respectively [36] (Figure A1). the cervical angle and shoulder angle were defined through three markers (tragus of ear, spinous process of the C7, acromion) attached to the participants' anatomical landmarks. Images were collected by a 16-megapixel camera (SM-N976N, Samsung, Suwon, Korea) with an acromion height of 1.5 m, located perpendicular to the ground by a spirit level. The collected images were processed through the MATLAB (version 2019b, Mathworks, Inc., Natick, MA, USA). The cervical angle is formed when a line drawn from the tragus of the ear to the C7 vertebra intersects a horizontal line, and the shoulder angle is formed when a horizontal line passing through the lateral shoulder meets the line drawn from C7 to the lateral shoulder.

2.5. Statistical Analysis

Data analyses were performed using IBM SPSS Statistics 25.0. (IBM-SPSS Inc, Chicago, IL, USA) The statistician was blinded to group allocation for all analyses. An independent t-test and the χ^2 test was performed in order to compare general characteristics between the two groups. Repeated measures ANOVA was used to analyze the changes in variables between groups over time and main effect comparisons were performed. Post-hoc analysis was performed through independent t-test and paired t-test using Bonferroni methods. A p-value of < 0.05 was considered statistically significant.

3. Results

3.1. Participant Characteristics

A total of 53 participants were recruited, all of whom were women. Fifteen individuals were excluded from participating; 13 did not meet the inclusion criteria and two declined to participate. Because individuals scheduled their problems, in the intervention group, one individual did not participate in the final assessment. In the control group, two individuals declined to participate after allocation. However, there were no complaints or dropout due to the intensity of the intervention except for those who were dropped out for the above reasons. A total of 35 patients completed the study. Figure 1 shows the participant flow through the enrollment, allocation, assessment, and analysis stages.

There were no significant differences between the intervention and control groups in terms of the general participant characteristics (age, height, weight, and body mass index) (Table 1). Additionally, there are no significant differences in the baseline values of the outcome variables assessed in this study between the two groups.

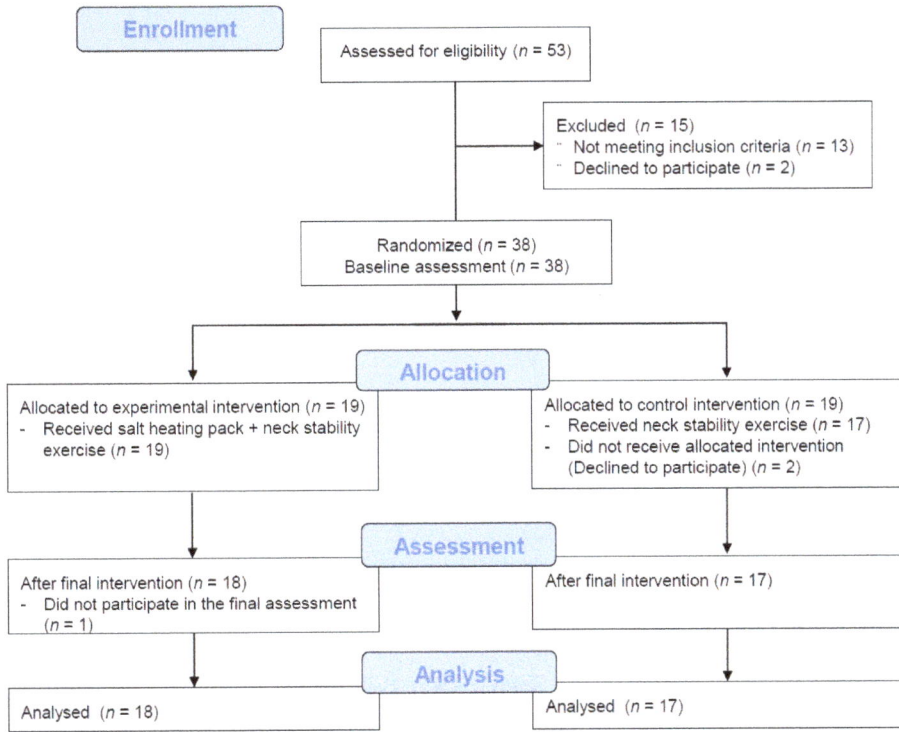

Figure 1. Flow diagram of study participants.

Table 1. General characteristics of the participants.

Variable	Intervention Group (n = 18)	Control Group (n = 17)	P
Age (years)	68.06 ± 4.71	66.24 ± 4.71	0.261
Height (m)	1.54 ± 0.04	1.53 ± 0.03	0.299
Weight (kg)	58.92 ± 7.52	57.34 ± 4.68	0.457
BMI (kg/m^2)	24.73 ± 2.93	24.5 ± 1.80	0.780
VAS at rest (cm)	4.78 ± 1.11	4.53 ± 1.37	0.560
Onset duration (month)	15.33 ± 7.76	14.29 ± 7.74	0.694
Job context [†]			
Working	13 (72.22)	11 (64.71)	0.632
Non-working	5 (27.78)	6 (35.29)	

Data are expressed as mean ± standard deviation or number (%) [†]. BMI, body mass index; P, p-value; VAS, visual analogue scale.

3.2. Primary Outcomes

3.2.1. Pain Intensity

As shown in Table 2, compared to neck stabilization exercise alone, salt pack therapy combined with neck stabilization exercise significantly improved pain intensity over time at rest ($p < 0.001$) and during movement ($p < 0.001$). The intervention group showed a significantly decreased pain intensity at rest ($p < 0.001$) and during movement ($p < 0.001$) after the intervention. The control group also showed a significantly decreased pain intensity at rest ($p = 0.009$) and during movement ($p = 0.001$).

Table 2. The changes in pain intensity, pain pressure threshold, and neck disability.

Outcome/Group	Baseline	Two Weeks Post-Treatment	P (Pairwise Comparison)	P (T * G)
VAS at rest(cm)				
Intervention group	4.78 ± 1.11	1.17 ± 1.04	<0.001	<0.001
Control group	4.53 ± 1.37	3.41 ± 1.28	0.009	
VAS during movement(cm)				
Intervention group	6.75 ± 1.06	2.28 ± 1.41	<0.001	<0.001
Control group	6.06 ± 1.14	4.53 ± 1.37	0.001	
PPT_Upper trapezius (kg)				
Intervention group	2.41 ± 0.50	4.28 ± 1.38	<0.001	0.002
Control group	2.56 ± 0.75	3.22 ± 0.87	0.014	
PPT_Levator scapula (kg)				
Intervention group	2.07 ± 0.51	4.12 ± 1.18	<0.001	<0.001
Control group	2.38 ± 0.89	2.99 ± 0.83	0.018	
PPT_Splenius capitis (kg)				
Intervention group	2.56 ± 0.93	4.52 ± 0.84	<0.001	0.001
Control group	2.90 ± 0.87	3.55 ± 0.78	0.015	
NDI (%)				
Intervention group	36.11 ± 12.88	16.56 ± 10.56	<0.001	0.005
Control group	33.65 ± 11.92	27.29 ± 10.79	0.052	

Data are expressed as mean ± standard deviation. P, p-value; T * G, time and group interaction; VAS, visual analog scale; PPT, pain pressure threshold; NDI, neck disability index.

3.2.2. Pain Pressure Threshold

A significant increase in the PPT for the upper trapezius ($p = 0.002$), levator scapula ($p < 0.001$), and splenius capitis ($p < 0.001$) was observed in the groups over time (Table 2). In comparison with the control, the intervention group showed a significant improvement in PPT for the upper trapezius ($p = 0.002$), levator scapula ($p < 0.001$), and splenius capitis ($p = 0.001$). Both thermotherapy with neck stabilization exercise (upper trapezius, $p < 0.001$; levator scapula, $p < 0.001$; splenius capitis, $p < 0.001$) and neck stabilization exercise alone (upper trapezius, $p = 0.014$; levator scapula, $p = 0.018$; splenius capitis, $p = 0.015$) significantly increased PPT after treatment.

3.2.3. Neck Disability

Significant improvement in disability due to neck pain was observed in groups over time ($p = 0.005$, Table 2). Interestingly, salt pack with neck stabilization exercise yielded significant improvements in disability due to neck pain in comparison with the improvements obtained with neck stability exercise alone ($p = 0.005$). The intervention group showed significant increases in NDI scores ($p < 0.001$). However, the control group did not show a significant change in NDI after neck stability exercise.

3.3. Secondary Outcomes

3.3.1. Muscle Properties

In comparison with the control group, the intervention group showed a significant improvement over time in muscle tone (upper trapezius, $p = 0.021$), stiffness (upper trapezius, $p = 0.017$; levator scapula, $p = 0.025$; splenius capitis, $p = 0.012$), and elasticity (levator scapula, $p = 0.035$) (Table 3). The intervention group also showed significant differences in muscle tone (upper trapezius, $p < 0.001$; levator scapula, $p = 0.003$; splenius capitis, $p = 0.006$), stiffness (upper trapezius, $p < 0.001$; levator scapula, $p < 0.001$; splenius capitis, $p < 0.001$), and elasticity (upper trapezius, $p = 0.001$; levator scapula, $p < 0.001$; splenius capitis, $p = 0.001$) after the intervention. However, the control group did not show significant improvements in muscle tone, stiffness, and elasticity after neck stabilization exercise.

Table 3. The changes in muscle characteristics.

Outcome/Group.	Baseline	Two Weeks Post-Treatment	P (Pairwise Comparison)	P (T * G)
Upper trapezius				
		Tone (Hz)		
Intervention group	13.71 ± 2.25	11.64 ± 0.91	<0.001	0.021
Control group	14.19 ± 2.72	13.88 ± 3.43	0.552	
		Stiffness (N/m)		
Intervention group	255.56 ± 19.25	229.83 ± 27.64	<0.001	0.017
Control group	260.94 ± 11.33	254.88 ± 32.14	0.288	
		Elasticity (logarithm)		
Intervention group	1.69 ± 0.26	1.97 ± 0.42	0.001	0.079
Control group	1.59 ± 0.23	1.67 ± 0.31	0.328	
Levator scapula				
		Tone (Hz)		
Intervention group	19.03 ± 1.89	17.04 ± 2.23	0.003	0.129
Control group	20.11 ± 2.66	19.48 ± 3.10	0.331	
		Stiffness (N/m)		
Intervention group	335.78 ± 48.50	280.06 ± 53.92	<0.001	0.025
Control group	345.00 ± 48.90	333.35 ± 54.75	0.393	
		Elasticity (logarithm)		
Intervention group	1.42 ± 0.17	1.65 ± 0.23	<0.001	0.035
Control group	1.38 ± 0.14	1.44 ± 0.25	0.325	
Splenius capitis				
		Tone (Hz)		
Intervention group	21.01 ± 1.65	19.07 ± 2.69	0.006	0.094
Control group	21.18 ± 2.47	20.88 ± 3.5	0.655	
		Stiffness (N/m)		
Intervention group	388.56 ± 48.13	332.22 ± 52.88	<0.001	0.012
Control group	395.24 ± 51.39	385.59 ± 59.32	0.449	
		Elasticity (logarithm)		
Intervention group	1.49 ± 0.15	1.64 ± 0.23	0.001	0.101
Control group	1.48 ± 0.15	1.53 ± 0.24	0.296	

Data are expressed as mean ± standard deviation. P, p-value; T * G, time and group interaction.

3.3.2. Cervical and Shoulder Alignments

In assessments of neck posture correction, cervical ($p = 0.016$) and shoulder ($p < 0.001$) alignments significantly improved in the groups over time (Table 4). As shown in Table 4, cervical ($p < 0.001$) and shoulder ($p < 0.001$) angles significantly improved after salt pack therapy with neck stabilization exercise. However, the control group did not show significant improvements in cervical and shoulder angles. Salt pack combined with neck stabilization exercise was not significantly more effective than neck stabilization exercise only.

Table 4. The changes in cervical and shoulder alignment.

Outcome/Group	Baseline	Two Weeks Post-Treatment	P (Pairwise comparison)	P (T * G)
		Cervical angle (degree)		
Intervention group	48.06 ± 6.31	50.26 ± 6.22	<0.001	0.016
Control group	50.12 ± 4.62	50.59 ± 5.43	0.352	
		Shoulder angle (degree)		
Intervention group	60.49 ± 4.57	65.86 ± 4.64	<0.001	<0.001
Control group	62.18 ± 5.49	62.97 ± 6.30	0.293	

Data are expressed as mean ± standard deviation. P, p-value; T * G, time and group interaction.

4. Discussion

This study aimed to compare the effects of thermotherapy combined with neck stabilization exercise to those of neck stabilization exercise alone on chronic nonspecific neck pain. This study is the first investigation to demonstrate that 10 sessions of salt pack thermotherapy plus neck stabilization exercise provide benefits that are superior to those of neck stability exercise alone on pain intensity, PPT, neck disability, muscle properties, and body alignment in individuals with chronic nonspecific neck pain. These results may provide evidence to use salt pack therapy plus neck stabilization exercise as a complementary intervention for relief from nonspecific neck pain.

Previous studies have reported the effects of therapeutic exercise, including neck stabilization exercise, with or without thermotherapy on nonspecific musculoskeletal pain and disability [8–12,34,37–39]. Our study also demonstrated that both thermotherapy using a salt pack plus neck stabilization exercise and neck stabilization exercise alone had significant effects in reducing pain intensity, increasing PPT, and improving disability. Interestingly, in comparison with neck stabilization exercise alone, the intervention group also showed significantly better neck pain control. In the study by Cramor et al. [12] both the thermotherapy and non-thermotherapy groups received their usual medication and physical therapy regimens during the study period, with the thermotherapy group receiving thermotherapy using mud packs; their findings suggested that the additional thermotherapy significantly alleviated nonspecific neck pain. Thermotherapy has been shown to effectively alleviate pain and improve somatosensory function in individuals with chronic neck pain [12]. The results of previous studies that applied thermotherapy with exercise for low back pain control support our findings [11]. In addition to the thermal effect, it appears that there is also the effect of FIR emitted from the bay salt. FIR can provide pain control and increased blood flow [40]. This effect of FIR may contribute to pain reduction and changes in muscle characteristics. The superiority of the intervention group may be explained by a reduction in pain intensity [11,12,37] and improvement in muscle flexibility [41] as a result of thermotherapy prior to neck stabilization exercise. These changes in pain intensity and PPT may have resulted in the decreased neck disability evidenced by the NDI results.

This study showed significant time and group interactions of PPT, and both intervention and control groups showed significant improvements in PPT. Prior studies have also reported that thermotherapy has a greater influence on PPT in comparison with other treatments for chronic neck pain [38,42]. However, a previous study [12] reported no significant change in PPT after thermotherapy application. That study explained that with hyperalgesia pressure is maintained by central sensitization in patients with chronic neck pain [43] and that thermotherapy had no effect on central sensitization. The discrepancies between the findings of our study and that study may be attributable to the alteration of pain memories associated with central sensitization in patients with chronic musculoskeletal pain via exercise [44]. A previous study [9] reported significant improvement in the PPT on the middle point of the upper trapezius in patients with nonspecific neck pain after neck stabilization exercise, which supports our results for PPT.

This study also examined the changes in muscle properties of the neck/shoulder in both groups. The intervention group demonstrated significantly decreased muscle tone, stiffness and elasticity, but the control group did not show significant changes in muscle properties. Thermotherapy increases the temperature of and blood flow to the muscle and reduces muscle fatigue [14–16], which may decrease muscle tone, stiffness, and elasticity. In addition, significant recovery of these muscle properties and neck pain may be associated with the significant differences in the effects on cervical and shoulder alignment between the two groups. Previous studies have reported that the high tone of the upper trapezius is associated with the forward neck [45,46], and that increased tone and stiffness of the neck and shoulder muscles can be a major physical factor for neck pain [47,48]. Our results showed a significant reduction in tone and stiffness of the neck and shoulder muscles, neck pain, and forward neck and round shoulder in the intervention group. These results showed that changes in muscle characteristics due to thermotherapy combined with neck stabilization exercise had a significant effect on neck and shoulder alignment and neck pain.

In the intervention group of this study, the intervention time for one session is more than one hour, which may be burdensome to the body. The participant's condition was continuously checked during and after the intervention, and there were no adverse symptoms such as pain, fatigue, and delayed onset muscle soreness. Moreover, there were no complaints about the interventions, and no participants dropped out due to problems with interventions. It seems that there was no problem because active intervention (neck stabilization exercise) was performed for only 40 min and then thermos-intervention was performed for 30 min.

There are some limitations to the present study. First, since the current study assessed the findings only after 10 sessions applied over 5 days, a thorough understanding of the effects of repeated thermotherapy with neck stability exercises over longer periods is necessary to evaluate the clinical use of salt pack interventions. Second, all participants in this study were women, even though sex was not an inclusion/exclusion criterion in this study. To obtain more generalizable conclusions relating to the efficacy of the salt pack combined with neck stabilization exercise for chronic nonspecific neck pain, further studies with suitable sex ratios may be needed. Third, although this feasibility study showed significant effects on pain intensity, PPT, muscle properties, and aliment in individuals with chronic nonspecific neck pain, the small sample size may limit the generalizability of these results.

5. Conclusions

According to the results of this study, salt pack thermotherapy combined with neck stabilization exercise is superior to neck stabilization exercise alone for chronic nonspecific neck pain control. However, to generalize the clinical use of this intervention for management of nonspecific neck pain, further studies with larger sample sizes and longer periods of application are needed.

Author Contributions: Conceptualization, S.-C.H., H.-Y.C.; Data curation, H.-J.S., S.-H.K.; Investigation, H.-J.S., S.-H.K.; Formal analysis, S.-C.H.; Funding acquisition, H.-Y.C.; Project administration, S.-C.H.; Methodology, S.-C.H., H.-J.S., S.-H.K.; Visualization, H.-J.S., S.-H.K.; Writing–original draft, H.-J.S., S.-H.K.; Writing–review and editing, S.-C.H. All authors have read and agreed to the published version of the manuscript.

Funding: This research was a part of the project entitled "The base study to discover and to commercialize for the resources of sea healing to activate marine industry", funded by the Ministry of Oceans and Fisheries, Republic of Korea (20170242).

Conflicts of Interest: The authors of this study have no conflicts of interest to declare.

Appendix A

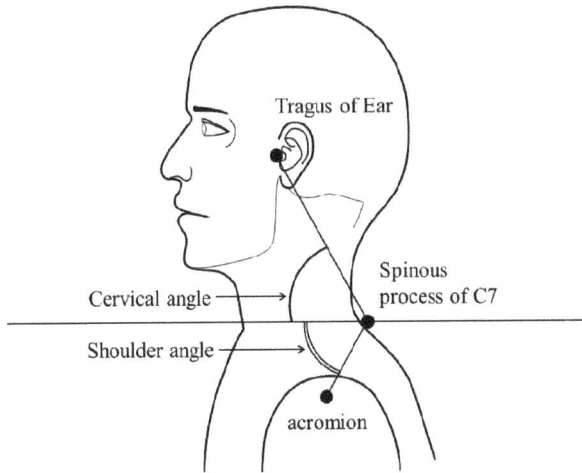

Figure A1. Cervical and shoulder angles.

Table A1. Emissivity and emission power of the far infrared radiation by 45 °C bay salt.

Emissivity (5~20 μm)	Emission Power (W/m²·μm)
0.9000	3.89×10^2

References

1. Fejer, R.; Kyvik, K.O.; Hartvigsen, J. The prevalence of neck pain in the world population: A systematic critical review of the literature. *Eur. Spine J.* **2006**, *15*, 834–848. [CrossRef] [PubMed]
2. Son, K.M.; Cho, N.H.; Lim, S.H.; Kim, H.A. Prevalence and risk factor of neck pain in elderly Korean community residents. *J. Korean Med. Sci.* **2013**, *28*, 680–686. [CrossRef] [PubMed]
3. Binder, A. The diagnosis and treatment of nonspecific neck pain and whiplash. *Eur. Med.* **2007**, *43*, 79–89.
4. Tsakitzidis, G.; Remmen, R.; Peremans, L.; Van Royen, P.; Duchesnes, C.; Paulus, D.; Eyssen, M. Non-Specific neck pain: Diagnosis and treatment. *Good Clin. Pract.* **2009**. KCE Reports 119C. D/2009/10.273/56.
5. Gross, A.R.; Haines, T.; Goldsmith, C.H.; Santaguida, L.; McLaughlin, L.M.; Peloso, P.; Burnie, S.; Hoving, J. Knowledge to action: A challenge for neck pain treatment. *J. Orthop. Sports Phys. Ther.* **2009**, *39*, 351–363. [CrossRef] [PubMed]
6. Graham, N.; Gross, A.R.; Carlesso, L.C.; Santaguida, P.L.; Macdermid, J.C.; Walton, D.; Ho, E. An ICON Overview on Physical Modalities for Neck Pain and Associated Disorders. *Open Orthop. J.* **2013**, *7*, 440–460. [CrossRef] [PubMed]
7. O'Riordan, C.; Clifford, A.; Van De Ven, P.; Nelson, J. Chronic neck pain and exercise interventions: Frequency, intensity, time, and type principle. *Arch. Phys. Med. Rehabil.* **2014**, *95*, 770–783. [CrossRef]
8. Celenay, S.T.; Kaya, D.O.; Akbayrak, T. Cervical and scapulothoracic stabilization exercises with and without connective tissue massage for chronic mechanical neck pain: A prospective, randomised controlled trial. *Man. Ther.* **2016**, *21*, 144–150. [CrossRef]
9. Celenay, S.T.; Akbayrak, T.; Kaya, D.O. A Comparison of the Effects of Stabilization Exercises Plus Manual Therapy to Those of Stabilization Exercises Alone in Patients With Nonspecific Mechanical Neck Pain: A Randomized Clinical Trial. *J. Orthop. Sports Phys. Ther.* **2016**, *46*, 44–55. [CrossRef]
10. Dusunceli, Y.; Ozturk, C.; Atamaz, F.; Hepguler, S.; Durmaz, B. Efficacy of neck stabilization exercises for neck pain: A randomized controlled study. *J. Rehabil. Med.* **2009**, *41*, 626–631. [CrossRef]
11. Hahm, S.C.; Shin, H.J.; Lee, M.G.; Lee, S.J.; Cho, H.Y. Mud Therapy Combined with Core Exercise for Chronic Nonspecific Low Back Pain: A Pilot, Single-Blind, Randomized Controlled Trial. *Evid. Based Complement. Alternat. Med.* **2020**, *2020*, 7547452. [CrossRef] [PubMed]
12. Cramer, H.; Baumgarten, C.; Choi, K.E.; Lauche, R.; Saha, F.J.; Musial, F.; Dobos, G. Thermotherapy self-treatment for neck pain relief—A randomized controlled trial. *Eur. J. Integr. Med.* **2012**, *4*, e371–e378. [CrossRef]
13. Nadler, S.F.; Weingand, K.; Kruse, R.J. The physiologic basis and clinical applications of cryotherapy and thermotherapy for the pain practitioner. *Pain Physician* **2004**, *7*, 395–399. [PubMed]
14. Erasala, G.; Rubin, J.; Tuthill, T.; Fowlkes, J.; de Drue, S.; Hengehold, D.; Weingand, K.J. The effect of topical heat treatment on trapezius muscle blood flow using power Doppler ultrasound. *Phys. Ther.* **2001**, *81*, A5.
15. Nadler, S.F.; Deprince, M.L.; Stitik, T.P.; Hendgehold, D.; Weingand, K. Experimentally induced trapezius fatigue and the effects of topical heat on the EMG power density spectrum. *Am. J. Phys. Med. Rehab.* **1999**, *80*, 1123.
16. Mulkern, R.; McDannold, N.; Hynynen, K.; Fielding, J.; Panych, L.; Jolesz, F.; Weingand, K. Temperature Distribution Changes in Low Back Muscles during Applied Topical Heat: A Magnetic Resonance Thermometry Study. In Proceedings of the 7th Annual Meeting of the International Society of Magnetic Resonance, in Medicine, Philadelphia, PA, USA, 22–28 May 1999; p. 1054.
17. Strickler, T.; Malone, T.; Garrett, W.E. The effects of passive warming on muscle injury. *Am. J. Sports Med.* **1990**, *18*, 141–145. [CrossRef] [PubMed]
18. Petrofsky, J.; Laymon, M.; Lee, H. Local heating of trigger points reduces neck and plantar fascia pain. *J. Back Musculoskelet. Rehabil.* **2020**, *33*, 21–28. [CrossRef] [PubMed]

19. Petrofsky, J.S.; Laymon, M.; Alshammari, F.; Khowailed, I.A.; Lee, H. Use of low level of continuous heat and Ibuprofen as an adjunct to physical therapy improves pain relief, range of motion and the compliance for home exercise in patients with nonspecific neck pain: A randomized controlled trial. *J. Back Musculoskelet. Rehabil.* **2017**, *30*, 889–896. [CrossRef]
20. Robertson, V.J.; Ward, A.R.; Jung, P. The effect of heat on tissue extensibility: A comparison of deep and superficial heating. *Arch. Phys. Med. Rehabil.* **2005**, *86*, 819–825. [CrossRef]
21. Knight, C.A.; Rutledge, C.R.; Cox, M.E.; Acosta, M.; Hall, S.J. Effect of superficial heat, deep heat, and active exercise warm-up on the extensibility of the plantar flexors. *Phys. Ther.* **2001**, *81*, 1206–1214. [CrossRef]
22. Oshima-Saeki, C.; Taniho, Y.; Arita, H.; Fujimoto, E. Lower-limb warming improves sleep quality in elderly people living in nursing homes. *Sleep Sci.* **2017**, *10*, 87–91. [CrossRef] [PubMed]
23. Saeki, Y. Effect of local application of cold or heat for relief of pricking pain. *Nurs. Health Sci.* **2002**, *4*, 97–105. [CrossRef] [PubMed]
24. Vakilinia, S.R.; Vaghasloo, M.A.; Aliasl, F.; Mohammadbeigi, A.; Bitarafan, B.; Etripoor, G.; Asghari, M. Evaluation of the efficacy of warm salt water foot-bath on patients with painful diabetic peripheral neuropathy: A randomized clinical trial. *Complement. Ther. Med.* **2020**, *49*, 102325. [CrossRef] [PubMed]
25. Tishler, M.; Shoenfeld, Y. The medical and scientific aspects of spa therapy. *Isr. J. Med. Sci.* **1996**, *32*, S8–S10.
26. Cerezo-Téllez, E.; Torres-Lacomba, M.; Fuentes-Gallardo, I.; Perez-Muñoz, M.; Mayoral-Del-Moral, O.; Lluch-Girbés, E.; Prieto-Valiente, L.; Falla, D. Effectiveness of dry needling for chronic nonspecific neck pain: A randomized, single-blinded, clinical trial. *Pain* **2016**, *157*, 1905–1917. [CrossRef]
27. Cohen, J. *Statistical Power Analysis for the Behavioral Sciences*; Academic Press: New York, NY, USA, 2013.
28. Kim, J.; Shin, W. How to do random allocation (randomization). *Clin. Orthop. Surg.* **2014**, *6*, 103–109. [CrossRef]
29. Garra, G.; Singer, A.J.; Leno, R.; Taira, B.R.; Gupta, N.; Mathaikutty, B.; Thode, H.J. Heat or cold packs for neck and back strain: A randomized controlled trial of efficacy. *Acad. Emerg. Med.* **2010**, *17*, 484–489. [CrossRef]
30. Crichton, N. Visual analogue scale (VAS). *J. Clin. Nurs.* **2001**, *10*, 697–706.
31. Lauche, R.; Cramer, H.; Langhorst, J.; Michalsen, A.; Dobos, G.J. Reliability and validity of the pain on movement questionnaire (POM) in chronic neck pain. *Pain Med.* **2014**, *15*, 1850–1856. [CrossRef]
32. Hahm, S.-C.; Suh, H.R.; Cho, H.Y. The effect of transcutaneous electrical nerve stimulation on pain, muscle strength, balance, and gait in individuals with dementia: A double blind, pilot randomized controlled trial. *Eur. J. Integr. Med.* **2019**, *29*, 100932. [CrossRef]
33. Cleland, J.A.; Fritz, J.M.; Whitman, J.M.; Palmer, J.A. The reliability and construct validity of the Neck Disability Index and patient specific functional scale in patients with cervical radiculopathy. *Spine* **2006**, *31*, 598–602. [CrossRef] [PubMed]
34. Lluch, E.; Arguisuelas, M.D.; Coloma, P.S.; Palma, F.; Rey, A.; Falla, D. Effects of deep cervical flexor training on pressure pain thresholds over myofascial trigger points in patients with chronic neck pain. *J. Manip. Physiol. Ther.* **2013**, *36*, 604–611. [CrossRef] [PubMed]
35. Gapeyeva, H.; Vain, A. *Methodical Guide: Principles of Applying Myoton in Physical Medicine and Rehabilitation*; Muomeetria Ltd.: Tartu, Estonia, 2008.
36. Singla, D.; Veqar, Z.; Hussain, M.E. Photogrammetric Assessment of Upper Body Posture Using Postural Angles: A Literature Review. *J. Chiropr. Med.* **2017**, *16*, 131–138. [CrossRef] [PubMed]
37. Koyuncu, E.; Ökmen, B.M.; Özkuk, K.; Taşoğlu, Ö.; Özgirgin, N. The effectiveness of balneotherapy in chronic neck pain. *Clin. Rheumatol.* **2016**, *35*, 2549–2555. [CrossRef] [PubMed]
38. Cramer, H.; Lauche, R.; Hohmann, C.; Lüdtke, R.; Haller, H.; Michalsen, A.; Langhorst, J.; Dobos, G. Randomized-controlled trial comparing yoga and home-based exercise for chronic neck pain. *Clin. J. Pain* **2013**, *29*, 216–223. [CrossRef] [PubMed]
39. Lansinger, B.; Larsson, E.; Persson, L.C.; Carlsson, J.Y. Qigong and exercise therapy in patients with long-term neck pain: A prospective randomized trial. *Spine* **2007**, *32*, 2415–2422. [CrossRef]
40. Vatansever, F.; Hamblin, M.R. Far infrared radiation (FIR): Its biological effects and medical applications. *Photonics Lasers Med.* **2012**, *4*, 255–266. [CrossRef]
41. Lentell, G.; Hetherington, T.; Eagan, J.; Morgan, M. The use of thermal agents to influence the effectiveness of a low-load prolonged stretch. *J. Orthop. Sports Phys. Ther.* **1992**, *16*, 200–207. [CrossRef]
42. Hohmann, C.; Lauche, R.; Choi, K.E.; Saha, F.; Rampp, T.; Dobos, G.; Musial, F. Quantitative sensory testing in patients with chronic neck pain before and after the application of the acupressure pad—A randomized, controlled pilot study. *Eur. J. Integr. Med.* **2009**, *1*, 212–213. [CrossRef]

43. Sterling, M. Testing for sensory hypersensitivity or central hyperexcitability associated with cervical spine pain. *J. Manip. Physiol. Ther.* **2008**, *31*, 534–539. [CrossRef]
44. Nijs, J.; Lluch Girbés, E.; Lundberg, M.; Malfliet, A.; Sterling, M. Exercise therapy for chronic musculoskeletal pain: Innovation by altering pain memories. *Man. Ther.* **2015**, *20*, 216–220. [CrossRef] [PubMed]
45. Yip, C.H.; Chiu, T.T.; Poon, A.T. The relationship between head posture and severity and disability of patients with neck pain. *Man. Ther.* **2008**, *13*, 148–154. [CrossRef] [PubMed]
46. Fernández-de-Las-Peñas, C.; Cuadrado, M.L.; Pareja, J.A. Myofascial trigger points, neck mobility and forward head posture in unilateral migraine. *Cephalalgia* **2006**, *26*, 1061–1070. [CrossRef] [PubMed]
47. Ijmker, S.; Huysmans, M.A.; Blatter, B.M.; van der Beek, A.J.; van Mechelen, W.; Bongers, P.M. Should office workers spend fewer hours at their computer? A systematic review of the literature. *Occup. Environ. Med.* **2007**, *64*, 211–222. [CrossRef] [PubMed]
48. Wahlström, J. Ergonomics, musculoskeletal disorders and computer work. *Occup. Med.* **2005**, *55*, 168–176. [CrossRef]

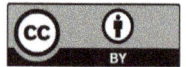

© 2020 by the authors. Licensee MDPI, Basel, Switzerland. This article is an open access article distributed under the terms and conditions of the Creative Commons Attribution (CC BY) license (http://creativecommons.org/licenses/by/4.0/).

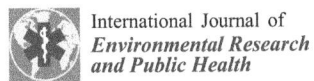

Article

The Prevalence of Anticholinergic Drugs and Correlation with Pneumonia in Elderly Patients: A Population-Based Study in Taiwan

Chien-Ying Lee [1,2], Yih-Dih Cheng [3,4], Wei-Yuan Cheng [5], Tung-Han Tsai [6] and Kuang-Hua Huang [6,*]

1. Department of Pharmacology, Chung Shan Medical University, Taichung 40201, Taiwan; cshd015@csmu.edu.tw
2. Department of Pharmacy, Chung Shan Medical University Hospital, Taichung 40201, Taiwan
3. School of pharmacy, China Medical University, Taichung 40402, Taiwan; tovis168@gmail.com
4. Department of Pharmacy, China Medical University Hospital, Taichung 40402, Taiwan
5. Taso-Tun Psychiatric Center, Ministry of Health and Welfare, Nantou 54249, Taiwan; continentaln78005@gmail.com
6. Department of Health Services Administration, China Medical University, Taichung 40402, Taiwan; dondon0525@gmail.com
* Correspondence: khhuang@mail.cmu.edu.tw

Received: 30 May 2020; Accepted: 25 August 2020; Published: 28 August 2020

Abstract: Anticholinergic drugs may increase the risk of serious respiratory infection, especially in the elderly. The study aims to investigate the prevalence of anticholinergic drugs and the correlation of incident pneumonia associated with the use of anticholinergic drugs among the elderly in Taiwan. The study population was 275,005 elderly patients aged ≥65 years old, selected from the longitudinal health insurance database (LHID) in 2016. Among all the elderly patients, about 60% had received anticholinergic medication at least once. Furthermore, the study selected elderly patients who had not been diagnosed with pneumonia and had not received any anticholinergic drugs in the past year in order to evaluate the correlation between pneumonia and anticholinergic drugs. The study excluded elderly patients who died or had received related drugs of incident pneumonia during the study period and selected elderly patients receiving anticholinergic drugs as the case group. Propensity score matching (PSM) on a 1:1 scale was used to match elderly patients that were not receiving any anticholinergic drugs as the control group, resulting in a final sample of 32,215 patients receiving anticholinergic drugs and 32,215 patients not receiving any anticholinergic drugs. Conditional logistic regression was used to estimate the association between anticholinergic drugs and pneumonia after controlling for potential confounders. Compared with patients not receiving anticholinergic drugs, the adjusted odds ratio of patients receiving anticholinergic drugs was 1.33 (95% confidence interval: 1.18 to 1.49). Anticholinergic medication is common among elderly patients in Taiwan. Elderly patients receiving anticholinergic drugs may increase their risk of incident pneumonia. The safety of anticholinergic drugs in the elderly should be of concern in Taiwan.

Keywords: anticholinergic drugs; pneumonia; elderly; potentially inappropriate medication; pharmacoepidemiology

1. Introduction

Anticholinergic drugs act centrally and peripherally on muscarinic acetylcholine receptors. Cimetidine, metoclopramide, and ranitidine are commonly employed in the treatment of the urinary bladder, the respiratory tract, and gastroesophageal disease via the intervention of the muscarinic receptor [1]. The peripheral anticholinergic complaint of dry mouth can promote mucosal damage and increase the risk for serious respiratory infection, secondary to losing the effect of the antimicrobial activity of saliva [2]. Owing to the nonselective nature of this muscarinic receptor antagonist, elderly patients are particularly susceptible to anticholinergic drugs because of age-related changes in pharmacokinetic and pharmacodynamic properties [3].

Anticholinergic drugs are one of the risk factors for pneumonia in elderly patients. It can increase the risk of pneumonia in elderly patients, although the strength of the muscarinic blockade of every anticholinergic drug is different [4,5]. One of the mechanisms for pneumonia is that dry mouth caused by anticholinergic drugs may lead to oropharyngeal and esophageal swallowing impairments and result in aspiration pneumonia [6,7]. The impairment of airway mucociliary transport in patients can prolong bacterial stay in the lungs and eventually contribute to respiratory infections; in addition, lower esophageal sphincter pressure can lead to acid reflux and cause aspiration [8]. The central effects of anticholinergic drugs may increase the risk of pharyngeal aspiration, including sedation and altered mental status, then lead to the incident pneumonia. This can more likely result in bacterial pneumonia when aspirated bacteria are not effectively cleared [9,10]. Sedation and altered mental status have also been associated with poor pulmonary hygiene and may lead to viral respiratory infection. It may also contribute to pneumonia [11]. Another mechanism that could be involved in anticholinergic-induced pneumonia is low levels of mucous secretions, which may increase the risk of incident pneumonia because of bacterial growth [6]. Previous literature suggests that oropharyngeal aspiration is a prominent etiologic factor for pneumonia in elderly adults with swallowing disorders and weak cough reflexes [9–11].

Many elderly patients suffer from multiple chronic diseases and commonly take different prescription medications for multiple conditions. It is known that changes in drug metabolism in the elderly occur with age. There is a common finding in elderly patients, where the use of multiple drugs may cause serious side effects. Many age-related diseases and disease-related conditions may predispose geriatric patients to anticholinergic intoxication [2]. In clinical practice, medications with anticholinergic effects are considered potentially inappropriate when used on the elderly [12,13]. Consequently, anticholinergic rating scales (ARS) are used to express the grade of anticholinergic effect in clinical practice, ranging from limited or none (Level 0), moderate (Level 1), strong (Level 2), and very strong (Level 3) [14,15], while the correlation between anticholinergic gradation and incident pneumonia is inconsistent. Some studies have indicated that the risk of incident pneumonia is not related to high potency anticholinergic drugs (Level 3) [6]. Previous studies have identified several drugs with anticholinergic properties we should be aware of, namely, the possibility of side effects in elderly patients, including respiratory system medicines (cetirizine, loratadine, pseudoephedrine), psychotropic medicines (paroxetine, quetiapine), alimentary tract medicines (cimetidine, ranitidine), and neurological disorder medications (larbidopa–levodopa, levodopa) [15–17].

To date, few studies have been conducted using a nationwide database to evaluate the correlation between pneumonia and anticholinergic drugs in elderly patients, especially in Taiwan [6,18]. It is essential to understand the risk of pneumonia in elderly patients receiving anticholinergic drugs. Therefore, this study was conducted to investigate the prevalence of anticholinergic drugs and the risk factors related to pneumonia and, moreover, estimate the correlation of incident pneumonia associated with the use of anticholinergic drugs among the elderly by using a nationwide database in Taiwan.

2. Materials and Methods

2.1. Data Source

The study is secondary data analysis, from 2015 to 2016, based on the longitudinal health insurance database (LHID) released by the Health and Welfare Data Science Center, Ministry of Health and Welfare (HWDC, MOHW; Registration No. H107175). LHID randomly selected two million beneficiaries from the Taiwan National Health Insurance (NHI) program. The information in LHID included detailed clinical records of the outpatient department and hospitalization, diagnostic codes, and prescribing information. The NHI program is nationwide social insurance that has enrolled up to 99% of citizens since 1995. Hence, the database is a nationally representative health database for Taiwan. HWDC provides scrambled random identification numbers for insured patients to protect the privacy of beneficiaries. This study protocol was approved as a completely ethical review by the Institutional Review Board of China Medical University Hospital, Taiwan (No. CMUH107-REC2-004). The database is anonymous; therefore, the requirement for informed consent was waived.

2.2. Study Subjects

Figure 1 lists the flowchart of the selected patients for inclusion. The study population was 275,005 elderly patients aged ≥65 years old, selected from LHID on 1 January 2016 to investigate the prevalence of anticholinergic drugs. Furthermore, the elderly patients who had not been diagnosed with pneumonia and had not received any anticholinergic drugs in the past year were enrolled in the study to evaluate the correlation between pneumonia and anticholinergic drugs. We also excluded 10,532 patients who died and the 33,189 patients who had received related drugs of incident pneumonia in the study period in order to improve the validity of the study results. The related drugs of incident pneumonia contained amiodarone, angiotensin-converting enzyme inhibitors (ACEIs), amantadine, and steroids [12–17]. Moreover, the study classified elderly patients according to their medication records in 2016 and selected elderly patients who were receiving anticholinergic drugs as the case group. In the study, there were a total of 49 drugs with the potential to cause anticholinergic adverse effects [17], including psychotropic medicines (e.g., paroxetine, quetiapine, trazodone), alimentary tract and metabolism medicines (e.g., cimetidine, metoclopramide, ranitidine, loperamide), respiratory system and allergy medicines (e.g., cetirizine, loratadine, pseudoephedrine), and neurological disorder medications (e.g., carbidopa–levodopa, levodopa) (see Table A1). Furthermore, to reduce the potential confounding caused by unbalanced covariates in nonexperimental settings, we used propensity score matching (PSM) on a 1:1 scale to match elderly patients not receiving any anticholinergic drugs as the control group, resulting in a final sample of 32,215 patients receiving anticholinergic drugs and 32,215 patients not receiving any anticholinergic drugs. The propensity score of the study is the probability of patients receiving anticholinergic drugs, calculated by gender, age, insured salary, urbanization, and the Charlson comorbidity index (CCI).

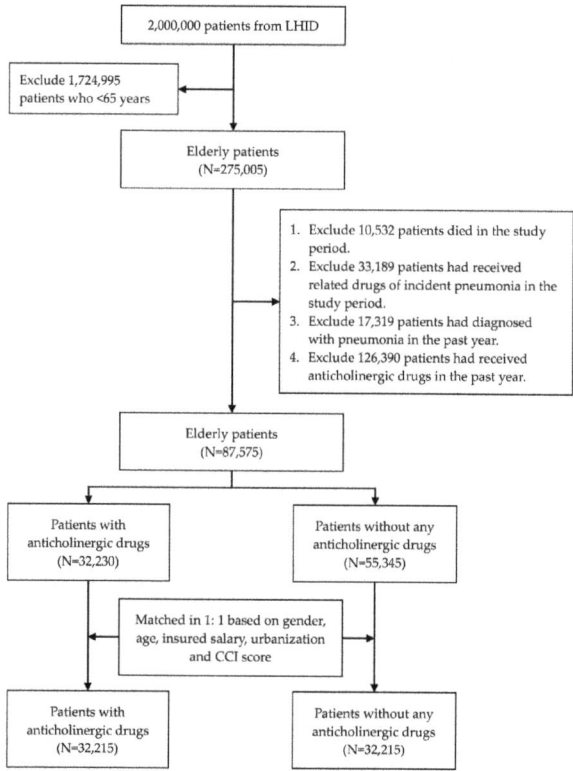

Figure 1. Flowchart of the study subject selection process. (Abbreviations: LHID, longitudinal health insurance database; CCI, Charlson comorbidity index)

2.3. Study Design

The study is a retrospective study to investigate the prevalence of anticholinergic drugs among elderly patients in Taiwan. Furthermore, the study design is divided into three phases to assess the correlation between anticholinergic drugs and pneumonia. The first phase was the exclusion period, from 1 January to 31 December 2015, in which to select the study subjects. The second phase was the observation period, from 1 January to 30 November 2016, in which to estimate the correlation between anticholinergic drugs and pneumonia. Patients were followed-up 30 days after anticholinergic drug prescriptions in order to observe the incidence of pneumonia. The third phase was in December 2016 to ensure the follow-up period. Thus, the patients receiving anticholinergic drugs in this phase would not be enrolled as study subjects. The study design diagram is exhibited in Figure 2.

The definition of incident pneumonia in the study was according to the principal diagnosis code in J12–J18, based on the International Classification of Diseases, Tenth Revision, Clinical Modification (ICD-10-CM). The study investigated the association between anticholinergic drugs and pneumonia via conditional logistic regression. Control variables in the study contained gender, age, insured salary, urbanization, CCI scores, and comorbidities related to pneumonia. Comorbidities contained diabetes mellitus (DM; ICD-10-CM: E08-E13), Alzheimer's disease (AD; ICD-10-CM: G30, F00), stroke (ICD-10-CM: I60-I69), Parkinson's disease (PD; ICD-10-CM: G20), major depression disorder (MDD; ICD-10-CM: F32.9, F33.9), chronic kidney disease (CKD; ICD-10-CM: N18), asthma (ICD-10-CM: J45), chronic obstructive pulmonary disease (COPD; ICD-10-CM: J40-J44, J47), heart failure (HF; ICD-10-CM: I50), upper respiratory infection (URI; ICD-10-CM: J00-J06), gastroesophageal reflux disease (GERD; ICD-10-CM: K21), and epilepsy (ICD-10-CM: G40-G41). The definition of comorbidities was with diagnosis at least three times a year, except epileptic seizure. Epileptic seizure was defined by diagnosis once a year.

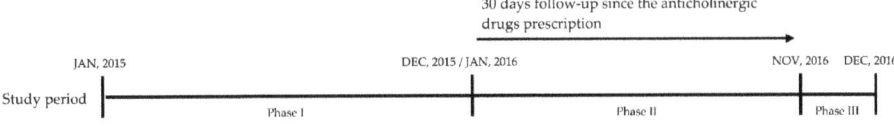

Figure 2. The study design diagram.

2.4. Statistical Analysis

Descriptive statistics were used to summarize distributions of the prevalence of anticholinergic drugs in the elderly in Taiwan. We used the standardized mean difference to examine the balance of case and control groups after matching. We further used conditional logistic regression to estimate the association between anticholinergic drugs and pneumonia after controlling for potential confounders. SAS software version 9.4 (SAS Institute Inc., Cary, NC, USA) was used for statistical analysis in the study, and the statistical significance was defined as p-value < 0.05.

3. Results

3.1. The Prevalence of Anticholinergic Drugs

Table 1 presents the prevalence of anticholinergic drugs in elderly patients. There was a total of 967,887 prescriptions with anticholinergic drugs, about 12.96%, out of all prescriptions. The most frequency anticholinergic prescriptions were cimetidine (2.54%), cetirizine (1.19%), pseudoephedrine (1.15%), metoclopramide (1.13%), ranitidine (0.83%), quetiapine (0.80%), carbidopa–levodopa (0.66%), loratadine (0.65%), trazodone (0.54%), and loperamide (0.51%), sequentially. To elderly patients, there were 165,262 patients (60.09%) who had received anticholinergic medication at least once out of all elderly patients.

Table 1. The distribution of prescriptions in elderly patients.

Prescriptions	No. of Prescriptions		No. of Patients Had Received	
	N	%	N	%
Total	7,467,908	100.00	275,005	100.00
Without anticholinergic drugs	6,500,021	87.04	109,743	39.91
With anticholinergic drugs	967,887	12.96	165,262	60.09
Most frequency anticholinergic drugs				
Cimetidine	189,862	2.54	53,171	19.33
Cetirizine	88,587	1.19	33,987	12.36
Pseudoephedrine	86,201	1.15	36,453	13.26
Metoclopramide	84,483	1.13	30,241	11.00
Ranitidine	61,831	0.83	16,066	5.84
Quetiapine	59,961	0.80	8126	2.95
Carbidopa–Levodopa	49,145	0.66	6371	2.32
Loratadine	48,793	0.65	20,132	7.32
Trazodone	40,079	0.54	6875	2.50
Loperamide	38,237	0.51	20,527	7.46

3.2. The Baseline Characteristics Distribution of Study Subjects

After subject selection, there was a total of 64,430 elderly patients in the study, and both groups, with and without anticholinergic drugs, had 32,215 patients. The mean age of patients receiving anticholinergic drugs was 73.58 ± 7.35 years, 51.77% were female, and 72.74% were in highly urbanization areas. As in Table 2, baseline characteristics were well balanced between elderly patients with and without anticholinergic drugs after matching. Among patients receiving anticholinergic drugs, there were 8614 patients (26.74%) with DM, 3457 patients (10.73%) with stroke, 317 patients with Parkinson's disease (0.98%), 3684 patients with CKD (11.43%), 1928 patients with asthma (5.98%), 2781 patients with COPD (8.63%), 1076 patients with HF (3.34%), 18,688 patients with URI (58.01%), 862 patients with GERD (2.68%), and 120 patients with epilepsy (0.37%).

Table 2. The baseline characteristics distribution of study subjects after matching.

Variables	Crude Data						After Matching					
	Anticholinergic Drugs				SMD[3]	p-Value[1]	Anticholinergic Drugs				SMD[3]	p-Value[1]
	Without		With				Without		With			
	N	%	N	%			N	%	N	%		
Total	55,345	100.00	32,230	100.00			32,215	100.00	32,215	100.00		
Gender[2]					0.08	<0.001					0	0.969
Female	27,610	49.89	17,337	53.79			17,317	53.75	17,322	53.77		
Male	27,735	50.11	14,893	46.21			14,898	46.25	14,893	46.23		
Age (year)[2]	73.28±7.42		73.58±7.35		0.05	<0.001	73.59±7.42		73.58±7.35		0	0.981
65–70	25,432	45.95	14,034	43.54			13,992	43.43	14,034	43.56		
71–75	11,619	20.99	6881	21.35			6878	21.35	6878	21.35		
76–80	8317	15.03	5322	16.51			5344	16.59	5310	16.48		
>80	9977	18.03	5993	18.59			6001	18.63	5993	18.60		
Insured salary[3]					0.06	<0.001					0	0.994
<20,008	18,342	33.14	9070	28.14			9046	28.08	9070	28.15		
20,008–22,800	19,850	35.87	13,174	40.87			13,184	40.93	13,159	40.85		
22,801–50,600	11,176	20.19	6632	20.58			6621	20.55	6632	20.59		
>50,600	5977	10.80	3354	10.41			3364	10.44	3354	10.41		
Urbanization[2]					0.07	<0.001					0	0.903
Urban	42,143	76.15	23,434	72.71			23,480	72.89	23,434	72.74		
Suburban	8781	15.87	5759	17.87			5729	17.78	5747	17.84		
Rural	4421	7.99	3037	9.42			3006	9.33	3034	9.42		
CCI[2,3]					0.22	<0.001					0	0.989
0	32,820	59.30	15,617	48.45			15,626	48.51	15,617	48.48		
1–2	18,210	32.90	13,155	40.82			13,138	40.78	13,155	40.84		
≥3	4315	7.80	3458	10.73			3451	10.71	3443	10.69		
DM[3]					−0.14	<0.001					−0.02	0.015
No	43,788	79.12	23,605	73.24			23,872	74.10	23,601	73.26		
Yes	11,557	20.88	8625	26.76			8343	25.90	8614	26.74		
AD[3]					−0.04	<0.001					−0.03	<0.001
No	55,148	99.64	32,012	99.32			32,076	99.57	31,997	99.32		
Yes	197	0.36	218	0.68			139	0.43	218	0.68		
Stroke					−0.11	<0.001					−0.04	<0.001
No	51,081	92.30	28,768	89.26			29,131	90.43	28,758	89.27		
Yes	4264	7.70	3462	10.74			3084	9.57	3457	10.73		
PD[3]					−0.08	<0.001					−0.08	<0.001
No	55,175	99.69	31,913	99.02			32,101	99.65	31,898	99.02		
Yes	170	0.31	317	0.98			114	0.35	317	0.98		
MDD[3]					−0.06	<0.001					−0.05	<0.001
No	54,660	98.76	31,579	97.98			31,773	98.63	31,564	97.98		
Yes	685	1.24	651	2.02			442	1.37	651	2.02		
CKD[3]					−0.13	<0.001					−0.08	<0.001
No	51,169	92.45	28,540	88.55			29,312	90.99	28,532	88.57		
Yes	4176	7.55	3690	11.45			2903	9.01	3683	11.43		
Asthma					−0.14	<0.001					−0.11	<0.001
No	53,685	97.00	30,302	94.02			31,048	96.38	30,287	94.02		
Yes	1660	3.00	1928	5.98			1167	3.62	1928	5.98		
COPD[3]					−0.19	<0.001					−0.15	<0.001
No	53,077	95.90	29,448	91.37			30,653	95.15	29,434	91.37		
Yes	2268	4.10	2782	8.63			1562	4.85	2781	8.63		

Table 2. Cont.

Variables	Crude Data					After Matching				
	Anticholinergic Drugs						Anticholinergic Drugs				
	Without		With		SMD [3]	p-Value [1]	Without		With		SMD [3]	p-Value [1]
	N	%	N	%			N	%	N	%		
HF [3]					−0.08	<0.001					−0.05	<0.001
No	54,226	97.98	31,150	96.65			31,429	97.56	31,139	96.66		
Yes	1119	2.02	1080	3.35			786	2.44	1076	3.34		
URI [3]					−0.63	<0.001					−0.59	<0.001
No	39,636	71.62	13,536	42.00			22,565	70.05	13,527	41.99		
Yes	15,709	28.38	18,694	58.00			9650	29.95	18,688	58.01		
GERD [3]					−0.12	<0.001					−0.11	<0.001
No	54,765	98.95	31,368	97.33			31,849	98.86	31,353	97.32		
Yes	580	1.05	862	2.67			366	1.14	862	2.68		
Epilepsy					−0.02	0.004					−0.01	0.075
No	55,199	99.74	32,109	99.62			32,121	99.71	32,095	99.63		
Yes	146	0.26	121	0.38			94	0.29	120	0.37		

[1] Chi-square test. [2] The matching variables and the unit of insured salary are in New Taiwan dollars (NTD). [3] Abbreviations: SMD, Standardized mean difference; CCI, Charlson comorbidity index; DM, diabetes mellitus; AD, Alzheimer's disease; PD, Parkinson's disease; MDD, major depression disorder; CKD, chronic kidney disease; COPD, chronic obstructive pulmonary disease; HF, heart failure; URI, upper respiratory infection; GERD, gastroesophageal reflux disease.

3.3. The Incidence Rate of Pneumonia in Elderly Patients

Table 3 indicates that among all participants, 1519 patients had occurred pneumonia, and the incidence rate was 23.58 cases per 1000 elderly patients. The incidence rate of patients receiving anticholinergic drugs was 33.23 cases per 1000 elderly patients. Compared with patients not receiving anticholinergic drugs, the risk ratio was 2.18 times of incident pneumonia. Compared with patients without DM, patients with DM had 1.31 times the risk of incident pneumonia. Additionally, compared with patients without comorbidities, patients with comorbidities had a higher risk of incident pneumonia, including stroke (2.21 times), PD (2.89 times), CKD (1.85 times), asthma (5.54 times), COPD (6.77 times), HF (2.75 times), URI (1.98 times), GERD (2.15 times), and epilepsy (4.61 times).

Table 3. The incidence rate of pneumonia in elderly patients.

Variables	Pneumonia		Risk Ratio
	N	Incident Rate (‰)	
Total	1519	23.58	
Anticholinergic drugs			
Without	529	15.27	
With	990	33.23	2.18
Diabetes mellitus			
No	1036	21.82	
Yes	483	28.48	1.31
Alzheimer's disease			
No	1507	23.52	
Yes	12	33.61	1.43
Stroke			
No	1215	20.99	
Yes	304	46.48	2.21
Parkinson's disease			
No	1490	23.28	
Yes	29	67.29	2.89

Table 3. Cont.

Variables	Pneumonia		Risk Ratio
	N	Incident Rate (‰)	
Major depression disorder			
No	1493	23.57	
Yes	26	23.79	1.01
Chronic kidney disease			
No	1255	21.70	
Yes	264	40.09	1.85
Asthma			
No	1187	19.35	
Yes	332	107.27	5.54
Chronic obstructive pulmonary disease			
No	1020	16.98	
Yes	499	114.90	6.77
Heart failure			
No	1404	22.44	
Yes	115	61.76	2.75
Upper respiratory infection			
No	594	16.46	
Yes	925	32.64	1.98
Gastroesophageal reflux disease			
No	1458	23.07	
Yes	61	49.67	2.15
Epilepsy			
No	1496	23.30	
Yes	23	107.48	4.61

3.4. Correlation between Anticholinergic Drugs and Pneumonia

Table 4 points out that patients receiving anticholinergic drugs increased their risk of incident pneumonia (adjusted odds ratio [OR]: 1.33; 95% confidence interval [CI]: 1.18 to 1.49) after controlling for potential confounders. DM increased the risk of incident pneumonia (aOR: 1.44; 95% CI: 1.26 to 1.65). AD also increased the risk of incident pneumonia, but had no statistical significance (aOR: 1.20; 95% CI: 0.66 to 2.17). aORs of incident pneumonia in patients with comorbidities were all significantly higher than patients without, including stroke (aOR: 2.02; 95% CI: 1.75 to 2.33), PD (aOR: 1.94; 95% CI: 1.28 to 2.94), CKD (aOR: 1.57; 95% CI: 1.35 to 1.82), asthma (aOR: 1.57; 95% CI: 1.31 to 1.87), COPD (aOR: 4.93; 95% CI: 4.21 to 5.78), HF (aOR: 1.64; 95% CI: 1.32 to 2.04), URI (aOR: 1.79; 95% CI: 1.60 to 2.00), GERD (aOR: 1.52; 95% CI: 1.15 to 2.01), and epilepsy (aOR: 3.11; 95% CI: 1.92 to 5.03).

Table 4. Comparing the risk of incident pneumonia between elderly patients with and without anticholinergic drugs.

Variables	aOR [1,2]	95% Confidence Interval		p-Value
Anticholinergic agent	1.33	1.18–1.49		<0.001
DM [1]	1.44	1.26–1.65		<0.001
AD [1]	1.20	0.66–2.18		0.561
Stroke	2.02	1.75–2.33		<0.001
PD [1]	1.94	1.28–2.94		0.002
MDD [1]	0.74	0.49–1.12		0.158
CKD [1]	1.57	1.35–1.82		<0.001
Asthma	1.57	1.31–1.87		<0.001
COPD [1]	4.93	4.21–5.78		<0.001
HF [1]	1.64	1.32–2.04		<0.001
URI [1]	1.79	1.60–2.00		<0.001
GERD [1]	1.52	1.15–2.01		0.003
Epilepsy	3.11	1.92–5.03		<0.001

[1] Abbreviations: aOR, adjusted odds ratio; DM, diabetes mellitus; AD, Alzheimer's disease; PD, Parkinson's disease; MDD, major depression disorder; CKD, chronic kidney disease; COPD, chronic obstructive pulmonary disease; HF, heart failure; URI, upper respiratory infection; GERD, gastroesophageal reflux disease. [2] The conditional logistic regression model, stratified by matching variables, was used to estimate the risk.

4. Discussion

Our study results indicate that about 60% of elderly patients had received anticholinergic medication at least once, and the most frequent anticholinergic prescriptions in Taiwan were cimetidine, cetirizine, pseudoephedrine, metoclopramide, and ranitidine. These drugs are used to treat URI and excessive secretions of gastric acid in primary care clinics in Taiwan. A previous study indicated that most frequent anticholinergic drugs were ranitidine, trazodone, paroxetine, oxybutynin, and nortriptyline [19]. Those were used to treat cardiovascular and neurological disorders. This indicates that there is a wide disparity in the prescription pattern of anticholinergic drugs between other countries and Taiwan. It may be related to the difference in medical care-seeking behavior caused by the health care system.

Pneumonia is a life-threatening infectious disease where age is one of the strongest risk factors. Our study demonstrates that anticholinergic drugs are related to incident pneumonia in the elderly. A population-based case–control study by Paul et al. [10] expressed that anticholinergic medication use is associated with pneumonia risk, compared with no use. Moreover, both acute and chronic use of anticholinergic drugs were associated with a higher risk for pneumonia, whereas there was no association with previous use. Another case–control study in America by Chatterjee et al. [6] estimated anticholinergic drug exposure and the risk of pneumonia. The overall use of anticholinergic drugs was associated with the risk of pneumonia, while the effect of anticholinergic drugs was not related to pneumonia. It indicated that even low-potency anticholinergic drugs may cause a significant risk of pneumonia. A nationwide study in Finland had a similar result [18]. Most of the low-potency anticholinergic drugs are cardiovascular drugs, and the risk may be partially explained by comorbidity. The main purpose of our study was to explore the potential relationship between the risk of pneumonia and anticholinergic drug use in the elderly in Taiwan. To enhance the accuracy of the study results, our study used PSM to obtain control groups for each elderly patient receiving anticholinergic drugs. A propensity score is a unit with certain characteristics that is assigned to each elderly patient receiving anticholinergic drugs. The scores can be used to reduce or eliminate selection bias in observational studies by the characteristics of elderly patients with and without anticholinergic drugs [20–23]. Compared with previous studies, our study design and methodology are more rigorous. Our study was inappropriate for further analysis regarding the effect of different levels of anticholinergic drugs due to the elderly subjects in our study being matched based on whether they received anticholinergic drugs rather than different levels of anticholinergic drugs. To our knowledge, there has been no related population-based study to estimate the relationship between incident pneumonia and anticholinergic drug use in Taiwan. Our study was not aimed at exploring the mechanisms between anticholinergic drugs and increased pneumonia risk, but the association between anticholinergic drugs and pneumonia in the elderly was clear. Although the incident rate of pneumonia caused by anticholinergic drugs is relatively rare, future studies should develop more well-designed prospective population trials to be carried out to ascertain the relationship.

The comorbidities may also predispose elderly patients to an increased risk of pneumonia. Our study results were consistent with previous studies that noted that comorbidities, including DM, stroke, PD, CKD, asthma, COPD, HF, URI, and GERD, were risk factors of pneumonia. The elderly with COPD or asthma are a high-risk population of bacterial infection, and one of the major infections is caused by streptococcus pneumoniae bacteria. It can cause many types of illnesses that contained pneumonia, meningitis, and septicemia. Therefore, COPD and asthma are both associated with a greater risk of incident pneumonia in the elderly [24–26]. DM may also increase the pneumonia risk in the elderly due to poor glycemic control. Aging is associated with a progressive decline in respiratory system function, and poor glycemic control can cause microvascular complications of lung capillaries [27–29]. Moreover, previous studies have documented that the elderly with stroke, dementia, or Parkinson's disease have a higher risk of incident pneumonia [26,27,30]. It was possibly attributable to dysphagia, difficulty swallowing, and cough reflexes. Oropharyngeal dysphagia is also one of the risk factors for pneumonia in elderly patients [31–33]. Renal disease in the elderly is clinically important. Previous studies have described that there is a positive direction in the association between predialysis CKD and acute community-acquired infection [34]. Hypoimmunity of the elderly patient with CKD may predispose the patient to acute lower respiratory infections. Another study demonstrated that cardiovascular function declined in elderly patients with heart disease, which would affect the mucociliary clearance functions that trap and remove particulates and pathogens from the airways, leading to an increased risk of incident pneumonia [35]. Furthermore, a population-based cohort study indicated that GERD is associated with a long-term risk of pneumonia, especially in GERD with proton pump inhibitors (PPIs) for a longer treatment than four months [36]. There is a relationship between gastric acid suppressants and an increased risk of pneumonia [37]. Authors have suggested that the inhibition of gastric acid secretion by acid-suppressive therapy allows pathogen colonization from the upper gastrointestinal tract [24].

The major strength of the study is that it is based on a nationwide database, avoiding bias such as selection, nonresponse, and poor recall. Big data analysis is a new trend in modern healthcare research. LHID has completeness in recording prescriptions and clinical diagnosis. Moreover, the study was not only adjusted for potential confounding factors but also used PSM to avoid bias in the selection of study subjects. Therefore, the study indicates the correlation between anticholinergic drugs and pneumonia with a narrower and statistically significant confidence interval.

There were also a few limitations to the study. Some pneumonia-related variables, such as medication adherence, tobacco consumption behavior, and laboratory parameters, cannot be obtained from LHID. Additionally, the study only used the ICD code to define disease without any medical procedure codes. There may be overdiagnosis. Although our study indicated the correlation between anticholinergic drugs and pneumonia, the strength of the anticholinergic effect may also be related to pneumonia. We will explore the risk of incident pneumonia with different anticholinergic drugs in further study. Finally, this study is a type of observational study that analyzes data from a population database. The study result can only provide evidence to demonstrate that anticholinergic drugs are related to incident pneumonia. It is essential to obtain more information from other databases to analyze the cause–effect relation in future research.

5. Conclusions

The use of anticholinergic drugs is common in the elderly in Taiwan because these medications are prescribed for the symptomatic management of medical conditions. Elderly patients receiving anticholinergic drugs may increase their risk of incident pneumonia. Moreover, DM, stroke, PD,

CKD, asthma, COPD, HF, URI, and GERD were also associated with incident pneumonia in the elderly. Anticholinergic drugs can have many beneficial effects, but these drugs need to be balanced against potential harm. Drugs with anticholinergic properties can be problematic, especially for the elderly population. Prescribers should consider dose reductions and monitoring when prescribing anticholinergic drugs to elderly patients to reduce the risks of adverse outcomes. Furthermore, randomized clinical trials are warranted to determine the effectiveness and safety of anticholinergic drugs in the elderly.

Author Contributions: Conceptualization, C.-Y.L. and K.-H.H.; formal analysis, W.-Y.C. and T.-H.T.; methodology, C.-Y.L., Y.-D.C., W.-Y.C., and K.-H.H.; validation, K.-H.H.; writing—original draft, C.-Y.L., Y.-D.C., and K.-H.H.; writing—review and editing, K.-H.H. All authors have read and agreed to the published version of the manuscript.

Funding: This research was funded by the Ministry of Science and Technology Taiwan (MOST 107-2410-H-039-007), Chung Shan Medical University Taiwan (CSMU-INT-108-14), and China Medical University Taiwan (CMU108-MF-100).

Acknowledgments: We are grateful to Chung Shan Medical University, Taiwan, China Medical University, Taiwan, Asia University, Taiwan, and the Health Data Science Center, China Medical University Hospital, for providing administrative, technical, and funding support that has contributed to the completion of this study. This study is based, in part, on data released by the Health and Welfare Data Science Center, Ministry of Health and Welfare. The interpretation and conclusions contained herein do not represent those of the Ministry of Health and Welfare.

Conflicts of Interest: The authors declare no conflict of interest.

Appendix A

Table A1. The list of anticholinergic drugs.

Anticholinergic Drugs
Amitriptyline hydrochloride
Atropine products
Benztropine mesylate
Carisoprodol
Chlorpheniramine maleate
Chlorpromazine hydrochloride
Cyproheptadine hydrochloride
Dicyclomine hydrochloride
Diphenhydramine hydrochloride
Fluphenazine hydrochloride
Hydroxyzine hydrochloride and hydroxyzine pamoate
Hyoscyamine products
Imipramine hydrochloride
Meclizine hydrochloride
Oxybutynin chloride
Perphenazine
Promethazine hydrochloride
Thioridazine hydrochloride
Thiothixene
Tizanidine hydrochloride
Trifluoperazine hydrochloride
Amantadine hydrochloride
Baclofen
Cetirizine hydrochloride
Cimetidine
Clozapine
Cyclobenzaprine hydrochloride
Desipramine hydrochloride
Loperamide hydrochloride

Table A1. Cont.

Anticholinergic Drugs
Loratadine
Nortriptyline hydrochloride
Olanzapine
Prochlorperazine maleate
Pseudoephedrine hydrochloride-triprolidine hydrochloride
Tolterodine tartrate
Carbidopa-levodopa
Entacapone
Haloperidol
Metocarbamol
Metoclopramide hydrochloride
Mirtazapine
Paroxetine hydrochloride
Pramipexole dihydrochloride
Quetiapine fumarate
Ranitidine hydrochloride
Risperidone
Selegiline hydrochloride
Trazodone hydrochloride
Ziprasidone hydrochloride

Source: Rudolph, J.L.; Salow, M.J.; Angelini, M.C.; McGlinchey, R.E. The anticholinergic risk scale and anticholinergic adverse effects in older persons. *Arch. Intern. Med.* **2008**, *168*, 508–513.

References

1. Soukup, O.; Winder, M.; Killi, U.K.; Wsol, V.; Jun, D.; Ramalho, T.D.C.; Tobin, G. Acetylcholinesterase Inhibitors and Drugs Acting on Muscarinic Receptors-Potential Crosstalk of Cholinergic Mechanisms during Pharmacological Treatment. *Curr. Neuropharmacol.* **2017**, *15*, 637–653. [CrossRef] [PubMed]
2. Feinberg, M. The Problems of Anticholinergic Adverse Effects in Older Patients. *Drugs Aging* **1993**, *3*, 335–348. [CrossRef]
3. Tune, L.E. Anticholinergic effects of medication in elderly patients. *J. Clin. Psychiatry* **2001**, *62*, 11–14. [PubMed]
4. Gutiérrez, F.; Masiá, M. Improving Outcomes of Elderly Patients with Community-Acquired Pneumonia. *Drugs Aging* **2008**, *25*, 585–610. [CrossRef] [PubMed]
5. Stupka, J.E.; Mortensen, E.M.; Anzueto, A.; Restrepo, M.I. Community-acquired pneumonia in elderly patients. *Aging Health* **2009**, *5*, 763–774. [CrossRef] [PubMed]
6. Chatterjee, S.; Carnahan, R.M.; Chen, H.; Holmes, H.M.; Johnson, M.L.; Aparasu, R.R. Anticholinergic Medication Use and Risk of Pneumonia in Elderly Adults: A Nested Case-Control Study. *J. Am. Geriatr. Soc.* **2016**, *64*, 394–400. [CrossRef]
7. Venkatesan, P.; Gladman, J.R.F.; Macfarlane, J.T.; Barer, D.; Berman, P.; Kinnear, W.; Finch, R.G. A hospital study of community acquired pneumonia in the elderly. *Thorax* **1990**, *45*, 254–258. [CrossRef] [PubMed]
8. Riquelme, R.; Torres, A.; El-Ebiary, M.; De La Bellacasa, J.P.; Estruch, R.; Mensa, J.; Fernández-Solà, J.; Hernández, C.; Rodriguez-Roisin, R. Community-acquired pneumonia in the elderly: A multivariate analysis of risk and prognostic factors. *Am. J. Respir. Crit. Care Med.* **1996**, *154*, 1450–1455. [CrossRef]
9. Huxley, E.J.; Viroslav, J.; Gray, W.R.; Pierce, A.K. Pharyngeal aspiration in normal adults and patients with depressed consciousness. *Am. J. Med.* **1978**, *64*, 564–568. [CrossRef]
10. Paul, K.J.; Walker, R.L.; Dublin, S. Anticholinergic Medications and Risk of Community-Acquired Pneumonia in Elderly Adults: A Population-Based Case-Control Study. *J. Am. Geriatr. Soc.* **2015**, *63*, 476–485. [CrossRef]
11. Marik, P.E.; Kaplan, D. Aspiration Pneumonia and Dysphagia in the Elderly. *Chest* **2003**, *124*, 328–336. [CrossRef]
12. Fick, D.M.; Cooper, J.W.; Wade, W.E.; Waller, J.L.; MacLean, J.R.; Beers, M.H. Updating the Beers criteria for potentially inappropriate medication use in older adults: Results of a US consensus panel of experts. *Arch. Intern. Med.* **2003**, *163*, 2716–2724. [CrossRef] [PubMed]

13. Shrank, W.; Polinski, J.M.; Avorn, J. Quality Indicators for Medication Use in Vulnerable Elders. *J. Am. Geriatr. Soc.* **2007**, *55*, S373–S382. [CrossRef] [PubMed]
14. Gorup, E.; Rifel, J.; Šter, M.P. Anticholinergic burden and most common anticholinergic-acting medicines in older general practice patients. *Slov. J. Public Health* **2018**, *57*, 140–147. [CrossRef] [PubMed]
15. Salahudeen, M.; Duffull, S.B.; Nishtala, P. Anticholinergic burden quantified by anticholinergic risk scales and adverse outcomes in older people: A systematic review. *BMC Geriatr.* **2015**, *15*, 31. [CrossRef]
16. Sittironnarit, G.; Ames, D.; Bush, A.I.; Faux, N.G.; Flicker, L.; Foster, J.; Hilmer, S.N.; Lautenschlager, N.T.; Maruff, P.; Masters, C.L.; et al. Effects of Anticholinergic Drugs on Cognitive Function in Older Australians: Results from the AIBL Study. *Dement. Geriatr. Cogn. Disord.* **2011**, *31*, 173–178. [CrossRef]
17. Rudolph, J.L.; Salow, M.J.; Angelini, M.C.; McGlinchey, R.E. The Anticholinergic Risk Scale and Anticholinergic Adverse Effects in Older Persons. *Arch. Intern. Med.* **2008**, *168*, 508. [CrossRef]
18. Lampela, P.; Tolppanen, A.; Tanskanen, A.; Tiihonen, J.; Hartikainen, S.; Taipale, H. Anticholinergic Exposure and Risk of Pneumonia in Persons with Alzheimer's Disease: A Nested Case-Control Study. *J. Alzheimer Dis.* **2017**, *56*, 119–128. [CrossRef]
19. Miyashita, N.; Yamauchi, Y. Bacterial Pneumonia in Elderly Japanese Populations. *Jpn. Clin. Med.* **2018**, *9*, 1179670717751433. [CrossRef]
20. Lee, T.-Y.; Hsu, Y.-C.; Tseng, H.-C.; Yu, S.-H.; Lin, J.-T.; Wu, M.-S.; Wu, C.-Y. Association of Daily Aspirin Therapy With Risk of Hepatocellular Carcinoma in Patients With Chronic Hepatitis B. *JAMA Intern. Med.* **2019**, *179*, 633–640. [CrossRef]
21. Cheng, Y.-T.; Cheng, C.-T.; Wang, S.-Y.; Wu, V.C.-C.; Chu, P.-H.; Chou, A.-H.; Chen, C.-C.; Ko, P.-J.; Liu, K.-S.; Chen, S.-W. Long-term Outcomes of Endovascular and Open Repair for Traumatic Thoracic Aortic Injury. *JAMA Netw. Open* **2019**, *2*, e187861. [CrossRef]
22. Wang, C.J.; Cheng, S.H.; Wu, J.-Y.; Lin, Y.-P.; Kao, W.-H.; Lin, C.-L.; Chen, Y.-J.; Tsai, S.-L.; Kao, F.-Y.; Huang, A.T. Association of a Bundled-Payment Program With Cost and Outcomes in Full-Cycle Breast Cancer Care. *JAMA Oncol.* **2017**, *3*, 327–334. [CrossRef] [PubMed]
23. Wei, K.-C.; Bee, Y.-S.; Wang, W.-H.; Huang, Y.-T.; Lu, T.-H. Incidence of Cataract Surgery in Patients After Percutaneous Cardiac Intervention in Taiwan. *JAMA Intern. Med.* **2016**, *176*, 710. [CrossRef] [PubMed]
24. Woodhead, M. Inhaled corticosteroids cause pneumonia or do they? *Am. J. Respir. Crit. Care Med.* **2007**, *176*, 111–112. [CrossRef]
25. Farr, B.; Woodhead, M.; Macfarlane, J.; Bartlett, C.; McCracken, J.; Wadsworth, J.; Miller, D. Risk factors for community-acquired pneumonia diagnosed by general practitioners in the community. *Respir. Med.* **2000**, *94*, 422–427. [CrossRef] [PubMed]
26. Almirall, J.; Bolíbar, I.; Serra-Prat, M.; Roig, J.; Hospital, I.; Carandell, E.; Agustí, M.; Ayuso, P.; Estela, A.; Torres, A.; et al. New evidence of risk factors for community-acquired pneumonia: A population-based study. *Eur. Respir. J.* **2008**, *31*, 1274–1284. [CrossRef] [PubMed]
27. Jackson, M.L.; Neuzil, K.M.; Thompson, W.W.; Shay, D.; Yu, O.; Hanson, C.A.; Jackson, L.A. The Burden of Community-Acquired Pneumonia in Seniors: Results of a Population-Based Study. *Clin. Infect. Dis.* **2004**, *39*, 1642–1650. [CrossRef]
28. Bouter, K.; Diepersloot, R.J.; Van Romunde, L.K.; Uitslager, R.; Masurel, N.; Hoekstra, J.B.; Erkelens, D.W. Effect of epidemic influenza on ketoacidosis, pneumonia and death in diabetes mellitus: A hospital register survey of 1976–1979 in The Netherlands. *Diabetes Res. Clin. Pract.* **1991**, *12*, 61–68. [CrossRef]
29. Martin, J.-J.; Boavida, J.M.; Raposo, J.F.; Froes, F.; Nunes, B.; Ribeiro, R.T.; Macedo, M.; Penha-Gonçalves, C. Diabetes hinders community-acquired pneumonia outcomes in hospitalized patients. *BMJ Open Diabetes Res. Care* **2016**, *4*, e000181. [CrossRef]
30. Kalf, J.; De Swart, B.; Bloem, B.R.; Munneke, M. Prevalence of oropharyngeal dysphagia in Parkinson's disease: A meta-analysis. *Park. Relat. Disord.* **2012**, *18*, 311–315. [CrossRef]
31. Loeb, M.; Neupane, B.; Walter, S.D.; Hanning, R.; Carusone, S.C.; Lewis, D.; Krueger, P.; Simor, A.E.; Nicolle, L.; Marrie, T.J. Environmental Risk Factors for Community-Acquired Pneumonia Hospitalization in Older Adults. *J. Am. Geriatr. Soc.* **2009**, *57*, 1036–1040. [CrossRef] [PubMed]
32. Almirall, J.; Rofes, L.; Serra-Prat, M.; Icart, R.; Palomera, E.; Arreola, V.; Clavé, P. Oropharyngeal dysphagia is a risk factor for community-acquired pneumonia in the elderly. *Eur. Respir. J.* **2012**, *41*, 923–928. [CrossRef] [PubMed]

33. Chang, Y.-P.; Yang, C.-J.; Hu, K.-F.; Chao, A.-C.; Chang, Y.-H.; Hsieh, K.-P.; Tsai, J.-H.; Ho, P.-S.; Lim, S.-Y. Risk factors for pneumonia among patients with Parkinson's disease: A Taiwan nationwide population-based study. *Neuropsychiatr. Dis. Treat.* **2016**, *12*, 1037–1046. [CrossRef]
34. McDonald, H.; Thomas, S.L.; Nitsch, R. Chronic kidney disease as a risk factor for acute community-acquired infections in high-income countries: A systematic review. *BMJ Open* **2014**, *4*, e004100. [CrossRef]
35. Bornheimer, R.; Shea, K.M.; Sato, R.; Weycker, D.; Pelton, S.I. Risk of exacerbation following pneumonia in adults with heart failure or chronic obstructive pulmonary disease. *PLoS ONE* **2017**, *12*, e0184877. [CrossRef]
36. Hsu, W.-T.; Lai, C.-C.; Wang, Y.-H.; Tseng, P.-H.; Wang, K.; Wang, C.-Y.; Chen, L. Risk of pneumonia in patients with gastroesophageal reflux disease: A population-based cohort study. *PLoS ONE* **2017**, *12*, e0183808. [CrossRef]
37. Laheij, R.J.; Sturkenboom, M.C.J.M.; Hassing, R.-J.; Dieleman, J.; Stricker, B.H.C.; Jansen, J.B.M.J. Risk of Community-Acquired Pneumonia and Use of Gastric Acid–Suppressive Drugs. *JAMA* **2004**, *292*, 1955–1960. [CrossRef]

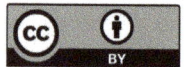

© 2020 by the authors. Licensee MDPI, Basel, Switzerland. This article is an open access article distributed under the terms and conditions of the Creative Commons Attribution (CC BY) license (http://creativecommons.org/licenses/by/4.0/).

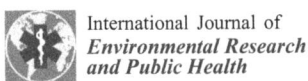

Article

Thermal Sensation in Older People with and without Dementia Living in Residential Care: New Assessment Approaches to Thermal Comfort Using Infrared Thermography

Charmaine Childs [1,*], Jennifer Elliott [1], Khaled Khatab [1], Susan Hampshaw [2], Sally Fowler-Davis [1], Jon R. Willmott [3] and Ali Ali [4]

[1] College of Health, Wellbeing and Life Sciences, Sheffield Hallam University, Sheffield S10 2BP, UK; jennifer@centralmedicalservices.co.uk (J.E.); k.khatab@shu.ac.uk (K.K.); s.fowler-davis@shu.ac.uk (S.F.-D.)
[2] School of Health and Related Research (SCHARR), University of Sheffield, Sheffield S10 2TN, UK; s.hampshaw@sheffield.ac.uk
[3] Electronic and Electrical Engineering Department, University of Sheffield, Sheffield S10 2TN, UK; j.r.willmott@sheffield.ac.uk
[4] Sheffield Teaching Hospitals, National Institute for Health Research (NIHR), Biomedical Research Centre, Sheffield S10 2JF, UK; ali.ali@sheffield.ac.uk
* Correspondence: c.childs@shu.ac.uk; Tel.: +44-0-114-225-2282

Received: 14 August 2020; Accepted: 18 September 2020; Published: 22 September 2020

Abstract: The temperature of the indoor environment is important for health and wellbeing, especially at the extremes of age. The study aim was to understand the relationship between self-reported thermal sensation and extremity skin temperature in care home residents with and without dementia. The Abbreviated Mental Test (AMT) was used to discriminate residents to two categories, those with, and those without, dementia. After residents settled and further explanation of the study given (approximately 15 min), measurements included: tympanic membrane temperature, thermal sensation rating and infrared thermal mapping of non-dominant hand and forearm. Sixty-nine afebrile adults (60–101 years of age) were studied in groups of two to five, in mean ambient temperatures of 21.4–26.6 °C (median 23.6 °C). Significant differences were observed between groups; thermal sensation rating ($p = 0.02$), tympanic temperature ($p = 0.01$), fingertip skin temperature ($p = 0.01$) and temperature gradients; fingertip-wrist $p = 0.001$ and fingertip-distal forearm, $p = 0.001$. Residents with dementia were in significantly lower air temperatures ($p = 0.001$). Although equal numbers of residents per group rated the environment as 'neutral' (comfortable), resident ratings for 'cool/cold' were more frequent amongst those with dementia compared with no dementia. In parallel, extremity (hand) thermograms revealed visual temperature demarcation, variously across fingertip, wrist, and forearm commensurate with peripheral vasoconstriction. Infrared thermography provided a quantitative and qualitative method to measure and observe hand skin temperature across multiple regions of interest alongside thermal sensation self-report. As an imaging modality, infrared thermography has potential as an additional assessment technology with clinical utility to identify vulnerable residents who may be unable to communicate verbally, or reliably, their satisfaction with indoor environmental conditions.

Keywords: infrared thermography; cutaneous temperature; skin blood flow; dementia; body temperature; thermal sensation; thermal comfort; imaging; mapping; environmental temperature; frailty

1. Introduction

To experience a thermally comfortable indoor environment, an older person living in residential care relies almost entirely upon decisions made by others. This is typically the care home staff who will regulate the temperature of the communal spaces and bedrooms. For those residents with dementia, simple interventions to adjust the physical stimuli of light, noise and temperature can improve a person's quality of life [1] experience [2] and behaviour [3]. Thermal comfort, therefore, becomes an important aspect of wellbeing and quality of life, which may require a different set of indoor thermal adjustments (including clothing) than required for active younger people.

A fundamental starting point is to understand the definition of thermal comfort; a condition of mind which expresses satisfaction with the immediate environment [4]. As a subjective experience, it may well differ amongst groups of people sharing the same environment at the same time.

The international standard, EN ISO 7730 [5] covering the evaluation of moderate thermal environments (developed in parallel with the revised American Society of Heating, Refrigerating and Air-Conditioning Engineers (ASHRAE, standard 55) specifies methods for measurement and evaluation of thermal environments. Thermal sensation is predominately related to heat balance and is influenced by physical activity, clothing and the indoor environmental factors of air temperature, mean radiant temperature, humidity and air velocity [5]. By seeking to provide a comfortable thermal environment for the majority, building and architectural sciences have led the way in finding solutions to achieve thermal comfort for the built environment. A subjective seven-point thermal sensation scale [4] developed originally from the work of Bedford [6] is completed by each individual. It is a scale widely used in thermal surveys and field trials [7] and forms the basis to calculate the average thermal sensation vote of large groups of individuals exposed to the same environment, along with an index of those dissatisfied i.e., people who vote feeling too hot, warm, cool or cold.

Whilst international standards are available, their use has largely been focused on determining thermal comfort of the workforce in offices and factories. Much less is known about thermal comfort in the old and very old living in residential care [8–10]. The need for new perspectives on thermal sensation and thermal comfort in older age is now appreciated [3,11–13] particularly given that the changes that occur in the nervous system associated with ageing leads to a decrease ('blunting') of thermal sensitivity and thermal perception [14] especially in response to cold stimuli [15] which is most pronounced at the extremities and follows a distal-proximal pattern [16]. Furthermore, due to a diminished cutaneous vasoconstrictor response to body cooling [17], older people may lose both their perception of the environment and their ability to conserve heat at the extremities. They may therefore (a) not perceive themselves as cold and (b) have a reduced physiological efficiency to conserve heat and are therefore at an increased risk of 'symptomless cooling' [14,18] putting the older person at greater risk of chilling or worse still, hypothermia [16].

As evidence emerges [11] that the existing analytical models for determination and interpretation of thermal comfort are not appropriate in older age, opportunities open up to investigate multidimensional approaches to thermal comfort, specifically of relevance to older people.

The aims of this study therefore, were to (i) identify the range of thermal sensation self-reports amongst groups of care-home residents, with and without dementia, sharing the same indoor environmental conditions (ii) use objective, long-wave infrared (LWIR) thermography to map extremity skin temperature and (iii) determine the correspondence between thermal sensation self-report and the extremity thermal map.

2. Materials and Methods

2.1. Study Design

Prospective observational feasibility investigation.

Inclusion Criteria: residents living in residential care aged 60 years or over.

Exclusion criteria: residents unable to communicate or lacking capacity to respond to simple questions.

2.2. Sample Size

As a feasibility study, the target population is 70 participants. Assuming attrition, the revised target is 60 participants. With this number, there will be 90% power, at significance level 0.05, to detect one value or unit (°C) change in temperature with 1.4 SD difference between the two groups.

2.3. Participants

Adults living in residential care homes within the South Yorkshire and Derbyshire counties of the UK were recruited over 12 months.

2.4. Screening and Recruitment Pathway

Older adults were invited to give their written informed consent to participate in the study after first reading the participant information sheet. Screening for capacity was undertaken by research nurses of the clinical research network (CRN) for the Yorkshire-Humber and Derbyshire National Health Service (NHS regions). The manager of each residence was first contacted and information was provided verbally and via leaflets for the care home staff to retain. If the manager was interested in the objectives of the study, a researcher returned to the care home to discuss the specific details of the study. The care home manager identified those residents considered to have capacity to give their own informed consent as a study participant using a 'Noticeable Problems Checklist'. For those residents with a medical diagnosis of dementia, or those considered by the care staff to have fluctuating capacity, the relative (or independent clinician) was provided with study information, by letter, and asked to consider willingness to give their signed consent on behalf of the resident. Once consent had been obtained, a mutually convenient date for recruitment was made to obtain signed consent from the resident or appropriate authority.

2.5. Recruitment

On the day of study, and with consent obtained, a further screening for capacity was undertaken using the Abbreviated Mental Test (AMT) [19], a 10-point scale used as a guide to screening for dementia in those without a formal dementia diagnosis. A score below 8 indicates a level of cognitive impairment warranting 'assignment' to the dementia category (D). Residents with AMT score of ≥8 were assigned to a 'no dementia' category (ND).

2.6. Data Collection

2.6.1. Demographic Data

Demographic data was collected to include, age, gender, ethnicity, years in residence, 'handedness'.

2.6.2. Frailty Assessment

The level of clinical frailty was assessed on a seven-point, clinical frailty scale (version 2007–2009 Dalhousie University, Halifax, NS, Canada) [20].

2.6.3. Body Temperature Measurement

Body temperature was measured at the tympanum (T_{tymp}) using a Thermoscan device (Model LF 40, Braun, Lausanne, Switzerland) before thermography commenced.

2.6.4. Past Medical History (PMH) and Current Medications

For each older resident, a brief medical history was obtained along with co-morbid condition/s and medication history, including polypharmacy. Past medical history (PMH) and medication type may influence: (a) the individuals' thermal 'perception' and (b) heat distribution at the extremities; the former influencing feelings of thermal comfort and the latter, the appearance of the heat signature (i.e., the appearance of the thermal map).

PMH with potential to affect thermal comfort perception includes thyroid dysfunction, impaired neurological perception (e.g., learning difficulties, stroke, dementia, including Alzheimer's disease, peripheral neuropathy). A PMH likely to affect heat distribution at the extremities (and thus the thermal map) is linked to vascular compromise. Pre-existing conditions were documented and include all forms of diabetes, hypertension, vasculitis, peripheral vascular disease, heart failure and Raynaud's disease. Current medication/s and dose was also documented with drugs having potential thermoregulatory effects assigned to the following categories: (a) vasoconstrictor effects, (b) vasodilator effects, (c) neurological effects, (d) diuretic effects.

2.6.5. Indoor Environment

Residents were studied in groups of two or more sitting in their usual daytime communal room. Responses were sought under 'real world' conditions of the care home. The study was scheduled to commence at least one hour after breakfast. This gave sufficient time to complete imaging before lunch was served. Recommendations for measurement of ambient conditions (EN ISO 7730) [5] were made for air temperature, (T_a °C), relative humidity (RH%) and air velocity ($m \cdot s^{-1}$) measured using a Kestrel environmental monitor (Kestrel 3000, Kestrel Instruments, Boothwyn, PA, USA).

2.6.6. Clothing

An approximation of clothing fabric insulation for each garment worn by the resident was made using available reference values [21]. Insulation of clothing is expressed as a 'Clo' unit. Clothing 'ensembles' were estimated from a weighted valuation:

$$0.676 \sum I_{cl,i} + 0.117 \qquad (1)$$

where $\sum I_{cl}$ refers to the sum of individual clothing items worn. A pragmatic approach to clothing category produced three groups: 0–0.50 Clo, 0.51–1.00 Clo, >1.0 Clo for light, medium and heavy clothing ensembles respectively. A Clo score of 0 corresponds to a person, nude. A Clo score of 1.0, the value of clothing insulation needed to maintain a person in comfort, sitting at 21 °C with air movement, 0.1 $m \cdot s^{-1}$, relative humidity (RH) $\leq$ 50%, the example used being a person wearing a business suit [21].

2.6.7. Imaging-Long Wave Infrared (LWIR) Thermography

Infrared thermography was undertaken using an uncooled microbolometer detector, (model A-600 series, FLIR, Täby, Sweden) with image resolution 640 × 320 pixels, mounted on a tripod (Vanguard, Alta Pro 264AT, Dorset, UK) and connected to a laptop computer. The LWIR detector system was positioned such that the seated participants were comfortable. In the sitting position, acral region (both hands) were positioned, first with the dorsum followed by palmar surface upwards resting upon a paper 'hand template' (Figure 1) overlying an insulated tile.

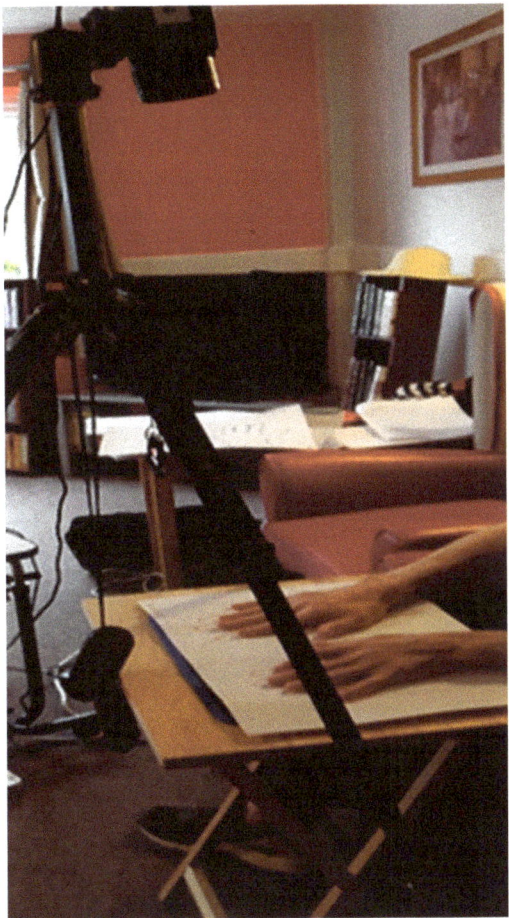

Figure 1. Long wave infrared imaging detector mounted on a tripod. The figure shows the participant during imaging with hands positioned upon a paper 'hand template' overlying an insulated tile. The portable table was used throughout the study to ensure consistency of the imaging set-up.

This provided visual orientation to the participants for the placement of fingers and hands in a consistent position and to obtain a clear field of view (FOV). After checking detector focus and distance, a maximum of three images were obtained. Colour thermal maps were obtained using a proprietary FLIR software (FLIR Systems AB, Täby, Sweden) and colour palette (see Figure 2).

In this paper, data were reported of the dorsum of the hand as this was the most comfortable position for older participants. The colour palette, with temperature key, shows darkest colours (indigo/blue) representing the lowest skin temperature and bright colour (white/yellow) highest temperatures (Figure 2).

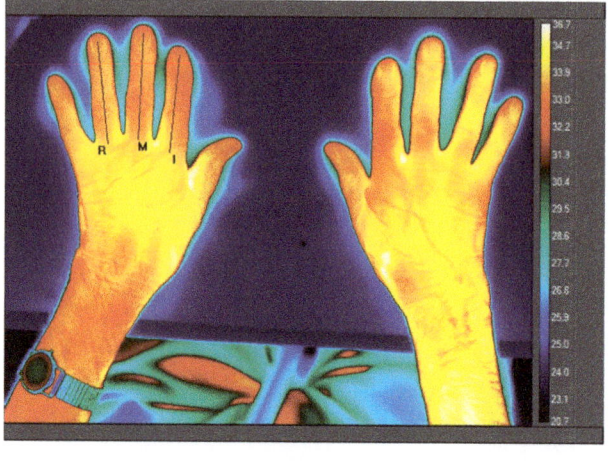

(A)

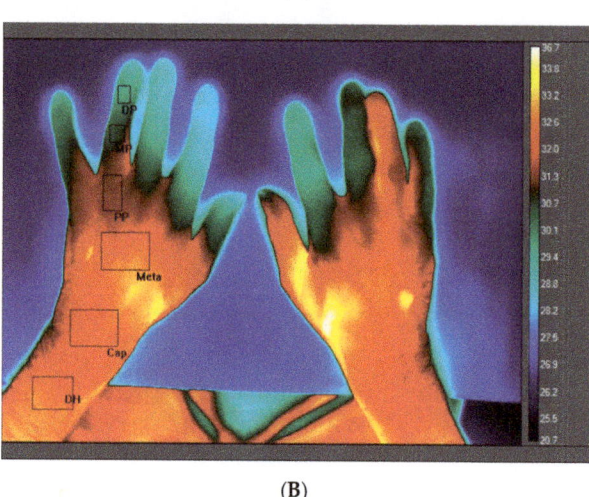

(B)

Figure 2. (**A**): Thermal map of left and right hand positioned upon an insulated tile. The region of interest (ROI, non-dominant hand) displayed as a vertical line constructed centrally for ring (R), middle (M) and index (I) fingers. Selection of the finger with greatest variability was used to construct six 'box' ROIs from which mean ROI values were obtained (B) and with data from the selected finger used in subsequent analyses. (**B**) shows anatomical ROI positions for temperature (°C) of distal phalange (T_{DP}), middle phalange (T_{Tmp}), proximal phalange (T_{PP}), metacarpal (T_{Meta}), capitate bones (T_{Cap}) and distal humerus (T_{DH}).

2.6.8. LWIR Region of Interest (ROI) and Image Processing

Emissivity was set to 0.98 for all images; temperature span 16 °C; range 20.7–36.7 °C. A 'first-pass' review of thermal maps for temperature variability across ring (R), middle (M) and index (I) finger was made. Thermograms showed that fingers typically appeared 'non-uniform' in temperature distribution. Thus, for each participant, a vertical 'line' ROI was constructed (Figure 2A) for each of R, M and I fingers. The finger with the greatest skin temperature value S.D (an indication of temperature variability) was used in subsequent analyses. For the selected finger, a series of six vertical 'box' ROIs (Figure 2B) were constructed (manually) traversing the centre of each finger of the non-dominant hand and using pre-defined dimensions; fingertip (distal phalange, T_{DP}), wrist (capitate bones, T_{Cap}) and forearm (distal humerus/ulnar T_{DH}). Thee ROI dimensions were used throughout the post-processing of LWIR images; T_{DP}, (280 pixels) T_{Cap}, (2436 pixels) and T_{DH}, (1900 pixels). On occasions, the anatomical ROI did not conform well to the finger (e.g., the hand was too slim for the size of the ROI or the hands were 'gnarled' by arthritis, preventing the 'flat' placement of the hands, so the ROI dimension was adjusted slightly to 'fit' ROI to finger anatomy. Mean temperature difference (°C) across the extremities were calculated as: $T_{DP} - T_{Cap}$ (ΔT_1) and $T_{DP} - T_{DH}$ (ΔT_2). The mean temperature difference between T_{DP} and tympanic temperature is given as ΔT_3.

2.6.9. Calibration

Calibration of the FLIR thermal camera was undertaken against a black-body source (P80P, Ametek-Land, Dronfield, UK) to determine temperature accuracy and thermal camera performance across a 20 °C environmental temperature range (20–40 °C).

2.6.10. Warmth Sensation Rating

After adjusting to the study environment, each participant was asked to rate their thermal sensation using the 7-point thermal sensation scale with options ranging from −3 (cold), −2 (cool), −1 (slightly cool), 0 (neutral), +1 (slightly warm), +2 (warm), +3 (hot) [4]. The McIntyre scale [22] for thermal preference (thermal vote, TV) was used to obtain a response to the question "I would like to be": options include (a) cooler (b) no change (c) warmer.

2.6.11. Statistical Analyses

All computations have been carries out with SPSS version 24 (IBM, Armonk, NY, USA). The associated factors analysed in participants over 60 years are presented as numbers, percentage, mean (standard deviation, SD), with *p*-value. Chi-Square tests were used for categorical data. Anova tests were performed for comparison of mean values of independent variables amongst the two participant groups: ND and D. ANOVA was used to determine whether there were any statistically significant differences between the means of two independent groups (Table 1).

Table 1. Characteristic of care home residents, clothing ensemble, ambient conditions and core and skin temperature values (°C) with temperature difference (ΔT). Table shows descriptive analysis that focused on associations between key variables.

Categorical Factor	Dementia Diagnosis/AMT < 8 Group D n = (%)		AMT 8–10 Group ND n = (%)		p Value
Male	10 (45.5)		12 (54.5)		0.43
Female	24 (51.5)		23 (48.9)		
Age: years					
60–70	2 (33.3)		4 (66.7)		
71–80	9 (69.2)		4 (30.8)		0.25
81–90	16 (51.6)		15 (48.4)		
Over 90	7 (36.8)		12 (63.2)		
Ethnicity					
White British	33 (50)		33 (50)		
White European	0		2 (100)		0.22
White	1 (100)		0		
Frailty Score					
Well	0		1 (100)		
Managing Well	6 (75)		2 (25)		
Vulnerable	1 (10)		9 (90)		0.028
Mildly Frail	1 (50)		1 (50)		
Moderately Frail	9 (40.9)		13 (59.1)		
Severely Frail	17 (65.4)		9 (34.6)		
Dominant Hand					
Right	31 (49.2)		32 (50.8)		
Left	3 (60)		2 (40)		0.4
Ambidextrous	0		1 (100)		
Finger with greatest SD					
Left ring	11 (68.8)		5 (31.2)		
Left middle	5 (38.5)		8 (61.5)		
Left index	14 (43.8)		18 (56.2)		0.34
Right ring	1 (100)		0		
Right middle	0		1 (100)		
Right index	2 (40)		3 (60)		
Clothing ensemble (Clo unit)					
Light	6 (30)		14 (70)		
Medium	26 (55.3)		21 (44.7)		0.05
Heavy	2 (100)		0		
Thermal sensation rating					
−2	1 (100)		0		
−1	10 (76.9)		3 (23.1)		
0	21 (48.8)		22 (51.2)		0.02
1	0		7 (100)		
1.5	1 (100)		0		
2	1 (33.3)		2 (66.7)		
Thermal Vote					
Cooler	1 (16)		5 (84)		
No change	27 (49.1)		28 (50.9)		0.09
Warmer	6 (75)		2 (25)		
Temperature	n = (%)	Mean (SD)	n = (%)	Mean (SD)	
Air temperature (°C)	34 (49.3)	23.1 (0.2)	35 (50.7)	24.1 (0.17)	0.001
Relative Humidity (%RH)	34 (49.3)	49 (1.1)	35 (50.7)	52.1 (1.6)	0.2
ROI: mean DP (°C)	33 (48.5)	30.0 (0.46)	35 (51.5)	31.6 (0.4)	0.01
ROI: mean Cap (°C)	33 (48.5)	31.7 (0.25)	35 (51.5)	32.0 (0.25)	0.4
ROI: mean DH (°C)	33 (48.5)	31.9 (0.19)	35 (51.5)	32.0 (0.24)	0.1
ΔT_1 (mean DP- mean CAP) °C	33 (48.5)	−1.7 (0.29)	35 (51.5)	−0.43 (0.24)	0.001
ΔT_2 (mean DP-mean DH) °C	33 (48.5)	−1.8 (0.34)	35 (51.5)	−0.39 (0.26)	0.001
Tympanic temperature (°C)	34 (50)	36.6 (0.07)	34 (50)	36.8 (0.6)	0.01

ROI—region of interest; DP—distal phalange; CAP—capitate bones; DH—distal humerus.

2.7. Ethics Approval, Screening and Recruitment

All subjects gave their informed consent for inclusion before they participated in the study. The study was conducted in accordance with the Declaration of Helsinki, and the protocol was approved by the East Midlands (Derby, UK) research ethics committee and Health Research Authority (HRA) (16/EM/0483).

3. Results

3.1. Characteristics of Older Adults Living in Residential Care

Seventy-three residents gave their consent to the study. Data was analysed from 69 people aged 60–101 (mean 84) years; 47 were female. Participants were recruited from 15 English residences. All were white British, Irish or European. Sixty residents had mild, moderate, or severe frailty. Nine residents only, were 'well' or 'managing well' on the frailty score. There was a significant difference concerning frailty with more residents in the dementia (D) group being severely frail ($p = 0.028$) (Table 1).

AMT ranged from 0–10 (median 8). Thirty-four residents were assigned to 'dementia' category, (D) and 35 residents, (ND) (Table 1). Residents were studied in groups of two to five at each imaging session (median three residents per session) in still air (<0.1 m·sec^{-1}) T_a 21.4–26.6 °C (mean 23.6 °C) RH 32–78% (mean 51%). Under these indoor ambient conditions, a variety of clothing ensembles were worn (Clo range 0.26–1.54, mean 0.61 Clo) corresponding to light ($n = 20$) medium ($n = 47$) heavy ($n = 2$) clothing ensembles respectively.

3.2. Thermal Sensation (TS) Self-Rating

Of the 68 of 69 participants who provided a TS self-report, the majority rated the environment 'comfortable' (TS score 0, $n = 43$, 63%). For the remainder, responses raged from +2 ($n = 3$), +1 ($n = 7$), −1 ($n = 13$), −2 ($n = 1$) corresponding to 'warm', 'slightly warm', 'slightly cool', 'cool' respectively with a range of different TS ratings between residents across individual care homes (Table 2). None of the residents rated −3 (cold) or +3 (hot). Overall, 92% of residents rated TS −1 to +1. Most residents ($n = 55$, 80%) on providing a TV did not wish to change the temperature of the environment whereas eight (11%) would have preferred a warmer temperature and six (9%) a lower air temperature.

Table 2. Individual thermal sensation ratings reported by residents sharing the same environmental conditions at each imaging session in groups of two to five. Study undertaken over a period of 12 calendar months at 15 residential care sites. Residents with dementia who participated in the imaging sessions are identified by highlighted and emboldened text. Four residential care sites (6,9,11,12) were visited twice.

Site ID	Month/Day of Study	Mean T_a (°C)	Mean RH %	Thermal Sensation Rating				
				Resident 1	Resident 2	Resident 3	Resident 4	Resident 5
1	7 June	24.3	60	**0**	missing	0		
2	13 July	24.0	47	0	0	0	−1	
3	12 July	24.3	56	0	1	1	1	
4	28 July	22.5	54	0	0			
5	6 September	24.6	60	0	0	0		
6	28 September	25.8	52	0	1	1	0	
6	6 October	23.6	38	0	−1	0	**0**	
7	12 October	23.1	57	**2**	**0**			
8	20 October	24.2	60	0	1	0	0	
9	7 November	22.0	53	−1	−1			
9	8 December	24.0	32	1	0			
10	11 April	22.0	55	**0**	1.5			
11	17 April	24.5	48	−1	0	**0**		
11	24 April	21.8	44	0	0	−1		
12	11 May	25.3	37	−1	0			
13	16 May	22.6	45	0	0	0	0	
14	18 May	24.2	46	0	0	0		
12	21 May	22.7	50	−1	0	0	−1	−1
11	12 June	22.0	53	−1	0	0		
15	14 June	23.6	54	0	−2	−1	0	2
11	19 June	22.1	54	0	−1	**0**		
6	19 June	24.0	58	0	2			

RH—relative humidity, emboldened text within highlighted cells indicates the residents with a confirmed diagnosis of dementia or Abbreviated Mental Test (AMT) < 8.

3.3. Thermal Sensation Ratings and Clothing Insulation

When sharing the same room (and thus same T_a), differences in TS rating and TV were reported. A significant difference in TS rating was noted between residents (D vs. ND) ($p = 0.02$, Table 1). Residents (D) more frequently expressed feeling 'slightly cool' or 'cool' ($n = 11$) compared with ND residents ($n = 3$; Table 1). By contrast, residents without dementia more frequently expressed feelings of being 'slightly warm' or 'warm' ($n = 9$) compared to those with dementia ($n = 2$). Throughout the months during which the study was conducted, clothing worn by the majority of residents (Table 1) provided light to medium insulation; differences in clothing insulation tending towards medium to heavy Clo units for residents with dementia (borderline significance, $p = 0.05$).

3.4. Core (Tympanic) Temperature

Residents were afebrile, T_{tymp} 35.5–37.5 °C (mean 36.7 °C). A statistical but not clinically significant difference was observed between ND vs. D groups ($p = 0.01$, Table 1). Differences ($T_{DP} − T_{tymp}$) were consistently negative for all older adults; ΔT_3 range −12.5 °C to −2.3 °C.

3.5. Skin Extremity Temperature

Right hand was dominant in 63 of 69 residents (91%). Thermal mapping and data analysis of 'non-dominant' finger/hand ROIs were therefore performed predominately for left hand. Individual extremity skin temperature values for T_{DP}, T_{Cap}, T_{DH} for all residents are lowest for T_{DP}. Mean vales for T_{DP}, T_{Cap}, T_{DH} were 30.9 °C (2.6 °C), 31.9 °C (1.5 °C), 31.9 °C (1.3 °C) respectively. Mean T_{DP} was significantly lower ($p = 0.01$) for residents with dementia compared to ND (Table 1; Figure 3).

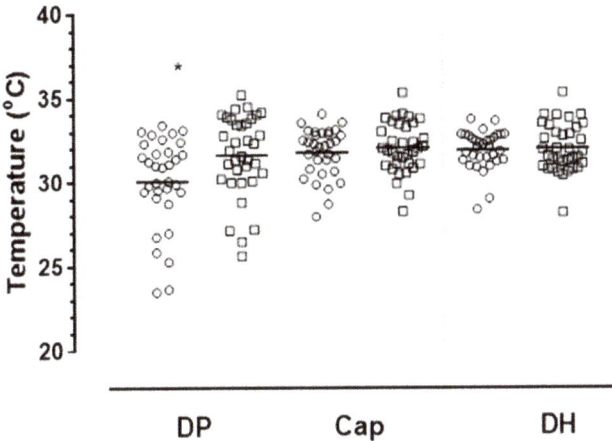

Figure 3. Mean skin temperature at each of three ROI regions represented by finger-tip (distal phalange, T_{DP}), capitate bones (T_{Cap}) and forearm at distal humerus/ulner (T_{DH}) of residents with dementia/AMT < 8 (D) (open circles, O) and residents without a confirmed diagnosis of dementia/AMT ≥ 8 (ND) (open square □). * Significant difference between mean temperature for T_{DP} of residents D vs. ND group ($p = 0.01$). Horizonal bars represent mean values.

3.6. Comparisons Between Groups

D vs. ND: Air, extremity skin and tympanic temperature: T_a of the communal rooms where residents were sitting was, on average, 1.0 °C lower ($p = 0.001$) in D compared to the ND group (Table 1; Figure 4).

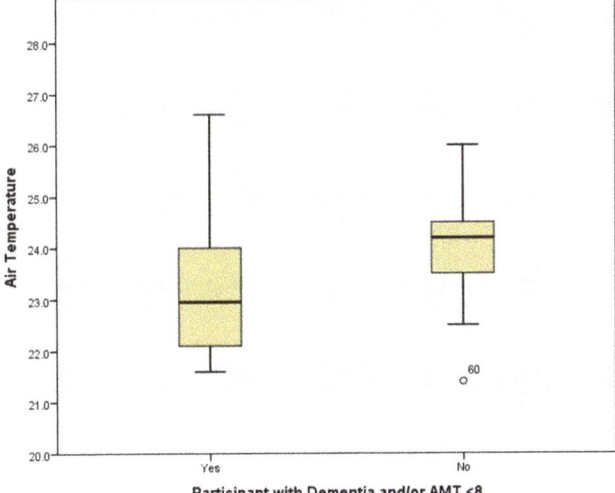

Figure 4. Distribution of air temperature (°C) within care homes by group: dementia or an AMT < 8 (yes/no) showing median, lower and upper quartiles, and lower and upper extremes of air temperature. Outlier: participant studied at lowest T_a, 21.4 °C.

A wide range of ROI temperature differences were recorded at each ROI (Figure 5) and from these values the temperature gradient, delta T (ΔT) calculated for ΔT_1 ($T_{DP} - T_{Cap}$) and ΔT_2 ($T_{DP} - T_{DH}$)

with respect to TS rating. Figure 6 shows the mean temperature (°C) at each of the three ROIs with respect to each residents' reported TS rating.

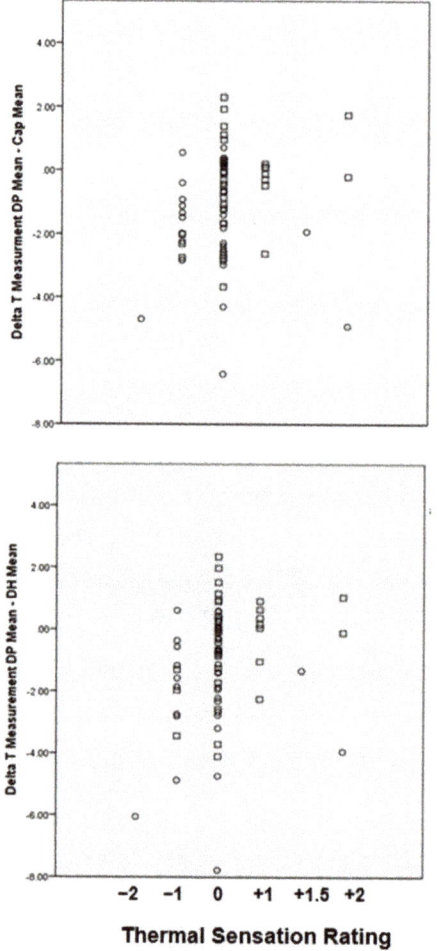

Figure 5. Upper panel: extremity temperature difference between fingertip to wrist ΔT_1 (mean T_{DP}- mean T_{Cap}) and lower panel: fingertip to forearm, ΔT_2 (mean T_{DP} − T_{DH}) by group and TS ratings; dementia (O); no dementia (ND).

For ΔT_1, mean difference, 0.43 °C (0.24) (ND) vs. −1.7 °C (0.29 °C) (D) $p = 0.001$. For ΔT_2, mean difference, 0.39 °C (0.26 °C) (ND) vs. −1.8 °C (−0.34 °C) (D) $p = 0.001$ (Table 1) The range of temperature differences, ΔT_1 for residents with dementia ranged from −6.4 °C to −1.5 °C and for residents without dementia, −3.7 °C to 2.3 °C. The range of temperature differences, ΔT_2, −7.7 °C to 0.6 °C and −4.1 °C to 2.3 °C for D vs. ND respectively. A significant difference (mean 0.2 °C) for tympanic temperature ($p = 0.01$) was observed between groups ND and D.

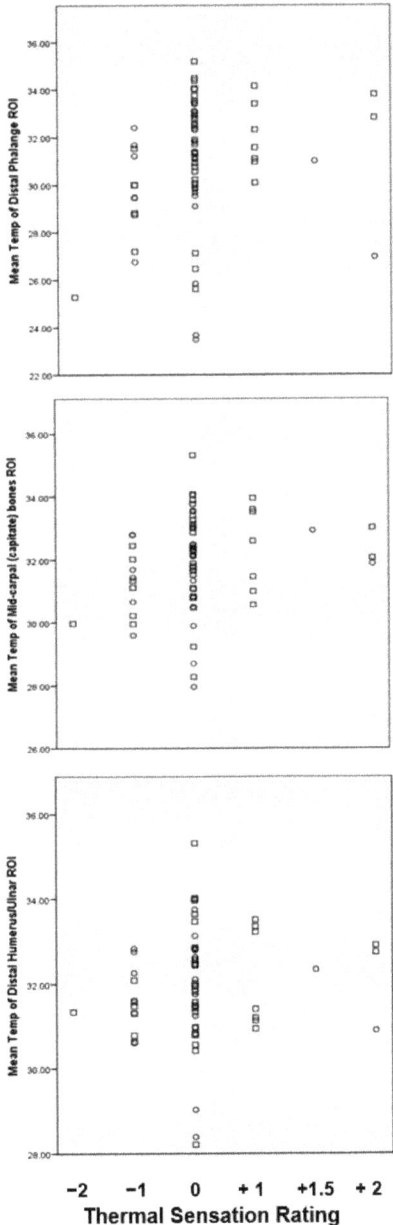

Figure 6. Mean extremity temperature values at three ROIs; distal phalange T_{DP} (upper panel); capitate bones, T_{Cap} (middle); distal humerus, T_{DH} (lower) by group and TS rating. dementia (O), no dementia (□) for each reported thermal sensation rating.

3.7. Extremity Temperature Values and Thermal Sensation Rating

On further exploration of thermal sensation for T_{DP}, residents who were dissatisfied with the environment provided ratings of −2 and −1 (slightly cool, cool, respectively), 11 were residents with dementia (D) and 4 did not have dementia (ND). Eleven residents (9 ND, 2 D) were also dissatisfied with the environment perceiving it as slightly warm (+1, +1.5) or warm (+2).

3.8. Thermal Mapping of Extremities: Correspondence Between the Thermal Map and Thermal Sensation Report

Qualitative review of hand thermograms, showed the visual appearance of skin temperature for ΔT_1 and ΔT_2 of all residents in the environment of their cluster groups:

(A) 'Cold hands': LWIR thermogram appearance was not consistent with thermal sensation report. Thirteen residents (9 in D category) showed the visible appearance of 'cold hands' mean $T_{DP} < 30$ °C (range 23.5–29.9 °C; median 26.5 °C) in air temperatures ranging from 21.4 °C to 25.6 °C (median 23.5 °C) (Figure 7). Thermal sensation ratings were variable ranging from −2 (cool $n = 1$), −1 (slightly cool, $n = 3$), 0 (comfortable/neutral, $n = 8$) to +2 (warm $n = 1$). For cold hands, the temperature difference for ΔT_1 ranged from −6.4 °C to −2.0 °C (median −2.8 °C) and for ΔT_2 −7.8 °C to −1.3 °C (median −3.8 °C). A clear demarcation in temperature across the hands was observed such that areas were 'invisible' against ambient temperature on the thermal map. 'Thermal amputation' was evident visually for the digits in 4 residents with (D) where ΔT_1 was −6.4 °C, −4.7 °C, −4.3 °C ($n = 1$ data missing).

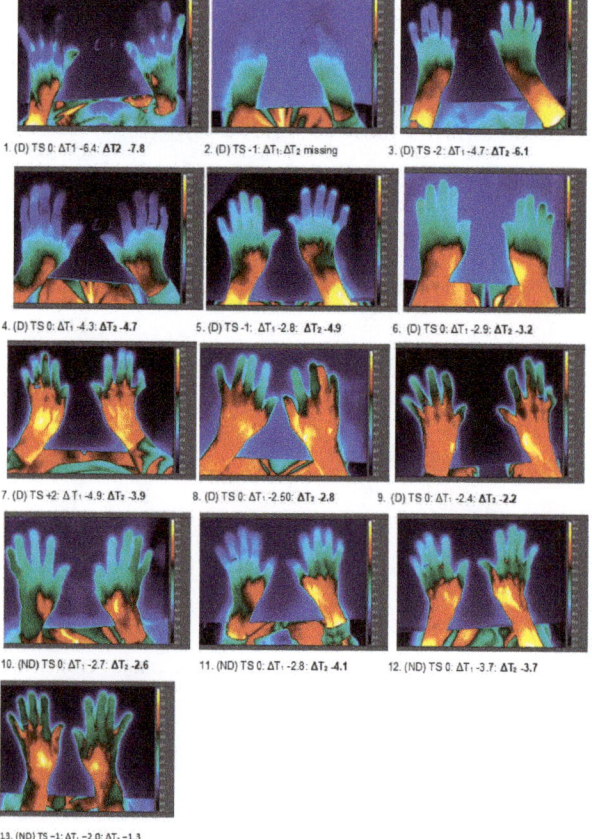

Figure 7. Thermal maps of hand and forearm of 13 residents with the visual appearance of 'cold' hands. Figure shows the study group; dementia (D) or no dementia (ND), thermal sensation (TS) rating and the individual temperature difference (°C) for ΔT_1 and for ΔT_2.

(B) 'Warm hands': By contrast (Figure 8) the brightest colour appearance visually on thermograms corresponded with highest hand temperatures in 10 residents (5 D; 5 ND) (mean T_{DP} 31.7–35.2 °C; median 33.7 °C) across air temperature of 21.9 °C to 25.3 °C (median 22.9 °C) i.e., similar air temperature to those with cold hands. Individual thermal sensation ratings for this group were: −1 (slightly cool, $n = 1$); 0 (comfortable/neutral, $n = 7$), 1 (slightly warm, $n = 1$) and 2 (warm, $n = 1$). Temperature difference across the hands for ΔT_1 ranged from −1.1 °C to +1.9 °C (median 0.3 °C). Similarly, for ΔT_2, mean temperature differences between ROIs was small: range −1.2 °C to +2.34 °C (median 0.45 °C).

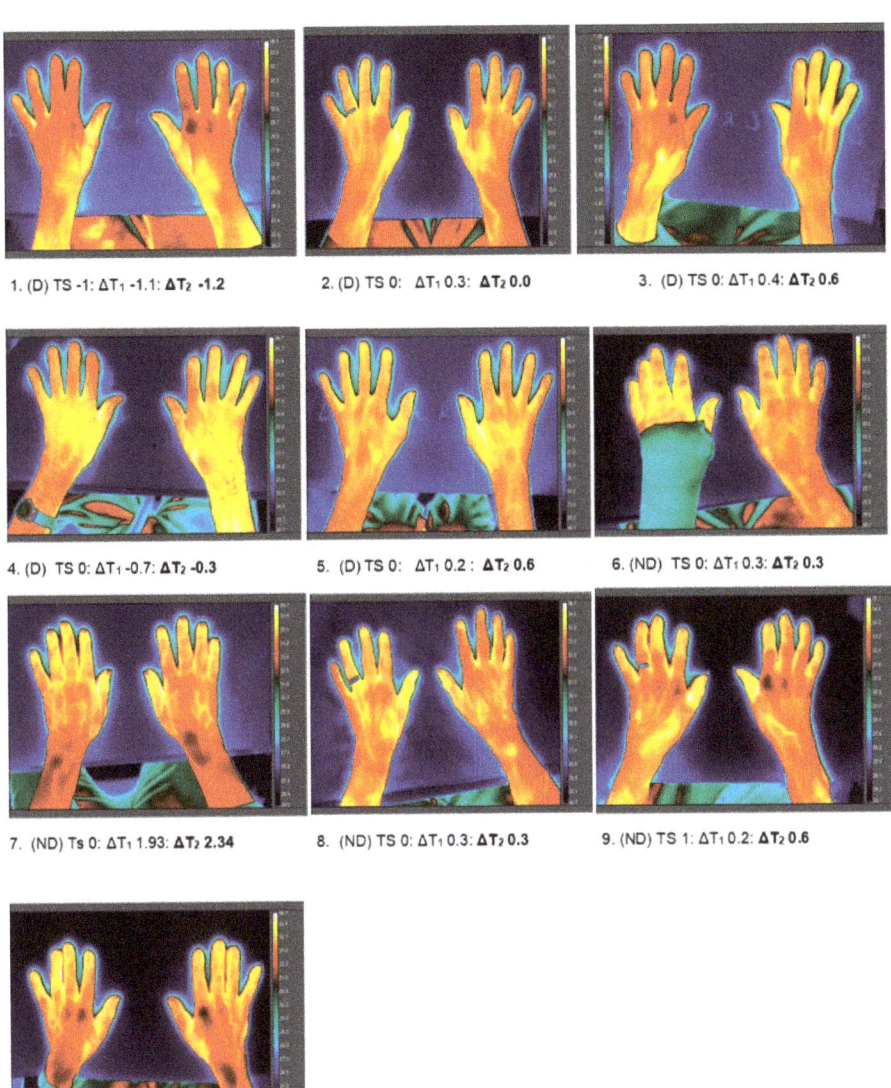

Figure 8. Thermal maps of hand and forearm of 10 residents with the visual appearance of 'warm' hands. Figure shows the study group; dementia (D) or no dementia (ND), thermal sensation (TS) rating and temperature difference (°C) for ΔT_1 and for ΔT_2.

3.9. Medical History and Medications with Potential Influence on Perception of Temperature and Thermal Appearance

None of the residents had a past medical history of Raynaud's disease. There was however, a significant difference in the number of current medications between the residents with and without dementia ($p = 0.001$). However, with respect to medication with known vasoconstrictor or vasodilator effects which might be expected to have an effect on the distribution of blood flow (and temperature) at the extremities, there was no significant difference between the groups, neither were there significant difference in the medications given with known effects on neurological function known to impact on perception of thermal comfort. No other significant difference in medication type was noted for the remaining classes of prescribed drugs.

4. Discussion

The majority of care home residents in this study were in the older-old age group; 27% aged 90 years or more and with approximately half of the group with cognitive deficits. Studies of thermal comfort are typically performed under controlled conditions of a climate chamber e.g., [13,23]. Whilst Soebarto et al. [24] did undertake studies (of young and old people) in a climate chamber in both young and older people, the authors comment that this is not practical for the very old and frail. Undertaking the current study under the 'real-world' conditions of the care home provides a true representation of an individual's day to day indoor environment and associated thermoregulatory responses. In seeking to understand the responses of older people to their environment, we recognise that identifying those with cognitive deficits (vascular cognitive impairment, Alzheimer's prodrome) often falls short of an exact medical diagnosis [25]. This makes disease classification for research [26] to two binary groups ('dementia' vs. 'no dementia') rather more 'nuanced' because age-related cognitive decline follows a continuum across the boundary between normal cognition to the severely demented [26]. It was therefore not possible to assign residents accurately to two groups based on diagnostic differentiation using neuropathology or amyloid biomarkers [27] so the AMT score was used as a pragmatic alternative in the absence of a confirmed diagnosis.

Conducted across 15 English residential care homes, the overarching finding was that older people exposed to the same environmental conditions sense thermal comfort quite differently from one another and this carriers an important message for their carers, alerting them to the potential that residents will experience both satisfaction and dissatisfaction under the same indoor conditions.

Thermal comfort is just one aspect of the environment that exerts an effect on older people [11,28] especially those with dementia [29]. It is clear from the work of Walker et al. [10] that during cold weather, carers and managers are concerned about keeping residents warm and comfortable but see this as challenging due to the diversity of co-morbid conditions, frailty, and different levels of activity of people who live together. The same concerns hold for keeping residents cool in hot weather [3]. However, in the absence of any established method or consensus on how best to provide thermal comfort for the majority, it is likely that those residents in thermal discomfort (whether too cold or too hot) will be overlooked, especially if they are unable to communicate effectively.

Many researchers [30–33] have explored skin temperature (the physiological interface with the environment) as a predictor of thermal comfort. For example Wu et al. [34] investigated upper skin extremity temperature (finger, wrist, hand, forearm) and the conditions required for indoor thermal comfort in an office environment using the same 7-point thermal sensation scale as for the current study. In mean air temperature of 26.8 °C, 60% of adults rated thermal sensation 0 ('neutral') and 90%, rated TS from −1 to +1 (slightly cool, neutral, slightly warm). Similar results were observed in the older aged residents in this study, 63% and 92% rating TS 0 (neutral) and −1 to +1 respectively, albeit in mean air temperature 2 °C lower than the office-based adults. As for upper extremity temperatures in the older residents, mean finger-tip (30.9 °C), wrist (31.9 °C) and forearm (31.9 °C) temperatures were 2 °C lower than reported by Wu et al. [34] where corresponding regions (fingertip, wrist, forearm temperatures) were 33.4 °C 33.7 °C and 33.7 °C respectively. Of interest therefore is that whilst older adults had lower mean skin temperatures and were in lower indoor temperatures, a comparable percentage of residents were satisfied with the environment and rated their TS as 0 (neutral/comfortable). The possibility that the older person's thermal perception of the environment is 'blunted' is consistent with the biological consequences of ageing on thermogenesis and decline in thermosensitivity [35]. This blunting of thermal sensation can occur similarly as in other types of sensory perception loss with age [36]; hearing, vision, taste and smell being additional examples. We have observed features of thermal blunting in the older residents, particularly those with dementia where we observed residents with low extremity (digit) temperatures corresponding to 'cold hands' reporting thermal sensation as neutral (or comfortable) even with obvious visual 'thermal amputation' on the thermal map and even where environmental temperature was within the thermoneutral range [37,38].

In the thermoneutral zone, skin blood flow in the hands is tonically active and vasomotor tone of skin capillaries operates as the primary 'controller' of deep body temperature. Hands (and feet) represent 'radiator' organs [39] losing heat to the environment as well as retaining and conserving body heat. Skin temperature therefore varies with changes in vasomotor tone. Capillaries of non-glabrous skin, along with arterio-venous anastomoses (AVAs) of glabrous (hairless) skin of hands and feet are continuously adjusting (cycling) blood flow to extremity skin to balance heat loss with heat retention [38,40]. These physiological measures, independent of an individual's TS perception may provide a more robust indicator of temperature derangement than achieved through thermal comfort scales, especially under conditions where there is a risk of 'symptomless cooling' [14,18]. If it is possible to measure and/or 'see' the consequences of marked vasoconstriction (or vasodilation) at the extremities this may provide a more reliable indicator of thermal risk; 'cooling without noticing'. We have shown previously [8], as have others [41], that the feeling of being chilled tends to start in the hands or feet. Harazin et al. [42] report finger skin temperature (at a 'cut-off' temperature below 29 °C) in adults (with vibrotactile perception disorders consequent on peripheral neuropathy) as a characteristic of 'cold hands' even in air temperature above 21 °C.

In addition, Pathak et al. [23] have shown that skin temperature gradients are significantly related to resting metabolic rate such that air temperature of 25 °C may serve as an objective measure for the conditions to maintain homeothermy. Looking further at both extremity skin temperature, Wu et al. [34] report finger temperature above 30 °C (and finger-forearm temperature gradients close to 0 °C) to represent a significant threshold for an overall sensation of thermal comfort. Furthermore, at mean air temperature of 26.8 °C, Wu et al. [34] report temperature gradients between fingertip to wrist and fingertip to forearm ranging from −3.5 to 0.3 °C and −4.0 °C to −0.3 °C respectively; the negative temperature gradient serving as an indicator of a 'cool' TS response.

In the current study, older adults showed peripheral vasoconstriction as evidenced by the temperature gradients across the extremities; more intense in those with D than ND for both fingertip to wrist (ΔT_1) and fingertip to distal forearm (ΔT_2). At mean air temperature of 23 °C (Group D) and 24 °C (group ND) this air temperature is within the thermoneutral (comfort) zone (23–27 °C) for light to moderately clothed adults [23] yet older residents show evidence of extremes of thermoregulation as evidenced by both marked peripheral vasoconstriction and vasodilation in hand ROIs observable on the thermal maps.

Being able to take temperature measurements using conventional thermometry and across multiple areas of the skin surface in the setting of care homes presents a significant challenge in routine care. However, with infrared thermography, a quick visual assessment of the physiological response to the environment can be made by imaging of the extremities. Heat maps reflect the net effect of changes in vasomotor tone on skin temperature. As far as it is possible to tell, this is the first report of an independent imaging technology to map 'what we see' on LWIR thermography with 'what people say' about their thermal comfort. In other words, can we 'see' signs of thermal discomfort using thermal imaging and is there a potential benefit in doing so? Although other techniques; laser Doppler imaging [43], laser speckle imaging [44] or venous occlusion plethysmography [45] are available, they are rather less practical for the conditions of the care home whereas LWIR thermography offers an 'at a glance' imaging solution about thermal conditions of the 'radiator' organs, the most obvious exposed skin site being the hands. What we see on thermal imaging is the distribution of heat at the extremities which, at least for digit skin temperature (where metabolically active tissue is minimal) is entirely due to blood flow.

On qualitative review of thermal maps, the appearance of 'cold' and 'warm' hands emerged based on colour coding across a temperature span of 16 °C. For residents with 'cold hands', fingertip temperature (T_{DP}) was, in all cases <30 °C with fingertips consistently colder than wrist and forearm and with a wide (negative) skin temperature gradients for ΔT_1 and ΔT_2 irrespective of TS rating. These results support the work of both Pathak and Wu [23,34] (albeit studying younger, healthy adults) that fingertip temperature below a cut-off, together with wide (negative) temperature gradient (fingertip-wrist and fingertip-forearm) occur across the thermoneutral range. As we have observed, on review of the hand thermograms, this powerful vasoconstrictor response, which can decrease skin blood essentially to zero [46], is not always accompanied by a sensation equivalent to thermal discomfort.

Whilst commonly used models for thermal comfort are based on Fanger's work [47], such models were developed from studies in young, healthy adults in the workplace. That these models are inappropriate for older people is now recognized because changes in the structure of the nervous system as people age means that thermal sensitivity and perception decreases [14]. In the older group of residents, we have seen how varied the thermal comfort responses of older people are, even under the same environmental temperature. Shahzad et al. [48] have shown that neutral thermal sensation does not guarantee thermal comfort; 36% of participants in their study did not want to feel 'neutral' as their comfort condition, preferring a non-neutral thermal sensation. This finding supports the work of de Dear [49] in differentiating thermal 'pleasure' from thermal 'neutrality'; some people finding a cool environment more 'pleasing' than a neutral position which, apart from personal preference may also be influenced by cultural and social factors. For example, Florez-Duquet et al. [50] showed that older subjects generally did not report, or complain, of cold even during an entire cold exposure test whereas young adults did. Taylor et al. [15] showed that older people require a more intense stimulus, starting at the extremities before they 'feel' cold. Consequently, older people are being exposed to intense thermoregulatory challenges that will go unnoticed under the 'normal' indoor temperatures of the care home.

As the focus for long-term care has shifted from processes of care (safety, medical concerns) towards improving outcomes for residents [1] opportunities arise to meet this new challenge; to improve quality of life through considerations of the care home environment [51].

Whilst the majority of residents (both groups), expressed satisfaction with the environment by rating 0 on the thermal sensation scale, many did not; rating the environment too cool or even too warm. The first impression therefore, would be that residents were not in their comfort zone even in warm conditions but is this truly a measure of true satisfaction with the environment? Further evidence of the validity of the thermal sensation report can be explored by investigating concomitant changes in physiological factors, notably the degree of peripheral skin vasomotor tone.

Finally, of importance, in the context of determining the health and thermal comfort of older people in residential care, is not only in the ability to spot the vulnerable person at risk of chilling (or overheating) but in finding a practical solution to the variability in thermal sensation responses to the indoor environment in this older population, many of whom are immobile. Personal thermal comfort approaches could include 'smart' garments and local climate 'bubbles'. Our next step will be in tackling the best approaches to determine a range of approaches that are practical and feasible within the care home. What is clear, due to the COVID-19 pandemic, is that assessing residents by touch will now be excluded for any thermal comfort assessment for the near future.

5. Conclusions

What we have observed by undertaking this feasibility study, perhaps more useful to those involved in the care of older people than relying on a persons reported thermal sensation rating, is in being able to 'see' the physiological responses to the environment in which they live. It is recognised that in older age, cultural factors as well as decline in neurosensory function can have an impact on sensory perception such that these senses may be blunted. This further confounds the value of thermal comfort rating scales in older people. The quick, relatively inexpensive, technique of thermal imaging, allows an immediate assessment of 'live' efferent thermoregulatory activity without the need for absolute measurements per se, so providing a new aspect of multi-dimensional thermal assessment. Thus, from the physiological 'first responders' of thermoregulation: skin extremity temperature (and concomitant extremity skin perfusion), the technique of infrared thermography could, in the future, provide technology-driven approaches to thermal assessment. Thermographic mapping of extremities as a prodromal thermal signature of incipient chilling (or overheating) could offer a better biomarker of thermal satisfaction and temperature safety within the environment than an older person's own temperature sensibility. The future for this challenging field of health care will be in designing solutions to promote personalised thermal comfort involving interdisciplinary collaborations across medical, engineering, design and the built environment.

Author Contributions: Conceptualization, C.C.; data curation, J.E., C.C. and K.K.; formal analysis, C.C. and K.K.; funding acquisition, Principal Investigator C.C.; investigation, C.C., J.E., S.F.-D., J.R.W. and A.A.; methodology, C.C., K.K. and A.A.; project administration, J.E.; visualization, C.C., S.H.; writing—original draft, C.C.; review & editing, K.K., S.H., S.F.-D., J.R.W. and A.A. All authors have read and agreed to the published version of the manuscript.

Funding: This study was funded with a grant from the Dunhill Medical Trust (R507/0716).

Acknowledgments: We would also like to express our sincere thanks to the Trustees of the Dunhill Medical Trust for funding the study. Their support has been invaluable to the delivery of this work. We also thank The Dowager Countess Eleanor Peel Trust for the purchase of an infrared thermal imaging detector. We also thank the managers and care staff of the many residences we visited. They generously gave of their time to assist and support the study. We acknowledge the support of the Clinical Research Networks, who provided assistance in screening participants, especially the significant contribution of Graham Spencer, Derbyshire CRN. Our thanks also go to our colleagues Lee Pearse and Andrew Pearse of Heeley City Farm, Sheffield for their support, advice and experience of dementia care in the community. Finally, our thanks go to the residents who participated in the study, without whom this study would not have been possible.

Conflicts of Interest: The funding body had no role in the design of the study, collection or analysis. The datasets generated and or analysed during the current study are not publicly available due to issue of intellectual property. Data can be available from the corresponding author on reasonable request.

Abbreviations

AMT	Abbreviated Mental Test
ASHRAE	American Society of Heating, Refrigerating and Air-Conditioning Engineers
CIT	Cold induced thermogenesis
Clo	clothing insulation unit
CRN	clinical research network
Icl	overall insulation of assembly in Clo units (Clo)
FOV	field of view
LWIR	long wave infrared thermography
PMH	past medical history
RH	relative humidity
ROI	region of interest
SD	standard deviation
T_a	air temperature
T_r	rectal temperature
T_{DP}	distal phalange skin temperature
T_{CAP}	capitate bones skin temperature
T_{DH}	distal humerus/ulnar skin temperature
T_{tymp}	tympanic membrane temperature
TV	thermal vote
Δ	delta
ΔT	temperature difference
UK	United Kingdom of Great Britain and Northern Ireland
TC	thermal comfort
TS	thermal sensation

References

1. Garre-Olmo, J.; Lopez-Pousa, S.; Turon-Estrada, A.; Juvinya, D.; Ballester, D.; Vilalta-Franch, J. Environmental determinants of quality of life in nursing home residents with severe dementia. *J. Am. Geriatr. Soc.* **2012**, *60*, 1230–1236. [CrossRef] [PubMed]
2. Bills, R.; Soebarto, V.; Williamson, T. Thermal experiences of older people during hot conditions in Adelaide. In *Fifty Years Later: Revisiting the Role of Architectural Science in Design and Practice: 50th International Conference of the Architectural Science Association, Adelaide, Australia, 6–9 December 2016*; School of Architecture and Built Environment, The University of Adelaide: Adelaide, Australia, 2016; pp. 657–664.
3. Van Hoof, J.H.B.; Hansen, A.; Kazak, J.K.; Soebarto, V. The living environment and thermal behaviours of older south Australians. *Int. J. Environ. Public Health Res.* **2019**, *16*, 935. [CrossRef] [PubMed]
4. ASHRAE: Standard 55-2013. *Thermal Environmental Conditions for Human Occupancy*; The American Society of Heating, Refrigerating and Air-Conditioning Engineers: Atlanta, GA, USA, 2013.
5. International Standards Organisation (ISO). *Ergonomics of the Thermal Environment–Analytical Determination and Interpretation of Thermal Comfort Using Calculation of the PMV And PPD Indices and Local Thermal Comfort Criteria*; ISO 7730; ISO Standardization: Geneva, Switzerland, 2015.
6. Bedford, T. The Warmth Factor in Comfort at Work. In *A Physiological Study of Heating and Ventilation*; H.M.S.O.: London, UK, 1936.
7. Parsons, K.C. Human response to thermal environments Principles and methods. In *Evaluation of Human Work*; Wilson, J.R., Corlett, E.N., Eds.; Taylor and Francis: London, UK, 1990.
8. Childs, C.; Gwilt, A.; Sherriff, G.; Homer, C. Old and Cold: Challenges in the Design of Personalised Thermal Comfort at Home. In Proceedings of the 3rd European Conference on Design4Health, Sheffield, UK, 13–16 July 2015; ISBN 978-1-84387-385-3.
9. Cleary, M.; Raeburn, T.; West, S.; Childs, C. The environmental temperature of the residential care home: Role in thermal comfort and mental health. *Contemp. Nurse* **2019**, *55*, 38–46. [CrossRef] [PubMed]
10. Walker, G.; Brown, S.; Neven, L. Thermal comfort in care homes: Vulnerability, responsibility and 'thermal care'. *Build. Res. Inf.* **2016**, *44*, 135–146. [CrossRef]
11. Van Hoof, J.; Schellen, L.; Soebarto, V.; Wong, J.K.W.; Kazak, J.K. Ten questions concerning thermal comfort and ageing. *Build. Environ.* **2017**, *120*, 123–133. [CrossRef]
12. Iommi, M.; Barbera, E. Thermal Comfort for older adults. An experimental study on the thermal requirements for older adults. In Proceedings of the CISBAT Conference, Lausanne, Switzerland, 9–11 September 2015; pp. 357–362.
13. Schellen, L.; van Marken Lichtenbelt, W.; Loomans, M.G.L.C.; Frijns, A.; Toftum, J.; deWit, M. Thermal comfort physiological responses and performance of elderly during exposure to a moderate temperature drift. In Proceedings of the 9th International Conference and Exhibition on Healthy Buildings 2009 (HB09), Syracuse, NY, USA, 13–17 September 2009.
14. Szekely, M.; Garai, J. Thermoregulation and age. In *Handbook of Clinical Neurology; Thermoregulation: From basic Neuroscience to Clinical Neurology Part 1*; Romanovsky, A., Ed.; Elsevier B.V.: Amsterdam, The Netherlands, 2018; Volume 156, pp. 715–725.
15. Taylor, N.A.S.; Allsopp, N.K.; Parkes, D.G. Preferred Room Temperature of Young vs. Aged Males: The Influence of Thermal Sensation, Thermal Comfort, and Affect. *J. Gerontol. Ser. A* **1995**, *50*, M216–M221. [CrossRef]
16. Blatteis, C.M. Age-dependent changes in temperature regulation—A mini review. *Gerontology* **2012**, *58*, 289–295. [CrossRef]
17. Holowatz, L.A.; Thompson-Torgerson, C.; Kenney, W.L. Aging and the control of human skin blood flow. *Front. Biosci.* **2010**, *15*, 718–739. [CrossRef]
18. Lloyd, E.L. *Hypothermia and Cold Stress*; Croom Helm: London, UK, 1986.
19. Hodkinson, H.M. Evaluation of a mental test score for assessment of mental impairment in the elderly. *Age Ageing* **1972**, *1*, 233–238. [CrossRef]
20. Rockwood, K.; Song, X.; MacKnight, C.; Bergman, H.; Hogan, D.B.; McDowell, I.; Mitnitski, A. A global clinical measure of fitness and frailty in elderly people. *CMAJ* **2005**, *173*, 489–495. [CrossRef]
21. Parsons, K. The thermal properties of clothing. In *Human Thermal Environments*; CRC Press: London, UK, 2014.

22. McIntyre, D.A. Thermal sensation. A comparison of rating scales and cross modality matching. *Int. J. Biometeorol.* **1976**, *20*, 295. [CrossRef] [PubMed]
23. Pathak, K.; Calton, E.K.; Soares, M.J.; Zhao, Y.; James, A.P.; Keane, K.; Newsholme, P. Forearm to fingertip skin temperature gradients in the thermoneutral zone were significantly related to resting metabolic rate: Potential implications for nutrition research. *Eur. J. Clin. Nutr.* **2017**, *71*, 1074–1079. [CrossRef] [PubMed]
24. Soebarto, V.; Zhang, H.; Schiavon, S. A thermal comfort environmental chamber study of older and younger people. *Build. Environ.* **2019**, *155*, 1–14. [CrossRef]
25. Stephan, B.C.; Matthews, F.E.; Khaw, K.T.; Dufouil, C.; Brayne, C. Beyond mild cognitive impairment: Vascular cognitive impairment, no dementia (VCIND). *Alzheimer's Res. Ther.* **2009**, *1*, 1–9. [CrossRef]
26. Vos, S.J.; Verhey, F.; Frölich, L.; Kornhuber, J.; Wiltfang, J.; Maier, W.; Peters, O.; Rüther, E.; Nobili, F.; Morbelli, S.; et al. Prevalence and prognosis of Alzheimer's disease at the mild cognitive impairment stage. *Brain* **2015**, *138*, 1327–1338. [CrossRef]
27. Blennow, K.; Zetterberg, H. Biomarkers for Alzheimer's disease: Current status and prospects for the future. *J. Intern. Med.* **2018**, *284*, 643–663. [CrossRef]
28. Tartarini, F.; Cooper, P.; Fleming, R.; Batterham, M. Indoor air temperature and agitation of nursing home residents with dementia. *Am. J. Alzheimer's Dis. Dement.* **2017**, *32*, 272–281. [CrossRef]
29. Day, K.; Carreon, D.; Stump, C. The Therapeutic Design of Environments for People with Dementia: A Review of the Empirical Research. *Gerontology* **2000**, *40*, 397–416.
30. Wang, Z.; He, Y.; Hou, J.; Jiang, L. Human skin temperature and thermal responses in asymmetrical cold radiation environments. *Build. Environ.* **2013**, *67*, 217–223. [CrossRef]
31. Liu, W.; Lian, Z.; Deng, Q. Use of mean skin temperature in evaluation of individual thermal comfort for a person in a sleeping posture under steady thermal environment. *Indoor Built Environ.* **2014**, *24*, 489–499. [CrossRef]
32. Sakoi, T.; Tsuzuki, K.; Kato, S.; Ooka, R.; Song, D.; Zhu, S. Thermal comfort, skin temperature distribution, and sensible heat loss distribution in the sitting posture in various asymmetric radiant fields. *Build. Environ.* **2007**, *42*, 3984–3999. [CrossRef]
33. Wang, D.; Zhang, H.; Arens, E.; Huizenga, C. Observations of upper-extremity skin temperature corresponding overall-body thermal sensations and comfort. *Build. Environ.* **2007**, *42*, 3933–3943. [CrossRef]
34. Wu, Z.; Li, N.; Cui, H.; Peng, J.; Chen, H.; Liu, P. Using Upper Extremity Skin Temperatures to Assess Thermal Comfort in Office Buildings in Changsha, China. *Int. J. Environ. Res. Public Health* **2017**, *14*, 1092.
35. Horvath, S.; Radcliffe, C.E.; Hutt, B.K.; Spurr, G.B. Metabolic response of old people to a cold environment. *J. Appl. Physiol.* **1955**, *8*, 45–148. [CrossRef] [PubMed]
36. Cavazzana, A.; Röhrborn, A.; Garthus-Niegel, S.; Larsson, M.; Hummel, T.; Croy, I. Sensory-specific impairment among older people. An investigation using both sensory thresholds and subjective measures across the five senses. *PLoS ONE* **2018**, *13*, e0202969. [CrossRef]
37. Savage, M.V.; Brengelmann, G.L. Control of skin blood flow in the neutral zone of human body temperature regulation. *J. Appl. Physiol. (1985)* **1996**, *80*, 1249–1257. [CrossRef]
38. Walløe, L. Arterio-venous anastomoses in the human skin and their role in temperature control. *Temperature* **2016**, *3*, 92–103. [CrossRef]
39. Romanovsky, A.A. The thermoregulation system and how it works. *Handb. Clin. Neurol.* **2018**, *156*, 3–43.
40. Wilson, T.E.; Zhang, R.; Levine, B.D.; Crandall, C.D. Dynamic autoregulation of cutaneous circulation: Differential control in glabrous versus nonglabrous skin. *Heart Circ. Physiol.* **2005**, *289*, H385–H391. [CrossRef]
41. Cheung, S.S. Responses of the hands and feet to cold exposure. *Temperature* **2005**, *2*, 105–120. [CrossRef]
42. Harazin, B.; Harazin-Lechowska, A.; Kalamarz, J. Effect of individual finger skin temperature on vibrotactile perception threshold. *Int. J. Occup. Med. Environ. Health* **2013**, *26*, 930–939. [CrossRef] [PubMed]
43. Murray, A.K.; Herrick, A.L.; King, T.A. Laser Doppler imaging: A developing technique for application in the rheumatic diseases. *Rheumatology* **2004**, *43*, 1210–1218. [CrossRef] [PubMed]
44. Wilkinson, J.D.; Leggett, S.A.; Marjanovic, E.J.; Moore, T.L.; Allen, J.; Anderson, M.E.; Britton, J.; Buch, M.H.; Del Galdo, F.; Denton, C.P.; et al. A Multicenter Study of the Validity and Reliability of Responses to Hand Cold Challenge as Measured by Laser Speckle Contrast Imaging and Thermography: Outcome Measures for Systemic Sclerosis-Related Raynaud's Phenomenon. *Arthritis Rheumatol.* **2018**, *70*, 903–911. [CrossRef] [PubMed]

45. Mathiassen, O.N.; Buus, N.H.; Olsen, H.W.; Larsen, M.L.; Mulvany, M.J.; Christensen, K.L. Forearm plethysmography in the assessment of vascular tone and resistance vasculature design: New methodological insights. *Acta Physiol.* **2006**, *188*, 91–101. [CrossRef]
46. Charkoudian, N. Skin blood flow in adult human thermoregulation: How it works, when it does not, and why. *Mayo Clin. Proc.* **2003**, *78*, 603–612. [CrossRef]
47. Fanger, P.O. Assessment of man's thermal comfort in practice. *Br. J. Ind. Med.* **1973**, *30*, 313–324. [CrossRef]
48. Shahzad, S.; Brennan, J.; Theodossopoulos, D.; Calautit, J.K.; Hughes, B. Does a neutral thermal sensation determine thermal comfort? *Build. Serv. Eng. Res. Technol.* **2018**, *39*, 183–195. [CrossRef]
49. De Dear, R. Revisiting an old hypothesis of human thermal perception: Alliesthesia. *Build. Res. Inf.* **2011**, *39*, 108–117. [CrossRef]
50. Florez-Duquet, M.; McDonald, R.B. Cold-induced thermogenesis and biological aging. *Physiol. Rev.* **1998**, *78*, 339–358. [CrossRef]
51. White-Chu, E.F.; Graves, W.J.; Godfrey, S.M.; Bonner, A.; Sloane, P. Beyond the medical model: The culture change revolution in long-term care. *J. Am. Med Dir. Assoc.* **2009**, *10*, 370–378. [CrossRef]

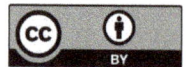

© 2020 by the authors. Licensee MDPI, Basel, Switzerland. This article is an open access article distributed under the terms and conditions of the Creative Commons Attribution (CC BY) license (http://creativecommons.org/licenses/by/4.0/).

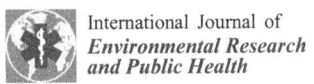

Article

Depressive Symptoms, Fatigue and Social Relationships Influenced Physical Activity in Frail Older Community-Dwellers during the Spanish Lockdown due to the COVID-19 Pandemic

Laura M. Pérez [1,2,*], Carmina Castellano-Tejedor [1,2,3], Matteo Cesari [4,5], Luis Soto-Bagaria [1,2], Joan Ars [1,2], Fabricio Zambom-Ferraresi [6], Sonia Baró [2,7], Francisco Díaz-Gallego [8], Jordi Vilaró [9], María B. Enfedaque [10], Paula Espí-Valbé [2] and Marco Inzitari [1,2,11]

1. Parc Sanitari Pere Virgili, Area of Intermediate Care, 08023 Barcelona, Spain; ccastellano@perevirgili.cat (C.C.-T.); lsoto@perevirgili.cat (L.S.-B.); jars@perevirgili.cat (J.A.); minzitari@perevirgili.cat (M.I.)
2. RE-FiT Barcelona Research Group, Vall d'Hebron Institute of Research & Parc Sanitari Pere Virgili, 08023 Barcelona, Spain; sbaro@perevirgili.cat (S.B.); pespi@perevirgili.cat (P.E.-V.)
3. GIES Research Group, Basic Psychology Department, Autonomous University of Barcelona, 08193 Bellaterra, Spain
4. Geriatric Unit, IRCCS Istituti Clinici Scientifici Maugeri, 20138 Milano, Italy; matteo.cesari@unimi.it
5. Department of Clinical Sciences and Community Health, Università di Milano, 20138 Milano, Italy
6. Navarrabiomed, Complejo Hospitalario de Navarra (CHN), Universidad Pública de Navarra (UPNA), IdiSNA, 31008 Pamplona, Navarra, Spain; fabricio.zambom.ferraresi@navarra.es
7. Primary Healthcare Center Larrard, Atenció Primària Parc Sanitari Pere Virgili, 08023 Barcelona, Spain
8. Primary Healthcare Center Bordeta-Magòria, Institut Català de la Salut, 08014 Barcelona, Spain; fdiazg.bcn.ics@gencat.cat
9. Department of Health Sciences, Blanquerna—Ramon Llull University, 08022 Barcelona, Spain; jordivc@blanquerna.url.edu
10. Institut Català de la Salut, Gerència de Barcelona, 08007 Barcelona, Spain; menfedaque.bcn.ics@gencat.cat
11. Department of Medicine, Autonomous University of Barcelona, 08035 Barcelona, Spain
* Correspondence: lperez@perevirgili.cat; Tel.: +34-932-594000

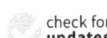

Citation: Pérez, L.M.; Castellano-Tejedor, C.; Cesari, M.; Soto-Bagaria, L.; Ars, J.; Zambom-Ferraresi, F.; Baró, S.; Díaz-Gallego, F.; Vilaró, J.; Enfedaque, M.B.; et al. Depressive Symptoms, Fatigue and Social Relationships Influenced Physical Activity in Frail Older Community-Dwellers during the Spanish Lockdown due to the COVID-19 Pandemic. IJERPH 2021, 18, 808. https://doi.org/10.3390/ijerph 18020808

Received: 21 December 2020
Accepted: 13 January 2021
Published: 19 January 2021

Publisher's Note: MDPI stays neutral with regard to jurisdictional claims in published maps and institutional affiliations.

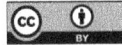

Copyright: © 2021 by the authors. Licensee MDPI, Basel, Switzerland. This article is an open access article distributed under the terms and conditions of the Creative Commons Attribution (CC BY) license (https://creativecommons.org/licenses/by/4.0/).

Abstract: Due to the dramatic impact of the COVID-19 pandemic, Spain underwent a strict lockdown (March–May 2020). How the lockdown modified older adults' physical activity (PA) has been poorly described. This research assesses the effect of the lockdown on PA levels and identifies predictors of sufficient/insufficient PA in frail older community-dwellers. Community-dwelling participants from the +ÀGIL Barcelona frailty intervention program, suspended during the pandemic, underwent a phone-assessment during the lockdown. PA was measured before and after the lockdown using the Brief Physical Activity Assessment Tool (BPAAT). We included 98 frail older adults free of COVID-19 (mean age = 82.7 years, 66.3% women, mean Short Physical Performance Battery = 8.1 points). About one third of participants (32.2%) were not meeting sufficient PA levels at the end of the lockdown. Depressive symptoms (OR = 0.12, CI95% = 0.02–0.55) and fatigue (OR = 0.11, CI95% = 0.03–0.44) decreased the odds of maintaining sufficient PA, whereas maintaining social networks (OR = 5.07, CI95% = 1.60–16.08) and reading (OR = 6.29, CI95% = 1.66–23.90) increased it. Living alone was associated with the reduction of PA levels (b = −1.30, CI95% = −2.14–−0.46). In our sample, pre-lockdown mental health, frailty-related symptoms and social relationships were consistently associated with both PA levels during-lockdown and pre-post change. These data suggest considering specific plans to maintain PA levels in frail older community-dwellers.

Keywords: COVID-19; frailty; aging; physical activity; mental health; social relationships

1. Introduction

The COVID-19 global pandemic has had a dramatic impact on the population's health, especially for older adults [1]. To mitigate the quick spread of infection, several measures have been undertaken around the globe. In Spain, one of the most affected countries, these measures included a strict lockdown (14 March to 2 May 2020). During this period, citizens were not allowed to leave their homes except to attend work, essential medical appointments, shop for food and take care of vulnerable or dependent individuals. A steady phase of de-escalation was then implemented until 21 June 2020, when mobility restrictions were finally removed.

Frailty, a dynamic state of increased vulnerability to internal or external stressors, determines a higher risk of negative health outcomes, such as disability, falls, fractures, institutionalization and death [2]. Therefore, its identification and the development of individualized prevention strategies are mandatory [3–5]. In order to promote a more comprehensive and life-course assessment of older adults, the World Health Organization (WHO) introduced the concept of functional ability (i.e., having the capabilities that enable all people to be and do what they value), which is determined by the interaction between intrinsic capacity (i.e., composite of all physical and mental capacities) and the environment [3]. This latter was clearly altered by the COVID-19 pandemic, and the consequent preventative restrictions. Although lockdowns and mobility restrictions are crucial public health countermeasures, these caused a radical and sudden change in people's lifestyles, in particular regarding physical activity (PA) levels [6,7].

PA has been previously described as a risk factor for frailty [8–10] and a key component of interventions to prevent or reduce the development and progression of frailty [3,11–13]. It has been estimated that the preventive measures applied during the COVID-19 pandemic led to a 25% reduction of PA in the general population [6,14–17], and more than 45% in older adults [6,14–16,18,19]. Despite these data, the possible determinants of this reduction in PA levels have not been explored yet. This might be relevant to design future strategies to resume PA and prevent frailty and disability. Comprehensive geriatric assessment (CGA) includes measures pertaining to different domains, such as functional, physical, cognitive, mood, nutritional and social, which usually interact to determine negative health outcomes for older adults [20]. Variables of the CGA might help predict the change or decrease in PA levels in older adults during the lockdown.

Among the heterogeneous group of older adults, the COVID-19 pandemic posed particular challenges to community-dwelling frail older adults' approach and care. Nevertheless, the impact and consequences of decreased daily activities and social contacts limitations in this vulnerable group, including community-dwelling, frail older adults with a relatively preserved autonomy before the pandemic, has been poorly described. Focusing on this population group is particularly relevant due to the increased risk of accelerated disability. Therefore, it is crucial to appropriately target at-risk individuals to implement individualized post-pandemic plans to recover PA.

In this paper, we describe PA changes due to mobility restrictions in community-dwelling, frail older persons who had not been diagnosed with COVID-19 from a running program, to delay or revert frailty in community-dwelling older adults of Barcelona. Taking advantage of the extensive CGA pre-lockdown, which also included a standardized measure of PA, we explored factors associated with the improvement or maintenance of sufficient PA levels during the lockdown.

2. Materials and Methods

2.1. Study Population

The study population was derived from the +ÀGIL Barcelona project, an implemented, ongoing, real-life multidimensional intervention program, based on integrating primary care, geriatrics and other community resources. Models and results of the initiative have been previously published [11,21]. In brief, the program enrolls nondisabled frail older adults [22] based on the comprehensive geriatric assessment (CGA) performed by a geriatric multidisciplinary team in collaboration with primary care professionals for designing a person-tailored community intervention. Pillars of the intervention include a 10-week boost of multicomponent physical exercise, aiming to empower participants to perform PA, complemented with home sessions based on the validated ViviFrail platform [23]. After the boost, the continuation of PA in existing resources in the community is pursued. Promotion of the Mediterranean diet, health education and optimization of pharmacological therapies are also part of the intervention. After the initial CGA, the geriatrician repeats an assessment at three months (and occasionally six months) to revise and adapt the intervention. +ÀGIL Barcelona has been continuously running from July 2016 until March 2020 (enrolling 100 participants/year). Due to the COVID-19 pandemic, face-to-face assessments were temporarily suspended, replaced by phone calls during the follow-up procedure and data collection.

In May 2020, at the end of the Spanish lockdown applied by the Spanish Government (14 March to 2 May), a follow-up visit via phone was performed with each participant in the +ÀGIL Barcelona program who had been assessed face-to-face during the 12 months prior to the lockdown (either as the baseline, three or six-month visit). In case the participant could not complete the phone call assessment, a self-identified proxy or caregiver answered the follow-up interview. The interviews lasted around 20 min and were performed by two trained physiotherapist researchers.

2.2. Measure of Physical Activity

During the phone survey, the level of PA was assessed with the Brief Physical Activity Assessment Tool (BPAAT), the same tool used in all the routine visits pre-lockdown [24,25]. The BPAAT is a two-question tool. The first item explores the frequency and duration of PA at vigorous intensity, and the second item assesses the frequency and PA duration at moderate-intensity during a typical week. The BPPAT scoring algorithm was designed to identify whether patients meet or not PA recommendations through the combination of both questions. Its total score ranges from 0 to 8, allowing the ability to distinguish sufficiently active (20 min of vigorous-intensity $\geq$ 3 times/week or 30 min of moderate-intensity $\geq$ 5 times/week or $\geq$5 times/week of any combination of moderate or vigorous PA, scores 4–8 points) from insufficiently active participants (who do not meet any previous recommendation, scores 0–3 points). Previous studies report a reliability of 0.76 and construct validity of 0.71 [25]. The outcomes of interest were: (1) total PA during the lockdown (BPAAT total score at the phone survey); (2) improvement (from insufficient to sufficient) or maintenance of sufficient PA vs reduction (from sufficient or insufficient) or maintenance of insufficient PA, according to BPAAT total score. Qualitative aspects related to PA during the lockdown were also part of the phone interview (e.g., self-reported maintenance of pre-lockdown PA level, use of +ÀGIL Barcelona strategies to maintain physical activity).

2.3. Covariates

Data from the last face-to-face CGA pre-lockdown were considered as covariates. These included sociodemographic data (age, sex, education, living alone), clinical characteristics including the Charlson Comorbidity Index [26] and current treatment, functional independence for basic (ADLs) and instrumental activities for daily living (IADLs), nutrition, depression, physical function and frailty. Functional independence for ADLs was assessed by the Barthel index, an ordinal scale range from 0–100 points (total dependent-independent) [27]. The Lawton index was used to measure the independence for IADLs; it ranges from 0–8 points (total dependent-independent) [28]. Nutrition was assessed by the Mini Nutritional Assessment–Short Form, a validated screening tool to identify older adults who are malnourished or at risk of malnutrition; it ranges from 0–12 points (normal nutrition status: 14–12 points, at risk malnutrition: 11–8 points, malnourish: 0–7 points) [29]. The Mini-cog© (Washington, DC, USA), a 3-min instrument was used for cognitive impairment screening, range from 0–5 points (<3 points increase the likelihood of dementia or cognitive impairment) [30,31]. The screening of depression symptoms was assessed by the Yesavage Geriatric Depression Scale, a simple and valid tool for discriminating depressive symptoms; it ranges from 0–15 points (≥6 points: moderate depression) [32,33]. The physical function was measured with the Short Physical Performance Battery (SPPB), a tool that combines the results of the gait speed, chair stand and balance tests, with a range from 0–12 points (<10 points high likelihood of frailty) [34]. Finally, the frailty degree was assessed according to the Clinical Frailty Scale (CFS), a clinical judgement-based frailty tool, which summarizes the CGA results and generates a frailty score range from very-fit to terminally ill [35]. The validity and reliability of all the scales used have been assessed previously.

Data collected by semi-structured phone interview during the lockdown, included sociodemographic data (cohabitation, support at home, social relations with family or other persons, tools to maintain social contact and frequency), COVID-19 related variables (COVID-19 diagnosis on relatives, new onset of acute clinical events and self-reported fatigue, considered a frailty-related symptom [36], health visits canceled due to the pandemic, communication with healthcare professional, and activities to stay active during the lockdown.

2.4. Statistical Analysis

Characteristics of the sample before the lockdown are presented as mean values and standard deviation (SD), or median values and interquartile range (IQR) for continuous variables, as applicable, and frequency and percentages for categorical variables. The pre-post lockdown PA level was analyzed by a paired sample t-test for repeated samples when total BPAAT score was taken into account, and McNemar's test for a repeated sample when the change in PA categories was analyzed (sufficient vs insufficient PA level). Differences among participants with improvement or sufficient PA level and those with reduction or insufficient PA level, were analyzed using the Student's t-test or the Mann-Whitney U-test and Chi-square test, as appropriate. Variables showing an association with the outcomes (p-value < 0.05) and those considered clinically relevant, or to have a potential influence on the outcomes, were included in a stepwise multivariable logistic (dichotomous outcome of change) and stepwise linear regression models (total PA during the lockdown), as appropriate, to obtain final parsimonious models (with age, gender and education locked into the models for being relevant predictors of PA or proxy of socio-economic status). All analyses were performed using Stata version 14.

2.5. Ethical Aspects

The +ÀGIL Barcelona program and study protocol were approved by the Clinical Research Ethics Committee of the Institut Universitari d'Investigació en Atenció Primaria, Jordi Gol i Gorina (20/048-P). Before starting the telephone interview, oral informed consent was obtained from all participants or, if the participant could not provide such consent, from a proxy.

3. Results

Out of 117 contacted participants from +ÀGIL, 107 (91.5%) agreed to answer the phone survey. To ensure the homogeneity of the population, those previously diagnosed with SARS-COVID-19 (n = 4), or with incomplete PA data (n = 5), were excluded. Finally, we included in the analyses 98 participants (mean age = 82.4 SD 6.1 years; 66.3% women; mean time since last face-to-face visit 8.1 SD 3.7 months). The vast majority (88.8%) of the phone interviews were answered by the participants. There were no significant differences in terms of age, sex and time since the last face-to-face assessment between those who participated and those who refused to participate or were excluded from the survey.

A general decrease in PA level during the lockdown (BPAAT total score: $-1.1/8$ (95 CI% 0.6; 1.5) points; $p < 0.001$)) and reduction of participants reporting sufficient PA (-32.2%; $p = 0.003$) was reported (Figure 1). Overall, 22% of the sample continued to follow the personalized PA recommendations designed and delivered through the +ÀGIL Barcelona program.

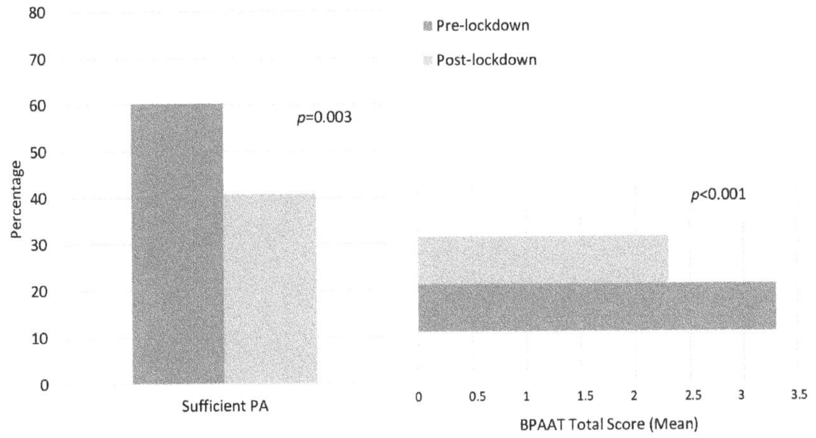

Figure 1. Effect of the strict lockdown due to COVID-19 pandemic on physical activity. The McNemar's test for repeated samples was used for categorical variables. Paired sample *t*-test for repeated samples was used for continuous variables. Brief Physical Activity Assessment score ranged from 0–8 (≥4 points: sufficient active, 0–3: insufficient active).

Participants with reduced or insufficient PA presented higher pre-lockdown IADLs disability and comorbidity, more prevalent depressive symptoms and previous diagnosis or positive screening for cognitive impairment/dementia than those who improved or maintained sufficient PA (Table 1). This same group, with reduced or insufficient PA level, also reported more fatigue, more health concerns and less social contact with friends or other people outside the family during the lockdown (Table 2). On the other hand, participants who improved or maintained sufficient PA were more likely to follow PA-related recommendations from the +ÀGIL Barcelona program during the lockdown and to perform other leisure activities, such as reading, as a strategy to stay physically or mentally active.

Table 1. Characteristics of the sample before the lockdown due to COVID-19.

Baseline Characteristics	Included $n = 98$	Reduction or Insufficient PA, $n = 58$ [a]	Improvement or Sufficient PA, $n = 40$ [a]	*p*-Value
Age, mean (SD)	82.4 (6.1)	82.2 (5.5)	82.8 (6.8)	0.606
Woman, % (*n*)	66.3 (65)	62.1 (36)	72.5 (29)	0.283
Lives alone, % (*n*)	54.1 (54)	56.9 (33)	50.0 (20)	0.501
Education, % (*n*)				
Illiterate	8.3 (8)	7.0 (4)	10.0 (4)	
Primary school	39.2 (38)	43.9 (25)	32.5 (13)	0.476
Secondary school	38.1 (37)	38.6 (22)	37.5 (15)	
University degree	14.4 (14)	10.5 (6)	20.0 (8)	
Falls in the last year, % (*n*)	28.6 (28)	27.6 (16)	30.0 (12)	0.795
Lawton Index [b], median (IQR)	5 (3–8)	4.5 (2–7)	7 (4–8)	0.012
Barthel Index [c], median (IQR)	95 (85–100)	92.5 (85–95)	95 (90–100)	0.091
Malnutrition risk [d], % (*n*)				
Normal nutrition status	79.0 (75)	73.2 (41)	87.2 (34)	
At risk of malnutrition	19.0 (20)	25.0 (14)	12.8 (5)	0.227
Malnourished	1.1 (1)	1.8 (1)	0.0 (0)	

Table 1. Cont.

Baseline Characteristics	Included $n = 98$	Reduction or Insufficient PA, $n = 58$ [a]	Improvement or Sufficient PA, $n = 40$ [a]	p-Value
Depressive symptoms [e], % (n)	21.9 (21)	30.4 (17)	10.0 (4)	0.017
Charlson Comorbidity Index, median (IQR)	2 (1–3)	2 (1–3)	1 (0–2)	0.041
Previous cognitive impairment or positive screening [f], % (n)	36.1 (35)	45.6 (26)	22.5 (9)	0.020
Number of drugs, mean (SD)	7.4 (3.5)	7.7 (3.4)	7.0 (3.5)	0.368
Clinical Frailty Scale—vulnerable or any degree of frailty, % (n)	63.3 (62)	67.2 (39)	57.5 (23)	0.326
SPPB [g], mean (SD)	8.3 (3.1)	7.9 (3.2)	8.8 (2.9)	0.202
Gait speed, median (IQR)	0.75 (0.58–0.92)	0.72 (0.66–0.77)	0.79 (0.72–0.86)	0.175
Sufficient physical activity, % (n)	60.2 (59)	51.7 (30)	72.5 (29)	0.039

PA: Physical Activity. IQR: interquartile range, SD: standard deviation. Student's t-test or the Mann-Whitney U-test were used for continuous variables as appropriate and Chi-square test for categorical. [a] Change in PA level: Improve an insufficient or maintain a sufficient PA level vs. reduction or maintain insufficient PA level. Brief PA Assessment score, range from 0–8 (≥ 4 points: sufficient active, 0–3: insufficient active). [b] Independence for activities of daily living, Barthel index: range from 0–100. [c] Independence for instrumental activities of daily living, Lawton index: range from 0–8. [d] Mini-Nutritional Assessment Short form score: range from 0–14 points (0–7: Malnourished, 8–11: At risk of malnutrition, 12–14: Normal). [e] Geriatric Depression Scale Yesavage: range from 0–15 points (>5 points: depression). [f] Previous diagnosis of cognitive impairment or dementia or positive screening performed with Minicog©. Minicog© range 0–5 (<3 positive screening for cognitive impairment). [g] Short Physical Performance Battery, range from 0–12 (<10 points: frailty).

In multivariable models, living alone before the lockdown (ß= −1.30, 95%CI −2.14−−0.46, $p = 0.003$), previous depressive symptoms (ß= −1.15, 95%CI −1.89−−0.41, $p = 0.003$) and self-reported fatigue during the COVID-19 outbreak (ß= −1.25, 95%CI −1.87−−0.63, $p < 0.001$) were inversely associated with PA levels (BPAAT total score) during the lockdown. Having social contact with people different from family (ß = 0.99, 95%CI 0.41–1.57, $p = 0.001$) and performing reading activities during the lockdown (ß = 0.74, 95%CI 0.08–1.39, $p = 0.028$) were associated with higher BPAAT scores during the lockdown (Table 3). Neither physical function measures (SPPB, gait speed), nor frailty (CFS) or cognitive impairment were associated with the amount of PA during the lockdown or with the change in PA levels.

Table 2. Description of characteristics of the sample during the lockdown due to COVID-19.

Baseline Characteristics	Included $n = 98$	Reduction or Insufficient PA, $n = 58$ [a]	Improvement or Sufficient PA, $n = 40$ [a]	p-Value
Lives alone, % (n)	38.1 (37)	38.6 (22)	37.5 (15)	0.913
Maintained daily social contact (any type), % (n)	79.6 (78)	75.9 (44)	85.0 (34)	0.270
Social contact different than family, % (n)	46.9 (46)	37.9 (22)	60.0 (24)	0.031
Any new health concerns [b], % (n)	39.8 (39)	48.3 (28)	27.5 (11)	0.039
Sought medical attention, % (n)	56.4 (22)	57.1 (16)	54.6 (6)	0.883
Following +ÀGIL PA recommendation, % (n)	22.5 (22)	8.6 (5)	42.5 (17)	<0.001
Obstacles to desired PA, % (n)				
Apathy	30.3 (10)	29.6 (8)	33.3 (2)	
Falls	3.0 (1)	3.7 (1)	0.0 (0)	
Fatigue	15.2 (5)	18.5 (5)	0.0 (0)	
Functional impairment	3.0 (1)	3.7 (1)	0.0 (0)	0.362
Lockdown situation	15.2 (5)	11.0 (3)	33.3 (2)	
Medical condition incident	21.2 (7)	25.9 (7)	0.0 (0)	
No time	12.2 (4)	7.4 (2)	33.3 (2)	
Vigorous PA (one-twice/wk) [c]	5.2 (5)	3.5 (2)	7.7 (3)	0.354
Moderate PA [d], % (n)				
≥ 5 times/wk	39.8 (39)	0.0 (0)	97.5 (39)	
3–4 times/wk	19.4 (19)	31.0 (18)	2.5 (1)	<0.001
1–2 times/wk	26.5 (26)	44.8 (26)	0.0 (0)	
Never	14.3 (14)	24.1 (14)	0.0 (0)	

Table 2. *Cont.*

Baseline Characteristics	Included n = 98	Reduction or Insufficient PA, n = 58 [a]	Improvement or Sufficient PA, n = 40 [a]	*p*-Value
Self-reported fatigue	38.1 (37)	49.1 (28)	22.5 (9)	0.008
Activities to stay active during the lockdown [e], % (*n*)				
Housework	45.9 (45)	37.9 (22)	57.5 (23)	0.056
Leisure activities [f]	36.7 (36)	32.8 (19)	42.5 (17)	0.326
Music/TV	69.4 (68)	74.1 (43)	62.5 (25)	0.219
Provide care	5.1 (5)	8.6 (5)	0.0 (0)	0.057
Reading	26.5 (26)	17.2 (10)	40.0 (16)	0.012
Social contact	10.2 (10)	8.6 (5)	12.5 (5)	0.533
Use of technology	5.1 (5)	1.7 (1)	10.0 (4)	0.067

PA: Physical activity. Wk: week. Chi-square test was performed to analyze the difference between categorical variables. [a] Change in PA level: Improve insufficient or maintain sufficient PA level vs reduction or maintain insufficient PA level. Brief Physical Activity Assessment score, range from 0–8 (≥4 points: sufficient active, 0–3: insufficient active). [b] Acute health concern: diarrhea, urinary infection, allergies. [c] ≥20 min or more of jogging (mainly in the house), heavy lifting, etc. [d] ≥30 min walking that increases heart rate or breath harder than normal. [e] Not mutually exclusive. [f] Painting, crafts, table games, urban gardening.

Table 3. Association of pre-lockdown characteristics and total physical activity [a] during the lockdown or pre-post improvement or maintenance of sufficient physical activity [a].

Prelockdown Characteristics (from the Last Available Assessment)	Linear Regression BPAAT during-Lockdown Total Score [a]			Logistic Regression Improve or Maintain Sufficient PA during vs. Prelockdown [b]		
	B	(95% CI)	*p*	OR	(95% CI)	*p*
Age	0.01	−0.04; 0.05	0.752	1.03	0.95; 1.12	0.494
Female	0.30	−0.31; 0.91	0.336	2.61	0.85; 8.04	0.094
Education	0.03	−0.13, 0.18	0.705	0.87	0.65; 1.17	0.370
Depressive symptoms (pre-lockdown) [c]	−1.15	−1.89; −0.41	0.003	0.12	0.02; 0.55	0.006
Social contact different than family (during the lockdown)	0.99	0.41; 1.57	0.001	5.07	1.60; 16.08	0.006
Self-reported fatigue	−1.25	−1.87; −0.63	<0.001	0.11	0.03; 0.44	0.002
Reading to stay active (during the lockdown)	0.74	0.08; 1.39	0.028	6.29	1.66; 23.90	0.007
Lives alone (pre-lockdown)	−1.30	−2.14; −0.46	0.003	-	-	-
Lives alone (during the lockdown)	−0.78	−1.74; 0.07	0.073	-	-	-
Diagnosis of cognitive impairment (pre-lockdown) [d]	-	-	-	0.29	0.08; 1.06	0.061

Stepwise multivariable linear and logistic regression were performed as appropriate. Age, sex and education level were set as lockterm in both cases. Variables with empty cells were not included in the final model. PA: Physical Activity. [a] Brief Physical Activity Assessment score, range from 0–8. [b] Change in physical activity level: Improve insufficient or maintain sufficient physical activity level vs reduction or maintain insufficient physical activity level. [c] Geriatric Depression Scale Yesavage: range from 0–15 points (>5 points: depression). [d] Previous diagnosis of cognitive impairment or dementia or last Minicog© assessment <3. Minicog© range 0–5 (<3 positive screening for cognitive impairment).

Looking at the pre-post change in PA levels, multivariable models showed consistent results for pre-lockdown depressive symptoms (OR= 0.12, 95%CI 0.02–0.55, p = 0.006) and self-reported fatigue (OR = 0.11, 95%CI 0.03–0.44; p = 0.002), which were negatively associated with improvement/maintenance of sufficient PA, as well as for social contacts with people different from family networks (friends or neighbors), which increased the odds for a positive outcome (OR = 5.07, 95%CI 1.60–16.08; p = 0.006). In this model, reading during the lockdown (OR = 6.29, 95%CI 1.66–23.90; p = 0.007) was positively associated with improving/maintaining sufficient PA (Table 3).

4. Discussion

In our population of community-dwelling frail older adults, strict home lockdown due to the COVID-19 pandemic determined a generalized decrease in PA, although a remarkable proportion maintained or improved PA. Regarding pre-lockdown characteristics, higher depressive symptoms were associated with total PA during the outbreak and change in PA, and participants living alone performed less PA during the outbreak. On the other hand, social relationships and leisure activities during the outbreak were directly associated with PA levels and pre-post change, whereas self-reported fatigue had an inverse association with PA levels.

During the first months of the outbreak, Spain adopted a strict home lockdown motivated by the pandemic's severe impact [37]. Previous studies from Italy and Japan also reported a decrease in PA [6,14–19,38]; or a rising prevalence of inactive older persons [18,19]. Despite the similarities in the mobility restriction measures among the three countries, the study populations are different: the Italian study used a cohort that underwent the implantation of a cardio meter-defibrillator before the pandemic [14,18] whereas the one enrolled by Suzuki et al. [18] was discharged from a rehabilitation setting; both samples were significantly younger than ours. Compared with the study by Yamada et al., which showed a relevant prevalence of frailty (25%) [18,19], our population was older and frailer. The impact on the mental and physical health status of preventive social distancing measures in frail community-dwelling older adults has been poorly described. Targeting such a vulnerable group is particularly relevant due to its higher risk of progressing to disability. Moreover, our study offers unique pre-post lockdown measures of PA.

Among the several public health challenges driven from the COVID-19 pandemic, promoting PA is particularly complex due to strict mobility restrictions, including access to public space (e.g., gyms, parks, civic centers, etc.), and social-distancing measures. These regulations precluded free and low-cost options to perform PA and might decrease motivation, hampering PA adherence. Interestingly, despite a long time since the last face-to-face visit, a remarkable proportion of our sample followed the personalized PA recommendations derived from the +ÀGIL Barcelona program. This reinforces the need of community-based programs to empower older adults for self-care [39].

The association between depressive symptoms and low PA levels has been previously described [40] and could be explained by generalized reduced activity, both in the cognitive/affective and behavioral realms. Depression negatively impacts lifestyle choices, and individuals with depressive symptoms tend to be less motivated, more sedentary and less physically fit than non-depressed ones [41,42]. In previous Spanish surveys during the lockdown, older persons showed less emotional distress and higher resilience to the pandemic than younger adults [43]. However, the profile of resilient individuals seemed to be characterized by more optimistic personality traits [44], a regular practice of vigorous and moderate PA, positive self-perceptions of ageing, less depressive symptoms [45,46] as well as less perceived loneliness during the lockdown [47]. It is possible that, in these surveys, vulnerable responders were not sufficiently represented. We also cannot exclude a bidirectional association between depressive symptoms and PA, because higher PA is associated with better physical and cognitive function [48], lower rates of frailty [49] and less depressive symptoms in community-dwelling older adults [50,51].

We also found a negative, independent association between fatigue and total PA levels and its improvement or maintenance during the lockdown. Fatigue, a subjective self-reported global tiredness and lack of energy [52], has been associated with lower physical and mental function, disability and mortality [53–55], and is one of the pillars of the frailty pre-disability concept [36,56]. Self-perceived fatigue can be a symptom of an underlying disease (e.g., cardiovascular, respiratory, psychiatric, etc.), but it has also been associated with an inactive lifestyle [57], so that a bidirectional causality, in the association between fatigue and PA, cannot be excluded, moreover because both fatigue and PA were collected in the same timeframe at the moment of the telephonic interview.

Social relationships are pivotal for healthy aging [58] and have been previously associated with a higher chance of maintaining physical health and longevity [59]. On the other hand, loneliness is a risk factor for physical and mental illness, fatigue and physical inactivity [60]. Consequently, social connections are essential to foster activity and PA in older adults and are an important component of PA group programs success [11,61]. Although during the first COVID-19 outbreak the population, especially older adults, may have progressively adapted to the new daily routines and limitations, this situation has a clear negative impact on social relationships and loneliness [62–64]. Tackling loneliness and social relationships requires specific implementation strategies [65], and these need to be adapted and implemented to promote the adherence to exercise programs [23,66], particularly in these challenging times. In summary, the complex interaction between depressive symptoms, physical function, social participation and activity deserves special attention in older adults [67], and this should be kept in mind for the post-lockdown and post-COVID-19 recovery plans.

Reading is a complex activity, which combines both cognitive and mental functions. Previous studies have reported that reading has a positive impact on stress, insomnia, depression symptoms and dementia development. Indeed, all of them related negatively with levels of physical activity [68]. Surprisingly, in our sample, although the group with preserved PA showed better physical function (either SPPB score or gait speed) and frailty (CFS), the association between frailty and PA was not significant in the multivariable models. Similarly, we found no association between previous cognitive impairment and PA. These negative findings might be attributable to the sample's relative homogeneity enrolled in the +ÀGIL Barcelona program, where the frailty screening was an inclusion criterion [21].

Limitations and Future Research Recommendations

We acknowledge the different limitations of our study. First, our pre-lockdown assessment cannot completely reflect the situation immediately pre-lockdown because of the time elapsed since the last face-to-face visit to the telephonic interview. However, it provides the added value of a longitudinal design. Second, the sample size was relatively small, although representing almost 50% of the whole +ÀGIL Barcelona sample. As for strengths, PA levels were assessed by the BPAAT scale, a short validated scale, with good psychometric properties, that was already part of the +ÀGIL Barcelona assessment, allowing us to track pre-post changes. In this same line, the study population had an extended pre-lockdown assessment, which offered a comprehensive sample characterization. The telephone interview was short, which is important for such a vulnerable population, who could get tired easily.

Considering that reduced PA is a key risk factor to increased frailty and disability, our results highlight the need to design and adapt strategies for community and home-based PA in older adults, particularly in challenging situations such as the ongoing COVID-19 pandemic. These strategies should likely take into account multifactorial contributors to reduced PA, such as mental status, social relationships and frailty-related symptoms such as fatigue. In light of COVID-19 pandemics, we also believe that there is an increased need for adapted digital solutions to provide PA in the community. These should be adapted through a broad system thinking strategy, particularly for vulnerable older adults with such multidomain contributors to inadequate PA.

5. Conclusions

In our sample, strict home lockdown due to the COVID-19 pandemic had determined a decrease in PA levels. Moreover, pre-lockdown mental health, frailty-related symptoms and social relationships were consistently associated with both PA levels during-lockdown and pre-post change. Our data could be used to design specific person-centered plans to maintain PA levels in frail older community-dwellers. However, larger population studies including dwelling older adults are needed to confirm our results.

Author Contributions: Conceptualization, L.M.P., C.C.-T., M.C., F.Z.-F., J.V., M.B.E. and M.I.; data curation, L.M.P., L.S.-B., J.A. and P.E.-V.; formal analysis, L.M.P.; investigation, M.I.; methodology, L.M.P., C.C.-T., M.C., J.V. and M.I.; project administration, C.C.-T. and M.I.; resources, F.Z.-F., S.B., F.D.-G., J.V. and M.B.E.; software, P.E.-V.; supervision, M.C. and M.I.; writing—original draft, L.M.P., C.C.-T. and M.I.; writing—review & editing, L.M.P., C.C.-T., M.C., L.S.-B., J.A., F.Z.-F., S.B., F.D.-G., J.V., M.B.E., P.E.-V. and M.I. All authors have read and agreed to the published version of the manuscript.

Funding: This research project was partially supported by Subvencions de L'institut de Cultura de Barcelona per a Projectes de Recerca i Innovació del Pla Barcelona Ciència 2019 (ID 19S01576-006).

Institutional Review Board Statement: The study was conducted according to the guidelines of the Declaration of Helsinki, and approved by the Jordi Gol i Gorina Ethics Committee (code: 20/048-P, date 25 March 2020).

Informed Consent Statement: Informed consent was obtained from all subjects involved in the Study.

Data Availability Statement: The data presented in this study are available on request from the corresponding author. The data are not publicly available due to ethical reasons.

Acknowledgments: The authors of the present research wish to thank the collaboration of all the participants who voluntarily and selflessly participated in the study.

Conflicts of Interest: Pérez has received honoraria for teaching activities by Nestlé, unrelated with the topic of the present work. Cesari and Inzitari have also received honoraria by Nestlé for presenting at scientific meetings and serving as members of expert advisory boards, unrelated to the present work.

References

1. CDC Older Adults. Available online: https://www.cdc.gov/coronavirus/2019-ncov/need-extra-precautions/older-adults.html#:~{}:text=Among%20adults%2C%20the%20risk%20for,or%20they%20may%20even%20die (accessed on 12 November 2020).
2. Cesari, M.; Calvani, R.; Marzetti, E. Frailty in Older Persons. *Clin. Geriatr. Med.* **2017**, *33*, 293–303. [CrossRef] [PubMed]
3. World Health Organization. *World Report on Ageing and Health*; World Health Organization: Geneva, Switzerland, 2015; ISBN 9789241565042.
4. Ruiz, J.G.; Dent, E.; Morley, J.E.; Merchant, R.A.; Beilby, J.; Beard, J.; Tripathy, C.; Sorin, M.; Andrieu, S.; Aprahamian, I.; et al. Screening for and Managing the Person with Frailty in Primary Care: ICFSR Consensus Guidelines. *J. Nutr. Health Aging* **2020**, *24*, 920–927. [CrossRef] [PubMed]
5. Morley, J.E.; Vellas, B.; van Kan, G.A.; Anker, S.D.; Bauer, J.M.; Bernabei, R.; Cesari, M.; Chumlea, W.C.; Doehner, W.; Evans, J.; et al. Frailty Consensus: A Call to Action. *J. Am. Med. Dir. Assoc.* **2013**, *14*, 392–397. [CrossRef] [PubMed]
6. Ammar, A.; Brach, M.; Trabelsi, K.; Chtourou, H.; Boukhris, O.; Masmoudi, L.; Bouaziz, B.; Bentlage, E.; How, D.; Ahmed, M.; et al. Effects of COVID-19 Home Confinement on Eating Behaviour and Physical Activity: Results of the ECLB-COVID19 International Online Survey. *Nutrients* **2020**, *12*, 1583. [CrossRef]
7. De Biase, S.; Cook, L.; Skelton, D.A.; Witham, M.; Ten Hove, R. The COVID-19 rehabilitation pandemic. *Age Ageing* **2020**, *49*, 696–700. [CrossRef]
8. Savela, S.L.; Koistinen, P.; Stenholm, S.; Tilvis, R.S.; Strandberg, A.Y.; Pitkala, K.H.; Salomaa, V.V.; Strandberg, T.E. Leisure-Time Physical Activity in Midlife Is Related to Old Age Frailty. *J. Gerontol. Ser. A Biol. Sci. Med. Sci.* **2013**, *68*, 1433–1438. [CrossRef]
9. Da Silva, V.D.; Tribess, S.; Meneguci, J.; Sasaki, J.E.; Garcia-Meneguci, C.A.; Carneiro, J.A.O.; Virtuoso, J.S., Jr. Association between frailty and the combination of physical activity level and sedentary behavior in older adults. *BMC Public Health* **2019**, *19*, 709. [CrossRef]
10. Zhang, X.; Tan, S.S.; Franse, C.B.; Bilajac, L.; Alhambra-Borrás, T.; Garcés-Ferrer, J.; Verma, A.; Williams, G.; Clough, G.; Koppelaar, E.; et al. Longitudinal Association Between Physical Activity and Frailty Among Community-Dwelling Older Adults. *J. Am. Geriatr. Soc.* **2020**, *68*, 1484–1493. [CrossRef]
11. Pérez, L.M.; Enfedaque-Montes, M.B.; Cesari, M.; Soto-Bagaria, L.; Gual, N.; Burbano, M.P.; Tarazona-Santabalbina, F.J.; Casas, R.M.; Díaz, F.; Martín, E.; et al. A Community Program of Integrated Care for Frail Older Adults: +AGIL Barcelona. *J. Nutr. Health Aging* **2019**, *23*, 710–716. [CrossRef]
12. Giné-Garriga, M.; Roqué-Fíguls, M.; Coll-Planas, L.; Sitjà-Rabert, M.; Salvà, A. Physical Exercise Interventions for Improving Performance-Based Measures of Physical Function in Community-Dwelling, Frail Older Adults: A Systematic Review and Meta-Analysis. *Arch. Phys. Med. Rehabil.* **2014**, *95*, 753–769.e3. [CrossRef]
13. Mañas, A.; Del Pozo-Cruz, B.; Rodríguez-Gómez, I.; Leal-Martín, J.; Losa-Reyna, J.; Rodríguez-Mañas, L.; García-García, F.J.; Ara, I. Dose-response association between physical activity and sedentary time categories on ageing biomarkers. *BMC Geriatr.* **2019**, *19*, 270. [CrossRef] [PubMed]
14. Malanchini, G.; Malacrida, M.; Ferrari, P.; Leidi, C.; Ferrari, G.; Racheli, M.; Senni, M.; de Filippo, P. Impact of the Coronavirus Disease-19 Outbreak on Physical Activity of Patients With Implantable Cardioverter Defibrillators. *J. Card. Fail.* **2020**, *26*, 898–899. [CrossRef] [PubMed]

15. Castañeda-Babarro, A.; Arbillaga-Etxarri, A.; Gutiérrez-Santamaria, B.; Coca, A. Impact of COVID-19 confinement on the time and intensity of physical activity in the Spanish population. *Res. Sq.* **2020**. [CrossRef]
16. Dunton, G.F.; Wang, S.D.; Do, B.; Courtney, J. Early Effects of the COVID-19 Pandemic on Physical Activity Locations and Behaviors in Adults Living in the United States. *Prev. Med. Rep.* **2020**, *20*, 101241. [CrossRef] [PubMed]
17. Cheval, B.; Sivaramakrishnan, H.; Maltagliati, S.; Fessler, L.; Forestier, C.; Sarrazin, P.; Orsholits, D.; Chalabaev, A.; Sander, D.; Ntoumanis, N.; et al. Relationships between changes in self-reported physical activity, sedentary behaviour and health during the coronavirus (COVID-19) pandemic in France and Switzerland. *J. Sports Sci.* **2020**, 1–6. [CrossRef] [PubMed]
18. Suzuki, Y.; Maeda, N.; Hirado, D.; Shirakawa, T.; Urabe, Y. Physical Activity Changes and Its Risk Factors among Community-Dwelling Japanese Older Adults during the COVID-19 Epidemic: Associations with Subjective Well-Being and Health-Related Quality of Life. *Int. J. Environ. Res. Public Health* **2020**, *17*, 6591. [CrossRef]
19. Yamada, M.; Kimura, Y.; Ishiyama, D.; Otobe, Y.; Suzuki, M.; Koyama, S.; Kikuchi, T.; Kusumi, H.; Arai, H. Effect of the COVID-19 Epidemic on Physical Activity in Community-Dwelling Older Adults in Japan: A Cross-Sectional Online Survey. *J. Nutr. Health Aging* **2020**, *24*, 948–950. [CrossRef]
20. Ellis, G.; Gardner, M.; Tsiachristas, A.; Langhorne, P.; Burke, O.; Harwood, R.H.; Conroy, S.P.; Kircher, T.; Somme, D.; Saltvedt, I.; et al. Comprehensive geriatric assessment for older adults admitted to hospital. *Cochrane Database Syst. Rev.* **2017**, *9*, CD006211. [CrossRef]
21. Inzitari, M.; Pérez, L.M.; Enfedaque, M.B.; Soto, L.; Díaz, F.; Gual, N.; Martín, E.; Orfila, F.; Mulero, P.; Ruiz, R.; et al. Integrated primary and geriatric care for frail older adults in the community: Implementation of a complex intervention into real life. *Eur. J. Intern. Med.* **2018**, *56*, 57–63. [CrossRef]
22. Vellas, B.; Balardy, L.; Gillette-Guyonnet, S.; Abellan Van Kan, G.; Ghisolfi-Marque, A.; Subra, J.; Bismuth, S.; Oustric, S.; Cesari, M. Looking for frailty in community-dwelling older persons: The Gérontopôle Frailty Screening Tool (GFST). *J. Nutr. Health Aging* **2013**, *17*, 629–631. [CrossRef]
23. Izquierdo, M.; Vivifrail Investigators Group; Rodriguez-Mañas, L.; Sinclair, A.J. What is new in exercise regimes for frail older people—How does the Erasmus Vivifrail Project take us forward? *J. Nutr. Health Aging* **2016**, *20*, 736–737. [CrossRef] [PubMed]
24. Puig Ribera, A.; Peña Chimenis, O.; Romaguera Bosch, M.; Duran Bellido, E.; Heras Tebar, A.; Solà Gonfaus, M.; Sarmiento Cruz, M.; Cid Cantarero, A. How to identify physical inactivity in primary care: Validation of the Catalan and Spanish versions of 2 short questionnaires. *Aten. Primaria* **2012**, *44*, 485–493. [CrossRef] [PubMed]
25. Marshall, A.L. Reliability and validity of a brief physical activity assessment for use by family doctors: Commentary. *Br. J. Sports Med.* **2005**, *39*, 294–297. [CrossRef] [PubMed]
26. Charlson, M.E.; Pompei, P.; Ales, K.L.; MacKenzie, C.R. A new method of classifying prognostic comorbidity in longitudinal studies: Development and validation. *J. Chronic Dis.* **1987**, *40*, 373–383. [CrossRef]
27. Mahoney, F.I.; Barthel, D.W. Functional evaluation: The barthel index. *Md. State Med. J.* **1965**, *14*, 61–65.
28. Lawton, M.P.; Brody, E.M. Assessment of Older People: Self-Maintaining and Instrumental Activities of Daily Living. *Gerontologist* **1969**, *9*, 179–186. [CrossRef]
29. Kaiser, M.J.; MNA-International Group; Bauer, J.M.; Ramsch, C.; Uter, W.; Guigoz, Y.; Cederholm, T.; Thomas, D.R.; Anthony, P.; Charlton, K.E.; et al. Validation of the Mini Nutritional Assessment short-form (MNA®-SF): A practical tool for identification of nutritional status. *J. Nutr. Health Aging* **2009**, *13*, 782–788. [CrossRef]
30. Carnero-Pardo, C.; Cruz-Orduña, I.; Espejo-Martínez, B.; Martos-Aparicio, C.; López-Alcalde, S.; Olazarán, J. Utility of the mini-cog for detection of cognitive impairment in primary care: Data from two spanish studies. *Int. J. Alzheimers. Dis.* **2013**, *2013*, 285462. [CrossRef]
31. Borson, S.; Scanlan, J.M.; Chen, P.; Ganguli, M. The Mini-Cog as a Screen for Dementia: Validation in a Population-Based Sample. *J. Am. Geriatr. Soc.* **2003**, *51*, 1451–1454. [CrossRef]
32. De la Iglesia, J.M.; de la Iglesia, J.M.; Onís Vilches, M.C.; Dueñas Herrero, R.; Albert Colomer, C.; Aguado Taberné, C.; Luque Luque, R. Versión española del cuestionario de Yesavage abreviado (GDS) para el despistaje de depresión en mayores de 65 años: Adaptación y validación. *Medifam* **2002**, *12*, 620–630.
33. Yesavage, J.A.; Sheikh, J.I. 9/Geriatric Depression Scale (GDS): Recent Evidence and Development of a Shorter Version. *Clin. Gerontol.* **1986**, *5*, 165–173. [CrossRef]
34. Guralnik, J.M.; Simonsick, E.M.; Ferrucci, L.; Glynn, R.J.; Berkman, L.F.; Blazer, D.G.; Scherr, P.A.; Wallace, R.B. A Short Physical Performance Battery Assessing Lower Extremity Function: Association with Self-Reported Disability and Prediction of Mortality and Nursing Home Admission. *J. Gerontol.* **1994**, *49*, M85–M94. [CrossRef] [PubMed]
35. Rockwood, K.; Song, X.; MacKnight, C.; Bergman, H.; Hogan, D.B.; McDowell, I.; Mitnitski, A. A global clinical measure of fitness and frailty in elderly people. *CMAJ* **2005**, *173*, 489–495. [CrossRef] [PubMed]
36. Pérez, L.M.; Roqué, M.; Glynn, N.W.; Santanasto, A.J.; Ramoneda, M.; Molins, M.T.; Coll-Planas, L.; Vidal, P.; Inzitari, M. Validation of the Spanish version of the Pittsburgh Fatigability Scale for older adults. *Aging Clin. Exp. Res.* **2019**, *31*, 209–214. [CrossRef] [PubMed]
37. Khafaie, M.A.; Rahim, F. Cross-Country Comparison of Case Fatality Rates of COVID-19/SARS-COV-2. *Osong Public Health Res. Perspect.* **2020**, *11*, 74–80. [CrossRef] [PubMed]

38. Gallè, F.; Sabella, E.A.; Ferracuti, S.; De Giglio, O.; Caggiano, G.; Protano, C.; Valeriani, F.; Parisi, E.A.; Valerio, G.; Liguori, G.; et al. Sedentary Behaviors and Physical Activity of Italian Undergraduate Students during Lockdown at the Time of CoViD-19 Pandemic. *Int. J. Environ. Res. Public Health* **2020**, *17*, 6171. [CrossRef] [PubMed]
39. Courel-Ibáñez, J.; Pallarés, J.G.; García-Conesa, S.; Buendía-Romero, Á.; Martínez-Cava, A.; Izquierdo, M. Supervised Exercise (Vivifrail) Protects Institutionalized Older Adults Against Severe Functional Decline After 14 Weeks of COVID Confinement. *J. Am. Med. Dir. Assoc.* **2020**, [CrossRef]
40. Gomes, M.; Figueiredo, D.; Teixeira, L.; Poveda, V.; Paúl, C.; Santos-Silva, A.; Costa, E. Physical inactivity among older adults across Europe based on the SHARE database. *Age Ageing* **2017**, *46*, 71–77. [CrossRef]
41. Craft, L.L.; Perna, F.M. The Benefits of Exercise for the Clinically Depressed. *Prim. Care Companion J. Clin. Psychiatry* **2004**, *6*, 104–111. [CrossRef]
42. Schuch, F.B.; Morres, I.D.; Ekkekakis, P.; Rosenbaum, S.; Stubbs, B. A critical review of exercise as a treatment for clinically depressed adults: Time to get pragmatic. *Acta Neuropsychiatr.* **2017**, *29*, 65–71. [CrossRef]
43. García-Fernández, L.; Romero-Ferreiro, V.; López-Roldán, P.D.; Padilla, S.; Rodriguez-Jimenez, R. Mental Health in Elderly Spanish People in Times of COVID-19 Outbreak. *Am. J. Geriatr. Psychiatry* **2020**, *28*, 1040–1045. [CrossRef] [PubMed]
44. Fundació La Caixa. Apuntes Programa Personas Mayores COVID19. Available online: https://fundacionlacaixa.org/documents/10280/1477443/apuntes-programa-personas-mayores-covid19.pdf (accessed on 25 November 2020).
45. Beard, J.R.; Officer, A.; de Carvalho, I.A.; Sadana, R.; Pot, A.M.; Michel, J.-P.; Lloyd-Sherlock, P.; Epping-Jordan, J.E.; (Geeske) Peeters, G.M.E.E.; Mahanani, W.R.; et al. The World report on ageing and health: A policy framework for healthy ageing. *Lancet* **2016**, *387*, 2145–2154. [CrossRef]
46. Carriedo, A.; Cecchini, J.A.; Fernandez-Rio, J.; Méndez-Giménez, A. COVID-19, Psychological Well-being and Physical Activity Levels in Older Adults during the Nationwide Lockdown in Spain. *Am. J. Geriatr. Psychiatry* **2020**, *28*, 1146–1155. [CrossRef] [PubMed]
47. Losada-Baltar, A.; Jiménez-Gonzalo, L.; Gallego-Alberto, L.; del Sequeros Pedroso-Chaparro, M.; Fernandes-Pires, J.; Márquez-González, M. "We Are Staying at Home." Association of Self-perceptions of Aging, Personal and Family Resources, and Loneliness with Psychological Distress during the Lock-Down Period of COVID-19. *J. Gerontol. Ser. B* **2020**. [CrossRef] [PubMed]
48. Benedict, C.; Brooks, S.J.; Kullberg, J.; Nordenskjöld, R.; Burgos, J.; Le Grevès, M.; Kilander, L.; Larsson, E.-M.; Johansson, L.; Ahlström, H.; et al. Association between physical activity and brain health in older adults. *Neurobiol. Aging* **2013**, *34*, 83–90. [CrossRef]
49. Vermeulen, J.; Neyens, J.C.L.; van Rossum, E.; Spreeuwenberg, M.D.; de Witte, L.P. Predicting ADL disability in community-dwelling elderly people using physical frailty indicators: A systematic review. *BMC Geriatr.* **2011**, *11*, 33. [CrossRef]
50. Penninx, B.W.J.H.; Rejeski, W.J.; Pandya, J.; Miller, M.E.; Di Bari, M.; Applegate, W.B.; Pahor, M. Exercise and depressive symptoms: A comparison of aerobic and resistance exercise effects on emotional and physical function in older persons with high and low depressive symptomatology. *J. Gerontol. B Psychol. Sci. Soc. Sci.* **2002**, *57*, P124–P132. [CrossRef]
51. Worrall, C.; Jongenelis, M.; Pettigrew, S. Modifiable Protective and Risk Factors for Depressive Symptoms among Older Community-dwelling Adults: A Systematic Review. *J. Affect. Disord.* **2020**, *272*, 305–317. [CrossRef]
52. Alexander, N.B.; Taffet, G.E.; Horne, F.M.; Eldadah, B.A.; Ferrucci, L.; Nayfield, S.; Studenski, S. Bedside-to-Bench conference: Research agenda for idiopathic fatigue and aging. *J. Am. Geriatr. Soc.* **2010**, *58*, 967–975. [CrossRef]
53. Hardy, S.E.; Studenski, S.A. Fatigue Predicts Mortality in Older Adults. *J. Am. Geriatr. Soc.* **2008**, *56*, 1910–1914. [CrossRef]
54. Vestergaard, S.; Nayfield, S.G.; Patel, K.V.; Eldadah, B.; Cesari, M.; Ferrucci, L.; Ceresini, G.; Guralnik, J.M. Fatigue in a Representative Population of Older Persons and Its Association With Functional Impairment, Functional Limitation, and Disability. *J. Gerontol. Ser. A Biol. Sci. Med. Sci.* **2009**, *64A*, 76–82. [CrossRef] [PubMed]
55. Penner, I.-K.; Paul, F. Fatigue as a symptom or comorbidity of neurological diseases. *Nat. Rev. Neurol.* **2017**, *13*, 662–675. [CrossRef] [PubMed]
56. Fried, L.P.; Tangen, C.M.; Walston, J.; Newman, A.B.; Hirsch, C.; Gottdiener, J.; Seeman, T.; Tracy, R.; Kop, W.J.; Burke, G.; et al. Frailty in older adults: Evidence for a phenotype. *J. Gerontol. A Biol. Sci. Med. Sci.* **2001**, *56*, M146–M157. [CrossRef] [PubMed]
57. Soyuer, F.; Şenol, V. Fatigue and Physical Activity Levels of 65 and Over Older People Living in Rest Home. *Int. J. Gerontol.* **2011**, *5*, 13–16. [CrossRef]
58. Holt-Lunstad, J.; Smith, T.B.; Layton, J.B. Social relationships and mortality risk: A meta-analytic review. *PLoS Med.* **2010**, *7*, e1000316. [CrossRef]
59. Holt-Lunstad, J. Why Social Relationships Are Important for Physical Health: A Systems Approach to Understanding and Modifying Risk and Protection. *Annu. Rev. Psychol.* **2018**, *69*, 437–458. [CrossRef]
60. Giné-Garriga, M.; Jerez-Roig, J.; Coll-Planas, L.; Skelton, D.; Inzitari, M.; Booth, J.; Souza, D. Is loneliness a predictor of the modern geriatric giants? Analysis from the survey of health, ageing, and retirement in Europe. *Maturitas* **2021**. [CrossRef]
61. Newsom, J.T.; Denning, E.C.; Shaw, B.A.; August, K.J.; Strath, S.J. Older adults' physical activity-related social control and social support in the context of personal norms. *J. Health Psychol.* **2020**, 1359105320954239. [CrossRef]
62. Kotwal, A.A.; Holt-Lunstad, J.; Newmark, R.L.; Cenzer, I.; Smith, A.K.; Covinsky, K.E.; Escueta, D.P.; Lee, J.M.; Perissinotto, C.M. Social Isolation and Loneliness Among San Francisco Bay Area Older Adults During the COVID-19 Shelter-in-Place Orders. *J. Am. Geriatr. Soc.* **2020**. [CrossRef]

63. Heidinger, T.; Richter, L. The Effect of COVID-19 on Loneliness in the Elderly. An Empirical Comparison of Pre-and Peri-Pandemic Loneliness in Community-Dwelling Elderly. *Front. Psychol.* **2020**, *11*, 585308. [CrossRef]
64. Sepúlveda-Loyola, W.; Rodríguez-Sánchez, I.; Pérez-Rodríguez, P.; Ganz, F.; Torralba, R.; Oliveira, D.V.; Rodríguez-Mañas, L. Impact of Social Isolation Due to COVID-19 on Health in Older People: Mental and Physical Effects and Recommendations. *J. Nutr. Health Aging* **2020**, *24*, 938–947. [CrossRef]
65. Perissinotto, C.; Holt-Lunstad, J.; Periyakoil, V.S.; Covinsky, K. A Practical Approach to Assessing and Mitigating Loneliness and Isolation in Older Adults. *J. Am. Geriatr. Soc.* **2019**, *67*. [CrossRef]
66. Gallucci, A.; Trimarchi, P.D.; Abbate, C.; Tuena, C.; Pedroli, E.; Lattanzio, F.; Stramba-Badiale, M.; Cesari, M.; Giunco, F. ICT technologies as new promising tools for the managing of frailty: A systematic review. *Aging Clin. Exp. Res.* **2020**. [CrossRef]
67. Ostir, G.V.; Ottenbacher, K.J.; Fried, L.P.; Guralnik, J.M. The Effect of Depressive Symptoms on the Association between Functional Status and Social Participation. *Soc. Indic. Res.* **2007**, *80*, 379–392. [CrossRef]
68. Kourkouta, L.; Iliadis, C.; Frantzana, A.; Vakalopoulou, V. Reading and Health Benefits. *J. Healthc. Commun.* **2018**, *3*, 39. [CrossRef]

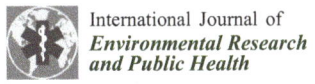

Article

Association of Social Frailty with Physical Health, Cognitive Function, Psychological Health, and Life Satisfaction in Community-Dwelling Older Koreans

Hana Ko [1] and SuJung Jung [2],*

[1] College of Nursing, Gachon University, Incheon 21936, Korea; hanago11@gachon.ac.kr
[2] College of Nursing, Seoul National University, Seoul 03080, Korea
* Correspondence: tnwjdpeach@snu.ac.kr

Abstract: Social frailty affects various aspects of health in community-dwelling older adults. This study aimed to identify the prevalence of social frailty and the significance of its association with South Korean older adults' health status and life satisfaction. This study involved a secondary data analysis of the 2017 National Survey of Older Koreans. From the 10,299 respondents of the survey, 10,081 were selected with no exclusion criteria. Multiple regression analyses were conducted to identify the factors related to life satisfaction. Compared with the robust and social prefrailty groups, the social frailty group had higher nutritional risk (χ^2 = 312.161, p = 0.000), depressive symptoms (χ^2 = 977.587, p = 0.000), cognitive dysfunction (χ^2 = 25.051, p = 0.000), and lower life satisfaction (F = 1050.272, p = 0.000). The results of multiple linear regression, adjusted for sociodemographic and health-related characteristics, indicated that social frailty had the strongest negative association with life satisfaction (β = −0.267, p = 0.000). However, cognitive function was significantly positively associated with life satisfaction (β = 0.062, p = 0.000). Social frailty was significantly correlated with physical, psychological, and mental health as well as life satisfaction in community-dwelling older South Koreans. Therefore, accounting for the social aspect of functioning is an essential part of a multidimensional approach to improving health and life satisfaction in communities.

Keywords: social frailty; older adults; life satisfaction

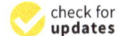

Citation: Ko, H.; Jung, S. Association of Social Frailty with Physical Health, Cognitive Function, Psychological Health, and Life Satisfaction in Community-Dwelling Older Koreans. *IJERPH* **2021**, *18*, 818. https://doi.org/10.3390/ijerph18020818

Received: 12 December 2020
Accepted: 17 January 2021
Published: 19 January 2021

Publisher's Note: MDPI stays neutral with regard to jurisdictional claims in published maps and institutional affiliations.

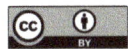

Copyright: © 2021 by the authors. Licensee MDPI, Basel, Switzerland. This article is an open access article distributed under the terms and conditions of the Creative Commons Attribution (CC BY) license (https://creativecommons.org/licenses/by/4.0/).

1. Introduction

The median age of the South Korean population is rapidly increasing; in 2019, individuals aged 65 and over accounted for 14.9% of the South Korean population, and this proportion has been projected to exceed 46.5% by 2067 [1]. Given this rapid increase in the older adult population, frailty and life satisfaction in this age group are becoming more critical than at any other age [2,3]. A high level of life satisfaction is an indicator of happiness and success in old age [4–6]. Life satisfaction, a subjective evaluation of contentment with one's life [4], is affected not only by intrinsic physical and mental capacities but also by functional abilities and environmental aspects such as social factors [7]. Therefore, the World Health Organization's initiative to create age-friendly cities includes measures to increase older adults' life satisfaction [8]. Creating age-friendly environments requires collaboration and coordination across multiple sectors and with diverse stakeholders, including older people. The foundation of such efforts is to allow older adults to have social relationships in their own life community.

Frailty is defined as a biological syndrome of extreme vulnerability to endogenous and exogenous stressors associated with multisystem decline in physiological reserve, resulting in increased risk of adverse outcomes including disability, hospitalization, and death [3,9]. This multidimensional concept has physical, cognitive, psychological, and social components [10].

Recently, the concept of "social frailty" has been increasingly emphasized. Based on a scoping review [4] and using the theory of social production function, a conceptual framework has been proposed. Social frailty is defined as a continuum of being at risk of losing, or having lost, resources that are important for fulfilling one or more basic social needs during the lifespan [11]. However, existing explorations of social frailty have been complicated by the interconnections of contextual, societal, and cultural considerations [10].

Previous studies have reported that social frailty is associated with muscle weakness [12] and cognitive function [2], and that social frailty can lead to disability and mortality [13]. In a study of homeless women, drug use, emotion regulation, and daily alcohol use were significant correlates of social frailty [14]. However, there have been few reports of the prevalence of social frailty and how it relates to older South Korean adults' health status and life satisfaction.

Thus, this study aims (1) to examine the differences in general and health status characteristics of community-dwelling older adults in South Korea according to social frailty status; (2) to examine the correlations among social frailty status, nutritional status, depression, cognitive function, and life satisfaction; and (3) to explore the health-related predictors associated with life satisfaction.

2. Materials and Methods

2.1. Participants

This cross-sectional study used secondary data from the 2017 National Survey of Older Koreans [15]. The National Survey of Older Koreans, conducted by the Ministry of Health and Welfare every three years, seeks to gather the data necessary to devise policy measures to improve quality of life and better manage population aging in this age group. The 2017 survey included 10,299 individuals aged 65 or older living in standard residential facilities or premises in 17 metropolitan cities and provinces across South Korea. The 2017 National Survey of Older Koreans sample was selected using a proportional two-stage stratified sampling method, which was first stratified and collected by 17 metropolitan cities and provinces across Korea and then again by neighborhoods in the nine provinces and Sejong (but not in the metropolitan cities) [15]. The Ministry of Health and Welfare research team applied various weights in the raw data to ensure the accuracy of estimations. The weight of the raw data was adjusted by considering the weights for households and individuals [15]. The data were obtained through in-person interviews in 934 survey areas from 12 June to 28 August 2017. The survey was conducted by 60 surveyors, trained by the research staff in advance. Surveyors checked the answered questionnaires for any omissions and errors and relayed their feedback to the research team. Raw data used in this study were obtained on 5 June 2020 after obtaining approval from the Health and Welfare Data Portal (https://data.kihasa.re.kr/). From the 10,299 respondents of the 2017 National Survey of Older Koreans, 10,081 were selected without any exclusion criteria; 218 were excluded for missing responses.

2.2. Measures

2.2.1. Sociodemographic and Health-Related Characteristics

Sociodemographic characteristics included age, gender, education level, economic status, and living conditions (living alone, living with partner, living with others). Economic status was sorted in ascending order by annual personal income and divided into five categories so that each group contained 20% of the participants. Then, only the bottom 20% of the group were used in the analysis, as they best suited our interests. Health-related characteristics included the number of prescription medications, diagnosis of chronic diseases, subjective health status (very healthy, healthy, average, in ill health, in very ill health), lower-extremity muscle (sitting and standing up), and lifestyle (smoking and physical activity).

2.2.2. Social Frailty

To identify and assess social frailty, we operationalized the concept into five categories based on a previous study [9]: going out (not participating in any leisure and social activities such as travel, hobbies, learning or studying, social clubs, networking, political and social groups, volunteering, senior citizen centers, community centers for older adults), visiting friends (no), feeling worthless (yes), living alone (yes), and contact with someone (no). Participants with none, one, and two or more of these components were classified into the robust, social prefrailty, and social frailty groups, respectively [9,16,17].

2.2.3. Nutritional Status

Nutritional status was measured using "Determine Your Nutritional Health," a tool developed by the Nutrition Screening Initiative [18]. Used to assess nutritional status in older adults, this instrument consists of 10 items, each of which is rated from 1 to 4. The range of possible scores is from 0 to 21; accordingly, nutritional status is categorized as good (0 to 2 points), moderate risk (3 to 5 points), and high risk (6 points or more). In this study, 3 points or more were classified into the nutritional risk group.

2.2.4. Depression

Depression was measured using the 15-item Geriatric Depression Scale-Short Form Korean Version (GDSSF-K) [19]. The GDSSF-K includes five positive items and 10 negative items in a yes/no response format. The total GDSSF-K score was obtained by counting the number of "yes" responses after the positive items were reverse coded so that higher scores indicated higher levels of depressive symptoms. The total scores ranged from 0 to 15. The criteria for determining depression were "normal" in the total score for less than 5 points, "moderate depression" for 6 to 9 points, and "depressed" for more than 10 points. In the 2017 National Survey of Older Koreans [15], people scoring more than 8 points were classified as "depressed", and this criterion was used in our analysis. There is evidence supporting the construct and criterion related validity of the GDSSF-K [19]; Cronbach's alpha was 0.88 in a previous study [19] and 0.89 in the present study.

2.2.5. Cognitive Function

Cognitive function was measured using the Mini-Mental State Examination for Dementia Screening (MMSE-DS) [20]. The 19-item MMSE-DS has a maximum score of 30 points, with higher scores indicative of higher cognitive function. This tool has been standardized by age, gender, and educational level for normative cognitive function assessment in older adults in South Korea [20]. There is evidence supporting the validity of the MMSE-DS [21]; Cronbach's alpha was 0.82 in a previous study and 0.93 in the present study.

2.2.6. Life Satisfaction

Life satisfaction was measured using the question "To what extent are you satisfied with the following aspects of your life: health status, economic status, relationship with spouse, relationship with children, leisure and cultural activities, and relationships with friends and society?" The response options were: 1 = very satisfied, 2 = satisfied, 3 = average, 4 = not satisfied, and 5 = not satisfied at all. Responses to all items were reverse coded, so that higher scores indicated higher levels of life satisfaction. The total scores ranged from 6 to 30; Cronbach's alpha was 0.61 in the present study.

2.3. Ethical Considerations

The 2017 National Survey of Older Koreans was approved by Statistics Korea (Approval No. 11771). For our study, after obtaining approval from the Korea Institute for Health and Social Affairs, we received raw data without personal identification information. Moreover, the study was approved by the Institutional Review Board (IRB No.: 1044396-202006-HR-110-01) of Gachon University, to which one of the researchers is affiliated.

2.4. Data Analyses

Sample characteristics were summarized using means and standard deviations (SDs) for continuous variables and proportions for categorical variables. To evaluate the differences in characteristics between participants from the three groups (robust, social prefrailty, and social frailty), we used Pearson's χ^2 test for categorical data and analysis of variance for continuous data. Then, we performed multiple regression analysis to identify the factors related to life satisfaction. Before running the multiple regression analysis, we conducted a correlation analysis, and the independent variables were tested for multicollinearity using tolerance value and variance inflation factor (VIF). Less than 10% of confirmed missing cases were excluded from the analysis by applying listwise deletion [22]. All statistical analyses were conducted using SPSS version 23.0 (IBM Corp., Armonk, NY, USA) with the two-tailed significance level set at 0.05. For effect size, we followed Cohen's criteria (0.10 = small, 0.25 = medium, 0.40 = large) [23] in analysis of variance, and Rea and Parker's criteria ($0.00 \leq x < 0.10$ = negligible, $0.10 \leq x < 0.20$ = weak, $0.20 \leq x < 0.40$ = moderate, $0.40 \leq x < 0.60$ = relatively strong, $0.60 \leq x < 0.80$ = strong, $0.80 \leq x \leq 1.00$ = very strong) [24] in Pearson's χ^2 test.

3. Results

3.1. General Characteristics of the Study Sample

The sample characteristics are shown in Table 1. Out of the 10,081 participants, 1292 (12.8%), 4281 (42.5%), and 4508 (44.7%) were classified into the robust, social prefrailty, and social frailty groups, respectively. The mean age in the robust, social prefrailty, and social frailty groups was 72.2 years, 73.9 years, and 75.6 years, respectively. Those in the social frailty group were older, had lower education level, economic status, and subjective health status, and were more likely to live alone compared with the robust and social prefrailty groups ($p = 0.000$). Regarding lifestyle, there was a difference in physical activity according to social frailty status ($p = 0.000$). However, there were no statistically significant differences between the three groups regarding smoking.

Additionally, the social frailty group had a higher proportion of participants with more than three diagnosed chronic diseases and a higher number of prescribed medications compared to those in the robust and social prefrailty groups.

Table 1. General characteristics of participants in the robust, social prefrailty, and social frailty groups.

Characteristic	Total $n = 10{,}081$	Robust $n = 1292$	Social Prefrailty $n = 4281$	Social Frailty $n = 4508$	χ^2/F (df)	p (E.S.)
Age, years Mean (SD)	74.5 (6.2)	72.2 (5.5)	73.9 (6.0)	75.6 (6.4)	180.424 [a] (2)	0.000 (0.139) [b]
Men n (%)	4046 (40.1)	598 (46.3)	1864 (43.5)	1584 (35.1)	87.868 (2)	0.000 (0.093) [c]
Education, years Mean (SD)	6.8 (4.6)	7.6 (4.3)	7.2 (4.5)	6.1 (4.7)	106.257 [a] (2)	0.000 (0.212) [b]
Low economic status n (%)	2037 (20.2)	53 (4.1)	488 (11.4)	1496 (33.2)	1063.055 (8)	0.000 (0.230) [c]
Living alone n (%)	2552 (25.3)	0 (0.0)	450 (10.5)	2102 (46.7)	2061.501 (4)	0.000 (0.320) [c]
More than 3 diagnosed chronic diseases n (%)	5326 (52.8)	556 (43.0)	2135 (49.9)	2635 (58.5)	137.111 (6)	0.000 (0.082) [c]
Number of prescribed medicines Mean (SD)	4.0 (3.4)	3.3 (3.2)	3.7 (3.2)	4.5 (3.5)	88.864 [a] (2)	0.000 (0.132) [b]

Table 1. Cont.

Characteristic	Total n = 10,081	Robust n = 1292	Social Prefrailty n = 4281	Social Frailty n = 4508	χ²/F (df)	p (E.S.)
Current smoker n (%)	950 (9.4)	129 (10.0)	368 (8.6)	453 (10.0)	5.975 (2)	0.050 (0.024) [c]
Weakness in lower-extremity muscles n (%)	2148 (21.3)	107 (8.3)	682 (15.9)	1359 (30.1)	414.594 (2)	0.000 (0.203) [c]
No physical activity n (%)	3346 (33.2)	289 (22.4)	1263 (29.5)	1794 (39.8)	183.198 (2)	0.000 (0.135) [c]
Subjective health status, very poor health n (%)	469 (4.7)	30 (2.3)	112 (2.6)	327 (7.3)	439.035 (8)	0.000 (0.148) [c]

Note: E.S. = effect size; [a] analysis of variance; [b] Effect size f; [c] Cramer's V.

3.2. Differences in Nutritional Status, Depression, Cognitive Function, and Life Satisfaction by Social Frailty Status

Table 2 displays the differences in nutritional status, depression, cognitive function, and life satisfaction by social frailty status, categorized into the three groups robust, social prefrailty, and social frailty. The prevalence of nutritional risk, depression, and lower cognitive function was highest in the social frailty group. Moreover, the social frailty group scored the lowest on all six categories of life satisfaction: health status, economic status, relationship with spouse, relationship with children, leisure and cultural activities, and relationships with friends and society.

Table 2. Prevalence of social frailty in different health domains.

Health Domain	Total n = 10,081	Robust n = 1292	Social Prefrailty n = 4281	Social Frailty n = 4508	χ²/F (df)	p (E.S.)
Nutritional status risk [a] n (%)	6213 (61.6)	623 (48.2)	2401 (56.1)	3189 (70.7)	312.161 (2)	0.000 (0.176) [e]
Depressed [b] n (%)	2177 (21.6)	73 (5.7)	495 (11.6)	1609 (35.7)	977.587 (2)	0.000 (0.311) [e]
Cognitive dysfunction [c] n (%)	260 (2.6)	10 (0.8)	104 (2.4)	146 (3.2)	25.051 (2)	0.000 (0.050) [e]
Life satisfaction Mean (SD)	18.81 (3.81)	21.14 (3.09)	19.89 (3.32)	17.06 (3.68)	1050.272 [d] (2)	0.000 (0.462) [f]

Note: [a] Determine Your Nutritional Health tool developed by the Nutrition Screening Initiative; [b] Geriatric Depression Scale-Short Form Korean Version (GDSSF-K); [c] Mini-Mental State Examination for Dementia Screening (MMSE-DS); [d] analysis of variance; [e] Cramer's V; [f] effect size f; df = degrees of freedom; E.S. = effect size.

3.3. Correlation of Predictors

Table 3 shows that the predictors were correlated. Depression and nutritional status had a high correlation (r = 0.455, p = 0.000). In addition, life satisfaction, which was the criterion variable, was significantly correlated with all predictors.

Table 3. Correlations between predictors and life satisfaction.

	Social Frailty	Nutritional Status	Depression	Cognitive Function
	r (p)	r (p)	r (p)	r (p)
Social frailty				
Nutritional status	0.236 (0.000)			
Depression	0.339 (0.000)	0.455 (0.000)		
Cognitive function	−0.175 (0.000)	−0.261 (0.000)	−0.273 (0.000)	
Life satisfaction	−0.408 (0.000)	−0.486 (0.000)	−0.545 (0.000)	0.339 (0.000)

3.4. Multiple Regression Analysis

Multiple linear regression analyses revealed that social frailty had the strongest negative association with life satisfaction ($\beta = -0.267$, $p = 0.000$) (Table 4). However, cognitive function was significantly positively associated with life satisfaction ($\beta = 0.062$, $p = 0.000$). The variance inflation factor (VIF) of predictors and the tolerance of predictors were 1.427–2.749 and 0.364–0.701 respectively, which suggests the absence of multicollinearity between the predictors.

Table 4. Factors related to the life satisfaction of older adults.

Predictors	Criterion: Life Satisfaction $R^2 = 0.49$, $p = 0.000$				
	β	SE	T	p	VIF
Social frailty	−0.267	0.091	−22.422	0.000	2.749
Depression	−0.224	0.008	−24.632	0.000	1.597
Nutritional status	−0.186	0.010	−21.718	0.000	1.427
Cognitive function	0.062	0.009	7.041	0.000	1.528

Note: n = 9833 (missing cases are excluded listwise); β = standardized coefficient; SE = standard error; VIF = variance inflation factor.

4. Discussion

The prevalence of social frailty in the sample was 44.7%. Further, the social frailty group displayed the highest prevalence of nutritional risk, depression, low cognitive function, and poor life satisfaction. Additionally, social frailty displayed the strongest negative association with life satisfaction. These findings suggest that social frailty may affect older adults' physical, cognitive, and psychological functions as well as life satisfaction.

The prevalence of social frailty in this study was higher than the rates reported by Tsutsumimoto et al. (11.1%) [9] and Yamada and Arai (18%) [13]. Our social frailty index was operationalized based on several previous studies [9,16,17]. Additionally, our study samples were composed of community-dwelling older adults without any exclusion criteria like disabilities in activities of daily living or severe diseases [9] and long-term care recipients [13]. Therefore, the major differences from previous studies are with regard to the items of the social frailty questionnaire and the study population. While the five-item social frailty assessment is popular [9,25–27], participants' culture and environment have not always been considered in existing research. Regarding other measures of social frailty, as in this study, many previous studies have used participants' living status (living alone or with someone) [9,12,13,16,17]. In Korea, the proportion of single-person households ages 65 or older is expected to be 36.6% in 2045, the highest compared to couple households

(30.2%) or couples and children (9.2%) [28]. Therefore, the country needs to prepare for social frailty caused by population aging and the rapid increase in the number of older adults living alone.

This study shows that older adults with social frailty tend to be more vulnerable to impairments in cognitive and psychological functions than their robust counterparts. This result is in line with those of several previous studies, which revealed that higher levels of social frailty were associated with cognitive dysfunction [9,25] and depressive symptoms [16,25]. Furthermore, deteriorations in social frailty status have been associated with worsening physical nutritional status. Malnutrition is considered one of the physical functions responsible for sarcopenia, osteoporosis, and impaired immune response [29]. In terms of physical functions, recent cohort studies have focused on the impact of social frailty on physical frailty [12] and disability [26,30]. Similarly, social frailty has been shown to be associated with cognitive impairment, depression, and physical functioning in China [25]. These findings confirm that older adults with poor social relationships and social engagement are at an increased risk of multidimensional dysfunctions. Future studies should further delineate the causal relationship between social frailty and multidimensional health functions.

To the best of our knowledge, this is the first study to examine the association between social frailty and life satisfaction in older adults. According to the results, social frailty had a stronger negative association with life satisfaction than with physical, psychological, and cognitive functions. Previous studies have revealed a negative relationship between depression levels and life satisfaction [31–33]. Further, in a longitudinal study, long-term life dissatisfaction predicted the onset of major depressive disorder [34]. In addition, cognition has been shown to be associated with life satisfaction [33]. Our study provides a starting point for examining the impact of social frailty on life satisfaction in older adults. Life satisfaction, a subjective cognitive evaluation of an individual's life [5], is a component and crucial indicator of quality of life [6]. The World Health Organization also emphasizes the importance of social relationships for older adults; the maintenance of social relationships is a prerequisite for healthy aging, bringing life satisfaction [8]. Especially, during the current coronavirus disease 2019 pandemic, social isolation may amplify the prevalence of social frailty in older adults [35]. Therefore, the result that social frailty had the strongest association with life satisfaction in older adults provides justification for preparing plans to increase life satisfaction by preventing social frailty and promoting social relationships.

The strengths of this study are the large sample size and the use of an operationalized assessment to identify social frailty. On the other hand, the large sample size can cause overpower problems in situations where there is little association between groups. It is necessary to pay attention to the interpretation of the results based on the effect size [23,24], which are reported in Tables 1 and 2. In the difference in characteristics according to social frailty status, the effect sizes of gender, chronic disease, age, number of prescribed medicines, physical activity, subjective health status, nutritional status, and cognitive function were lower than those of other characteristics [24]; however, there was a considerable difference in life satisfaction according to social frailty [23]. While the effect size can confirm the practical difference (or association) between groups [36], it has a limitation in that it is a relative value that can vary depending on the characteristics of the population or other variables [23]. Nevertheless, to our knowledge, the current study is the first to report an association between life satisfaction and social frailty.

However, this study also has some limitations. First, owing to the use of cross-sectional secondary data, causality could not be explored; this should be clarified in a future prospective study. Second, although Diener et al.'s Satisfaction with Life Scale [37] is the most widely used instrument in the field, we used the six categories of life satisfaction surveyed in the 2017 National Survey of Older Koreans. Third, the categories of social frailty were based on recent studies [9,16,17], not an established method. Therefore, future research on tool development to measure social frailty is needed. Lastly, social frailty can be affected by many environmental factors based on social context. Therefore, research is needed to identify the relationship between social frailty and life satisfaction in people of various ethnic groups.

5. Conclusions

Social frailty and its association with nutritional status, depression, cognitive function, and life satisfaction should be considered as an integrative comprehensive older adult care. Further studies are needed to develop of efficient social frailty intervention strategies to improve and enhance life satisfaction.

Author Contributions: Conceptualization, H.K. and S.J.; methodology, H.K. and S.J.; formal analysis, S.J.; writing—original draft preparation, H.K. and S.J.; writing—review and editing, H.K. and S.J.; supervision, H.K. All authors have read and agreed to the published version of the manuscript.

Funding: This work was supported by the Gachon University Research Fund of 2020 (GCU-2020-202002100001).

Institutional Review Board Statement: The study was approved by the Institutional Review Board (or Ethics Committee) of Gachon University (1044396-202006-HR-110-01 and 18 June 2020).

Informed Consent Statement: Not applicable.

Data Availability Statement: The authors have no authority over the data, and the data is provided upon request to the Ministry of Health and Welfare.

Acknowledgments: This study used the 2017 National Survey of Older Koreans sampling data from the Ministry of Health and Welfare.

Conflicts of Interest: The authors declare no conflict of interest.

References

1. Korea Institute for Health and Social Affairs, Survey of Korea Older Adults 2017. 30 November 2017. Available online: http://www.prism.go.kr/homepage/entire/retrieveEntireDetail.do?pageIndex=1&research_id=1351000-201700250&leftMenuLevel=160&cond_research_name=%EB%85%B8%EC%9D%B8%EC%8B%A4%ED%83%9C%EC%A1%B0%EC%82%AC&cond_research_start_date=&cond_research_end_date=&pageUnit=10&cond_order=3 (accessed on 1 May 2020).
2. Kim, S.; Lee, E.; Chung, S. Life satisfaction of older adults using hierarchical model analysis focused on individual and community factors. *J. Korea Gerontol Soc.* **2016**, *36*, 581–594.
3. Cesari, M.; Prince, M.; Thiyagarajan, J.A.; De Carvalho, I.A.; Bernabei, R.; Chan, P.; Gutierrez-Robledo, L.M.; Michel, J.-P.; Morley, J.E.; Ong, P.; et al. Frailty: An emerging public health priority. *J. Am. Med. Dir. Assoc.* **2016**, *17*, 188–192. [CrossRef]
4. Mannell, R.C.; Dupuis, S. Life Satisfaction; Birren, J.E., Ed.; Encyclopedia of Gerontology: San Diego, CA, USA, 1996; Volume 2.
5. Diener, E. Assessing participantive well-being: Progress and opportunities. *Soc. Indic. Res.* **1994**, *31*, 103–157. [CrossRef]
6. Moons, P.; Budts, W.; De Geest, S. Critique on the conceptualisation of quality of life: A review and evaluation of different conceptual approaches. *Int. J. Nurs. Stud.* **2006**, *43*, 891–901. [CrossRef] [PubMed]
7. World Health Organization. *World Report on Ageing and Health*; World Health Organization: Geneva, Switzerland, 2015.
8. World Health Organization. *The Global Network for Age-friendly Cities and Communities: Looking Back over the Last Decade, Looking Forward to the Next*; World Health Organization: Geneva, Switzerland, 2018.
9. Tsutsumimoto, K.; Doi, T.; Makizako, H.; Hotta, R.; Nakakubo, S.; Makino, K.; Suzuki, T.; Shimada, H. Association of social frailty with both cognitive and physical deficits among older people. *J. Am. Med. Dir. Assoc.* **2017**, *18*, 603–607. [CrossRef] [PubMed]
10. Pek, K.; Chew, J.; Lim, J.P.; Yew, S.; Tan, C.N.; Yeo, A.; Ding, Y.Y.; Lim, W.S. Social frailty is independently associated with mood, nutrition, physical performance, and physical activity: Insights from a theory-guided approach. *Int. J. Environ. Res. Public Health* **2020**, *17*, 4239. [CrossRef]
11. Bunt, S.; Steverink, N.; Olthof, J.; Van Der Schans, C.P.; Hobbelen, J.S.M. Social frailty in older adults: A scoping review. *Eur. J. Ageing* **2017**, *14*, 323–334. [CrossRef] [PubMed]
12. Makizako, H.; Shimada, H.; Doi, T.; Tsutsumimoto, K.; Hotta, R.; Nakakubo, S.; Makino, K.; Lee, S. Social frailty leads to the development of physical frailty among physically non-frail adults: A four-year follow-up longitudinal cohort study. *Int. J. Environ. Res. Public Health* **2018**, *15*, 490. [CrossRef] [PubMed]
13. Yamada, M.; Arai, H. Social frailty predicts incident disability and mortality among community-dwelling Japanese older adults. *J. Am. Med. Dir. Assoc.* **2018**, *19*, 1099–1103. [CrossRef] [PubMed]
14. Salem, B.E.; Brecht, M.-L.; Ekstrand, M.L.; Faucette, M.; Nyamathi, A. Correlates of physical, psychological, and social frailty among formerly incarcerated, homeless women. *Health Care Women Int.* **2019**, *40*, 788–812. [CrossRef] [PubMed]

15. Ministry of Health and Welfare and Korea Institute of Health and Social Affairs, 2017 National Survey of Older Koreans. 2018. Available online: https://meta.narastat.kr/metasvc/index.do?confmNo=117071 (accessed on 26 January 2020).
16. Tsutsumimoto, K.; Doi, T.; Makizako, H.; Hotta, R.; Nakakubo, S.; Kim, M.; Kurita, S.; Suzuki, T.; Shimada, H. Social frailty has a stronger impact on the onset of depressive symptoms than physical frailty or cognitive impairment: A 4-year follow-up longitudinal cohort study. *J. Am. Med. Dir. Assoc.* **2018**, *19*, 504–510. [CrossRef]
17. Yoo, M.; Kim, S.; Kim, B.; Yoo, J.; Lee, S.; Jang, H.; Cho, B.; Son, S.; Lee, J.; Park, Y.; et al. Moderate hearing loss is related with social frailty in a community-dwelling older adults: The Korean frailty and aging cohort study (KFACS). *Arch. Gerontol. Geriatr.* **2019**, *83*, 126–130. [CrossRef] [PubMed]
18. Posner, B.M.; Jette, A.M.; Smith, K.W.; Miller, D.R. Nutrition and health risks in the elderly: The Nutrition Screening Initiative. *Am. J. Public Health* **1993**, *83*, 972–978. [CrossRef] [PubMed]
19. Kee, B. A preliminary study for the standardization of geriatric depression scale short form-Korea version. *J. Korean Neurol. Assoc.* **1996**, *35*, 298–306.
20. Han, J.; Kim, T.; Jhoo, J.; Park, J.; Kim, J.; Ryu, S.; Moon, S.; Choo, I.; Lee, D.; Yoon, J.; et al. A Normative study of the Mini-Mental State Examination for dementia screening (MMSE-DS) and its short form (SMMSE-DS) in the Korean elderly. *J. Korean Geriatr. Psythiatry* **2010**, *14*, 27–37.
21. Kim, T.H.; Jhoo, J.H.; Park, J.H.; Kim, J.L.; Ryu, S.H.; Moon, S.W.; Choo, I.H.; Lee, D.W.; Yoon, J.C.; Do, Y.J.; et al. Korean version of mini mental status examination for dementia screening and its' short form. *Psychiatry Investig.* **2010**, *7*, 102–108. [CrossRef]
22. Hair, J.F.; Black, W.C.; Babin, B.J.; Anderson, R.E.; Tatham, R.L. *Multivariate Data Analysis*; Pearson Education, Inc.: Uppersaddle River, NJ, USA, 2006.
23. Cohen, J. *Statistical Power Analysis for the Behavioral Sciences*, 2nd ed.; Lawrence Erlbaum Publishers: Hillsdale, MI, USA, 1988; pp. 19–27.
24. Rea, L.M.; Parker, R.A. *Designing and Conducting Survey Research: A Comprehensive Guide*; Jossey-Bass Publishers: San Francisco, CA, USA, 1992.
25. Ma, L.; Sun, F.; Tang, Z. Social frailty is associated with physical functioning, cognition, and depression, and predicts mortality. *J. Nutr. Health Aging.* **2018**, *22*, 989–995. [CrossRef]
26. Makizako, H.; Shimada, H.; Tsutsumimoto, K.; Lee, S.; Doi, T.; Nakakubo, S.; Hotta, R.; Suzuki, T. Social frailty in community-dwelling older adults as a risk factor for disability. *J. Am. Med. Dir. Assoc.* **2015**, *16*, 1003.e7–1003.e11. [CrossRef]
27. Park, H.; Jang, Y., II; Lee, H.Y.; Jung, H.-W.; Lee, E.; Kim, D.H. Screening value of social frailty and its association with physical frailty and disability in community-dwelling older Koreans: Aging study of PyeongChang rural area. *Int. J. Environ. Res. Public Health* **2019**, *16*, 2809. [CrossRef]
28. Statistics Korea, Population projections for Korea 2019. 2019. Available online: https://kosis.kr/statHtml/statHtml.do?orgId=101&tblId=DT_1BPA003&vw_cd=MT_ETITLE&list_id=&scrId=&seqNo=&language=en&obj_var_id=&itm_id=&conn_path=A6&path=%252Feng%252F (accessed on 6 December 2019).
29. World Health Organization. *Integrated Care for Older People: Guidelines on Community-Level Interventions to Manage Declines in intrinsic Capacity*; World Health Organization: Geneva, Switzerland, 2017.
30. Teo, N.; Gao, Q.; Nyunt, M.S.; Wee, S.L.; Ng, T.P. Social frailty and functional disability: Findings from the Singapore Longitudinal Ageing Studies. *J. Am. Med. Dir. Assoc.* **2017**, *18*, 637.e13–637.e19. [CrossRef] [PubMed]
31. Strine, T.W.; Kroenke, K.; Dhingra, S.; Balluz, L.S.; Gonzalez, O.; Berry, J.T.; Mokdad, A.H. The associations between depression, health-related quality of life, social support, life satisfaction, and disability in community-dwelling US adults. *J. Nerv. Ment. Dis.* **2009**, *197*, 61–64. [CrossRef] [PubMed]
32. Gigantesco, A.; Fagnani, C.; Toccaceli, V.; Stazi, M.A.; Lucidi, F.; Violani, C.; Picardi, A. The Relationship Between Satisfaction with Life and Depression Symptoms by Gender. *Front. Psychiatry.* **2019**, *10*, 419. [CrossRef] [PubMed]
33. St John, P.D.; Montgomery, P.R. Cognitive impairment and life satisfaction in older adults. *Int. J. Geriatr. Psychiatry* **2010**, *25*, 814–821. [CrossRef] [PubMed]
34. Rissanen, T.; Viinamäki, H.; Honkalampi, K.; Lehto, S.M.; Hintikka, J.; Saharinen, T.; Koivumaa-Honkanen, H. Long term life dissatisfaction and subsequent major depressive disorder and poor mental health. *BMC Psychiatry* **2011**, *11*, 140. [CrossRef] [PubMed]
35. Steinman, M.A.; Perry, L.; Perissinotto, C.M. Meeting the care needs of older adults isolated at home during the COVID-19 pandemic. *JAMA Intern. Med.* **2020**, *180*, 819–820. [CrossRef]
36. Wilkinson, L.J.A. Statistical methods in psychology journals: Guidelines and explanations. *Am. Psychol.* **1999**, *54*, 594–604. [CrossRef]
37. Diener, E.; Emmons, R.A.; Larsen, R.J.; Griffin, S. The satisfaction with life scale. *J. Pers. Assess.* **1985**, *49*, 71–75. [CrossRef]

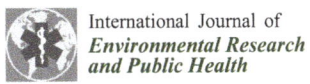

Article

Bibliometric Analysis on Research Trend of Accidental Falls in Older Adults by Using Citespace—Focused on Web of Science Core Collection (2010–2020)

Boyuan Chen [1,2] and Sohee Shin [2,*]

1   School of Physical Education (Main Campus), Zhengzhou University, Zhengzhou 450001, China; cby@haust.edu.cn
2   School of Sport and Exercise Science, University of Ulsan, 93 Daehak-ro, Nam-gu, Ulsan 44610, Korea
*   Correspondence: soheeshin@ulsan.ac.kr

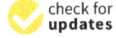

Citation: Chen, B.; Shin, S. Bibliometric Analysis on Research Trend of Accidental Falls in Older Adults by Using Citespace—Focused on Web of Science Core Collection (2010–2020). IJERPH 2021, 18, 1663. https://doi.org/10.3390/ijerph18041663

Academic Editors: Francisco José Tarazona Santabalbina, Sebastià Josep Santaeugènia Gonzàlez, José Augusto García Navarro and José Viña

Received: 23 December 2020
Accepted: 5 February 2021
Published: 9 February 2021

Publisher's Note: MDPI stays neutral with regard to jurisdictional claims in published maps and institutional affiliations.

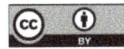

Copyright: © 2021 by the authors. Licensee MDPI, Basel, Switzerland. This article is an open access article distributed under the terms and conditions of the Creative Commons Attribution (CC BY) license (https:// creativecommons.org/licenses/by/ 4.0/).

Abstract: The present study aimed to identify the trends in research on accidental falls in older adults over the last decade. The MeSH (Medical Subject Headings) and entry terms were applied in the Web of Science Core Collection. Relevant studies in English within articles or reviews on falls in older adults were included from 2010 to 2020. Moreover, CiteSpace 5.6.R5 (64-bit) was adopted for analysis with scientific measurements and visualization. Cooper Cyrus, Stephen R Lord, Minoru Yamada, Catherine Sherrington, and others have critically impacted the study of falls in older adults. Osteoporosis, dementia, sarcopenia, hypertension, osteosarcopenia, traumatic brain injury, frailty, depression, and fear of falling would be significantly correlated with falls in older adults. Multiple types of exercise can provide effective improvements in executive cognitive performance, gait performance, quality of life, and can also lower the rates of falls and fall-related fractures. Fall detection, hospitalization, classification, symptom, gender, and cost are the current research focus and development direction in research on falls in older adults. The prevention of falls in older adults is one of the most important public health issues in today's aging society. Although lots of effects and research advancements had been taken, fall prevention still is uncharted territory for too many older adults. Service improvements can exploit the mentioned findings to formulate policies, and design and implement exercise programs for fall prevention.

Keywords: older adults; accidental falls; research hotspot; CiteSpace; knowledge domain visualization

1. Introduction

With aging, inactivity can lead to adverse and deep consequences, including health, economic, environmental, and social effects [1]. Many people are subject to multiple chronic diseases and drugs in their daily lives [2], which overall elevate the risk of falls for older adults. The annual incidence of falls for people aged over 65 is 30%–40%, and the incidence of falls for people aged over 80 is as high as 50% [3,4], which causes premature mortality, loss of independence, placement in assisted-living facilities, and death. A classification of fall risk factors has been proposed according to extrinsic and intrinsic factors. The extrinsic factors are related to surrounding space or environment-related, taking up to 30%–50% in most series [5], (e.g., tripping, slipping, walking on uneven surfaces, and inadequate illumination). The intrinsic or individual-related causes include advanced age, gait and balance impairment, concomitant chronic conditions (e.g., cardiovascular diseases, and sensory impairment), cognitive deficits, disorders of the central nervous system, severe osteoporosis with spontaneous fracture, and acute illness, drug side-effects, alcohol intake, anemia, hypothyroidism, unstable joints, and foot problems [6].

Falling always causes severe injuries, which is one of the costliest health conditions among older adults, imposing a heavy burden on the health care system [7]. An evidence-based fall prevention program can not only significantly reduce the incidence of fall-related injuries and medical costs but also improve the quality of life of older adults. As revealed from high-certainty evidence, exercise can prevent falls [8], which could reduce the rate of falls by 23% and down-regulate the number of people that experience one or more falls by 15% in community-dwelling older adults [9]. Furthermore, exercise-based interventions as a cost-effective treatment to prevent falls can benefit older adults substantially by improving their health, independence, and quality of life. Accordingly, regular screening for fall risk and care, and interventions, should be implemented in older adults.

Falls are usually multifactorial, effective prevention strategies are essential to reduce the public health burden on the increasing number of falls and fall-related mortality. Some countries recommend annual instability screening in people aged 65 or over, the geriatric specialists for coping with falls and other geriatric syndromes are increasingly demanded. To this end, it is necessary to conduct a comprehensive summary of the research about accidental falls in older adults over the last decade. An evidence-based fall prevention program can not only significantly reduce the incidence of fall-related injuries and medical costs, but also enhance the public's awareness, and improve the quality of life of older adults. Therefore, articles or reviews in English were downloaded from the Web of Science Core Collection from 2010 to 2020, and Citespace 5.6.R5 (64-bit) (Chaomei Chen, Philadelphia, PA, USA) was used for visualization and interpretation to identify the status and focus of studies regarding falls in older adults, presenting the development direction for following falls studies in older adults.

2. Method

2.1. Data Selected

The input data of this study was found using a combination of the research results from the multiple topic search queries into the Web of Science Core Collection. This study employed the MeSH and entry terms singularly or in combination (34,899, see Appendix A). First, we ensured that the data being used was from 2010 to 2020.

The second placed stress on older adults and falls. One of the topic terms included "accidental fall*", fall*, "fall*, accidental", "fall and slip", "slip and fall". This query produced 171,659 records as Set #6. Besides, another topic term consists of aged, elderly, this query led to 1,705,687 records as Set #9. At last, we combined Set #6 and Set #9 together and got the final dataset, Set #10, containing 34,899 records.

Similar queries #1–#10 were employed here to retrieve bibliographic records on the common data sources for science mapping, including PubMed (14,025, see Appendix B), Embase (15,588, see Appendix C), Scopus (33,624, see Appendix D). Books, documents, and research grants, or other types of data sources may be required to be considered. However, this review is only limited to the records of types of articles or reviews in English in the Web of Science Core Collection.

All bibliographic information was downloaded and saved as plain text files for subsequent data processing and analysis. Subsequently, the data were imported into the Citespace and the duplicate data were deleted to prepare for the next step of visualization.

2.2. Data Analysis Method

Citespace refers to an information visualization tool extensively applied in the field of knowledge graphs [10]. Visualization tools were adopted to display and analyze the knowledge context of a certain domain, and the development process and structural relationship in this domain were suggested. Therefore, this review adopted CiteSpace 5.6.R5 (64-bit) to achieve visualization to gain insights into this field of accidental falls in older adults and discover the research frontier and knowledge base of the field in considerable data.

Notably, when the clustering function was started, the Modularity Q and the Mean Silhouette scores critically impacted visualization, representing an overall structural characteristic of the network. Overall, $Q > 0.3$ displayed an overall significant structure. If $S > 0.5$ or higher, the cluster was usually considered to be reasonable [11].

3. Result
3.1. Analysis Results and Visualization
3.1.1. Basic Statistical Analysis

The number of papers published regarding falls in older adults was elevated from 2127 in 2010 to 4244 in 2020 (Figure 1). It is suggested that falls in older adults are attracting rising attention from researchers.

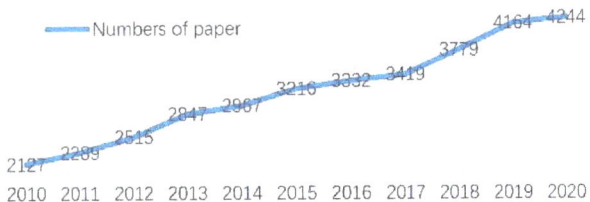

Figure 1. Papers regarding accidental falls in older adults (2010–2020).

3.1.2. Distribution of Journal Papers

Table 1 lists the top 10 journals that published the largest number of papers regarding falls in older adults from 2010 to 2020. PLoS One published about 609 papers, ranking the first. Overall, the specific subject scope comprises Geriatrics Gerontology, Medical General Internal, Public Environmental Occupational Health, Gerontology, Rehabilitation, Orthopedics, Clinical Neurology, Surgery, Neurosciences, Sport Sciences, and so on. In the listed top 10 journals, the highest impact factor is Age and Ageing, nearly 4.902.

Table 1. Top 10 journal published analysis (2010–2020).

No.	Journal Title	IF	Amount	Country	Research Area
1	PLoS One	2.740	609	USA	Science & Technology-Other Topics (Q2)
2	Gait & Posture	2.349	425	Ireland	Neuroscience & Neurology (Q3) Orthopedics (Q2) Sport Sciences (Q2)
3	BMC Geriatrics	3.077	366	England	Geriatrics & Gerontology (Q2)
4	Journal of the American Geriatrics Society	4.180	321	USA	Geriatrics & Gerontology (Q1)
5	Archives of Gerontology and Geriatrics	2.128	272	Ireland	Geriatrics & Gerontology (Q3)
6	Osteoporosis International	3.864	271	England	Endocrinology & Metabolism (Q2)
7	Aging Clinical and Experimental Research	2.697	264	Italy	Geriatrics & Gerontology (Q3)
8	BMJ Open	2.496	219	England	General & Internal Medicine (Q2)
9	Journal of the American Medical Directors Association	4.367	197	USA	Geriatrics & Gerontology (Q1)
10	Age and Ageing	4.902	196	England	Geriatrics & Gerontology (Q1)

3.1.3. Co-Institution Analysis

We ran CiteSpace, generating a network as usual: 2010–2020, Slice length: 1 year; Node Select the node type: Institution, Top N = 20, choice Pathfinder and Pruning the merged network. Other parameters were the default settings. Also, the Co-institutions knowledge mapping was generated, in which N = 60, E = 67 (density was 0.0379).

Figure 2 indicates that the main research strengths were in universities. The University of Sydney has published the most papers and has conducted strong scientific research in the study on falls in older adults. Furthermore, the greatest number of bursts in the study was Harvard Medical School, reaching 59.04. The University of Oxford was the institution with the strongest centrality, reaching 8. The highest-ranked by Sigma was the University of Pittsburgh.

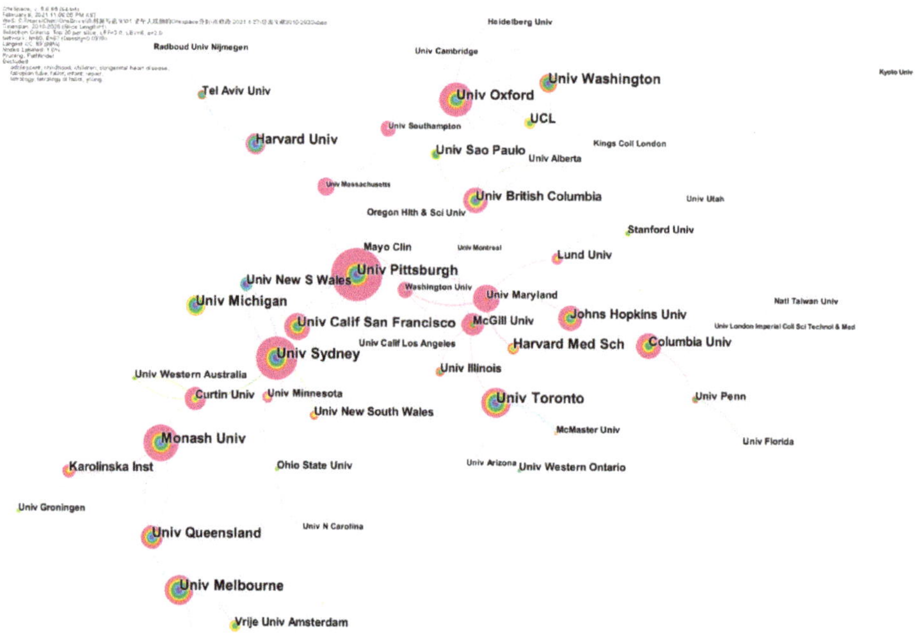

Figure 2. Co-institutions' network (2010–2020). The color of the circle represents when the article was published. The larger the node diameter, the more papers institutions have published. The thicker the line between the nodes, the closer the two institutions work together.

3.1.4. Co-Author Analysis

By analyzing the author, the cooperative relationship with others could be investigated. We ran CiteSpace, generating a network as usual: 2010–2020, Slice length: 1 year; Node Select the node type: Author, Top N = 20, and choice Pathfinder and Pruning the merged network, other parameter settings were likely to institutions. This study found knowledge mapping of the co-author with N = 186, E = 186 (a density of 0.0108) (Figure 3).

Table 2 shows that Stephen R. Lord ranked first in the number of citations, with 175 citations. The most obvious Burst referred to the Minoru Yamada, reaching 12.13. The strongest centripetal force was Cooper Cyrus, displaying a centripetal force of 8. The highest Sigma (Σ) was Catherine Sherrington, and the Sigma was 0.32.

Table 2. Author rank in different conditions.

No.	Co-Authorship Papers	Burst	Centrality	Sigma
1	Stephen R Lord	Minoru Yamada	Cooper Cyrus	Catherine Sherrington
2	Kim Delbaere	Koutatsu Nagai	Mirjam Pijnappels	Clemens Becker
3	Catherine Sherrington	Kazuki Uemura	Teresa Liu-Ambrose	Jacqueline C T Close
4	Keith D Hill	Anne-Marie Hill	Keith D Hill	Jorunn L Helbostad
5	Jacqueline CT Close	Noriaki Ichihashi	Jeffrey M Hausdorff	Lindy Clemson

Centrality represents the degree of nodes that are part of the path that connects any pair of nodes in the network. Burst refers to the specific time during which a sudden change in frequency occurs. Sigma measures a combination of structural and temporal characteristics of nodes.

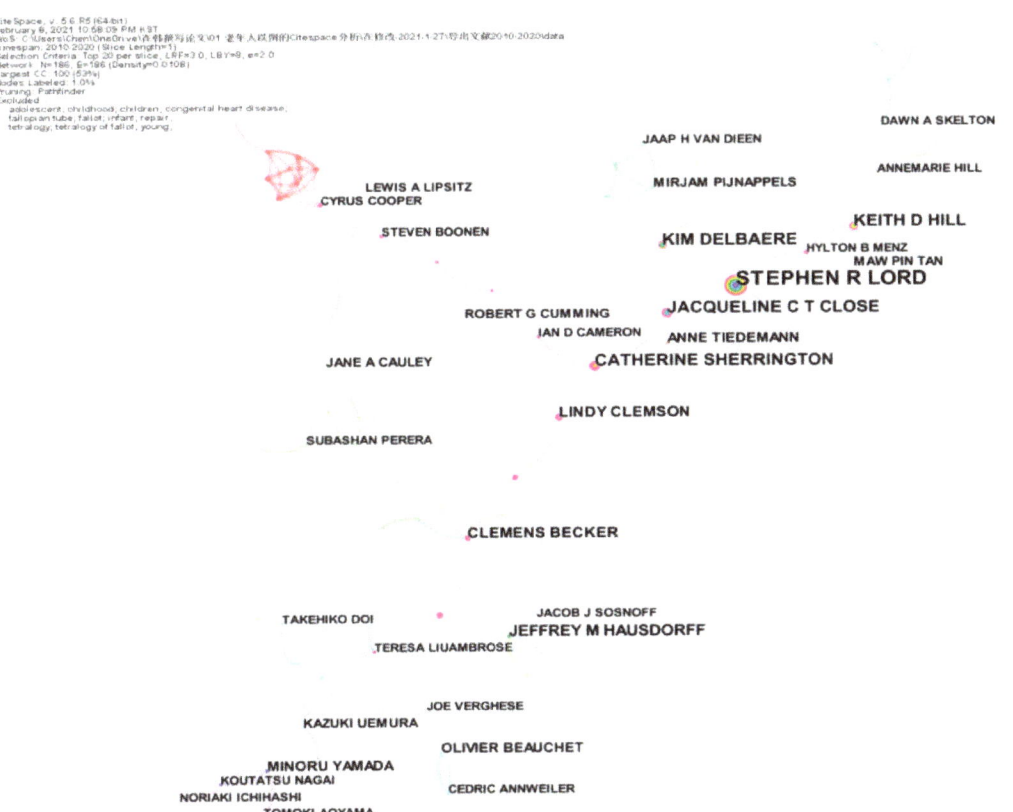

Figure 3. Co-authorship network (2010–2020). The color of the line represents the time the co-authors worked together. The larger the node diameter, the more papers the author has collaborated to publish. The thicker the line between the nodes, the closer the cooperation between the two authors.

The Web of Science was used (Table 3), and Cooper Cyrus's H-index was 144. Professor Cyrus leads an internationally competitive program of research into the epidemiology of musculoskeletal disorders, most notably osteoporosis. Stephen R Lord has published over 600 papers in the areas of balance, gait, falls in older people, and is acknowledged as a leading international researcher in his field. His research primarily focuses on two themes: the identification of physiological risk factors for falls and the development and evaluation of fall prevention strategies. Minoru Yamada's H-index was 28; cited 2501 times. Also, his research follows three main themes: the epidemiological study on sarcopenia and frailty; the effect of a care prevention program on healthy life expectancy; and the effect of physical activity on health outcomes in older adults. Catherine Sherrington's H-index reached 52; cited 11,623 times. Currently, she is leading the Physical Activity, Ageing, and Disability Research Stream within the Institute, and is focused on health, aging falls, and rehabilitation.

Table 3. Researchers' academic information.

Researcher	H-Index	Sum of Cited	Research Areas
Cooper Cyrus	144	106,019	Osteoporosis & Osteoarthritis & Epidemiology
Stephen R Lord	93	91,427	Falls in Older People
Jeffrey M Hausdorff	76	28,247	Gait & Neurodynamic
Catherine Sherrington	52	11,620	Health & Exercise & falls & Ageing & Rehabilitation
Keith D Hill	44	6778	Falls prevention & Exercise & Rehabilitation
Teresa Liu-Ambrose	41	5789	Fall prevention & Healthy aging
Jacqueline C T Close	40	6746	Gait & Gerontology & Geriatric Assessment
Kim Delbaere	38	4792	Ageing & Accidental falls & Fear of falling & Cognitive function
Clemens Becker	36	4654	Falls & Exercise & Rehabilitation
Jorunn L Helbostad	31	3476	Movement disorders and falls at old age
Minoru Yamada	28	2501	Gerontology & Rehabilitation
Mirjam Pijnappels	28	2787	The effects of aging on neuromuscular and cognitive aspects of mobility
Noriaki Ichihashi	26	2192	Rehabilitation & Physical therapy
Lindy Clemson	25	2972	Ageing & Occupational Therapy
Kazuki Uemura	23	1802	Rehabilitation & Welfare engineering
Koutatsu Nagai	17	816	Gerontology & Physical Therapy
Anne-Marie Hill	16	1043	Falls prevention & Patient education

3.2. Keyword Cluster Analysis

3.2.1. Keyword Analysis

Keyword frequency analysis helps clarify the research trends on falls in older adults. Risk, balance, mortality, and prevalence were relatively high with frequencies of more than 2000 times, and prevention, gait, injury, women, exercise, hip fracture, community, quality of life, exercise, fracture, care, and management were relatively high with frequencies over 1000 times.

3.2.2. Keyword Cluster Analysis

We ran CiteSpace, generating a network as usual: 2010–2020, Slice length: 1 year; Node Select the node type: Keyword; Top N = 100 and choice Pathfinder and Pruning the merged network. Given the co-occurrence of keywords, the nodes were revised, and the Log-likelihood (LLR) algorithm was adopted for clustering calculation. The visualization map obtained N = 147, E = 150 (density = 0.014), the Modularity Q score was 0.8423, the Mean Silhouette score was 0.6805, as presented in Figure 4.

There was a total of 20 clusters, mainly including 14 clusters, as listed in Table 4. Research topics regarding falls in older adults can be separated into two main topics. The first topic is risk factors that may cause accidental falls (e.g., #1 osteoporosis, #10 dementia, #13 fear of falling). The other one refers to intervention to prevent falls (e.g., #11 exercise, #12 vitamin D).

3.2.3. Research Hot Spots and Path Analysis

A timeline visualization depicts clusters along a horizontal timeline. The main 14 clusters are presented in Figure 5. Each one can indicate the evolution of research in the field on falls in older adults from 2010 to 2020.

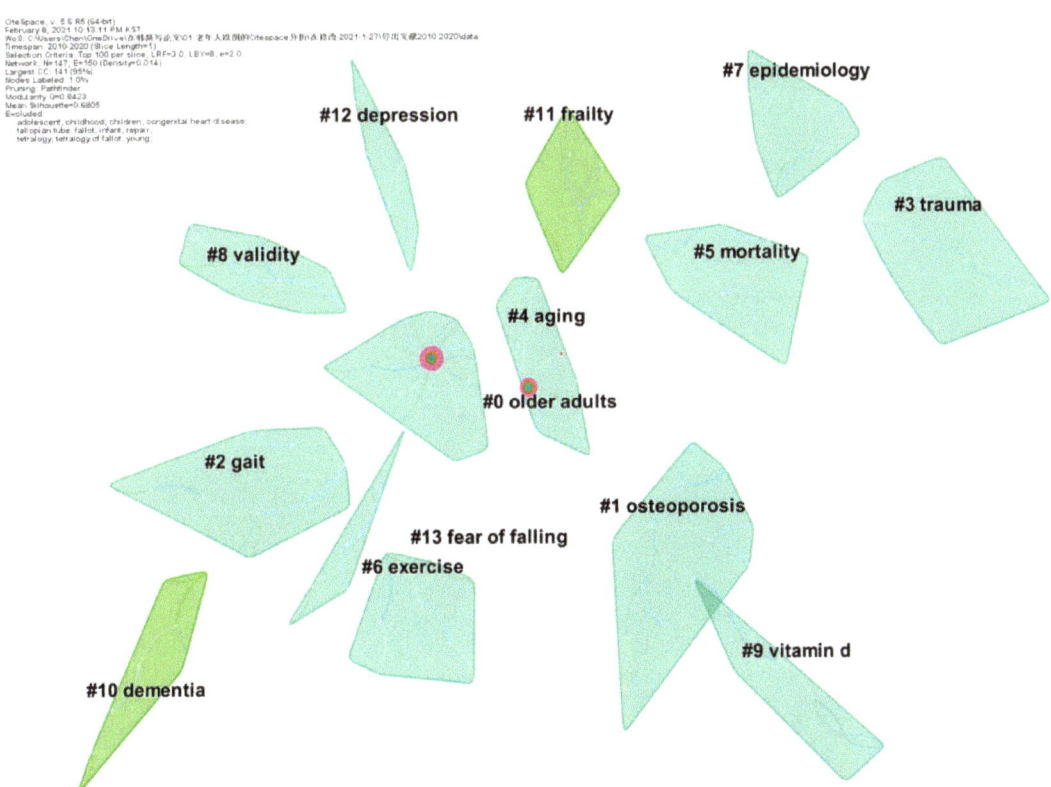

Figure 4. A landscape view of keyword cluster analysis generated by Top N = 100 per slice from 2010 to 2020. (LRF = 3, LBY = 8, and e = 2.0).

Table 4. Subjects of cluster analysis (2010–2020).

Clusters	Silhouette	Size	Log-Likelihood (LLR)
#0 older adults	15	1	Risk factor, mobility, pain, prevention, quality of life
#1 osteoporosis	14	0.968	Fall detection, bone mineral density, classification, machine learning, fracture, wearable sensors
#2 gait	13	0.985	Balance, walking, postural control, variability, parkinsons disease, gait analysis
#3 trauma	12	0.966	Injury, impact, emergency department, frailty, suicide
#4 aging	11	1	Hip fracture, falls, vitamin d supplementation, prescription, Romberg test
#5 mortality	11	1	Blood pressure, survival, surgery, hypertension, morbidity, disease
#6 exercise	10	0.971	Physical activity, health, intervention, randomized controlled trial, fitness, social participation
#7 epidemiology	9	0.956	Traumatic brain injury, management, trend, diagnosis, rehabilitation
#8 validity	9	0.967	Reliability, women health, knee pain, lower extremity, inertial sensors, practice guidelines
#9 vitamin d	8	1	Sarcopenia, fractures, physical performance, obesity, muscle strength, osteosarcopenia,
#10 dementia	8	0.966	Cognitive impairment, polypharmacy, motoric cognitive risk syndrome, attention, long-term care
#11 frailty	8	0.952	Care, quality, patient, comprehensive geriatric assessment, disability,
#12 depression	7	0.96	Prevalence, population, mental health, sleep quality, behavior, anxiety,
#13 fear of falling	6	0.918	Efficacy, safety, exercise, nurses, fear, physical activity monitoring

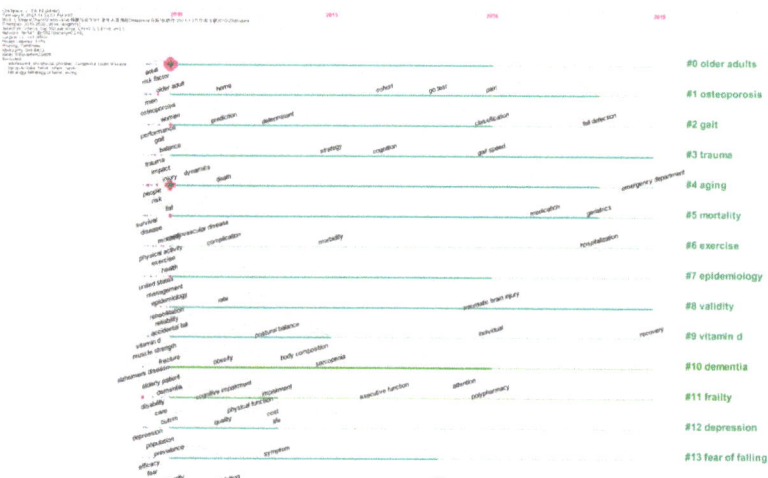

Figure 5. A timeline of the 14 largest clusters in accidental falls in older adults (2010–2020).

3.2.4. Keywords Citation Bursts Analysis

Citation burst refers to keywords appearing suddenly in a short period or which usage frequency increases sharply. Overall, it reveals the evolution of the research topic in different periods, as listed in Table 5.

Table 5. 38 Keywords with the strongest citation bursts (2010–2020).

Keywords	Year	Strength	Begin	End	2010–2020
vitamin d	2010	25.7615	2010	2013	
infection	2010	34.6606	2010	2012	
double blind	2010	22.0649	2010	2011	
growth	2010	4.5875	2010	2012	
history	2010	36.0171	2010	2013	
community	2010	10.2497	2010	2011	
guideline	2010	30.1278	2010	2013	
hypertension	2010	28.7127	2010	2015	
randomized controlled trial	2010	16.4364	2010	2011	
older people	2010	55.1187	2010	2014	
postmenopausal women	2010	16.4984	2010	2012	
bone mineral density	2010	2.6016	2010	2011	
older women	2010	31.0928	2010	2013	
dynamics	2010	26.5791	2011	2012	
home	2010	48.2979	2011	2014	
follow up	2010	16.818	2012	2017	
controlled trial	2010	23.878	2012	2013	
postural balance	2010	15.4265	2012	2017	
rate	2010	25.3309	2013	2014	
body composition	2010	32.8776	2013	2014	
prediction	2010	2.6749	2013	2014	
fall prevention	2010	25.6649	2013	2014	
consequence	2010	27.3192	2014	2015	
cohort	2010	43.2065	2014	2018	
safety	2010	28.2582	2015	2016	
attention	2010	33.7397	2016	2017	
experience	2010	13.7373	2016	2018	
pain	2010	28.5537	2016	2018	
individual	2010	33.4865	2016	2020	
trial	2010	9.7152	2016	2017	
symptom	2010	32.2689	2016	2020	
gait speed	2010	23.6379	2016	2017	
life	2010	16.1569	2017	2018	
classification	2010	37.0551	2018	2020	
fall detection	2010	48.4538	2018	2020	
cost	2010	16.6557	2018	2020	
hospitalization	2010	37.8174	2018	2020	
gender	2010	27.1045	2018	2020	

▬: shows which period the citation burst is the strongest. For instance, the postural balance has the longest period of burst from 2012 to 2017.

4. Discussion

4.1. Main Research Scholars' Views

Age-related anatomic and functional changes in perception, neuromuscular function, and cognitive systems impair the control of balance and gait. Targeted training can improve muscle strength, balance, gait, mobility, while preventing falls in older adults [12], so fall prevention programs should be tailored to older adults' level of physical well-being [13].

Postmenopausal women aged over 50 are at an increased risk of developing sarcopenia and osteoporosis. Accordingly, healthy lifestyle measures in women aged over 50 are essential for healthy aging [14]. Besides, the combination of optimal protein intake and exercise leads to a greater degree of benefit than either intervention alone.

Osteosarcopenia refers to a novel syndrome that often commonly appears in a frail subset of older adults. Combined with pharmacological, nutritional, and exercise-based interventions, it should enable a more comprehensive approach to mitigate osteosarcopenia in the future [15].

Exercise and fall prevention interventions should combine with special cultures and positively exploit the support from society, physicians, and families [16]. Health care professionals should routinely discuss fall prevention with older adults, provide evidence-based advice during consultations, and follow up with referrals [17]. In addition, dual-task training, cognitive-motor training, reactive step training, and multicomponent exercise programs can effectively improve executive cognitive, gait performance, and quality of life [18], as well as lower the rates of falls and fall-related fractures [19,20]. An environmental intervention perspective combined with adequate follow-up can successfully reduce community-dwelling older adults' falls [21].

4.2. Main Clusters Analysis

#1 Osteoporosis. Osteoporosis is a silent disease until a fracture occurs, which has widely developed as a worldwide health problem for men and women aged over 50. Lumbar muscle strength and the presence of osteoporosis are endogenous factors of the risk of falls [22]. Compared with women without osteoporosis, women with postmenopausal osteoporosis had a history of one or more falls in the past year and were at a higher risk of recurrent falls so that at-risk populations should be identified through early diagnosis and treatment [22]. Balance training may significantly reduce the frequency of falls in osteoporosis patients [23]. Activities aimed at developing muscle strength, body balance, and improving intrinsic receptive sensation should be encouraged [24]. The potential consequences of severe osteoporosis can be mitigated by pharmacological therapies and the proper selection of modalities [25].

#2 Gait and #13 Fear of falling. These are common with advancing age. Decreased attention while walking is a significant risk factor for falls among community-dwelling older adults. Impairments in balance and gait are critical to older adults because they jeopardize the independence and contribute to the risk of falls and injuries [26]. A cut-off gait speed of 1.0 m/s can be a useful tool to identify individuals who are high-risk individuals and evaluate preventive interventions [27]. The number of medications was associated with a decrease in gait performance. Each additional medication up-regulates the risk of gait decline by 12% to 16% [28]. A history of falls in the previous year was a good predictor of the fear of falling, and fear of falling is an independent risk factor for falls in older adults. Falls Efficacy Scale-International (FES-I) and Tinetti's Falls Efficacy Scale are reliable and valid to measure the fear of falling [29,30]. Whether exercise interventions reduce the fear of falling beyond the end of the intervention has been insufficiently evidenced [31].

#3 Trauma and #5 Mortality. Research on traumatic brain injury (TBI) has increased over the past two decades [32]. TBI is the main cause of emergency department visits in older adults, which is a significant part of the overall injury burden [33]. The major consequences of TBI are hip fractures and intracranial injury, which account for 46% of fatal falls in older adults [34]. Moreover, TBI arising from closed head trauma (CHT) significantly increases the risk of developing Alzheimer's disease (AD), Parkinson's disease

(PD), and chronic traumatic encephalopathy (CTE) [35], and these would increase the risk of fall-related injuries in older adults. The incidence of TBI may continue to increase over time. Trauma patients with these risk factors may require higher professional health care levels and should be enrolled in a formally fall prevention program [36]. Moreover, trauma in older adults should be addressed from a public health vision with improved social service quality and prevention. Falls are a significant cause of mortality in older adults [37]. Unintentional falls continued to be a major cause of death (29%) in China [38]. The trend in mortality from falls was similarly observed increasing among US and European data [39–42]. The fall-related mortality in Japanese older adults aged 65–74 years showed a more rapid and continuous decreasing trend, but men over 75 years did not decrease [43].

#4 Aging and #11 Frailty. With the increasing older adult population, frailty is an important health care topic for people with geriatric syndromes. The effect of satisfaction with aging as a potential protective mechanism against fall results in reducing the risk for falls [44]. Frailty and pre-frailness are significantly associated with a higher risk of fracture, disability, and falls [45]. The future fall risk attributed to frailty was suggested to be higher in men than in women [46]. Accordingly, older adults should be evaluated for the possibility of geriatric syndromes to lower the risk of falls, fractures, or death.

#6 Exercise and #9 Vitamin D. Exercise programs reduce the rate of falls. An exercise program primarily involves balance and functional training [9], while a program includes multiple types of exercise (usually balance and functional exercises and resistance exercises) [47]; Otago exercise program, high-intensity interval training (HIIT), or virtual reality (VR) will have more significantly reduced the fall rate [48–50]. The interaction of exercise and various nutrients, especially protein and some multi-nutritional supplements, influenced muscle and bone health in older adults. Low levels of vitamin D have been associated with increased fall rates. However, no consistent conclusion has been reached for the relationship between vitamin D deficiency and these broader health outcomes [51], including daily oral doses of vitamin D [52–54]. Subsequent research should be conducted to determine the role of vitamin D in the relationship with falls in older adults.

One point that needs to be emphasized is that most countries have taken active interventions to prevent falls in older adults, significantly reducing the rate of falls in older adults. However, our society still lacks awareness of sarcopenia (Table 4 #9). The underlying mechanism of sarcopenia remains unclear, and no widely accepted definitions are suitable for use in research and clinical settings, and methodological challenges and debates are ongoing [55]. Sarcopenia has been associated with aging and older adults, but the development of sarcopenia now can also possibly occur earlier in life [56], so this study attempted to give a brief introduction to sarcopenia.

In 1989, Irwin Rosenberg proposed the theory of sarcopenia. In 2016, the ICD-10-MC Diagnosis Code officially identified sarcopenia as a muscle disease [57]. In 2010, the European Working Group on Sarcopenia in Older People (EWGSOP) developed practical clinical definitions and consensus diagnostic criteria [56] and updated the definition of myasthenia gravis by exploiting the last decade's research and accumulated clinical evidence in 2018 [58]. The Asian Sarcopenia Working Group (AWGS) defined the diagnostic sarcopenia criteria by referencing Asian data in 2014 [59], while diagnostic procedures, protocols, and some metrics were revised in 2019 [60]. Both the Foundation for the National Institutes of Health (FNIH) and the International Working Group on Sarcopenia (IWGS) also have their definitions of sarcopenia. Thus, research based on different definitions may be misleading and difficult to interpret, such as cutoff point, diagnostic procedures, and so on.

Here, the definition of sarcopenia by the EWGSOP 2 is taken as an example. Sarcopenia is a progressive and generalized skeletal muscle disorder that is associated with an increased likelihood of adverse outcomes including falls, fractures, physical disability, and mortality [58]. Nutritional, inactivity, disease, iatrogenic may be the most frequent underlying causes of sarcopenia [61]. Specifically, sarcopenia is probable when low muscle strength is detected. A sarcopenia diagnosis is confirmed by the presence of low muscle quantity or quality. When low muscle strength, low muscle quantity/quality, and low physical performance are all detected, sarcopenia is considered severe. Subsequently, studies found that, when untreated, sarcopenia can bring a high personal, social, and economic burden [62]. For human health, sarcopenia can elevate the risk of falls and fractures [63], impairing the ability to perform activities of daily living [64], as well as raising the risk of hospitalization.

Lifestyle interventions, especially exercise and nutritional supplementation, prevail as mainstays of treatment. Subsequent research is required to investigate the potential long-term benefits of lifestyle interventions, nutritional supplements, or pharmacotherapy for sarcopenia. Moreover, several questions should be studied in-depth, including how to identify the high risk of sarcopenia early, what makes sarcopenia worse, which muscle indicators can be the most effective predictors of adverse outcomes, how we can optimally assess the muscle mass, how to determine effective critical value, which measurement tools are the most accurate, what interventions are available for sarcopenia, as well as which intervention should be the first choice.

#7 Epidemiology and #8 Validity. The incidence of falls and related complications increases with age. Furthermore, the epidemiology of falls in the incidence for women was higher than men. The rate of falls in community-dwelling adults is lower than in long-term care institutions. Most community-dwelling falls lead to about 5% fracture or hospitalization, and those in long-term institutions tend to more serious, with 10–25% of such falls resulting in fracture or laceration. Wrist fractures are common between the ages of 65 and 75, while hip fractures predominate after age 75 [5]. Wrist fractures usually result from falls forward or backward on an outstretched hand and hip fractures typically from falls to the side [65]. A lot of fall assessment tools have been developed and designed for different purposes over recent decades, most of them are targeted at assessing geriatric patients and have been available on reliability and validity [66]. But patient fall risk scales more focus on specific intrinsic and extrinsic factors, it could not fully assess a patient's current fall risk status, which needs more patient-centered assessments and interventions [67].

#10 Dementia and #12 Depression. People with various levels of cognitive impairment can benefit from supervised multimodal exercise to improve physical function [68]. With the incidence of dementia growing globally, people with dementia are at a higher risk of falls and fall-related injuries, while there is still an argument about the exercise intervention for dementia patients [69]. There is little evidence about the effect of specific types of exercise on dementia risk [70]. More high-quality intervention studies should be conducted to inform evidence-practice initiatives. Depression is associated with the incidence of dementia, with a variety of possibly psychological or physiological mechanisms. Depression and falls are common and co-exist. Geriatric depression score (GDs) was used as a significant predictor of older adults from falls. Depression treatment should be incorporated in fall prevention programs for older adults at a high risk of increasing/multiple falls. Based on the existing state of knowledge, exercise (especially tai chi) and cognitive behavioral therapy should be considered to treat mild depression in older fallers [71].

4.3. Keywords Citation Bursts

According to Table 5, hypertension and postmenopausal women have attracted widespread attention at first. In postmenopausal women, due to insufficient estrogen, osteoporosis affects bone formation and increases the risk of falls. Women have caught the attention of scholars, and studies had proved that exercise training for postmenopausal women is an effective approach to improve fall or fracture [72]. The studies conducted between 2010–2015 on links between hypertension and falls are also of high significance. It is known that the increased risk of falls due to hypertension is related to the use of antihypertensive drugs, vascular sclerosis, and poor gait performance. Accordingly, nursing and intervention guidance should be strengthened to prevent patients with hypertension falls. With studies conducted in-depth, bone mineral density, postural balance, and body composition became research hotspots, and then gradually turned to fall prevention and prediction. Note that fall detection, classification, hospitalization, cost, and gender are receiving more attention.

A fall detection system by exploiting the Internet of Things can reduce the serious consequences of falls [73], which has made important progress in novel sensors, technologies, and algorithms [74]. However, there are two main challenges facing fall detection systems. One is to identify when a serious fall takes place, the other one refers to the lack of real data on falls to improve the research. Furthermore, how to apply laboratory data to real life, how to protect user privacy, and how to shift from detecting falls to predicting falls are recognized as the novel directions of development [75]. The classification of falls and the incidence of falls in different settings, socio-demographic determinants, international trends, and the measurement of fall outcomes, including the costs of falls and fall-related injuries, are the hot topics [76]. Costs generated by falls are expected to increase with the rapid expansion of the aging population. These costs fall into two parts. One is direct costs including health care costs (e.g., medications), while the other is treatment and consultations for rehabilitation, i.e., losses in societal productivity of activities for individuals and caregivers [77]. Occupational therapy had the effectiveness and cost-effectiveness in improving functional ability and decrease hospital readmission for older adults [78]. Risk factors for falls vary with gender [79]. Gender should be considered in the design of fall prevention strategies [80].

5. Conclusions

First, studies on falls in older adults have been increasingly conducted in the 21st century; the number of papers published every year is increasing. The mentioned findings suggest that when setting the selection criteria for Top N = 20, Cooper Cyrus, Stephen R Lord, Minoru Yamada, and Catherine Sherrington play an important role in the study of falls in older adults. The University of Sydney (Australia) has published the largest number of papers on falls in older adults, and the most obvious burst in the present study is Harvard Medical School (USA). The University of Oxford (USA) was the most central institution. The highest Sigma ($\sum$) is The University of Pittsburgh (USA).

Second, Geriatrics Gerontology, Medical General Internal, Clinical Neurology, Clinical Neurology, Neurosciences, Orthopedics, Rehabilitation, Surgery, Sport Sciences, Public Environmental Occupational Health and Gerontology are considered the main research scopes involved in falls. The journals PloS One, Gait & Posture, and BMC Geriatrics were the top 3 journals regarding accidental falls in older adults.

Third, osteoporosis, dementia, sarcopenia, hypertension, traumatic brain injury, frailty, depression, fear of falling would be significantly correlated with falls in older adults. Nowadays, fall detection, hospitalization, classification, gender, and cost are the focus and direction of the development of falls in older adults.

Fourth, age-related changes in perception, neuromuscular, and cognitive systems interfere with the control of balance and gait. Fall prevention programs should be tailored to the older adult's level of physical well-being. Targeted training can improve muscle strength, balance, gait, and mobility while preventing falls in older adults. A program consisting of multiple types of exercise, HIIT, or VR may more significantly reduce the fall rate of older adults than a single exercise intervention.

Falling is a serious issue concerned with the health of older adults, which affects the physical and mental health and quality of life for themselves and their families. Only one-third of all older adults who fell have sought medical assistance; one possible reason is the lack of public awareness about the importance of fall prevention [81]. This study introduces the last decade of research results on fall-related factors from different aspects such as physiology, pathology, psychology, environment, and sports science expounds on the latest developments in this aspect of research and relevant experts' opinions are summarized, enabling more people to gain comprehensive insights into falls of older adults to prevent or reduce older adults from fall-related injuries. Moreover, a good peer view is presented for the study using scientific methods to find good methods to prevent, treat or reduce the risk of falls. There are some limitations to the study. For instance, the selected papers were only included in the Web of Science Core Collection, and searches are not selected in PubMed, Scopus, or other databases. Besides, the literature contains papers in English only; the status of research on falls in older adults in other language nations is not possible to determine. Lastly, CiteSpace analysis is biased towards quantitative analysis. In subsequent studies, the qualitative research method of the interview method should be adopted to remedy the defects of quantitative research. Though further research is needed, this preliminary result may give a new horizon for fall prevention.

Author Contributions: Conceptualization, B.C. and S.S.; methodology, B.C.; software, S.S.; validation, S.S.; investigation, S.S.; writing—original draft preparation, B.C.; writing—review and editing, S.S.; visualization, B.C.; supervision, S.S.; project administration, S.S. All authors have read and agreed to the published version of the manuscript.

Funding: This work was supported by the 2020 Research Fund of University of Ulsan.

Institutional Review Board Statement: Not applicable.

Informed Consent Statement: Not applicable.

Data Availability Statement: Not applicable.

Conflicts of Interest: The authors declare no conflict of interest.

Appendix A. Web of Science Core Collection

Table A1. Search history from Web of Science Core Collection.

Set	Results	
#10	34,899	#9 AND #6
		Indexes=SCI-EXPANDED, SSCI, A&HCI, CPCI-S, CPCI-SSH, BKCI-S, BKCI-SSH, ESCI, CCR-EXPANDED, IC Timespan=2010-2020
#9	1,834,798	#18 OR #17
		Indexes=SCI-EXPANDED, SSCI, A&HCI, CPCI-S, CPCI-SSH, BKCI-S, BKCI-SSH, ESCI, CCR-EXPANDED, IC Timespan=2010-2020
#8	134,166	TOPIC: (Elderly) AND DOCUMENT TYPES: (Article OR Review) AND LANGUAGE: (English)
		Indexes=SCI-EXPANDED, SSCI, A&HCI, CPCI-S, CPCI-SSH, BKCI-S, BKCI-SSH, ESCI, CCR-EXPANDED, IC Timespan=2010-2020
#7	1,784,189	TOPIC: (Aged) AND DOCUMENT TYPES: (Article OR Review) AND LANGUAGE: (English)
		Indexes=SCI-EXPANDED, SSCI, A&HCI, CPCI-S, CPCI-SSH, BKCI-S, BKCI-SSH, ESCI, CCR-EXPANDED, IC Timespan=2010-2020
#6	181,751	#5 OR #4 OR #3 OR #2 OR #1
		Indexes=SCI-EXPANDED, SSCI, A&HCI, CPCI-S, CPCI-SSH, BKCI-S, BKCI-SSH, ESCI, CCR-EXPANDED, IC Timespan=2010-2020
#5	73	TOPIC: ("Slip and Fall") AND DOCUMENT TYPES: (Article OR Review) AND LANGUAGE: (English)
		Indexes=SCI-EXPANDED, SSCI, A&HCI, CPCI-S, CPCI-SSH, BKCI-S, BKCI-SSH, ESCI, CCR-EXPANDED, IC Timespan=2010-2020
#4	3	TOPIC: ("Fall and Slip") AND DOCUMENT TYPES: (Article OR Review) AND LANGUAGE: (English)
		Indexes=SCI-EXPANDED, SSCI, A&HCI, CPCI-S, CPCI-SSH, BKCI-S, BKCI-SSH, ESCI, CCR-EXPANDED, IC Timespan=2010-2020
#3	16	TOPIC: ("Fall*, Accidental") AND DOCUMENT TYPES: (Article OR Review) AND LANGUAGE: (English)
		Indexes=SCI-EXPANDED, SSCI, A&HCI, CPCI-S, CPCI-SSH, BKCI-S, BKCI-SSH, ESCI, CCR-EXPANDED, IC Timespan=2010-2020
#2	181,751	TOPIC: (Fall*) AND DOCUMENT TYPES: (Article OR Review) AND LANGUAGE: (English)
		Indexes=SCI-EXPANDED, SSCI, A&HCI, CPCI-S, CPCI-SSH, BKCI-S, BKCI-SSH, ESCI, CCR-EXPANDED, IC Timespan=2010-2020
#1	1704	TOPIC: ("Accidental Fall*") AND DOCUMENT TYPES: (Article OR Review) AND LANGUAGE: (English)
		Indexes=SCI-EXPANDED, SSCI, A&HCI, CPCI-S, CPCI-SSH, BKCI-S, BKCI-SSH, ESCI, CCR-EXPANDED, IC Timespan=2010-2020

Appendix B. PubMed

Search: ((("Accidental Falls"[Mesh]) OR (((((((Falls[Title/Abstract]) OR (Falling[Title/Abstract])) OR ("Falls, Accidental"[Title/Abstract])) OR ("Falls, Accidental"[Title/Abstract])) OR ("Fall, Accidental"[Title/Abstract])) OR ("Slip[Title/Abstract] AND Fall"[Title/Abstract])) OR ("Fall[Title/Abstract] AND Slip"[Title/Abstract]))) AND ((("Aged"[Mesh]) OR (Elderly[Title/Abstract])) Filters: Journal Article, Review, English, Humans, from 2010/1/1–2020/12/31.

Appendix C. Embase

Table A2. Search history from Embase.

Set		Results
#8	#3 AND #6 AND ([article]/lim OR [review]/lim) AND [english]/lim AND [humans]/lim AND [2010–2020]/py	15,588
#7	#3 AND #6	33,343
#6	#4 OR #5	3,293,154
#5	'elderly':ab,ti	356,182
#4	'aged'/exp	3,213,541
#3	#1 OR #2	90,715
#2	'falls':ab,ti OR 'accidental falls':ab,ti OR 'falls, accidental':ab,ti OR 'accidental fall':ab,ti OR 'fall, accidental':ab,ti	67,327
#1	'falling'/exp	41,962

Appendix D. Scopus

((TITLE-ABS-KEY ("accidental fall*") OR TITLE-ABS-KEY (fall*) OR TITLE-ABS-KEY (falling) OR TI-TLE-ABS-KEY ("Fall*, Accidental") OR TITLE-ABS-KEY ("Slip and Fall") OR TITLE-ABS-KEY ("Fall and Slip"))) AND ((TITLE-ABS-KEY (aged) OR TITLE-ABS-KEY (elderly))) AND (LIMIT-TO (DOCTYPE, "ar") OR LIMIT-TO (DOCTYPE, "re")) AND (LIMIT-TO (PUBYEAR, 2020) OR LIMIT-TO (PUBYEAR, 2019) OR LIMIT-TO (PUBYEAR, 2018) OR LIMIT-TO (PUBYEAR, 2017) OR LIMIT-TO (PUBYEAR, 2016) OR LIMIT-TO (PUBYEAR, 2015) OR LIMIT-TO (PUBYEAR, 2014) OR LIMIT-TO (PUBYEAR, 2013) OR LIMIT-TO (PUBYEAR, 2012) OR LIMIT-TO (PUBYEAR, 2011) OR LIMIT-TO (PUBYEAR, 2010)) AND (LIMIT-TO (LANGUAGE, "English")) AND (LIMIT-TO (SRCTYPE, "j")) AND (LIM-IT-TO (EXACTKEYWORD, "Human") OR LIMIT-TO (EXACTKEYWORD, "Humans")).

References

1. Kohl, H.W., 3rd; Craig, C.L.; Lambert, E.V.; Inoue, S.; Alkandari, J.R.; Leetongin, G.; Kahlmeier, S.; Lancet Physical Activity Series Working, G. The pandemic of physical inactivity: Global action for public health. *Lancet* **2012**, *380*, 294–305. [CrossRef]
2. Qato, D.M.; Wilder, J.; Schumm, L.P.; Gillet, V.; Alexander, G.C. Changes in prescription and over-the-counter medication and dietary supplement use among older adults in the United States, 2005 vs. 2011. *JAMA Intern. Med.* **2016**, *176*, 473–482. [CrossRef]
3. Bergen, G.; Stevens, M.R.; Burns, E.R. Falls and Fall Injuries Among Adults Aged ≥ 65 Years—United States, 2014. *MMWR Morb. Mortal. Wkly. Rep.* **2016**, *65*, 993–998. [CrossRef] [PubMed]
4. Ambrose, A.F.; Paul, G.; Hausdorff, J.M. Risk factors for falls among older adults: A review of the literature. *Maturitas* **2013**, *75*, 51–61. [CrossRef] [PubMed]
5. Rubenstein, L.Z. Falls in older people: Epidemiology, risk factors and strategies for prevention. *Age Ageing* **2006**, *35*, 37–41. [CrossRef] [PubMed]
6. Boelens, C.; Hekman, E.E.G.; Verkerke, G.J. Risk factors for falls of older citizens. *Technol. Health Care* **2013**, *21*, 521–533. [CrossRef] [PubMed]
7. Florence, C.S.; Bergen, G.; Atherly, A.; Burns, E.; Stevens, J.; Drake, C. The medical costs of fatal falls and fall injuries among older adults. *J. Am. Geriatr. Soc.* **2018**, *66*, 693–698. [CrossRef] [PubMed]
8. Ng, C.; Fairhall, N.; Wallbank, G.; Tiedemann, A.; Michaleff, Z.A.; Sherrington, C. Exercise for falls prevention in community-dwelling older adults: Trial and participant characteristics, interventions and bias in clinical trials from a systematic review. *BMJ Open Sport Exerc. Med.* **2019**, *5*, e000663. [CrossRef]
9. Sherrington, C.; Fairhall, N.J.; Wallbank, G.K.; Tiedemann, A.; Michaleff, Z.A.; Howard, K.; Clemson, L.; Hopewell, S.; Lamb, S.E. Exercise for preventing falls in older people living in the community. *Cochrane Database Syst. Rev.* **2019**, *1*, CD012424. [CrossRef]
10. Jianhua, H.; Zhigang, H. Review on the application of citespace at home and abroad. *J. Mod. Inf. Ser.* **2013**, *33*, 99–103.
11. Chen, Y.; Chen, C.; Liu, Z.; Hu, Z.; Wang, X. The methodology function of CiteSpace mapping knowledge domains. *Stud. Sci. Sci.* **2015**, *33*, 242–253.
12. Lord, S.R.; Delbaere, K.; Sturnieks, D.L. Aging. *Handb. Clin. Neurol.* **2018**, *159*, 157–171. [CrossRef] [PubMed]
13. Yamada, M. Tailor-made programs for preventive falls. *Jpn. J. Clin. Med.* **2014**, *72*, 1821–1826.

14. Rizzoli, R.; Stevenson, J.C.; Bauer, J.M.; van Loon, L.J.; Walrand, S.; Kanis, J.A.; Cooper, C.; Brandi, M.L.; Diez-Perez, A.; Reginster, J.Y.; et al. The role of dietary protein and vitamin D in maintaining musculoskeletal health in postmenopausal women: A consensus statement from the European Society for Clinical and Economic Aspects of Osteoporosis and Osteoarthritis (ESCEO). *Maturitas* **2014**, *79*, 122–132. [CrossRef] [PubMed]
15. Paintin, J.; Cooper, C.; Dennison, E. Osteosarcopenia. *Br. J. Hosp. Med. (Lond.)* **2018**, *79*, 253–258. [CrossRef] [PubMed]
16. Jang, H.; Clemson, L.; Lovarini, M.; Willis, K.; Lord, S.R.; Sherrington, C. Cultural influences on exercise participation and fall prevention: A systematic review and narrative synthesis. *Disabil. Rehabil.* **2016**, *38*, 724–732. [CrossRef]
17. Lee, D.C.; Day, L.; Hill, K.; Clemson, L.; McDermott, F.; Haines, T.P. What factors influence older adults to discuss falls with their health-care providers? *Health Expect* **2015**, *18*, 1593–1609. [CrossRef]
18. Lord, S.R.; Close, J.C.T. New horizons in falls prevention. *Age Ageing* **2018**, *47*, 492–498. [CrossRef]
19. Kayama, H.; Okamoto, K.; Nishiguchi, S.; Yamada, M.; Kuroda, T.; Aoyama, T. Effect of a Kinect-based exercise game on improving executive cognitive performance in community-dwelling elderly: Case control study. *J. Med. Internet Res.* **2014**, *16*, e61. [CrossRef]
20. Yamada, M.; Aoyama, T.; Hikita, Y.; Takamura, M.; Tanaka, Y.; Kajiwara, Y.; Nagai, K.; Uemura, K.; Mori, S.; Tanaka, B. Effects of a DVD-based seated dual-task stepping exercise on the fall risk factors among community-dwelling elderly adults. *Telemed. J. E Health* **2011**, *17*, 768–772. [CrossRef]
21. Clemson, L.; Mackenzie, L.; Ballinger, C.; Close, J.C.; Cumming, R.G. Environmental interventions to prevent falls in community-dwelling older people: A meta-analysis of randomized trials. *J. Aging Health* **2008**, *20*, 954–971. [CrossRef]
22. Da Silva, R.B.; Costa-Paiva, L.; Morais, S.S.; Mezzalira, R.; Ferreira Nde, O.; Pinto-Neto, A.M. Predictors of falls in women with and without osteoporosis. *J. Orthop. Sports Phys. Ther.* **2010**, *40*, 582–588. [CrossRef] [PubMed]
23. Zhou, X.; Deng, H.; Shen, X.; Lei, Q. Effect of balance training on falls in patients with osteoporosis: A systematic review and meta-analysis. *J. Rehabil. Med.* **2018**, *50*, 577–581. [CrossRef] [PubMed]
24. Shier, V.; Trieu, E.; Ganz, D.A. Implementing exercise programs to prevent falls: Systematic descriptive review. *Inj. Epidemiol.* **2016**, *3*, 16. [CrossRef] [PubMed]
25. Miller, P.D. Management of severe osteoporosis. *Expert. Opin. Pharmacother.* **2016**, *17*, 473–488. [CrossRef] [PubMed]
26. Viswanathan, A.; Sudarsky, L. Balance and gait problems in the elderly. *Handb. Clin. Neurol.* **2012**, *103*, 623–634. [CrossRef] [PubMed]
27. Kyrdalen, I.L.; Thingstad, P.; Sandvik, L.; Ormstad, H. Associations between gait speed and well-known fall risk factors among community-dwelling older adults. *Physiother. Res. Int.* **2019**, *24*, e1743. [CrossRef]
28. Montero-Odasso, M.; Sarquis-Adamson, Y.; Song, H.Y.; Bray, N.W.; Pieruccini-Faria, F.; Speechley, M. Polypharmacy, gait performance, and falls in community-dwelling older adults. Results from the Gait and Brain Study. *J. Am. Geriatr. Soc.* **2019**, *67*, 1182–1188. [CrossRef] [PubMed]
29. Delbaere, K.; Close, J.C.; Mikolaizak, A.S.; Sachdev, P.S.; Brodaty, H.; Lord, S.R. The Falls Efficacy Scale International (FES-I). A comprehensive longitudinal validation study. *Age Ageing* **2010**, *39*, 210–216. [CrossRef] [PubMed]
30. Bosscher, R.J.; Raymakers, E.R.; Trompe, E.A.; Smit, J.H. Fear of falling: Psychometric aspects of Tinetti's Falls Efficacy Scale. *Tijdschr. Gerontol. Geriatr.* **2005**, *36*, 5–10. [CrossRef]
31. Kumar, A.; Delbaere, K.; Zijlstra, G.A.; Carpenter, H.; Iliffe, S.; Masud, T.; Skelton, D.; Morris, R.; Kendrick, D. Exercise for reducing fear of falling in older people living in the community: Cochrane systematic review and meta-analysis. *Age Ageing* **2016**, *45*, 345–352. [CrossRef]
32. Qi, B.; Jin, S.; Qian, H.; Zou, Y. Bibliometric Analysis of Chronic Traumatic Encephalopathy Research from 1999 to 2019. *Int. J. Environ. Res. Public Health* **2020**, *17*, 5411. [CrossRef] [PubMed]
33. Injury, G.B.D.T.B.; Spinal Cord Injury, C. Global, regional, and national burden of traumatic brain injury and spinal cord injury, 1990–2016: A systematic analysis for the Global Burden of Disease Study 2016. *Lancet Neurol.* **2019**, *18*, 56–87. [CrossRef]
34. Stevens, J.A.; Corso, P.S.; Finkelstein, E.A.; Miller, T.R. The costs of fatal and non-fatal falls among older adults. *Inj. Prev.* **2006**, *12*, 290–295. [CrossRef] [PubMed]
35. VanItallie, T.B. Traumatic brain injury (TBI) in collision sports: Possible mechanisms of transformation into chronic traumatic encephalopathy (CTE). *Metabolism* **2019**, *100*, 153943. [CrossRef]
36. Brown, C.V.; Ali, S.; Fairley, R.; Lai, B.K.; Arthrell, J.; Walker, M.; Tips, G. Risk factors for falls among hospitalized trauma patients. *Am. Surg.* **2013**, *79*, 465–469. [CrossRef] [PubMed]
37. Berkova, M.; Berka, Z. Falls: A significant cause of morbidity and mortality in elderly people. *Vnitr. Lek.* **2018**, *64*, 1076–1083. [PubMed]
38. Cheng, P.; Wang, L.; Ning, P.; Yin, P.; Schwebel, D.C.; Liu, J.; Qi, J.; Hu, G.; Zhou, M. Unintentional falls mortality in China, 2006–2016. *J. Glob. Health* **2019**, *9*, 010603. [CrossRef]
39. Hartholt, K.A.; Lee, R.; Burns, E.R.; van Beeck, E.F. Mortality from falls among us adults aged 75 years or older, 2000–2016. *JAMA* **2019**, *321*, 2131–2133. [CrossRef]
40. Hartholt, K.A.; van Beeck, E.F.; van der Cammen, T.J.M. Mortality from falls in dutch adults 80 years and older, 2000–2016. *JAMA* **2018**, *319*, 1380–1382. [CrossRef]
41. Padrón-Monedero, A.; Damián, J.; Pilar Martin, M.; Fernández-Cuenca, R. Mortality trends for accidental falls in older people in Spain, 2000–2015. *BMC Geriatr.* **2017**, *17*, 276. [CrossRef] [PubMed]

42. Kiadaliri, A.A.; Rosengren, B.E.; Englund, M. Fall-related mortality in southern Sweden: A multiple cause of death analysis, 1998–2014. *Inj. Prev.* **2019**, *25*, 129–135. [CrossRef] [PubMed]
43. Hagiya, H.; Koyama, T.; Zamami, Y.; Tatebe, Y.; Funahashi, T.; Shinomiya, K.; Kitamura, Y.; Hinotsu, S.; Sendo, T.; Rakugi, H.; et al. Fall-related mortality trends in older Japanese adults aged ≥65 years: A nationwide observational study. *BMJ Open* **2019**, *9*, e033462. [CrossRef] [PubMed]
44. Ayalon, L. Satisfaction with aging results in reduced risk for falling. *Int. Psychogeriatr.* **2016**, *28*, 741–747. [CrossRef] [PubMed]
45. Tom, S.E.; Adachi, J.D.; Anderson, F.A., Jr.; Boonen, S.; Chapurlat, R.D.; Compston, J.E.; Cooper, C.; Gehlbach, S.H.; Greenspan, S.L.; Hooven, F.H.; et al. Frailty and fracture, disability, and falls: A multiple country study from the global longitudinal study of osteoporosis in women. *J. Am. Geriatr. Soc.* **2013**, *61*, 327–334. [CrossRef] [PubMed]
46. Kojima, G. Frailty as a predictor of future falls among community-dwelling older people: A systematic review and meta-analysis. *J. Am. Med. Dir. Assoc.* **2015**, *16*, 1027–1033. [CrossRef]
47. Clemson, L.; Fiatarone Singh, M.A.; Bundy, A.; Cumming, R.G.; Manollaras, K.; O'Loughlin, P.; Black, D. Integration of balance and strength training into daily life activity to reduce rate of falls in older people (the LiFE study): Randomised parallel trial. *BMJ* **2012**, *345*, e4547. [CrossRef]
48. Mirelman, A.; Rochester, L.; Maidan, I.; Del Din, S.; Alcock, L.; Nieuwhof, F.; Rikkert, M.O.; Bloem, B.R.; Pelosin, E.; Avanzino, L.; et al. Addition of a non-immersive virtual reality component to treadmill training to reduce fall risk in older adults (V-TIME): A randomised controlled trial. *Lancet* **2016**, *388*, 1170–1182. [CrossRef]
49. Jiménez-García, J.D.; Hita-Contreras, F.; de la Torre-Cruz, M.; Fábrega-Cuadros, R.; Aibar-Almazán, A.; Cruz-Díaz, D.; Martínez-Amat, A. Risk of falls in healthy older adults: Benefits of high-intensity interval training using lower body suspension exercises. *J. Aging Phys. Act.* **2019**, *27*, 325–333. [CrossRef]
50. Thomas, S.; Mackintosh, S.; Halbert, J. Does the 'Otago exercise programme' reduce mortality and falls in older adults? A systematic review and meta-analysis. *Age Ageing* **2010**, *39*, 681–687. [CrossRef]
51. Holroyd, C.R.; Cooper, C.; Harvey, N.C. Vitamin D and the postmenopausal population. *Menopause Int.* **2011**, *17*, 102–107. [CrossRef] [PubMed]
52. Gallagher, J.C. Vitamin D and falls—The dosage conundrum. *Nat. Rev. Endocrinol.* **2016**, *12*, 680–684. [CrossRef] [PubMed]
53. Uusi-Rasi, K.; Patil, R.; Karinkanta, S.; Kannus, P.; Tokola, K.; Lamberg-Allardt, C.; Sievänen, H. Exercise and vitamin D in fall prevention among older women: A randomized clinical trial. *JAMA Intern. Med.* **2015**, *175*, 703–711. [CrossRef] [PubMed]
54. Bolland, M.J.; Grey, A.; Avenell, A. Effects of vitamin D supplementation on musculoskeletal health: A systematic review, meta-analysis, and trial sequential analysis. *Lancet Diabetes Endocrinol.* **2018**, *6*, 847–858. [CrossRef]
55. Dennison, E.M.; Sayer, A.A.; Cooper, C. Epidemiology of sarcopenia and insight into possible therapeutic targets. *Nat. Rev. Rheumatol.* **2017**, *13*, 340–347. [CrossRef]
56. Cruz-Jentoft, A.J.; Baeyens, J.P.; Bauer, J.M.; Boirie, Y.; Cederholm, T.; Landi, F.; Martin, F.C.; Michel, J.P.; Rolland, Y.; Schneider, S.M.; et al. Sarcopenia: European consensus on definition and diagnosis: Report of the european working group on sarcopenia in older people. *Age Ageing* **2010**, *39*, 412–423. [CrossRef]
57. Codes, I.-C. Sarcopenia. Available online: https://www.icd10data.com/ICD10CM/Codes/M00-M99/M60-M63/M62-/M62.84 (accessed on 1 October 2016).
58. Cruz-Jentoft, A.J.; Bahat, G.; Bauer, J.; Boirie, Y.; Bruyere, O.; Cederholm, T.; Cooper, C.; Landi, F.; Rolland, Y.; Sayer, A.A.; et al. Sarcopenia: Revised European consensus on definition and diagnosis. *Age Ageing* **2019**, *48*, 601. [CrossRef]
59. Chen, L.K.; Liu, L.K.; Woo, J.; Assantachai, P.; Auyeung, T.W.; Bahyah, K.S.; Chou, M.Y.; Chen, L.Y.; Hsu, P.S.; Krairit, O.; et al. Sarcopenia in Asia: Consensus report of the Asian Working Group for Sarcopenia. *J. Am. Med. Dir. Assoc.* **2014**, *15*, 95–101. [CrossRef]
60. Chen, L.K.; Woo, J.; Assantachai, P.; Auyeung, T.W.; Chou, M.Y.; Iijima, K.; Jang, H.C.; Kang, L.; Kim, M.; Kim, S.; et al. Asian Working Group for Sarcopenia: 2019 Consensus Update on Sarcopenia Diagnosis and Treatment. *J. Am. Med. Dir. Assoc.* **2020**, *21*, 300–307.e2. [CrossRef]
61. Cruz-Jentoft, A.J.; Sayer, A.A. Sarcopenia. *Lancet* **2019**, *393*, 2636–2646. [CrossRef]
62. Bischoff-Ferrari, H.A.; Orav, J.E.; Kanis, J.A.; Rizzoli, R.; Schlögl, M.; Staehelin, H.B.; Willett, W.C.; Dawson-Hughes, B. Comparative performance of current definitions of sarcopenia against the prospective incidence of falls among community-dwelling seniors age 65 and older. *Osteoporos Int.* **2015**, *26*, 2793–2802. [CrossRef] [PubMed]
63. Schaap, L.A.; van Schoor, N.M.; Lips, P.; Visser, M. Associations of sarcopenia definitions, and their components, with the incidence of recurrent falling and fractures: The longitudinal aging study amsterdam. *J. Gerontol. A Biol. Sci. Med. Sci.* **2018**, *73*, 1199–1204. [CrossRef] [PubMed]
64. Cawthon, P.M.; Lui, L.Y.; Taylor, B.C.; McCulloch, C.E.; Cauley, J.A.; Lapidus, J.; Orwoll, E.; Ensrud, K.E. Clinical definitions of sarcopenia and risk of hospitalization in community-dwelling older men: The osteoporotic fractures in men study. *J. Gerontol. A Biol. Sci. Med. Sci.* **2017**, *72*, 1383–1389. [CrossRef] [PubMed]
65. Nevitt, M.C.; Cummings, S.R. Type of fall and risk of hip and wrist fractures: The study of osteoporotic fractures. The Study of Osteoporotic Fractures Research Group. *J. Am. Geriatr. Soc.* **1993**, *41*, 1226–1234. [CrossRef] [PubMed]
66. Kulik, C. Components of a Comprehensive Fall-risk Assessment. In Special Supplement to American Nurse Today—Best Practices for Falls Reduction: A Practical Guide. 2011. Available online: http://www.americannursetoday.com/Article.aspx?id=7634&fid=7364. (accessed on 19 May 2014).

67. Avanecean, D.; Calliste, D.; Contreras, T.; Lim, Y.; Fitzpatrick, A. Effectiveness of patient-centered interventions on falls in the acute care setting compared to usual care: A systematic review. *JBI Database Syst. Rev. Implement Rep.* **2017**, *15*, 3006–3048. [CrossRef] [PubMed]
68. Toots, A.; Wiklund, R.; Littbrand, H.; Nordin, E.; Nordstrom, P.; Lundin-Olsson, L.; Gustafson, Y.; Rosendahl, E. The effects of exercise on falls in older people with dementia living in nursing homes: A randomized controlled trial. *J. Am. Med. Dir. Assoc.* **2019**, *20*, 835–842.e1. [CrossRef]
69. Peek, K.; Bryant, J.; Carey, M.; Dodd, N.; Freund, M.; Lawson, S.; Meyer, C. Reducing falls among people living with dementia: A systematic review. *Dementia* **2020**, *19*, 1621–1640. [CrossRef]
70. Livingston, G.; Huntley, J.; Sommerlad, A.; Ames, D.; Ballard, C.; Banerjee, S.; Brayne, C.; Burns, A.; Cohen-Mansfield, J.; Cooper, C.; et al. Dementia prevention, intervention, and care: 2020 report of the Lancet Commission. *Lancet* **2020**, *396*, 413–446. [CrossRef]
71. Iaboni, A.; Flint, A.J. The complex interplay of depression and falls in older adults: A clinical review. *Am. J. Geriatr. Psychiatry* **2013**, *21*, 484–492. [CrossRef]
72. Daly, R.M.; Dalla Via, J.; Duckham, R.L.; Fraser, S.F.; Helge, E.W. Exercise for the prevention of osteoporosis in postmenopausal women: An evidence-based guide to the optimal prescription. *Braz. J. Phys. Ther.* **2019**, *23*, 170–180. [CrossRef]
73. Gia, T.N.; Sarker, V.K.; Tcarenko, I.; Rahmani, A.M.; Westerlund, T.; Liljeberg, P.; Tenhunen, H. Energy efficient wearable sensor node for IoT-based fall detection systems. *Microprocess. Microsyst.* **2018**, *56*, 34–46.
74. Xu, T.; Zhou, Y.; Zhu, J. New advances and challenges of fall detection systems: A survey. *Appl. Sci.* **2018**, *8*, 418. [CrossRef]
75. Malasinghe, L.P.; Ramzan, N.; Dahal, K. Remote patient monitoring: A comprehensive study. *J. Ambient Intell. Humaniz. Comput.* **2019**, *10*, 57–76. [CrossRef]
76. Peel, N.M. Epidemiology of falls in older age. *Can. J. Aging* **2011**, *30*, 7–19. [CrossRef] [PubMed]
77. WHO. WHO Global Report on Falls Prevention in Older Age. Available online: https://www.who.int/ageing/publications/Falls_prevention7March.pdf?ua=1 (accessed on 23 December 2020).
78. Wales, K.; Clemson, L.; Lannin, N.A.; Cameron, I.D.; Salked, G.; Gitlin, L.; Rubenstein, L.; Barras, S.; Mackenzie, L.; Davies, C. Occupational therapy discharge planning for older adults: A protocol for a randomised trial and economic evaluation. *BMC Geriatr.* **2012**, *12*, 34. [CrossRef] [PubMed]
79. Gale, C.R.; Westbury, L.D.; Cooper, C.; Dennison, E.M. Risk factors for incident falls in older men and women: The English longitudinal study of ageing. *BMC Geriatr.* **2018**, *18*, 117. [CrossRef] [PubMed]
80. Gale, C.R.; Cooper, C.; Aihie Sayer, A. Prevalence and risk factors for falls in older men and women: The English Longitudinal Study of Ageing. *Age Ageing* **2016**, *45*, 789–794. [CrossRef] [PubMed]
81. Stevens, J.A.; Ballesteros, M.F.; Mack, K.A.; Rudd, R.A.; DeCaro, E.; Adler, G. Gender differences in seeking care for falls in the aged Medicare population. *Am. J. Prev. Med.* **2012**, *43*, 59–62. [CrossRef]

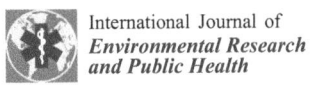

Review

Implementing Precision Medicine in Human Frailty through Epigenetic Biomarkers

José Luis García-Giménez [1,2,3,4], Salvador Mena-Molla [3,4], Francisco José Tarazona-Santabalbina [5], Jose Viña [6], Mari Carmen Gomez-Cabrera [6,*] and Federico V. Pallardó [1,2,3,4]

1. U733, Centre for Biomedical Network Research on Rare Diseases (CIBERER-ISCIII), 28029 Madrid, Spain; j.luis.garcia@uv.es (J.L.G.-G.); Federico.V.Pallardo@uv.es (F.V.P.)
2. Mixed Unit for Rare Diseases INCLIVA-CIPF, INCLIVA Health Research Institute, 46010 Valencia, Spain
3. Department of Physiology, Faculty of Medicine, University of Valencia, 46003 Valencia, Spain; salva.mena@uv.es
4. EpiDisease S.L., Parc Cientific de la Universitat de València, 46980 Paterna, Spain
5. Servicio de Geriatría, Hospital Universitario de la Ribera, CIBERFES, Alzira, 46010 Valencia, Spain; fjtarazonas@gmail.com
6. Freshage Research Group, Department of Physiology, Faculty of Medicine, Institute of Health Research-INCLIVA, University of Valencia and CIBERFES, 46010 Valencia, Spain; jose.vina@uv.es
* Correspondence: carmen.gomez@uv.es

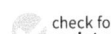

Citation: García-Giménez, J.L.; Mena-Molla, S.; Tarazona-Santabalbina, F.J.; Viña, J.; Gomez-Cabrera, M.C.; Pallardó, F.V. Implementing Precision Medicine in Human Frailty through Epigenetic Biomarkers. *IJERPH* 2021, *18*, 1883. https://doi.org/10.3390/ijerph18041883

Academic Editor: Paul B. Tchounwou

Received: 29 December 2020
Accepted: 9 February 2021
Published: 15 February 2021

Publisher's Note: MDPI stays neutral with regard to jurisdictional claims in published maps and institutional affiliations.

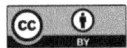

Copyright: © 2021 by the authors. Licensee MDPI, Basel, Switzerland. This article is an open access article distributed under the terms and conditions of the Creative Commons Attribution (CC BY) license (https://creativecommons.org/licenses/by/4.0/).

Abstract: The main epigenetic features in aging are: reduced bulk levels of core histones, altered pattern of histone post-translational modifications, changes in the pattern of DNA methylation, replacement of canonical histones with histone variants, and altered expression of non-coding RNA. The identification of epigenetic mechanisms may contribute to the early detection of age-associated subclinical changes or deficits at the molecular and/or cellular level, to predict the development of frailty, or even more interestingly, to improve health trajectories in older adults. Frailty reflects a state of increased vulnerability to stressors as a result of decreased physiologic reserves, and even dysregulation of multiple physiologic systems leading to adverse health outcomes for individuals of the same chronological age. A key approach to overcome the challenges of frailty is the development of biomarkers to improve early diagnostic accuracy and to predict trajectories in older individuals. The identification of epigenetic biomarkers of frailty could provide important support for the clinical diagnosis of frailty, or more specifically, to the evaluation of its associated risks. Interventional studies aimed at delaying the onset of frailty and the functional alterations associated with it, would also undoubtedly benefit from the identification of frailty biomarkers. Specific to the article yet reasonably common within the subject discipline.

Keywords: geriatric syndromes; healthy aging; exercise; histones; DNA methylation; non-coding RNA

1. Introduction

The concept of frailty has been evolving for more than 20 years. Since the publication of a validated phenotype of frailty as a medical syndrome in 2001 by Fried and colleagues [1], this geriatric condition has received growing interest due to its association with longevity and aging-related phenotypes (Figure 1). At the moment there is no consensus on the definition of frailty, but it is accepted that frailty reflects a state of increased vulnerability to stressors as a result of decreased physiologic reserves, and even dysregulation of multiple physiologic systems leading to adverse health outcomes for individuals of the same chronological age [2]. From a gerontological point of view, frailty is a stochastic, deleterious and dynamic process of deficit accumulation. Cellular deficits include: senescence and stem cell exhaustion, loss of proteostasis, decline in metabolism, inflammation, DNA damage and deficit in DNA repair, hormone dysregulation, and epigenetic alterations [3]. The accumulation of these deficits varies across life stages and some individuals are more predisposed to them [4]. Since cells are the primary sites of deficit accumulation, cellular frailty may be the major driver of the systemic physiological decline of tissues and organs [5], which may lead to late-onset multimorbidity.

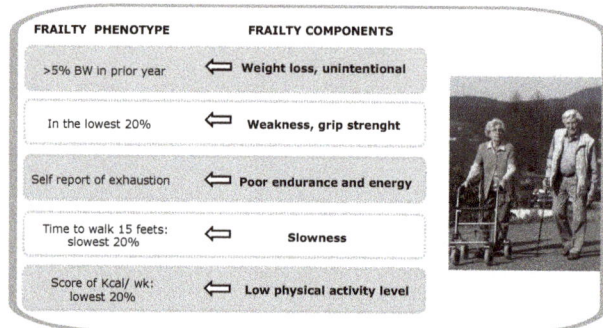

Figure 1. Frailty features contributing to the frailty phenotype during aging.

Frailty is the main determinant of longevity and quality of life in the elderly population and it has become a public health concern [6]. Among the causes of frailty, one of most important contributors is the adoption of unhealthy lifestyles (i.e., physical inactivity and/or sedentarism, malnutrition, smoking and alcohol intake) [7]. Frailty is a dynamic process, characterized by frequent transitions between states of frailty and towards disability and dependency. Disability is characterized by a functional limitation that increases the demand for long-term care services for the elderly, which infers high social-health and personal costs [8]. Frailty increases dramatically with age, with a prevalence of 5.2% in men and 9.6% in women over the age of 65 years [9]. These figures grow to 40% in adults aged 80 years and older. Frailty increases the risk of falls, delirium, disability and other geriatric syndromes [10,11]. It also increases vulnerability to age-related disorders, such as myocardial infarction, diabetes and hypertension in those who suffer from it [12].

In the past two decades, a large proportion of the global burden of disease has changed due to high rates of disability resulting from morbidity of non-communicable diseases. In fact, it is considered that disability increases health costs more than disease by itself [2]. In this scenario, we have to define phenotypic aging, which includes the changes in body composition and structures (i.e., loss of skeletal muscle mass), energetics, homeostatic mechanisms, and neuronal function that occur while we age and that may contribute to functional aging. Functional aging is referred to as the age-associated decline in physical, emotional, cognitive, and social functions leading to a decrease in the performance of basic activities of daily living and contributing to the loss of independence [13].

Recent research is helping to shed light on mechanisms underlying frailty, how frailty can influence disease onset and progression, and how new interventions can attenuate frailty to improve health status. Moreover, frailty helps to explain heterogeneity in aged people and it provides the basis to understand the differences between biological and chronological age.

The main physiological systems dysregulated in the frail patient include the endocrine [14], musculoskeletal [15], respiratory [16], renal, cardiovascular [17], immune [18], hematopoietic system [19], and also the nervous system [20]. Moreover, mounting evidence indicates that frailty may increase the risk of mild cognitive impairment and contribute to dementia [21]. This probably occurs because frailty and cognitive disorders may share common biological pathways. Thus, frail older adults may be at higher risk of incident cognitive disorders than robust ones.

Several predictive models related to frailty are available in the literature. Most of these predictive models are focused on defining and validating a frailty index, which is used as a predictor of disability, hospitalization, and mortality. There are also a smaller number of studies in which these indexes are used to predict the ability to perform activities of daily living (ADL), instrumental activities of daily living (IADL), or the risk of falls [22]. In any case, each of these indexes can improve the clinical management of frailty.

A key approach to overcoming the challenge of frailty is to implement precision medicine by using biological biomarkers to improve diagnostic accuracy and to optimize its management. Finding biomarkers would allow gerontologists to predict the functional trajectories of older adults at preclinical stages. This could help to develop early interventions aimed at preventing frailty and its natural progression to disability. Precision medicine was defined by the National Research Council's Toward Precision Medicine in 2008 as: "The tailoring of medical treatment to the individual characteristics of each patient . . . to classify individuals into subpopulations that differ in their susceptibility to a particular disease or their response to a specific treatment. Preventive and therapeutic interventions can then be concentrated on those patients who will benefit, sparing expense and side effects for those who will not".

Today we know, thanks to the "Human Genome Project" and the "Human Epigenome and the Human Epigenome Roadmap Projects", that genetics is not the only contributor to disease. In most complex diseases and human conditions genetics cannot, by itself, explain the deficits or molecular alterations related to the onset of the disease, its progression or even the response to a specific treatment. In fact, most human diseases are complex multifactorial pathologies, caused by genetic background and epigenetic inputs, which can modulate transcriptional programs and lead to adverse clinical outcomes.

Epigenetics is defined as the discipline that studies the regulation of gene expression by mechanisms not related to changes in the DNA sequence. These regulatory processes can be heritable and set the features of specific cell lineages and subpopulations. Many of these epigenetic mechanisms suffer the influence of environmental factors and are part of the adaptive homeostatic mechanisms of all organisms. Thus, the epigenetic regulatory mechanisms are continuously being implemented for surviving. Organisms with powerful adaptive mechanisms have developed an extremely complex epigenetic machinery and if the organism has a long-life span, like in humans, the epigenetic regulatory actions are expected to play a very important role.

Epigenetics is a rising discipline in biomedicine, which aims to improve predictive and precision medicine by discovering new mechanisms underlying diseases and providing new biomarkers in order to identify molecular targets that are modulable, for instance, by using epigenetic drugs [23–25]. Most human biological processes have complex multifactorial modulators that include polymorphisms and copy number variation in human genes, besides epigenetic mechanisms, that contribute to the modulation of gene expression [26].

According to Pal and Tyler [27] the main epigenetic features in aging are: (i) reduced bulk levels of core histones, (ii) altered pattern of histone post-translational modifications, (iii) changes in the pattern of DNA methylation, (iv) replacement of canonical histones with histone variants, and (v) altered expression of non-coding RNA. The consequence of these changes in the epigenetic regulation alters the local accessibility of the transcriptional and DNA repairing machinery to the genetic material, thus, producing among others, aberrant gene expression, reactivation of transposable elements and genomic instability [27]. Epigenetics is able to explain, in most cases, the importance of life style factors and the influence of the environment on the aging process.

We have defined an epigenetic biomarker as "any epigenetic mark or altered epigenetic mechanism which generally serves to evaluate health or disease status and is particularly stable and reproducible during sample processing and analysis" [25]. There is a current need to better understand the etiology of frailty to develop effective interventions for its prevention, amelioration, or even its reversion. The identification of potential sensitive and specific biomarkers may provide insights into the molecular, metabolic, cellular, and physiological alterations that lead human beings to frailty [28].

The present review aims to provide answers to some of the uncertainties regarding the role of epigenetic mechanisms in frailty development.

2. Materials and Methods

The present review was carried out by conducting an electronic search in OVID (Medline and Embase), combining the following MeSH keywords: "epigenomics" or "biomarkers", combined with "frailty". The search was limited to publications in the last ten years, in English, Spanish, and French. A total of 158 articles were obtained of which 87 were finally selected. The MeSH construction ("Epigenomics" [Mesh] OR "Epigenetic Repression" [Mesh] OR "Epigenesis, Genetic" [Mesh] OR "Biomarkers" [Mesh]) AND "Frailty" [Mesh] were used. Some additional instructions were added for certain specific objectives where necessary. In 14 cases, supplementary information was obtained in the form of references of the selected articles.

The articles were selected by the investigators based on the following inclusion criteria: randomized clinical trials, cohort studies, case-control studies, observational studies, and before and after analyses; population: older adults; outcome geriatric syndromes and frailty. The exclusion criteria were: letters to the editor, case reports, manuscripts with no available abstract or those with only the abstract published. All the published studies were re-evaluated by the authors of the review, and final inclusion was restricted to those of sufficient quality to afford information pertinent to the objectives of this review.

3. Results

Frailty has become a public health concern. A key approach to overcoming the challenge of frailty is to implement precision medicine by using biological biomarkers to improve diagnostic accuracy and to optimize its management. Finding epigenetic biomarkers would provide an excellent tool to predict the evolution of frailty to disability and dependency in older individuals as well as contribute to designing personalized pharmacological and non-pharmacological interventions.

3.1. Epigenetic Mechanisms Related to Aging and Frailty

Importantly, changes across cell generations accumulate genetic and epigenetic alterations [29]. Among the different generalized changes during aging in mammals, global DNA hypomethylation mainly in DNA repeats, as well as, local hypermethylation at specific gene promoters have been found [30]. These can result in gene expression silencing in DNA repair and anti-inflammatory genes [31]. It has also been suggested that other genes participating in the maintenance of muscle and nervous systems processes, chromatin remodeling, and transcription control may also be affected [32]. It has been proposed that these global changes in DNA methylation are associated with the incomplete restoration of epigenetic patterns after DNA replication or DNA repair [33], which contribute to the accumulation of epimutations in the bulk DNA. These changes in the methylation pattern together with other epigenetic related factors associated with aging were coined the "epigenetic drift [34]" by Veitia and coworkers since it was considered as a general and progressive epigenetic process directly related to senescence, which is especially important in tissue-specific stem cells. Among these adult stem cells, muscle satellite cells play a very important role in sarcopenia, which is one of the key features in frailty. The important changes that take place in satellite cells upon aging have been recently demonstrated in mouse muscle stem cells [35], underscoring the importance of skeletal muscle epigenetic regulation in the development of the frail phenotype.

3.1.1. DNA Methylation

Since its discovery, DNA methylation (DNAm) has been the best studied epigenetic modification. It affects the 5′ carbon position of cytosine, mostly in the context of CpG dinucleotide. There is a significant amount of work describing the analysis of DNA methylation and its role in human diseases. From a clinical point of view, DNA methylation harbors great potential value as a diagnostic and prognostic biomarker. The possibility of screening blood-circulating DNA or DNA extracted from leukocytes for alterations in DNA methylation also increases its value as an epigenetic biomarker.

It has been demonstrated that DNA methylation displays a strong correlation with age and age-related processes. In a pioneering work published in PNAS in 2005, global and locus-specific differences in DNA methylation in identical twins of various ages was found. Moreover, the authors demonstrated a correlation between DNA methylation and quality of life during aging and also that DNA methylation can be influenced by different environmental and lifestyle factors [33]. Seven years later, using DNA from peripheral blood cells, an association between global DNA methylation levels and age-related functional decline was reported [36]. The authors found lower global methylation levels in frail subjects than in those who had a better functional status such as pre-frail and non-frail [37]. This finding was accompanied by a longitudinal study to explore whether the methylation levels were sensitive to changes in the frailty status over time. It was found that the decrease in global DNA methylation was associated with functional decline and not to chronological age, at least after 65 years of age [36]. This led to the suggestion that biological age and aging acceleration can be predicted based on methylation patterns at specific CpG sites [38].

Epigenetic clocks, which are based on the use of specific DNA methylation patterns, can also be correlated to individuals' chronological ages to assess inter-individual and/or inter-tissue variability in the aging rate [38]. For a number of epigenetic clocks, the divergence between epigenetic age and chronological age reflects biological age acceleration. In this regard, epigenetic age acceleration has been associated with the risk of heart disease [39], breast cancer [40,41], lung cancer [42], neurodegenerative diseases such as Alzheimer's disease [43], and it has also been associated with differential susceptibility to death [44–47].

There are up to eleven epigenetic clocks [48], which incorporate a subset of CpGs (between 1 and 513) that are differentially weighted to estimate epigenetic age and predict age-related outcomes.

The most validated epigenetic clock was proposed by Horvath (the Horvath's clock) [40]. It uses the exact 353 CpG loci predictor to analyze DNAm age acceleration. Other epigenetic clocks are also gaining relevance, such as the Hannum's clock [49] or the clock proposed by Zhang and co-workers that was developed in 2017 as a predictor for all-cause mortality [47]. More recently, an epigenetic clock for lifespan and health span has been developed to differentiate same-aged individuals based on morbidity and mortality risk [45].

Over the years, additional approaches analyzing a lower number of CpG sites for an estimation of the epigenetic age have also been proposed [50,51]. Two clocks have been developed by Wolfgang Wagner's group: the 3 CpG model [50] and the 99 CpG model [52]. Weidner and co-workers selected 3 CpGs from DNAm in blood from array data of the 27K Illumina array, which were later validated by Lin and Wagner using the Infinium 450K Beadchip array (Illumina) [52]. This resulted in an age predictor with an average accuracy of 5.4 years. Vidal-Bralo et al. [51] developed an epigenetic clock analyzing the DNAm in 390 healthy subjects. This clock consists of an age predictor based on 8 CpG sites, out of a preselected list of the most informative CpGs (with an age correlation over 0.85). More recently, Liu and co-workers have also proposed a "Meta-Clock", consisting of a new approach by deconstructing the clocks into submodules and recombining them into a more robust epigenetic aging measurement [48]. This clock has demonstrated improved prediction for mortality and more robust aging associations with DNAm [48].

The influence of genetic and environmental factors as well as technical differences in the selected DNAm analysis methods have been highlighted as the main drawbacks of the age-related CpGs analysis [53].

Several studies have shown that epigenetic age acceleration is associated with frailty in older individuals [54,55]. Two laboratories have studied DNA methylation changes in frailty using the deficit accumulation method [56] and the frailty phenotype [55].

3.1.2. Histone Post-Translational Modifications and Histone Variants

Chromatin is organized by repeating arrays of nucleosomes, which consist of 145 bp of DNA wrapped around a histone octamer. Each histone octamer consists of two copies of each histone, H4, H3, H2A, and H2B. Histones can be chemically modified, producing histone post-translational modifications (PTMs) (i.e., acetylation, methylation, phosphorylation, butyrylation, hydroxybutyrylation, crotonylation, citrullination, formylation, glycosylation, O-GlcNAcylation, carbonylation, parsylation, and glutathionylation) [57]. These changes can modify the nucleosome structure and accessibility to different regions of the genome. Proper coordination between components of the epigenetic machineries is responsible for the introduction or removal of PTMs, which are essential for the correct control of epigenome function. Otherwise, mutations in epigenetic enzymes (i.e., writers and erasers) and/or in epigenetic readers, which alter the "histone code", can be translated into diseases.

Histone post-translational modifications are more difficult to map completely over the whole epigenome than DNA methylation, which makes them more difficult to analyze using high throughput technologies. However, several efforts have been made in order to explore histone metabolism, histone replacement, and histone PTMs introduction and removal. In this regard, Benayoun and co-workers have described reduced bulk levels of core histones, altered histone posttranslational modifications and cellular misregulation in the replacement of histone variants in aging [58].

In different histone post-translational modifications, phosphorylation of Ser139 in the histone variant H2AX, also known as γH2AX, is a key event that marks double strand breaks in the DNA [59], and therefore, DNA instability and DNA repair deficits. Importantly, elevated levels and persistence in time of γH2AX is considered an unrepairable double strand break [60], which may result in tumorigenesis, mitotic arrest or cell death.

3.1.3. Non-Coding RNA

Epigenetic regulation is also mediated by non-coding RNAs (ncRNAs), which are molecules that, despite being non-protein-coding RNAs, have important regulatory functions in gene expression. Generally, ncRNAs regulate gene expression at the transcriptional and post-transcriptional level. These ncRNAs include microRNAs (miRNAs) and long non-coding RNAs (lncRNAs). miRNAs are a large family of short RNA molecules with an average size of 17–25 nucleotides [61]. miRNAs can down-regulate gene expression by inhibiting mRNA translation when binding to its 3'-UTR or by degrading mRNA molecules, as well as increase mRNA translation of some targets [62] when miRNAs bind to 5'-UTR regions of the target mRNA. lncRNA transcripts are longer than 200 nucleotides and poorly conserved. lncRNAs are transcribed from all over the genome including intergenic regions, domains overlapping one or more exons of another transcript on the same strand (sense) or on the opposite strand (antisense), or intronic regions of protein-coding genes [63]. Many lncRNAs act by forming complexes with chromatin-modifying proteins and recruiting them to specific sites in the genome, thereby modifying chromatin states and influencing gene expression [64].

MiRNAs have gained relevance in recent years in research on aging due to their role in the control of several biological processes [65]. For instance, it has been suggested that miRNAs can control muscle metabolism and muscle wasting [66]. This opens up new avenues at different levels, such as the identification of the molecular targets to test miRNA-based interventions as a therapeutic strategy against sarcopenia [66].

Smith-Vikos and co-workers have proposed the analysis of circulating miRNAs in serum and plasma to screen for biomarkers of healthy aging and longevity [67]. Exosomes, small cell-derived vesicles found within extracellular fluids and originated from cellular multivesicular bodies fused with the plasma membrane, have also been identified as valuable biomarkers for a number of disease conditions. Exosomes can contain microRNA [68]. Inflamma-miRs, mitomiRs and myomiRs have been closely related with frailty [69] as we describe in the following section.

3.2. Epigenetic Biomarkers Associated with Aging and Frailty

A key approach to overcome the challenges of frailty is the development of biomarkers to improve early diagnostic accuracy and to predict clinical trajectories in older individuals. Furthermore, frailty biomarkers should allow us to stratify patients and distinguish those who will benefit from a specific therapeutic approach compared to those who will not benefit from a specific intervention, thus making frailty identification one of the pillars in decision-making in regard to older patients.

Epigenetic biomarkers should have the ability to detect early subclinical changes or deficits at the molecular and/or cellular level [70]. So, they can help to identify key dysregulated transcriptional programs, which may help to identify molecular targets for pharmacological and non-pharmacological interventions to prevent or delay the development of frailty, and also its consequences. Clinical validation of a candidate biomarker (Table 1) will provide support for the clinical diagnosis and monitoring of frailty or any of its associated risks.

It has been demonstrated that a biological epigenetic clock is better associated with frailty index [71] than the telomere length [54]. The DNA methylation patterns play a relevant role in explaining inter-individual differences in biological aging and frailty [36,72]. These studies suggest that an "accelerated" biological aging determined by epigenetic changes may be closely correlated to clinically relevant features related to frailty phenotypes [73].

3.2.1. DNA Methylation as a Frailty Biomarker

The first study performed to assess the potential relationship between epigenetic age acceleration and frailty-related characteristics was published in 2015. The authors performed a DNA methylation analysis in the Lothian Birth Cohort 1936 (LBC1936) and found significant correlation coefficients ranging from −0.05 to −0.07 between age acceleration based on the DNAm analysis and cognitive function, grip strength, or lung function [46].

Afterwards, Breitling and co-workers, studied the epigenetic clock developed by Horvath [40] in a cross-sectional observational study with 1820 subjects from two large subsets of community-dwelling older adults in the German ESTHER cohort study. These authors found that epigenetic age acceleration was correlated with clinically relevant aging-related phenotypes. More specifically, their results suggested one added functional deficit per 12 years of methylation age acceleration [54]. Importantly, in this study, the authors also found that telomere length measured in leukocytes, a well-studied parameter related with aging, was not associated with frailty index [54].

More recent studies have also explored the association between telomere length and DNAm with frailty. In the Berlin Aging Study II (BASE-II), a marginal association of age acceleration was found between leukocyte telomere length (rLTL) and DNAm [74]. However, in a recent work by Demuth et al., it was shown that neither DNAm age acceleration [51] nor rLTL were significantly associated with the Fried's Frailty Score or the functional assessments in the Berlin Aging Study II [75]. Interestingly, only one of the analyzed assessments, the clock drawing test, was significantly associated with DNAm age acceleration in older men, with an average of 1.9 years higher DNAm age acceleration [75]. This result seems important, because the clock drawing test is used to predict dementia and detect early-stage Alzheimer's disease [76]. The results reported by Demuth and co-workers seem contradictory to those described by Breitling's research group [54]. However, this might be the result of the different approaches used to measure frailty index and also the different methodologies used to measure DNAm age acceleration, the 353 CpG loci measurement according to the Hovarth's clock [40], and the seven-CpGs age acceleration method proposed by Vidal-Bralo and collaborators [51].

Further studies exploring the association of the "Meta-Clock" with frailty are needed to demonstrate its utility in assessing the relationship between epigenetic age acceleration and frailty-related phenotypes [48].

3.2.2. Histone PTMs and Histone Variants as Frailty Biomarkers

The implications of increased and decreased levels of histone acetylation in enhancing and constraining cognitive functions, particularly learning and memory have been demonstrated [77]. Accordingly, several histone deacetylase inhibitors (HDACis) have proven successful in rescuing cognitive deficits in animal models of neurodegeneration and cognitive decline such as Alzheimer's disease [77]. They might constitute a new strategy for pharmacological interventions against cognitive impairments by improving learning capacity, activating learning genes and mediating "cognitive epigenetic priming" [78]. "Cognitive epigenetic priming" is a theory that aims to explain the potential of histone acetylation to promote memory by facilitating the expression of neuroplasticity-related genes [78]. This is of special relevance, since cognitive impairment seems to be closely related with frailty, as we described above. Histone acetylation is closely related with other features associated with frailty such as sarcopenia. Global histone H3 methylation and acetylation decreases in muscle tissue with age, which may be linked to the well-known age-related type IIb fiber atrophy in skeletal muscle [79]. Walsh and collaborators demonstrated that the use of butyrate, an HDACi, increases the histone acetylation levels in skeletal muscle and prevents age-associated hindlimb muscle loss in female C57Bl/6 mice [80].

Measurement of the H2A histone family member X (H2AX) phosphorylation, at the amino acid Ser139, can provide information regarding frailty severity [81]. This was demonstrated in leukocytes and monocytes isolated from individuals classified as non-frail, pre-frail or frail depending on the Fried's frailty score [81]. The authors found that the percentage of γH2AX in the cells and the number of positive frailty criteria were significantly correlated ($r = 0.201$, $p < 0.01$). In addition, they performed a multivariate statistical analysis, adjusting by gender, age, and tobacco consumption (and alternatively adjusting by BMI), and confirmed previous results from univariate analyses on the influence of frailty. Therefore, frailty severity was accompanied by a progressive decrease in DNA repair capacity in lymphocytes ($p < 0.05$). Interestingly, the authors also independently studied the association of γH2AX with each one of the five Fried's frailty criteria: (i) unintentional weight loss; (ii) muscular weakness (grip strength); (iii) self-reported exhaustion; (iv) slow walking; and (v) low physical activity level [1] and found significantly higher γH2AX values in individuals positive for the low physical activity ($p < 0.001$), slow waking ($p < 0.01$) and low grip strength ($p < 0.01$) criteria. The main conclusion from this study is that the levels of γH2AX increase progressively according to frailty severity and that the use of the γH2AX levels, besides the micronucleus frequency in lymphocytes, could be a useful parameter to identify pre-frail and frail individuals [81]

3.2.3. Non-Coding RNAs as Frailty Biomarkers

Ipson and co-workers compared the differential expression of exosome-derived miRNAs from young adults by using small RNA sequencing (smallRNA-seq) in robust and frail individuals and identified eight enriched miRNAs associated with frailty: miR-10a-3p, miR-92a-3p, miR-185–3p, miR-194–5p, miR-326, miR-532–5p, miR-576–5p, and miR-760 [82].

Rusanova and collaborators [83] explored the expression of several miRNAs by RT-qPCR and found that robust subjects had higher expression of miR-146a, miR-223, and miR-483, while the frail ones showed higher expression of miR-21, miR-223, and miR-483 when compared to the control group. However, the authors found that miR-223 and miR-483 levels increased to a similar extent in robust and frail individuals matched by age, so both biomarkers should be considered as biomarkers of aging but not frailty. miR-223-5p targets BMI1, a transcript of a key gene involved in the self-renewal of bone marrow mesenchymal stem cells playing a critical role in promoting osteogenesis [84]. Further studies with bigger cohorts are needed to explore the potential of miR-223 as a candidate frailty biomarker due to its association with bone mass loss and osteoporosis [85].

Rusanova and coworkers have also reviewed different families of microRNAs linked to "inflammaging" (inflamma-miRs), to musculoskeletal health (myomiRs), and microRNAs that can directly or indirectly affect the mitochondrial function (mitomiRs) [69]. The list of miRNAs that can be considered as frailty biomarkers include: miR-1, miR-21, miR-34a, miR-146a, miR-185, and miR-206, miR-223 [69]. The importance of miR-21 as a potential frailty biomarker has also been suggested by other research groups [86].

Table 1. Epigenetic biomarkers to study frailty-related phenotypes.

Epigenetic Mechanism	Epigenetic Biomarker Associated to Frailty	Biospecimen	Association between the Epigenetic Change and Frailty	Reference
DNA methylation	Horvath's clock	Leukocytes	Epigenetic age acceleration was correlated with clinically relevant aging-related phenotypes	[54]
Histone PTMs	H3K9me3 and H3K9ac and H3K27ac decreases with age	Muscle samples in rat models	Muscle loss and sarcopenia	[79]
	γH2AX	Leukocytes	Significantly higher γH2AX values observed in individuals positive for low physical activity ($p < 0.001$), slow waking ($p < 0.01$), and low grip strength ($p < 0.01$) criteria	[81]
Non-coding RNAs	miR-10a-3p, miR-92a-3p, miR-185–3p, miR-194–5p, miR-326, miR-532–5p, miR-576–5p, miR-760	Plasma exosome-derived miRNAs	Associated to frailty	[82]
	miR-21, miR-223, miR-483	Plasma	Increased expression in frail subjects compared to control subjects	[83]
	miR-146a	Plasma	Low levels in frail subjects compared to robust old adults	[83]
	miR-1, miR-21, miR-34a, miR-146a, miR-185, miR-206, miR-223	Plasma	Increased levels in frail subjects compared to robust old adults	[69]
	miR-34a-5p miR-449b-5p	Muscle biopsy	Elevated in sarcopenic muscle compared with muscle tissue from controls	[87]

By using muscle biopsies and a microarray-based experimental approach, Zheng et al. found that miR-34a-5p and miR-449b-5p levels were elevated in sarcopenic muscles, highlighting their importance in muscle aging [87].

Further studies should be performed to increase the number of subjects and to provide reliable values for sensitivity and specificity, which may increase the validity of these miRNA as frailty biomarkers.

Regarding lncRNAs, in the LonGenity study, genome-wide association studies were used to explore whether variations in the 9p21–23 locus played a role in frailty in 637 community-dwelling older individuals [88]. The authors found associations between SNPs in the regulatory 9p21–23 region and the frailty phenotype; signifying the importance of this locus in aging [88]. Interestingly, the genomic locus 9p23 harbors several genes including ANRIL, a long non-coding RNA gene associated with cardiovascular diseases and strokes [89]. A polymorphism rs2811712 located in ANRIL gene has been associated with physical function in older people (65–80 years) with the minor allele being associated with reduced physical impairment [90]. However, although this SNP located into lncRNAs was indirectly associated with physical impairment, its expression levels have not yet been explored.

Other lncRNAs are feasible candidates to be investigated in elderly people to evaluate its contribution to frailty [91]. In this regard, lncRNA H19, is an interesting candidate because it plays a key role in myoblast differentiation during skeletal muscle regeneration by negatively regulating the bone morphogenetic protein (BMP) pathway [92]. Other lncRNAs that are related with muscle cells differentiation and proliferation are MALAT1, linc-MD1, and SIRT1 AS. lncRNA MALAT1 is downregulated by myostatin [93] and it suppresses the proliferation of myoblasts [94], suggesting that it may influence myogenesis during aging. Regarding linc-MD1, it is involved in the decline in skeletal muscle regeneration via HuR [95], a gene which is downregulated in differentiated muscle cells and contributes to sarcopenia. Another interesting lncRNA is SIRT1 AS, which is a natural antisense of the NAD-dependent deacetylase Sirt1. SIRT1 AS controls myogenic programs during muscle aging [96].

3.3. Epigenetic Biomarkers to Follow-up the Interventions in Frailty

There are two important characteristics regarding the frailty syndrome, firstly, if left unaddressed it will evolve into disability and eventually, death, and secondly, if it is properly treated, its onset can be delayed and the physiological condition of the subject can be improved [97].

The implementation of intervention programs in the elderly is not an easy task since it is a very heterogeneous population [98]. This heterogeneity is the basis of the previously mentioned field of personalized medicine, whose objective is to adapt interventions and treatments individually, considering the patient's lifestyle [99]. Interventional studies would undoubtedly benefit from the identification of frailty biomarkers, including epigenetic biomarkers.

There are no known pharmacologic interventions for the prevention of frailty [100]. However, because of major advances in understanding the molecular basis of aging, there is now tremendous interest and it is a very active area of investigation in the search for agents that may potentially modify human aging and health span. Delaying the onset of frailty is tightly correlated with improvement in health span. Although a single definition of health span is not available, a common definition is: "the period of life spent in good health, free from the chronic diseases and disabilities of aging" [101]. Several anti-aging interventions have potential translatability in the treatment and prevention of frailty [102]. Some of these interventions have been very well characterized in animal studies but they need to be tested in humans. The main pharmacological interventions in aging with potential translation to frailty are: caloric restriction mimetics such as (i) metformin, (ii) rapamycin, and (iii) resveratrol as well as more novel approaches that are emerging in the field such as (iv) nicotinamide adenine dinucleotide precursors, (v) synthetic activators of sirtuins such as SRT2104, and (vi) senolytics (dasatinib and quercetin) [102]. The ENRGISE (Enabling Reduction of Low-Grade Inflammation in Seniors) study deserves a comment in this section because it is an ongoing clinical trial (NCT02676466) that is examining the effect of fish oil and angiotensin receptor blockade on systemic inflammation and gait speed [100].

The main interventions developed to date to improve frailty-related health outcomes include lifestyle/behavioral factors: exercise, nutrition, multicomponent interventions, individually-tailored geriatric care models and cognitive health maintenance [32,100]. Among them, exercise is considered the most effective intervention in preclinical and clinical models of frailty [103,104].

In clinical practice, it has been shown that frailty can not only be delayed but also reversed by exercise training [105]. The use of an appropriate exercise program can delay or even reverse the physiological changes related to age that occur at the musculoskeletal level [97,106]. Multicomponent interventions have also proved beneficial to treat frailty. Multicomponent exercise is defined as a program of endurance, strength, coordination, balance, and flexibility exercises that have the potential to impact a variety of functional performance measurements. This type of exercise is a recommended alternative to more traditional exercise regimens, particularly due to its potential to impact functional performance outcomes in older adults [104,107–115].

One of the most successful multi-center intervention clinical trials with a one-year supervised physical activity program, "Lifestyle Interventions and Independence for Elders Pilot (LIFE-P) Study" (NCT00116194), established a 20% reduction in the prevalence of at least one criterion of frailty one year after the exercise program [116,117].

Exercise has an impact on several of the root mechanisms of aging also known as biological aging [118]. By doing so, it can delay phenotypic aging.

Despite the evidence of the benefits of physical exercise on health status, the prevalence of inactivity (35%) in subjects aged ≥75 years is worrisome [119]. Therefore, is very important to promote physical activity in this group of people. Several research groups have shown that supervised intervention programs aimed at improving the functionality of the elderly, fundamentally based on physical exercise, are more effective than those carried out autonomously in the subject's environment [109].

Physical exercise can influence fundamental epigenetic mechanisms such as DNA methylation in skeletal muscle. DNA methylation not only tracks chronological age in humans but also phenotypic changes along lifespan, predicting, for instance, cardiovascular mortality and other age-associated adverse outcomes [45]. Exercise-associated decrease in whole genome methylation has been found in muscle biopsies in healthy sedentary individuals after an acute bout of exercise [120,121]. This hypomethylation in specific promoters was accompanied by an increased expression of some genes involved in energy metabolism and mitochondrial function. These results suggest that DNA methylation changes can represent an active and adaptive response to skeletal muscle contraction. Methylation changes have also been analyzed in human skeletal muscle after a training program [122]. In this study the authors reported a significant modulation in DNA methylation in genes involved in structural changes of muscle tissue, inflammation, and immunological pathways after three months of endurance exercise training.

Lifelong physical activity is also able to induce hypomethylation in promoters of genes involved in resistance to oxidative stress, energy metabolism or myogenesis [123]. The exercise-induced epigenetic changes can be retained, and that DNA methylation could underpin the capacity of skeletal muscle to maintain information into later life and to respond differently to previous stimuli such as training [123].

Our current knowledge on how age-associated DNA methylation changes are related to frailty and the role of interventions such as exercise in epigenetic modifications is still sparse. Further research is needed because all the studies published up until now have been performed on young and healthy adults, and to date, no interventional studies have examined the effects of training on DNA methylation status in elderly people.

Apart from physical exercise, malnutrition and loneliness are other key aspects in the functional deterioration of the elderly. The prevalence of malnutrition in Western Europe in people over 65 is 23% on average and ranges between 6% and 51% [7]. This malnutrition, produced by a deficit of calories or protein, must be considered when proposing interventions aimed at improving the quality of life of our elderly.

4. Discussion and Conclusions

The identification of epigenetic biomarkers may contribute to the early detection of subclinical changes or deficits at the molecular and/or cellular level, to prevent or delay the development of frailty, and also its consequences. This will provide important support for the clinical diagnosis of frailty or any of its associated risks. Interventional studies would undoubtedly benefit from the search for biomarkers of frailty.

In addition, the identification of biomarkers can help to improve the health trajectory of the elderly, postponing and mitigating the appearance of functional problems. Improving the clinical follow-up of the elderly as well as predicting the future evolution of frailty and dependency in these people is a social and medical commitment. In this regard, it is necessary to orient research efforts in the design of personalized pharmacological and non-pharmacological interventions as a good example of personalized medicine.

Author Contributions: J.L.G.-G. drafted the manuscript and wrote it; S.M.-M. was involved in the literature search and analysis; M.C.G.-C. wrote sections of the manuscript and revised it; F.J.T.-S., J.V. and F.V.P. were involved in the conception and design of the review. They granted financial support and revised the manuscript. All authors have read and agreed to the published version of the manuscript.

Funding: This work was supported by FIS (PI16/01031) from the ISCIII, co-financed by European Regional Development Founds (ERDF). JLG-G is supported by the Spanish Ministry of Economy and Competitiveness and by the Instituto de Salud Carlos III through CIBERer (Biomedical Network Research Center for Rare Diseases and INGENIO2010). This project received funding from the program CREATEC-CV (IVACE) with the grant number IMCBTA/2018/29 and a grant from Agencia Valenciana de la Innovación (AVI) in the program "Incorporation of researchers for innovation projects in companies" (INNTA2/2020/4) from Generalitat Valenciana. J.L.G.-G. and S.M.-M. would like to thank IVACE for funding (IMIDTA/2020/54) through the program I+D PYME (PIDI-CV) 2020 and Ministerio de Ciencia e Innovación for PTQ2019-010552 through the program Torres Quevedo 2019. Work from FreshAge was supported by Instituto de Salud Carlos III CB16/10/00435 (CIBERFES), (PID2019-110906RB-I00/AEI/10.13039/501100011033) from the Spanish Ministry of Innovation and Science; 109_RESIFIT from Fundación General CSIC; PROMETEO/2019/097 de "Consellería, de Sanitat de la Generalitat Valenciana" and EU Funded H2020- DIABFRAIL-LATAM (Ref: 825546); European Joint Programming Initiative "A Healthy Diet for a Healthy Life" (JPI HDHL) and of the ERA-NET Cofund ERA-HDHL (GA N° 696295 of the EU Horizon 2020 Research and Innovation Programme). Part of the equipment employed in this work has been funded by Generalitat Valenciana and co-financed with ERDF funds (OP ERDF of Comunitat Valenciana 2014–2020).

Institutional Review Board Statement: Not applicable.

Informed Consent Statement: Not applicable.

Data Availability Statement: Not applicable.

Conflicts of Interest: The authors declare no competing interests.

References

1. Fried, L.P.; Tangen, C.M.; Walston, J.; Newman, A.B.; Hirsch, C.; Gottdiener, J.; Seeman, T.; Tracy, R.; Kop, W.J.; Burke, G.; et al. Frailty in Older Adults: Evidence for a Phenotype. *J. Gerontol. Ser. A Biol. Sci. Med. Sci.* **2001**, *56*, M146–M157. [CrossRef]
2. Rodriguez-Mañas, L.; Fried, L.P. Frailty in the clinical scenario. *Lancet* **2015**, *385*, e7–e9. [CrossRef]
3. Bisset, E.S.; Howlett, S.E. The biology of frailty in humans and animals: Understanding frailty and promoting translation. *Aging Med.* **2019**, *2*, 27–34. [CrossRef]
4. Rockwood, K. Conceptual Models of Frailty: Accumulation of Deficits. *Can. J. Cardiol.* **2016**, *32*, 1046–1050. [CrossRef] [PubMed]
5. van Deursen, J.M. The role of senescent cells in ageing. *Nature* **2014**, *509*, 439–446. [CrossRef] [PubMed]
6. Viña, J.; Tarazona-Santabalbina, F.J.; Pérez-Ros, P.; Martínez-Arnau, F.M.; Borras, C.; Olaso-Gonzalez, G.; Salvador-Pascual, A.; Gomez-Cabrera, M.C. Biology of frailty: Modulation of ageing genes and its importance to prevent age-associated loss of function. *Mol. Asp. Med.* **2016**, *50*, 88–108. [CrossRef]
7. Nascimento, C.M.; Ingles, M.; Salvador-Pascual, A.; Cominetti, M.R.; Gomez-Cabrera, M.C.; Viña, J. Sarcopenia, frailty and their prevention by exercise. *Free. Radic. Biol. Med.* **2019**, *132*, 42–49. [CrossRef]
8. Bock, J.-O.; König, H.-H.; Brenner, H.; Haefeli, W.E.; Quinzler, R.; Matschinger, H.; Saum, K.-U.; Schöttker, B.; Heider, D. Associations of frailty with health care costs—Results of the ESTHER cohort study. *BMC Health Serv. Res.* **2016**, *16*, 1–11. [CrossRef]
9. Collard, R.M.; Boter, H.; Schoevers, R.A.; Oude Voshaar, R.C. Prevalence of Frailty in Community-Dwelling Older Persons: A Systematic Review. *J. Am. Geriatr. Soc.* **2012**, *60*, 1487–1492. [CrossRef]
10. Eeles, E.M.P.; White, S.V.; O'Mahony, S.M.; Bayer, A.J.; Hubbard, R.E. The impact of frailty and delirium on mortality in older inpatients. *Age Ageing* **2012**, *41*, 412–416. [CrossRef] [PubMed]
11. Krishnan, M.; Beck, S.; Havelock, W.; Eeles, E.; Hubbard, R.E.; Johansen, A. Predicting outcome after hip fracture: Using a frailty index to integrate comprehensive geriatric assessment results. *Age Ageing* **2014**, *43*, 122–126. [CrossRef] [PubMed]
12. Hubbard, R.E.; Andrew, M.K.; Fallah, N.; Rockwood, K. Comparison of the prognostic importance of diagnosed diabetes, co-morbidity and frailty in older people. *Diabet. Med.* **2010**, *27*, 603–606. [CrossRef] [PubMed]

13. Sipila, S.; Taaffe, D.R.; Cheng, S.; Puolakka, J.; Toivanen, J.; Suominen, H. Effects of hormone replacement therapy and high-impact physical exercise on skeletal muscle in post-menopausal women: A randomized placebo-controlled study. *Clin. Sci.* **2001**, *101*, 147–157. [CrossRef]
14. Clegg, A.; Young, J.; Iliffe, S.; Rikkert, M.O.; Rockwood, K. Frailty in elderly people. *Lancet* **2013**, *381*, 752–762. [CrossRef]
15. Marzetti, E.; Leeuwenburgh, C. Skeletal muscle apoptosis, sarcopenia and frailty at old age. *Exp. Gerontol.* **2006**, *41*, 1234–1238. [CrossRef] [PubMed]
16. Vaz Fragoso, C.A.; Enright, P.L.; McAvay, G.; Van Ness, P.H.; Gill, T.M. Frailty and Respiratory Impairment in Older Persons. *Am. J. Med.* **2012**, *125*, 79–86. [CrossRef]
17. Lutski, M.; Haratz, S.; Weinstein, G.; Goldbourt, U.; Tanne, D. Impaired Cerebral Hemodynamics and Frailty in Patients with Cardiovascular Disease. *J. Gerontol. Ser. A* **2018**, *73*, 1714–1721. [CrossRef]
18. Drew, W.; Wilson, D.; Sapey, E. Frailty and the immune system. *J. Aging Res. Health* **2017**, *2*, 1–14. [CrossRef]
19. Abel, G.A.; Buckstein, R. Integrating Frailty, Comorbidity, and Quality of Life in the Management of Myelodysplastic Syndromes. *Am. Soc. Clin. Oncol. Educ. Book* **2016**, *36*, e337–e344. [CrossRef]
20. Walston, J.; Fedarko, N.; Yang, H.; Leng, S.; Beamer, B.; Espinoza, S.; Lipton, A.; Zheng, H.; Becker, K. The Physical and Biological Characterization of a Frail Mouse Model. *J. Gerontol. Ser. A Boil. Sci. Med. Sci.* **2008**, *63*, 391–398. [CrossRef]
21. Boyle, P.A.; Buchman, A.S.; Wilson, R.S.; Leurgans, S.E.; Bennett, D.A. Physical frailty is associated with incident mild cognitive impairment in community-based older persons. *J. Am. Geriatr. Soc.* **2010**, *58*, 248–255. [CrossRef]
22. Lipton, M.L.; Ifrah, C.; Stewart, W.F.; Fleysher, R.; Sliwinski, M.J.; Kim, M.; Lipton, R.B. Validation of HeadCount-2w for estimation of two-week heading: Comparison to daily reporting in adult amateur player. *J. Sci. Med. Sport* **2018**, *21*, 363–367. [CrossRef]
23. Beltrán-García, J.; Osca-Verdegal, R.; Mena-Mollá, S.; García-Giménez, J.L. Epigenetic IVD Tests for Personalized Precision Medicine in Cancer. *Front. Genet.* **2019**, *10*, 621. [CrossRef]
24. Garcia-Gimenez, J.L.; Sanchis-Gomar, F.; Lippi, G.; Mena, S.; Ivars, D.; Gomez-Cabrera, M.C.; Vina, J.; Pallardo, F.V. Epigenetic biomarkers: A new perspective in laboratory diagnostics. *Clin. Chim. Acta* **2012**, *413*, 1576–1582. [CrossRef] [PubMed]
25. García-Giménez, J.L.; Seco-Cervera, M.; Tollefsbol, T.O.; Romá-Mateo, C.; Peiró-Chova, L.; Lapunzina, P.; Pallardó, F.V. Epigenetic biomarkers: Current strategies and future challenges for their use in the clinical laboratory. *Crit. Rev. Clin. Lab. Sci.* **2017**, *54*, 529–550. [CrossRef]
26. Sandoval, J.; Peiró-Chova, L.; Pallardó, F.V.; García-Giménez, J.L. Epigenetic biomarkers in laboratory diagnostics: Emerging approaches and opportunities. *Expert Rev. Mol. Diagn.* **2013**, *13*, 457–471. [CrossRef]
27. Pal, S.; Tyler, J.K. Epigenetics and aging. *Sci. Adv.* **2016**, *2*, e1600584. [CrossRef] [PubMed]
28. Ferrucci, L.; Cavazzini, C.; Corsi, A.; Bartali, B.; Russo, C.R.; Lauretani, F.; Corsi, A.M.; Bandinelli, S.; Guralnik, J.M. Biomarkers of frailty in older persons. *J. Endocrinol. Investig.* **2002**, *25*, 10–15.
29. van der Graaf, A.; Wardenaar, R.; Neumann, D.A.; Taudt, A.; Shaw, R.G.; Jansen, R.C.; Schmitz, R.J.; Colomé-Tatché, M.; Johannes, F. Rate, spectrum, and evolutionary dynamics of spontaneous epimutations. *Proc. Natl. Acad. Sci. USA* **2015**, *112*, 6676–6681. [CrossRef] [PubMed]
30. Cruickshanks, H.A.; McBryan, T.; Nelson, D.M.; VanderKraats, N.D.; Shah, P.P.; van Tuyn, J.; Singh Rai, T.; Brock, C.; Donahue, G.; Dunican, D.S.; et al. Senescent cells harbour features of the cancer epigenome. *Nat. Cell Biol.* **2013**, *15*, 1495–1506. [CrossRef] [PubMed]
31. Jung, M.; Pfeifer, G.P. Aging and DNA methylation. *BMC Biol.* **2015**, *13*, 1–8. [CrossRef] [PubMed]
32. Gomez-Verjan, J.C.; Ramírez-Aldana, R.; Pérez-Zepeda, M.U.; Quiroz-Baez, R.; Luna-López, A.; Gutierrez Robledo, L.M. Systems biology and network pharmacology of frailty reveal novel epigenetic targets and mechanisms. *Sci. Rep.* **2019**, *9*, 10593. [CrossRef] [PubMed]
33. Fraga, M.F.; Ballestar, E.; Paz, M.F.; Ropero, S.; Setien, F.; Ballestar, M.L.; Heine-Suner, D.; Cigudosa, J.C.; Urioste, M.; Benitez, J.; et al. From The Cover: Epigenetic differences arise during the lifetime of monozygotic twins. *Proc. Natl. Acad. Sci. USA* **2005**, *102*, 10604–10609. [CrossRef]
34. Veitia, R.A.; Govindaraju, D.R.; Bottani, S.; Birchler, J.A. Aging: Somatic Mutations, Epigenetic Drift and Gene Dosage Imbalance. *Trends Cell Biol.* **2017**, *27*, 299–310. [CrossRef]
35. Sousa-Victor, P.; Gutarra, S.; García-Prat, L.; Rodriguez-Ubreva, J.; Ortet, L.; Ruiz-Bonilla, V.; Jardí, M.; Ballestar, E.; González, S.; Serrano, A.L.; et al. Geriatric muscle stem cells switch reversible quiescence into senescence. *Nature* **2014**, *506*, 316–321. [CrossRef]
36. Bellizzi, D.; D'Aquila, P.; Montesanto, A.; Corsonello, A.; Mari, V.; Mazzei, B.; Lattanzio, F.; Passarino, G. Global DNA methylation in old subjects is correlated with frailty. *AGE* **2012**, *34*, 169–179. [CrossRef] [PubMed]
37. Montesanto, A.; Lagani, V.; Martino, C.; Dato, S.; De Rango, F.; Berardelli, M.; Corsonello, A.; Mazzei, B.; Mari, V.; Lattanzio, F.; et al. A novel, population-specific approach to define frailty. *AGE* **2010**, *32*, 385–395. [CrossRef]
38. Horvath, S.; Raj, K. DNA methylation-based biomarkers and the epigenetic clock theory of ageing. *Nat. Rev. Genet.* **2018**, *19*, 371–384. [CrossRef] [PubMed]
39. Roetker, N.S.; Pankow, J.S.; Bressler, J.; Morrison, A.C.; Boerwinkle, E. Prospective Study of Epigenetic Age Acceleration and Incidence of Cardiovascular Disease Outcomes in the ARIC Study (Atherosclerosis Risk in Communities). *Circ. Genom. Precis. Med.* **2018**, *11*, e001937. [CrossRef] [PubMed]
40. Horvath, S. DNA methylation age of human tissues and cell types. *Genome Biol.* **2013**, *14*, R115. [CrossRef]

41. Ambatipudi, S.; Horvath, S.; Perrier, F.; Cuenin, C.; Hernandez-Vargas, H.; Le Calvez-Kelm, F.; Durand, G.; Byrnes, G.; Ferrari, P.; Bouaoun, L.; et al. DNA methylome analysis identifies accelerated epigenetic ageing associated with postmenopausal breast cancer susceptibility. *Eur. J. Cancer* **2017**, *75*, 299–307. [CrossRef]
42. Levine, M.E.; Hosgood, H.D.; Chen, B.; Absher, D.; Assimes, T.; Horvath, S. DNA methylation age of blood predicts future onset of lung cancer in the women's health initiative. *Aging* **2015**, *7*, 690–700. [CrossRef]
43. Levine, M.E.; Lu, A.T.; Bennett, D.A.; Horvath, S. Epigenetic age of the pre-frontal cortex is associated with neuritic plaques, amyloid load, and Alzheimer's disease related cognitive functioning. *Aging* **2015**, *7*, 1198–1211. [CrossRef]
44. Chen, B.H.; Marioni, R.E.; Colicino, E.; Peters, M.J.; Ward-Caviness, C.K.; Tsai, P.-C.; Roetker, N.S.; Just, A.C.; Demerath, E.W.; Guan, W.; et al. DNA methylation-based measures of biological age: Meta-analysis predicting time to death. *Aging* **2016**, *8*, 1844–1865. [CrossRef]
45. Levine, M.E.; Lu, A.T.; Quach, A.; Chen, B.H.; Assimes, T.L.; Bandinelli, S.; Hou, L.; Baccarelli, A.A.; Stewart, J.D.; Li, Y.; et al. An epigenetic biomarker of aging for lifespan and healthspan. *Aging* **2018**, *10*, 573–591. [CrossRef]
46. Marioni, R.E.; Shah, S.; McRae, A.F.; Ritchie, S.J.; Muniz-Terrera, G.; Harris, S.E.; Gibson, J.; Redmond, P.; Cox, S.R.; Pattie, A.; et al. The epigenetic clock is correlated with physical and cognitive fitness in the Lothian Birth Cohort 1936. *Int. J. Epidemiol.* **2015**, *44*, 1388–1396. [CrossRef] [PubMed]
47. Zhang, Y.; Wilson, R.; Heiss, J.; Breitling, L.P.; Saum, K.-U.; Schöttker, B.; Holleczek, B.; Waldenberger, M.; Peters, A.; Brenner, H. DNA methylation signatures in peripheral blood strongly predict all-cause mortality. *Nat. Commun.* **2017**, *8*, 14617. [CrossRef] [PubMed]
48. Liu, Z.; Leung, D.; Thrush, K.; Zhao, W.; Ratliff, S.; Tanaka, T.; Schmitz, L.L.; Smith, J.A.; Ferrucci, L.; Levine, M.E. Underlying features of epigenetic aging clocks in vivo and in vitro. *Aging Cell* **2020**, *19*, e13229. [CrossRef] [PubMed]
49. Hannum, G.; Guinney, J.; Zhao, L.; Zhang, L.; Hughes, G.; Sadda, S.; Klotzle, B.; Bibikova, M.; Fan, J.-B.; Gao, Y.; et al. Genome-wide Methylation Profiles Reveal Quantitative Views of Human Aging Rates. *Mol. Cell* **2013**, *49*, 359–367. [CrossRef] [PubMed]
50. Weidner, C.; Lin, Q.; Koch, C.; Eisele, L.; Beier, F.; Ziegler, P.; Bauerschlag, D.; Jöckel, K.-H.; Erbel, R.; Mühleisen, T.; et al. Aging of blood can be tracked by DNA methylation changes at just three CpG sites. *Genome Biol.* **2014**, *15*, R24. [CrossRef]
51. Vidal-Bralo, L.; Lopez-Golan, Y.; Gonzalez, A. Simplified Assay for Epigenetic Age Estimation in Whole Blood of Adults. *Front. Genet.* **2016**, *7*, 126. [CrossRef] [PubMed]
52. Lin, Q.; Wagner, W. Epigenetic Aging Signatures Are Coherently Modified in Cancer. *PLoS Genet.* **2015**, *11*, e1005334. [CrossRef]
53. Bergsma, T.; Rogaeva, E. DNA Methylation Clocks and Their Predictive Capacity for Aging Phenotypes and Healthspan. *Neurosci. Insights* **2020**, *15*, 263310552094222. [CrossRef]
54. Breitling, L.P.; Saum, K.-U.; Perna, L.; Schöttker, B.; Holleczek, B.; Brenner, H. Frailty is associated with the epigenetic clock but not with telomere length in a German cohort. *Clin. Epigenet.* **2016**, *8*, 1–8. [CrossRef] [PubMed]
55. Gale, C.R.; Marioni, R.E.; Harris, S.E.; Starr, J.M.; Deary, I.J. DNA methylation and the epigenetic clock in relation to physical frailty in older people: The Lothian Birth Cohort 1936. *Clin. Epigenet.* **2018**, *10*, 101. [CrossRef]
56. Kim, D.H.; Schneeweiss, S.; Glynn, R.J.; Lipsitz, L.A.; Rockwood, K.; Avorn, J. Measuring Frailty in Medicare Data: Development and Validation of a Claims-Based Frailty Index. *J. Gerontol. Ser. A* **2018**, *73*, 980–987. [CrossRef] [PubMed]
57. García-Giménez, J.L.; Romá-Mateo, C.; Pallardó, F.V. Oxidative post-translational modifications in histones. *BioFactors* **2019**, *45*, 641–650. [CrossRef] [PubMed]
58. Benayoun, B.A.; Pollina, E.A.; Brunet, A. Epigenetic regulation of ageing: Linking environmental inputs to genomic stability. *Nat. Rev. Mol. Cell Biol.* **2015**, *16*, 593–610. [CrossRef]
59. Siddiqui, M.S.; François, M.; Fenech, M.F.; Leifert, W.R. Persistent γH2AX: A promising molecular marker of DNA damage and aging. *Mutat. Res. Mutat. Res.* **2015**, *766*, 1–19. [CrossRef]
60. Sedelnikova, O.A.; Horikawa, I.; Redon, C.; Nakamura, A.; Zimonjic, D.B.; Popescu, N.C.; Bonner, W.M. Delayed kinetics of DNA double-strand break processing in normal and pathological aging. *Aging Cell* **2008**, *7*, 89–100. [CrossRef]
61. He, L.; Hannon, G.J. MicroRNAs: Small RNAs with a big role in gene regulation. *Nat. Rev. Genet.* **2004**, *5*, 522–531. [CrossRef] [PubMed]
62. Vasudevan, S.; Tong, Y.; Steitz, J.A. Switching from repression to activation: MicroRNAs can up-regulate translation. *Science* **2007**, *318*, 1931–1934. [CrossRef] [PubMed]
63. Ponting, C.P.; Oliver, P.L.; Reik, W. Evolution and functions of long noncoding RNAs. *Cell* **2009**, *136*, 629–641. [CrossRef]
64. Mercer, T.R.; Mattick, J.S. Structure and function of long noncoding RNAs in epigenetic regulation. *Nat. Struct. Mol. Biol.* **2013**, *20*, 300–307. [CrossRef]
65. Kobashigawa, J.; Dadhania, D.; Bhorade, S.; Adey, D.; Berger, J.; Bhat, G.; Budev, M.; Duarte-Rojo, A.; Dunn, M.; Hall, S.; et al. Report from the American Society of Transplantation on frailty in solid organ transplantation. *Am. J. Transplant.* **2019**, *19*, 984–994. [CrossRef] [PubMed]
66. Sannicandro, A.J.; Soriano-Arroquia, A.; Goljanek-Whysall, K. Micro(RNA)-managing muscle wasting. *J. Appl. Physiol.* **2019**, *127*, 619–632. [CrossRef] [PubMed]
67. Smith-Vikos, T.; Liu, Z.; Parsons, C.; Gorospe, M.; Ferrucci, L.; Gill, T.M.; Slack, F.J. A serum miRNA profile of human longevity: Findings from the Baltimore Longitudinal Study of Aging (BLSA). *Aging* **2016**, *8*, 2971–2987. [CrossRef] [PubMed]

68. Valadi, H.; Ekström, K.; Bossios, A.; Sjöstrand, M.; Lee, J.J.; Lötvall, J.O. Exosome-mediated transfer of mRNAs and microRNAs is a novel mechanism of genetic exchange between cells. *Nat. Cell Biol.* **2007**, *9*, 654–659. [CrossRef]
69. Rusanova, I.; Fernández-Martínez, J.; Fernández-Ortiz, M.; Aranda-Martínez, P.; Escames, G.; García-García, F.J.; Mañas, L.; Acuña-Castroviejo, D. Involvement of plasma miRNAs, muscle miRNAs and mitochondrial miRNAs in the pathophysiology of frailty. *Exp. Gerontol.* **2019**, *124*, 110637. [CrossRef]
70. García-Giménez, J.L. *Epigenetic Biomarkers and Diagnostics*; Academic Press: Amsterdam, The Netherlands, 2015.
71. Theou, O.; Sluggett, J.K.; Bell, J.S.; Lalic, S.; Cooper, T.; Robson, L.; Morley, J.E.; Rockwood, K.; Visvanathan, R. Frailty, Hospitalization, and Mortality in Residential Aged Care. *J. Gerontol. Ser. A* **2018**, *73*, 1090–1096. [CrossRef]
72. Collerton, J.; Gautrey, H.E.; van Otterdijk, S.D.; Davies, K.; Martin-Ruiz, C.; von Zglinicki, T.; Kirkwood, T.B.L.; Jagger, C.; Mathers, J.C.; Strathdee, G. Acquisition of aberrant DNA methylation is associated with frailty in the very old: Findings from the Newcastle 85+ Study. *Biogerontology* **2014**, *15*, 317–328. [CrossRef] [PubMed]
73. Mitnitski, A.; Rockwood, K. The rate of aging: The rate of deficit accumulation does not change over the adult life span. *Biogerontology* **2016**, *17*, 199–204. [CrossRef]
74. Vetter, V.M.; Meyer, A.; Karbasiyan, M.; Steinhagen-Thiessen, E.; Hopfenmüller, W.; Demuth, I. Epigenetic Clock and Relative Telomere Length Represent Largely Different Aspects of Aging in the Berlin Aging Study II (BASE-II). *J. Gerontol. Ser. A* **2019**, *74*, 27–32. [CrossRef] [PubMed]
75. Vetter, V.M.; Spira, D.; Banszerus, V.L.; Demuth, I. Epigenetic Clock and Leukocyte Telomere Length Are Associated with Vitamin D Status but not with Functional Assessments and Frailty in the Berlin Aging Study II. *J. Gerontol. Ser. A* **2020**, *75*, 2056–2063. [CrossRef] [PubMed]
76. Shulman, K.I. Clock-drawing: Is it the ideal cognitive screening test? *Int. J. Geriatr. Psychiatry* **2000**, *15*, 548–561. [CrossRef]
77. Gräff, J.; Tsai, L.H. Histone acetylation: Molecular mnemonics on the chromatin. *Nat. Rev. Neurosci.* **2013**, *14*, 97–111. [CrossRef]
78. Burns, A.M.; Gräff, J. Cognitive epigenetic priming: Leveraging histone acetylation for memory amelioration. *Curr. Opin. Neurobiol.* **2020**, *67*, 75–84. [CrossRef]
79. Yoshihara, T.; Machida, S.; Tsuzuki, T.; Kakigi, R.; Chang, S.W.; Sugiura, T.; Naito, H. Age-related changes in histone modification in rat gastrocnemius muscle. *Exp. Gerontol.* **2019**, *125*, 110658. [CrossRef]
80. Walsh, M.E.; Bhattacharya, A.; Sataranatarajan, K.; Qaisar, R.; Sloane, L.; Rahman, M.M.; Kinter, M.; Van Remmen, H. The histone deacetylase inhibitor butyrate improves metabolism and reduces muscle atrophy during aging. *Aging Cell* **2015**, *14*, 957–970. [CrossRef] [PubMed]
81. Valdiglesias, V.; Sánchez-Flores, M.; Marcos-Pérez, D.; Lorenzo-López, L.; Maseda, A.; Millán-Calenti, J.C.; Pásaro, E.; Laffon, B. Exploring Genetic Outcomes as Frailty Biomarkers. *J. Gerontol. Ser. A* **2019**, *74*, 168–175. [CrossRef]
82. Ipson, B.R.; Fletcher, M.B.; Espinoza, S.E.; Fisher, A.L. Identifying Exosome-Derived MicroRNAs as Candidate Biomarkers of Frailty. *J. Frailty Aging* **2018**, *7*, 100–103. [CrossRef]
83. Rusanova, I.; Diaz-Casado, M.E.; Fernández-Ortiz, M.; Aranda-Martínez, P.; Guerra-Librero, A.; García-García, F.J.; Escames, G.; Mañas, L.; Acuña-Castroviejo, D. Analysis of Plasma MicroRNAs as Predictors and Biomarkers of Aging and Frailty in Humans. *Oxidative Med. Cell. Longev.* **2018**, *2018*, 1–9. [CrossRef] [PubMed]
84. García-Giménez, J.L.; Rubio-Belmar, P.A.; Peiró-Chova, L.; Hervás, D.; González-Rodríguez, D.; Ibañez-Cabellos, J.S.; Bas-Hermida, P.; Mena-Mollá, S.; García-López, E.M.; Pallardó, F.V.; et al. Circulating miRNAs as diagnostic biomarkers for adolescent idiopathic scoliosis. *Sci. Rep.* **2018**, *8*, 2646. [CrossRef] [PubMed]
85. Greco, E.A.; Pietschmann, P.; Migliaccio, S. Osteoporosis and Sarcopenia Increase Frailty Syndrome in the Elderly. *Front. Endocrinol.* **2019**, *10*, 255. [CrossRef]
86. Wu, I.C.; Lin, C.C.; Hsiung, C.A. Emerging roles of frailty and inflammaging in risk assessment of age-related chronic diseases in older adults: The intersection between aging biology and personalized medicine. *Biomedicine* **2015**, *5*, 1. [CrossRef]
87. Zheng, Y.; Kong, J.; Li, Q.; Wang, Y.; Li, J. Role of miRNAs in skeletal muscle aging. *Clin. Interv. Aging* **2018**, *13*, 2407–2419. [CrossRef]
88. Sathyan, S.; Barzilai, N.; Atzmon, G.; Milman, S.; Ayers, E.; Verghese, J. Genetic Insights Into Frailty: Association of 9p21-23 Locus With Frailty. *Front. Med.* **2018**, *5*, 105. [CrossRef]
89. Pasmant, E.; Sabbagh, A.; Vidaud, M.; Bièche, I. ANRIL, a long, noncoding RNA, is an unexpected major hotspot in GWAS. *FASEB J.* **2011**, *25*, 444–448. [CrossRef]
90. Melzer, D.; Frayling, T.M.; Murray, A.; Hurst, A.J.; Harries, L.W.; Song, H.; Khaw, K.; Luben, R.; Surtees, P.G.; Bandinelli, S.S.; et al. A common variant of the p16(INK4a) genetic region is associated with physical function in older people. *Mech. Ageing Dev.* **2007**, *128*, 370–377. [CrossRef] [PubMed]
91. Kim, J.; Kim, K.M.; Noh, J.H.; Yoon, J.H.; Abdelmohsen, K.; Gorospe, M. Long noncoding RNAs in diseases of aging. *Biochim. Biophys. Acta* **2016**, *1859*, 209–221. [CrossRef]
92. Dey, B.K.; Pfeifer, K.; Dutta, A. The H19 long noncoding RNA gives rise to microRNAs miR-675-3p and miR-675-5p to promote skeletal muscle differentiation and regeneration. *Genes Dev.* **2014**, *28*, 491–501. [CrossRef]
93. McKay, B.R.; Ogborn, D.I.; Bellamy, L.M.; Tarnopolsky, M.A.; Parise, G. Myostatin is associated with age-related human muscle stem cell dysfunction. *FASEB J.* **2012**, *26*, 2509–2521. [CrossRef]
94. Watts, R.; Johnsen, V.L.; Shearer, J.; Hittel, D.S. Myostatin-induced inhibition of the long noncoding RNA Malat1 is associated with decreased myogenesis. *Am. J. Physiol. Cell Physiol.* **2013**, *304*, C995–C1001. [CrossRef] [PubMed]

95. Legnini, I.; Morlando, M.; Mangiavacchi, A.; Fatica, A.; Bozzoni, I. A feedforward regulatory loop between HuR and the long noncoding RNA linc-MD1 controls early phases of myogenesis. *Mol. Cell* **2014**, *53*, 506–514. [CrossRef]
96. Pardo, P.S.; Boriek, A.M. The physiological roles of Sirt1 in skeletal muscle. *Aging (Albany NY)* **2011**, *3*, 430–437. [CrossRef] [PubMed]
97. Viña, J.; Rodriguez-Mañas, L.; Salvador-Pascual, A.; Tarazona-Santabalbina, F.J.; Gomez-Cabrera, M.C. Exercise: The lifelong supplement for healthy ageing and slowing down the onset of frailty. *J. Physiol.* **2016**, *594*, 1989–1999. [CrossRef]
98. Arc-Chagnaud, C.; Millan, F.; Salvador-Pascual, A.; Correas, A.G.; Olaso-Gonzalez, G.; De la Rosa, A.; Carretero, A.; Gomez-Cabrera, M.C.; Viña, J. Reversal of age-associated frailty by controlled physical exercise: The pre-clinical and clinical evidences. *Sports Med. Health Sci.* **2019**, *1*, 33–39. [CrossRef]
99. Ramírez-Vélez, R.; Izquierdo, M. Editorial: Precision Physical Activity and Exercise Prescriptions for Disease Prevention: The Effect of Interindividual Variability Under Different Training Approaches. *Front. Physiol.* **2019**, *10*, 646. [CrossRef] [PubMed]
100. Espinoza, S.E.; Jiwani, R.; Wang, J.; Wang, C.P. Review of Interventions for the Frailty Syndrome and the Role of Metformin as a Potential Pharmacologic Agent for Frailty Prevention. *Clin. Ther.* **2019**, *41*, 376–386. [CrossRef] [PubMed]
101. Kaeberlein, M. How healthy is the healthspan concept? *Geroscience* **2018**, *40*, 361–364. [CrossRef] [PubMed]
102. Palliyaguru, D.L.; Moats, J.M.; Di Germanio, C.; Bernier, M.; de Cabo, R. Frailty index as a biomarker of lifespan and healthspan: Focus on pharmacological interventions. *Mech. Ageing Dev.* **2019**, *180*, 42–48. [CrossRef]
103. Garcia-Valles, R.; Gomez-Cabrera, M.C.; Rodriguez-Manas, L.; Garcia-Garcia, F.J.; Diaz, A.; Noguera, I.; Olaso-Gonzalez, G.; Vina, J. Life-long spontaneous exercise does not prolong lifespan but improves health span in mice. *Longev. Health* **2013**, *2*, 14. [CrossRef]
104. Gomez-Cabrera, M.C.; Garcia-Valles, R.; Rodriguez-Manas, L.; Garcia-Garcia, F.J.; Olaso-Gonzalez, G.; Salvador-Pascual, A.; Tarazona-Santabalbina, F.J.; Viña, J. A New Frailty Score for Experimental Animals Based on the Clinical Phenotype: Inactivity as a Model of Frailty. *J. Gerontol. A Biol. Sci. Med. Sci.* **2017**, *72*, 885–891. [CrossRef]
105. Tarazona-Santabalbina, F.J.; Gomez-Cabrera, M.C.; Perez-Ros, P.; Martinez-Arnau, F.M.; Cabo, H.; Tsaparas, K.; Salvador-Pascual, A.; Rodriguez-Manas, L.; Vina, J. A Multicomponent Exercise Intervention that Reverses Frailty and Improves Cognition, Emotion, and Social Networking in the Community-Dwelling Frail Elderly: A Randomized Clinical Trial. *J. Am. Med. Dir. Assoc.* **2016**, *17*, 426–433. [CrossRef] [PubMed]
106. Viña, J.; Salvador-Pascual, A.; Tarazona-Santabalbina, F.J.; Rodriguez-Mañas, L.; Gomez-Cabrera, M.C. Exercise training as a drug to treat age associated frailty. *Free. Radic. Biol. Med.* **2016**, *98*, 159–164. [CrossRef]
107. Marques, E.; Carvalho, J.; Soares, J.M.; Marques, F.; Mota, J. Effects of resistance and multicomponent exercise on lipid profiles of older women. *Maturitas* **2009**, *63*, 84–88. [CrossRef] [PubMed]
108. Cadore, E.L.; Casas-Herrero, A.; Zambom-Ferraresi, F.; Idoate, F.; Millor, N.; Gomez, M.; Rodriguez-Manas, L.; Izquierdo, M. Multicomponent exercises including muscle power training enhance muscle mass, power output, and functional outcomes in institutionalized frail nonagenarians. *Age (Dordr)* **2014**, *36*, 773–785. [CrossRef]
109. Gine-Garriga, M.; Roque-Figuls, M.; Coll-Planas, L.; Sitja-Rabert, M.; Salva, A. Physical exercise interventions for improving performance-based measures of physical function in community-dwelling, frail older adults: A systematic review and meta-analysis. *Arch. Phys. Med. Rehabil.* **2014**, *95*, 753–769.e753. [CrossRef]
110. Gudlaugsson, J.; Gudnason, V.; Aspelund, T.; Siggeirsdottir, K.; Olafsdottir, A.S.; Jonsson, P.V.; Arngrimsson, S.A.; Harris, T.B.; Johannsson, E. Effects of a 6-month multimodal training intervention on retention of functional fitness in older adults: A randomized-controlled cross-over design. *Int. J. Behav. Nutr. Phys. Act.* **2012**, *9*, 107. [CrossRef]
111. Jeon, M.Y.; Jeong, H.; Petrofsky, J.; Lee, H.; Yim, J. Effects of a randomized controlled recurrent fall prevention program on risk factors for falls in frail elderly living at home in rural communities. *Med. Sci. Monit.* **2014**, *20*, 2283–2291. [CrossRef] [PubMed]
112. Lee, H.C.; Chang, K.C.; Tsauo, J.Y.; Hung, J.W.; Huang, Y.C.; Lin, S.I.; Fall Prevention Initiatives in Taiwan (FPIT) Investigators. Effects of a multifactorial fall prevention program on fall incidence and physical function in community-dwelling older adults with risk of falls. *Arch. Phys. Med. Rehabil.* **2013**, *94*, 606–615.e601. [CrossRef]
113. Rosendahl, E.; Lindelöf, N.; Littbrand, H.; Yifter-Lindgren, E.; Lundin-Olsson, L.; Håglin, L.; Gustafson, Y.; Nyberg, L. High-intensity functional exercise program and protein-enriched energy supplement for older persons dependent in activities of daily living: A randomised controlled trial. *Aust. J. Physiother.* **2006**, *52*, 105–113. [CrossRef]
114. Serra-Rexach, J.A.; Bustamante-Ara, N.; Villarán, M.H.; Gil, P.G.; Ibáñez, M.J.S.; Bsc, N.B.S.; Bsc, V.O.S.; Bsc, N.G.S.; Bsc, A.B.M.P.; Gallardo, C.; et al. Short-term, light- to moderate-intensity exercise training improves leg muscle strength in the oldest old: A randomized controlled trial. *J. Am. Geriatr. Soc.* **2011**, *59*, 594–602. [CrossRef]
115. Zech, A.; Drey, M.; Freiberger, E.; Hentschke, C.; Bauer, J.M.; Sieber, C.C.; Pfeifer, K. Residual effects of muscle strength and muscle power training and detraining on physical function in community-dwelling prefrail older adults: A randomized controlled trial. *BMC Geriatr.* **2012**, *12*, 68. [CrossRef]
116. Cesari, M.; Vellas, B.; Hsu, F.C.; Newman, A.B.; Doss, H.; King, A.C.; Manini, T.M.; Church, T.; Gill, T.M.; Miller, M.E.; et al. A physical activity intervention to treat the frailty syndrome in older persons-results from the LIFE-P study. *J. Gerontol. A Biol. Sci. Med. Sci.* **2015**, *70*, 216–222. [CrossRef] [PubMed]
117. Fielding, R.A.; Guralnik, J.M.; King, A.C.; Pahor, M.; McDermott, M.M.; Tudor-Locke, C.; Manini, T.M.; Glynn, N.W.; Marsh, A.P.; Axtell, R.S.; et al. Dose of physical activity, physical functioning and disability risk in mobility-limited older adults: Results from the LIFE study randomized trial. *PLoS ONE* **2017**, *12*, e0182155. [CrossRef] [PubMed]

118. Ferrucci, L.; Levine, M.E.; Kuo, P.L.; Simonsick, E.M. Time and the Metrics of Aging. *Circ. Res.* **2018**, *123*, 740–744. [CrossRef] [PubMed]
119. Derbre, F.; Gratas-Delamarche, A.; Gomez-Cabrera, M.C.; Viña, J. Inactivity-induced oxidative stress: A central role in sarcopenia? *Eur. J. Sport Sci.* **2012**, *14*, S98–S108. [CrossRef] [PubMed]
120. Barrès, R.; Yan, J.; Egan, B.; Treebak, J.T.; Rasmussen, M.; Fritz, T.; Caidahl, K.; Krook, A.; O'Gorman, D.J.; Zierath, J.R. Acute exercise remodels promoter methylation in human skeletal muscle. *Cell Metab.* **2012**, *15*, 405–411. [CrossRef]
121. Lindholm, M.E.; Marabita, F.; Gomez-Cabrero, D.; Rundqvist, H.; Ekström, T.J.; Tegnér, J.; Sundberg, C.J. An integrative analysis reveals coordinated reprogramming of the epigenome and the transcriptome in human skeletal muscle after training. *Epigenetics* **2014**, *9*, 1557–1569. [CrossRef]
122. Sailani, M.R.; Halling, J.F.; Møller, H.D.; Lee, H.; Plomgaard, P.; Pilegaard, H.; Snyder, M.P.; Regenberg, B. Lifelong physical activity is associated with promoter hypomethylation of genes involved in metabolism, myogenesis, contractile properties and oxidative stress resistance in aged human skeletal muscle. *Sci. Rep.* **2019**, *9*, 3272. [CrossRef] [PubMed]
123. Gensous, N.; Bacalini, M.G.; Franceschi, C.; Meskers, C.G.M.; Maier, A.B.; Garagnani, P. Age-Related DNA Methylation Changes: Potential Impact on Skeletal Muscle Aging in Humans. *Front. Physiol.* **2019**, *10*, 996. [CrossRef] [PubMed]

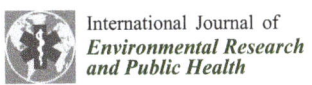

Review

Orthogeriatric Management: Improvements in Outcomes during Hospital Admission Due to Hip Fracture

Francisco José Tarazona-Santabalbina [1,2,*], Cristina Ojeda-Thies [3], Jesús Figueroa Rodríguez [4], Concepción Cassinello-Ogea [5] and José Ramón Caeiro [6]

1. Department of Geriatric Medicine, Hospital Universitario de la Ribera, Alzira, 46600 Valencia, Spain
2. CIBERFES, Centro de Investigación Biomédica en Red Fragilidad y Envejecimiento Saludable, Instituto Carlos III, 28029 Madrid, Spain
3. Department of Orthopaedic Surgery and Traumatology, Hospital Universitario 12 de Octubre, 28041 Madrid, Spain; cristina.ojeda@salud.madrid.org
4. Department of Physical Medicine and Rehabilitation, Complejo Hospitalario Universitario de Santiago de Compostela, 15706 Santiago de Compostela, Spain; jesfi@msn.com
5. Department of Anaesthesiology, Hospital Universitario Miguel Servet, 50009 Zaragoza, Spain; ccassinello@salud.aragon.es
6. Department of Orthopaedics and Traumatology, Complejo Hospitalario Universitario de Santiago de Compostela, 15706 Santiago de Compostela, Spain; jrcaeiro@telefonica.net
* Correspondence: Tarazona_frasan@gva.es

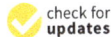

Citation: Tarazona-Santabalbina, F.J.; Ojeda-Thies, C.; Figueroa Rodríguez, J.; Cassinello-Ogea, C.; Caeiro, J.R. Orthogeriatric Management: Improvements in Outcomes during Hospital Admission Due to Hip Fracture. *IJERPH* **2021**, *18*, 3049. https://doi.org/10.3390/ijerph18063049

Academic Editor: Paul B. Tchounwou

Received: 20 February 2021
Accepted: 12 March 2021
Published: 16 March 2021

Publisher's Note: MDPI stays neutral with regard to jurisdictional claims in published maps and institutional affiliations.

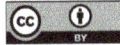

Copyright: © 2021 by the authors. Licensee MDPI, Basel, Switzerland. This article is an open access article distributed under the terms and conditions of the Creative Commons Attribution (CC BY) license (https://creativecommons.org/licenses/by/4.0/).

Abstract: Hip fractures are an important socio-economic problem in western countries. Over the past 60 years orthogeriatric care has improved the management of older patients admitted to hospital after suffering hip fractures. Quality of care in orthogeriatric co-management units has increased, reducing adverse events during acute admission, length of stay, both in-hospital and mid-term mortality, as well as healthcare and social costs. Nevertheless, a large number of areas of controversy regarding the clinical management of older adults admitted due to hip fracture remain to be clarified. This narrative review, centered in the last 5 years, combined the search terms "hip fracture", "geriatric assessment", "second hip fracture", "surgery", "perioperative management" and "orthogeriatric care", in order to summarise the state of the art of some questions such as the optimum analgesic protocol, the best approach for treating anemia, the surgical options recommendable for each type of fracture and the efficiency of orthogeriatric co-management and functional recovery.

Keywords: hip fractures; geriatric assessment; orthogeriatric care; functional recovery; geriatric syndromes; mortality; hip fracture surgery; multidisciplinary care

1. Introduction

Osteoporotic hip fractures are one of the main health problems of geriatric patients. Approximately 1.3 million hip fractures were diagnosed in 1990 worldwide [1], and this worldwide annual incidence is expected to increase to over 6 million globally by 2050 [2]. Nearly 80% of the fractures suffered by women and 50% of those in men occur after reaching the age of 70 years [3]. Ninety percent of the fractures occur after falls from standing height [4]. Mortality rates of 10% during acute hospital admission and 30% at one year [5,6] have been reported, but these figures can be reduced introducing an orthogeriatric team [7]. Orthogeriatric care can be defined as the collaboration between orthopedic surgeons and geriatricians to improve hip fracture patient outcomes during hospital admission [8].

Survival after hip fracture does not imply full recovery. Of those who survive, only half recover the functional level they had before the injury [9,10] and one quarter of previously independent patients require admission to an elderly care home [11]. The estimated socio-economic costs derived from treating hip fractures represent 0.1% of global health care costs worldwide increasing to 1.4% in more developed regions [1].

The advanced age, baseline functional status and the common presence of comorbidities such as chronic heart failure and cognitive impairment among patients with hip fracture are the main arguments in favor of orthogeriatric co-management, which reduces the risk of perioperative complications, functional decline, and mortality [12]. Joint geriatric trauma management was introduced in the United Kingdom in the mid-twentieth century [13]. The past two decades, however, have born an increase in the design and implementation of coordinated perioperative models [14], which have been shown to reduce in-hospital complications [15,16], hospital stay and readmissions [17], disability, and in-hospital mortality [16].

A narrative review published in 2016 [18] considered that geriatric medicine improved awareness of the extra-orthopedic issues complicating the patient's course and influenced treatment outcomes, improving length of stay, decreasing complication rates and reducing both in-hospital and mid-term mortality after discharge, as well as improving quality of care and reducing healthcare costs. Many questions remain to be answered this field. In addition to the traditional goals of the orthogeriatric team, another crucial objective is enrolling the patient in the most appropriate rehabilitation program, with the aims of reducing institutionalization and facilitating functional recovery and return to the patients' prefracture social situation [19]. To achieve these goals, correct assessment of the baseline functional situation and maximum potential of recovery are of vital importance. The high prevalence of disability following fracture can condition the patient referral process after hospital discharge [20], and in this sense the management plan does not conclude upon discharge from hospital but rather involves continuation of patient care beyond the in-hospital process. Thus, the scope of the orthogeriatric team goes beyond the hospital setting, expanding the benefits of integral geriatric care [19]. The role of orthogeriatric care has been defined best in the United Kingdom, largely as a consequence of the development of the best practice tariff introduced in 2010 in order to improve the care of patients with hip fracture [21]. Later, preoperative and postsurgical cognitive assessments were also included [22]. The National Institute for Health and Care Excellence issued a document on the quality care of patients with hip fracture that highlighted a number of quality standards to be met in order to maximise efficiency in the care of patients with hip fracture [23]. All orthogeriatric care models have in common the suitability of care provided by multidisciplinary teams proficient in geriatrics, the need of early surgery, the role of a case manager (in this case a geriatrician) throughout the whole process, pain control, avoidance of the appearance or worsening of geriatric syndromes, and adequate continuity of care after hospital discharge, with the aim of recovering baseline function [24]. Orthogeriatric care has been validated by a meta-analysis [8]. However, there are still areas of controversy in need of study and analysis, such as the ideal thromboprophylactic, anaesthetic and analgesic protocols, the assessment and management of cognitive impairment and malnutrition during acute hospitalisation, improvement of patient mobility, postoperative rehabilitation and the efficiency of the programs used in convalescence units or in home rehabilitation care [18,24]. Orthogeriatric co-management exists in several forms, with various types of structural collaboration between orthopedic trauma surgeons and multi-professional geriatric teams. The models are country-specific and there are still no clear recommendations on how this service should be best organized; further studies are needed to determine the best model and to define a uniform set of outcome parameters for use in future clinical studies [25].

The present review aims to provide answers to some of these questions regarding orthogeriatric management of patients with hip fracture, with the goal of clarifying which measures have improved outcomes.

2. Methods

The present review was carried out by conducting an electronic search in OVID (MedLine and Embase), combining the following MeSH keywords: "hip fractures" and "geriatric assessment", combined with "perioperative management" "surgery", "second hip fracture" and "orthogeriatric care". The MeSH construction [Hip fractures] AND ([Geriatric assessment] OR "perioperative management") OR "orthogeriatric care" OR "geriatric syndromes") was used. The search was limited to publications in the last 5 years; in English, Spanish, and French; and in human subjects.

A total of 783 articles were obtained, of which 124 were finally selected. Some additional instructions were added for certain specific objectives where necessary. In 9 cases, supplementary information was obtained in the form of references of the selected articles. Details of the evaluation and selection process of the items are shown in Figure 1. The articles were selected by four researchers based on the following inclusion criteria: (1) study type: randomized clinical trials, cohort studies, case–control studies, observational studies, and before–after analyses in orthogeriatric units; (2) population: geriatric patients with proximal femoral fracture; (3) intervention: orthogeriatric treatment initiated perioperatively; and (4) outcomes: surgical delay (defining delayed surgery as that occurring beyond the day after admission, as recommended by the UK's National Institute for Health and Care Excellence (NICE) clinical guideline for the management of hip fractures [23]), length of hospital stay, prognostic factors and mortality, functional recovery, geriatric syndromes, perioperative care such as renal function, anemia, and costs. The exclusion criteria were letters to the Editor, case reports, articles with no available abstract or those with only the abstract published, and studies meeting the inclusion criteria but with 50% of the study sample aged less than 65 years (i.e., predominantly non-geriatric). All selected studies were included in a database including an abstract of the main results reported. The authors of the review reevaluated all articles, and final inclusion was restricted to those of sufficient quality to provide information pertinent to the aims of this review. In case of discrepancy between the four authors, the fifth author determined including the study or not. The outcome measures examined were mortality, length of hospital stay, medical complications, discharge destination, functional status and recovery. The authors evaluated the different studies according the 12 outcomes parameters proposed by an Expert Roundtable [26].

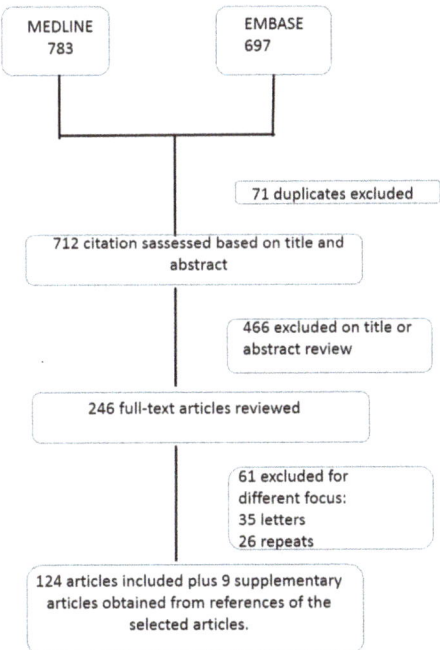

Figure 1. Flow chart of the study selection procedure used in the literature research.

3. Results

A total number of 133 studies we included in this review. Aspects such as race or sex-related differences in the outcomes were only taken into account when reported in the studies. A recent pre-post intervention observational study compared a retrospective control arm (Usual orthopedic care (UOC)) to two parallel arms, orthogeriatric co-management (OGC) and orthopedic team with the support of a geriatric consultant service (GCS). Patients in the OGC group were more likely to undergo surgery within 48 h after admission (OR 2.62; 95% Confidence Interval (CI): 1.40–4.91), but not those in the GCS group, compared with those who received UOC. OGC was also associated with lower length of stay (LOS) and 1-year mortality [27]. In spite of the available evidence, many hospitals still lack this model of care. Another important issue is the collection of data via national registries allowing for audit and comparison of outcomes between the traditional approach and orthogeriatric management, as well between the models available in different countries, in order to define the benefits of the different implemented models [28]. All variants agree in the need for early geriatric clinical care and early surgical management. A 24-h delay may be a threshold for an increased risk of complications and mortality. In a population-based, retrospective cohort study among 42,230 patients with hip fracture, patients who received surgery after 24 h had a significantly higher risk of 30-day mortality (% absolute RD, 0.79; 95%CI, 0.23–1.35) and the composite outcome of complications (myocardial infarction, deep vein thrombosis, pulmonary embolism, and pneumonia) (% absolute RD, 2.16; 95%CI, 1.43–2.89) [29]. Clinical stabilization of patients by the orthogeriatric teams, based on clinical recommendations and guidelines, can help reduce delays, increasing diagnostic precision and risk assessment of comorbidities. Thus, the role of an orthogeriatrician in an orthopaedic department who leads a multidisciplinary approach in the management of older patients with hip fractures is vital, ensuring that surgical delay is under 48 h after presentation, as well as reducing postoperative and total length of stay [30].

The orthogeriatric approach uses an important tool: The Comprehensive Geriatric Assessment (CGA). Two recent meta-analyses on the advantages of this tool in hip fractures patients showed a decrease in mortality and an improvement in activities of daily living [31], physical function and quality of life [32]. By adequately estimating perioperative risk, preventing complications and avoiding heterogeneity in the fulfilment of the goals of care; CGA leads to an important decrease of hospital stay and complications, and prioritizes the recovery of baseline functional and social status. The good results shown are made possible by a continuous improvement in quality of care, reduction of the length of stay in the emergency department, promotion of structured management, and inclusion of new evidence-based measures. Throughout this review, the authors will describe the newest evidence regarding the management of geriatric patients admitted for hip fractures.

3.1. Geriatric Syndromes
Delirium

The incidence of delirium among orthopedic surgery patients has been reported to be between 4.5 and 41.2%, according to a recent meta-analysis [33]; this wide range in the incidence reported is due to the different ages of the patients included in the studies, the screening tools employed, the types of settings and the surgical and anesthetic techniques used. Risk factors for delirium included advanced age, male sex, comorbidities, malnutrition, preoperative and postoperative haemoglobin levels, postoperative sodium levels, postoperative length of stay, hearing impairment, polypharmacy, antipsychotic drugs, opioid prescription, and cognitive impairment [33].

Analogously, four observational studies have shown an incidence of delirium of 15.7% [34], 22,09% [35], 24.2% [36] and 31.1% [37]. Poeran et al. associated postoperative delirium with long-acting and combined short and long-acting benzodiazepines and ketamine while neuraxial anaesthesia and opioid use were associated with lower risk [34]. Tao et al. identified baseline Barthel index, Mini-Mental State Examination (MMSE), instrumental activities of daily living (IADLs), and Geriatric Depression Scale (GDS) as risk factors for delirium [35]. Aldwikat et al. found that comorbidity and cognitive impairment were independent risk factors for the development of delirium [36]. Finally, Pioli et al. linked risk of delirium to older age, higher degree of comorbidity and functional impairment [37]. In addition, in the multivariate analysis, surgical delay was an independent risk factor for delirium, along with age, prefracture functional disability and cognitive impairment (mildly to moderately impaired versus cognitively healthy or severely impaired patients). All the described factors were included in the previously cited meta-analysis [33].

Another two meta-analyses identified risk factors already described in the one mentioned above. Yang et al. reported an incidence of delirium of 24.0 % and found preoperative cognitive impairment, advanced age, living in an institution, heart failure, total hip arthroplasty, multiple comorbidities and opioid usage as risk factors for delirium, while females were less likely to develop delirium after hip surgery [38]. Smith et al. found age 80 years and over, living in a care institution before the fracture and the pre-admission diagnosis of dementia to be factors associated with the appearance of delirium, which occurred in 31.2% [39].

Delirium is associated with increased mortality, with the aforementioned confounders responsible for the statistically significant association between incident postoperative delirium and mortality, as shown in a meta-analysis published in 2017 [40].

There is an overlap between the different geriatric syndromes, emphasizing the need of CGA in older patients admitted by hip fracture. Patients that were malnourished (OR = 2.98; 95%CI: 1.43–6.19), or at risk of malnutrition (OR = 2.42; 95%CI: 1.29–4.53) had an increased risk of delirium [41]. Other known risk factors for delirium are cognitive impairment and dementia. An observational study reported that 52% of patients developed delirium in addition to dementia, and as this overlap increased length of stay and short-term mortality [42]. A study published before the period included in this review already showed an overlap of geriatric syndromes between depressive symptoms and incidence of delirium (21.7% of patients); other syndromes overlapping with delirium in this study were vision impairment and lower cognitive function [43].

It is perhaps due to this overlap of geriatric syndromes that strategies for prevention and treatment of delirium based on proactive geriatric consultation have shown a decrease in the incidence of delirium. Two meta-analyses published in 2017 analysed the role of CGA in reducing the incidence of delirium. The first one found a significant reduction in delirium overall (relative risk [RR] = 0.81; 95% = 0.69–0.94) in the intervention group. Post-hoc subgroup analysis found this effect to be maintained in the team-based intervention group (RR = 0.77; 95%CI = 0.61–0.98) but not the ward-based group [44]. The second one showed that comprehensive geriatric care reduced the incidence of perioperative delirium (Odds ratio [OR] = 0.71; 95%CI = 0.57–0.89; p = 0.003) and that it was associated with better cognitive status during hospitalization or at 1-month follow-up (MD = 1.03; 95%CI, 0.93–1.13; $p \leq 0.00001$) but there was no significant difference in the duration of perioperative delirium between both groups (MD = -2.48; 95%CI = -7.36–2.40; p = 0.32) [45]. Most of the risk factors described for delirium are evaluated during the CGA process, and this assessment reduces delirium incidence by identifying potential risk factors and developing preventive strategies.

Another important strategy to decrease the incidence of delirium incidence is prompt surgery. Surgical delay is linked to delirium, as has been previously mentioned [37], but the duration of surgery is associated to delirium risk, too. A recent study reported that the risk for delirium was increased with surgical duration: every 30-min increase in the duration of surgery was associated with a 6% increase in the risk of delirium, and the risk was higher was in patients who had received general anaesthesia [46].

3.2. Cognitive Impairment

Both cognitive impairment and dementia are quite prevalent among patients with hip fractures. Furthermore, rather than maintaining their cognitive function, older patients with cognitive decline could further develop cognitive disorders after hospitalization following hip fracture. An observational study included 402 patients with hip fracture, 188 of whom were previously cognitively intact. Of these, 12 (6.4%) patients showed a cognitive decline in the 6 months following the fracture. Multivariate regression analysis showed that older age and the appearance of medical complications were significant independent risk factors for cognitive decline [47]. Older studies have reported from a 40% prevalence of some degree of cognitive impairment [48] to an 85% prevalence of dementia [49]. Dementia is underdiagnosed in older hospitalised patients, in spite of being an important risk factor for suffering hip fractures [49].

Detecting cognitive impairment is vital, as one of the most important risk factors of functional decline and mortality in hip fracture patients is concomitant dementia. A recent observational study found that patients with cognitive impairment showed a higher overall mortality, even after discharge from hospital [50]. This study reported that patients with dementia were more likely to suffer respiratory infections, urinary tract infections, sepsis, had a poorer baseline functional status, and worse ambulation at final follow-up [50]. The relationship between function and cognitive decline is well known [51]. Only 31% percent of hip fracture patients recovered previous activities of daily living (ADL) ability in an observational study, and recovery was less likely for those ≥85 years old, with dementia and with a Charlson Comorbidity Index > 2 [52]. Another study reported that hip fracture patients with worse scores in a cognition scale had less functional gain, but those who improved their cognitive score showed better recovery of gait ability [53], demonstrating the benefits of a dual cognitive and functional rehabilitation in these patients. For this reason, rehabilitation protocols for functional recovery in hip fracture patients with cognitive impairment or dementia should include cognitive stimulation programs, as well. As previously mentioned, the negative association between dementia in hip fracture patients and mortality can be attenuated by geriatric care. A study of 650 patients (mean age 86 years (standard deviation [SD]: 6 years)) identified 168 patients with dementia (DP), 400 patients without dementia (NDP) and 82 patients with in whom cognitive status was not determined (CSND). After adjusting for age, sex, comorbidities, polypharmacy, pre-fracture independence, time-to-surgery, and delirium, there were no significant differences between groups for mortality or for recovery of ambulation at 6 months, but DP and CSND were more likely to be newly institutionalized, being possible to attribute this absence of difference to the effect of a dedicated geriatric care pathway [54]. Thus, treatment of behavioral psychological symptoms of dementia (BPSD) during rehabilitation is crucial. A retrospective cohort study based on the Japan Rehabilitation Database showed that participants who presented BPSD when initiating rehabilitation but who had resolved their symptoms at the end of rehabilitation had better functional recovery [55]. Likewise, the goals of rehabilitation in hip fracture patients with dementia should focus not only on functional recovery, but rather add other objectives such as quality of life, decrease in the complication rate or optimization of social support [56].

Finally, a study among older veterans diagnosed with dementia suggested that acetyl-cholinesterase inhibitors (AChEI) could reduce the risk of fragility fractures by increasing bone density and quality, as well as improving bone healing after fracture [57]. Over an average of 4.6 years of follow-up, 20.1% suffered a fracture, and 42.3% of the cohort had been prescribed AChEIs. The hazard of suffering any fracture was significantly lower among AChEI users compared with those on other/no dementia medications in fully adjusted models (hazard ratio [HR] = 0.81; 95%CI: 0.75–0.88). After considering competing mortality risks, fracture risk remained 18% lower in veterans using AChEIs (HR = 0.82; 95%CI: 0.76–0.89) [57]. This is a field of interest for research to confirm if AChEI would be useful to prevent hip fracture or increase bone healing after surgery in patients with dementia.

3.3. Mood Disorders and Depression

The prevalence of mood disorders is high among hip fracture patients and depression and its treatment increase the risk of fractures and have a negative impact on functional recovery and mortality [58]. Van de Ree et al. reported a prevalence of psychological distress of 36% at 1 week to 31% at 1 year after hip fracture. Frailty at presentation for hip fracture was the most important prognostic factor for symptoms of depression (OR = 2.74; 95%CI = 1.41–5.34) and anxiety (OR = 2.60; 95%CI = 1.15–5.85) in the year following hip fracture [59]. Again, overlapping of geriatric syndromes overlap has important consequences for older patients with hip fractures and highlight CGA-based intervention strategies that involve early identification of geriatric syndromes and provision of appropriate and prompt treatments.

Depression is common among hip fracture elderly patients: a cross-sectional study reported and overall prevalence of 46%, significantly higher in women, persons over 81 years old, diabetics and those with anxiety [60]. These studies provide further proof of the need of routine geriatric assessment in older patients hospitalized after hip fracture. A secondary analysis of data from a randomized controlled trial comparing usual care with an interdisciplinary program evaluated differences in depressive symptoms using the Chinese version of the Geriatric Depression Scale short-form. Three trajectory groups were defined according to changes in depressive symptoms: a non-depressive group, a marginally depressive group and a persistently depressive group. Compared to patients who received usual care, those in the interdisciplinary program had a significantly lower risk of being in the persistently depressive group [61]. Women and those physically and cognitively more impaired were found to be more likely to be assigned to the marginally and persistently depressive groups. Screening of depression could contribute to managing it better and minimizing its negative impact on patient recovery.

3.3.1. Urinary Incontinence

Urinary incontinence (UI) is another highly prevalent geriatric syndrome among older patients with hip fracture. In a randomized clinical trial, 44% of study participants self-reported UI and four out of five reported nocturia at baseline [62]. A cohort study demonstrated that UI was associated to an increased risk of falls, but not of hip fractures [63]. Post-void residual (PVR) urine volume was elevated in 15.6% of patients included in a prospective observational study, and elevated PVR was more likely in the setting of urinary or fecal incontinence, difficulties in activities of daily living, malnutrition, poor performance on Timed Up and Go test and Elderly Mobility Scale. One-year mortality after hip fracture was significantly higher among those with elevated PVR. PVR deserves to be included in the CGA of frail older patients, including women [64]. Post-operative urinary retention (POUR) is common after hip fracture surgery, and is linked to opioid use and anticholinergic medication. The high incidence of asymptomatic POUR in older patients underscores the need of improved screening tools for early identification and treatment of this condition [65]. Half of the population was unable to recover their prefracture autonomy in a prospective cohort study. Risk factors for not recovering autonomy were increasing age, number of comorbidities, lower prefracture autonomy, increased use of an anti-decubitus mattress, more days with diapers, a urinary catheter or bed rails, a higher number of days with disorientation, failure to recover ambulation, and a nonintensive care pathway. Recovery of ambulation, treatment of disorientation and management of urinary incontinence are modifiable factors significantly associated with the functional recovery of autonomy [66]. Health professionals should be aware of the high prevalence of urinary problems in older adults with hip fractures, and screening tools and early management should be implemented in these patients.

3.3.2. Constipation

Constipation is also common among patients admitted due to hip fracture. I has been reported to be associated with immobilization, loss of intimacy, polypharmacy and treatments such as opioids. Approximately 70% of all patients develop constipation the first days after surgery, and 62% continue to suffer from it 1 month after surgery [67]. Some multicomponent interventions included in the CGA could reduce the incidence of constipation. A quasi-experimental study testing the efficacy of a nursing intervention based on active patient involvement including individualised nursing care plans reported significant lower rates of constipation in the intervention group, attributed to higher fibre and fluid intakes [68].

4. Malnutrition

Nutritional problems have a reported prevalence between 9 and 18,7% among older patients hospitalised due to hip fracture according to recent studies, and 50% of patients are at risk of malnutrition.

In a retrospective cohort study of 29,377 geriatric patients 45.9% had hypoalbuminemia, and the risk of mortality was inversely associated with serum albumin concentration as a continuous variable. Compared with normoalbuminemic patients, hypoalbuminemic patients had higher rates of death, sepsis and unplanned intubation, as well as a longer length of stay. Hypoalbuminemia is a powerful independent risk factor for mortality [69]. A systematic review including 44 articles and 26,281 subjects found a prevalence of malnutrition of 18.7% (using the Mini-Nutritional Assessment (MNA) (large or short form)) that increased to 45.7% when different criteria were used (such as Body Mass Index (BMI), weight loss, or albumin concentration). Low scores in anthropometric indices were associated with a higher risk of in-hospital complications and with poorer functional recovery. Despite improvement in the management of geriatric patients with hip fractures, mortality remained unacceptably high (30% at 1 year and up to 40% at 3 years) and malnutrition was associated with a higher risk of dying [70]. Nutritional assessment as part of the CGA including nutritional screening tools and serum parameters such as albumin is cost effective, improves nutritional status and functional recovery. At baseline, 9% patients were malnourished and 42% patients at risk of malnutrition among 472 hip fracture patients aged 65 years and older included in a population-based prospective study that used baseline Mini-Nutritional Assessment Short Form (MNA-SF) scores. Malnutrition was associated with mortality. Risk of malnutrition and malnutrition also predicted institutionalization, and the risk of malnutrition was associated with decline in mobility in the multivariate binary logistic regression analyses [71]. In a prospective study that included 509 patients (mean age 85.6 (SD 6.9) years, 79.2% female), 20.1% had a BMI lower than 22 kg/m^2; 81.2% had protein and 17.1% had both energy and protein malnutrition. Serum vitamin D was <30 ng/mL in 93% of patients and 17.1% were sarcopenic. There is an overlap between protein and energy malnutrition, vitamin D deficiency and sarcopenia [72].

Nutritional impairments, vitamin D deficiency and sarcopenia have been associated with functional decline, length of stay, complications such as sepsis and mortality. Furthermore, nutritional assessment has been reported to be cost-effective, and should be included in routine CGA in elderly patients admitted for hip fracture. The question regarding which is the best nutritional screening tool remains open. Three studies evaluated which best tool was best to diagnose malnutrition. Helminen et al. performed a prospective study in which 7% of patients were malnourished and 41% at risk of malnutrition at baseline, according to the MNA-SF. The MNA-SF predicted mortality, LOS and readmissions better than the NRS2002 (Nutritional Risk Score 2002), while both were ineffective in predicting changes in mobility and living arrangements [73]. Inoue et al. compared the MNA-SF, MUST (Malnutrition Universal Screening Tool), NRS-2002 and GNRI (Geriatric Nutritional Risk Index) in 205 patients. Multiple linear regression revealed that MNA-SF was associated with the motor-FIM (functional independence measure) at discharge, efficiency on the motor-FIM relative to length of stay and 10-m walking speed. The GNRI was associated with 10-m walking speed, but not motor-FIM or motor-FIM efficiency. MNA-SF was identified as the ideal nutritional screening tool predict functional outcomes during the acute postoperative phase in older hip fracture patients [74]. Finally, Koren-Hakim compared MNA-SF, MUST and NRS-2002 in 215 patients (71.6% female; mean age 83.5 (SD 6.09)) and found a.significant relationship between the nutritional groups of the three scores. For all screening tools, body mass index, weight loss and pre-admission food intake were related to the patients' nutritional status. Only the MNA-SF was able to detect the well-nourished patients that would have less readmissions in the 6 months after the fracture. Well-nourished patients according to the MNA-SF had lower mortality at 36 months than malnourished patients and those at risk of malnutrition. The association between the NRS-2002 patients' nutritional status and mortality was weaker [75]. According to these studies, the MNA could be the best nutritional screening tool for hip fracture patients and would offer the best prediction of survival and functional recovery.

Several studies have evaluated functional recovery among patients with nutritional impairments after hospital discharge. A retrospective observational cohort study divided patients into two groups based on MNA-SF scores at discharge vs. admission: improvement in nutritional status (IN group) and non-improvement in nutritional status (NN group). Patients in the IN group were younger and had higher admission FIM and MNA-SF scores. The median FIM score at discharge was significantly higher in the IN group than in the NN group. Multivariate analysis revealed a significant association between improvement in nutritional status and higher FIM scores at discharge [76]. Another retrospective cohort study analysing 107 rehabilitation patients aged ≥65 years and older reported that compared to lower-functioning patients, higher-functioning patients were younger, were hospitalised less time, and had lower Cumulative Illness Rating-Scale for Geriatrics (CIRS-G) scores with higher mean Mini-Mental Status Examination (MMSE) scores. The gain in FIM was significantly higher in patients at low risk of malnutrition (according to the Short Nutritional Assessment Questionnaire, SNAQ), in those who did not lose weight, had normal albumin, and lower CIES-G scores. Patients who achieved functional independence–discharge FIM ≥ 90–ate normally and experienced less "loss of appetite". Weight loss was the strongest negative predictor of the gain in FIM. Nutritional status, especially weight change, is an independent negative predictor for the success of rehabilitation [77]. A multicenter prospective cohort study evaluated nutritional status using the MNA-SF in 204 patients: 51 (25.0%) patients were malnourished, 98 (48.0%) were at risk of malnutrition, and 55 (27.0%) were well-nourished before the fracture. At discharge, FIM scores were higher in well-nourished patients than in those malnourished or at risk of malnutrition ($p < 0.01$). MNA-SF remained a significant independent predictor for FIM at discharge even after adjusted multiple regression. The baseline nutritional status was a significant independent predictor for functional status at discharge from acute admission [78]. Finally, a prospective observational cohort study of 254 geriatric patients undergoing surgery showed that most followed one of the five trajectories at one-year: (1) 30% (n = 63) returned home, (2) 11% (n = 22) returned to a nursing home, (3) 16% (n = 36) needed rehabilitation, (4) 13% (n = 28) were discharged to a location different from that prior to admission and (5) 18% (n = 37) had died. Patients following trajectory 1 were younger while those in trajectory 5 had lower MNA scores. Delay between discharge from the attending staff and true departure from the hospital was associated with low MNA scores, low MMSE scores and with the need for a rehabilitation centre (trajectory 3) [79]. Early assessment of nutritional status and early intervention are important for successful postoperative rehabilitation.

A subanalysis of a randomized controlled trial of orthogeriatric care included nutritional advice and supplementation in the intervention group (orthogeriatric care). Vitamin K1 and 25-(OH)-D levels were higher at 4 months in the intervention group than in controls. No difference was found in bone turnover markers between groups, but a substantial loss of weight and physical function was found in both groups [80].

4.1. Sarcopenia

Sarcopenia is partially dependent of nutritional status. The following risk factors of sarcopenia were identified in a multicenter prospective observational study: undernutrition (body mass index-BMI and Mini Nutritional Assessment-Short Form or MNA-SF), hand-grip strength and skeletal muscle index. During follow-up, 114 patients died (60.5% sarcopenic vs. 39.5% non-sarcopenic, p = 0.001). Cox regression analyses showed that sarcopenia and low hand-grip strength were associated with an increased risk of dying.

Older patients with undernutrition had a higher risk of developing sarcopenia during hospitalisation, and sarcopenic patients were almost twice as likely to die during follow-up after hip fracture [81]. Using the European Working Group on Sarcopenia in Older People Criteria (EWGSOP), a prospective study of 479 consecutive patients hospitalized for hip fracture identified sarcopenia in 17.1%. Sarcopenia was associated with living in nursing homes, older age, and having a lower body mass index, but only low body mass index was predictive of sarcopenia after adjustment in the multivariate analysis [82]. A third study assessed sarcopenia using the SARC-F self-reported questionnaire and found a prevalence of 63.5%. The sensitivity, specificity, positive predictive value, negative predictive value were 95.35 %, 56.94 %, 56.94%, 95.35%, and 71.3%, respectively versus the EWGSOP-2 criteria as the reference standard [83], suggesting SARC-F could be useful to identify sarcopenia in hip fracture patients. This is particularly important as sarcopenia is linked to poorer functional recovery. Another study diagnosed sarcopenia using the definition of the Foundation for National Institutes of Health (FNIH) criteria in 127 patients (mean age of 81.3 (SD 4.8) years, and 64.8% female) and identified sarcopenia in 33.9%. Participants with sarcopenia were less likely to have complete functional recovery and showed lower Barthel index scores at discharge from the rehabilitation unit [84].

In summary, sarcopenia is common among older patients with hip fractures, and is associated with a poorer nutritional status and lower likelihood of functional recovery in rehabilitation programs. These patients could benefit of the development of personalized treatment plans that include nutritional and functional interventions.

4.2. Frailty

Frailty is another geriatric syndrome highly prevalent in older patients with hip fracture and has been associated with the incidence of complications and length of stay. Of 696 patients aged 65 years and older included in a prospective cohort study, 53.3% were considered frail. Frailty was negatively associated with health status, self-rated health and capability well-being 1 year after hip fracture, even after adjusting for confounders [85]. Another study evaluated the value of the ASA (American Society of Anaesthesiologists) score and Edmonton frailty score in predicting the outcome of treatment of femoral neck fractures in older patients. The frailty index, calculated using Edmonton scoring index, showed that 49% had low frailty scores and 51% had high frailty scores. Patients with high frailty scores and ASA grade had a greater chance of developing wound infection, as well as higher morbidity and mortality following femoral neck fracture [86]. Frail patients had a significantly lower survival compared to nonfrail patients in a prospective observational cohort study [87]. The final study included in this subsection used the 7-point Clinical Frailty Scale to diagnosis frailty in 164 patients: 81 patients were 'not vulnerable' (frailty score 1–3) and 83 were 'vulnerable or frail' (frailty score $\geq$ 4). One month after surgery, 5% patients had died, all of them with frailty scores $\geq$ 4 ($p = 0.007$). Postoperative morbidity during the 28-day follow-up was less common among patients categorised as 'not vulnerable'. Postoperative length of stay was longer for 'vulnerable or frail' with scores $\geq$ 4 [88]. Frail patients also show a lower chance of functional recovery: in a study of 100 consecutive hip fracture patients (mean age 79.1 (SD 9.6) years), 37.8% had post-operative complications. Frailty, measured using the MFC (modified fried criteria) and REFS (reported Edmonton frail scale), was significantly associated with suffering complications using both scales (OR = 4.46, $p = 0.04$ and OR = 6.76, $p = 0.01$, respectively), which were the only significant predictors of post-operative complications on univariate analyses. However, only REFS (OR = 3.42, $p = 0.04$) predicted early post-operative complications in the hierarchical logistic regression model. REFS also significantly predicted [basic activities of daily living (BADL)] function at 6-month follow-up in the multivariable logistic regression models. (BADL, OR = 6.19, $p = 0.01$). Frailty, measured with the REFS, was a good predictor of early post-operative outcomes in this pilot study of older adults undergoing hip surgery, and it also predicted 6-month BADL function [89].

4.3. Pressure Sores

Pressure sores are a geriatric syndrome commonly presenting during hospitalisation after hip fracture. Proof of their importance is that national hip fracture audits include pressure sores as a variable. A study comparing the results reported by different national hip fracture registries described an incidence of pressure sores between 2 and 6.7% [28]. These rates are lower than those described in cohort studies and meta-analysis, as we shall discuss later. The difference can be possibly explained due to the fact that registries are based on health records and rely of the quality of this clinical information.

Pressure sores are more common in some diseases such as diabetes. A meta-analysis reported that 15.1% of diabetics had pressure sores, compared to 7.5% among hip fracture patients without diabetes. The risk of pressure ulcers during hospitalisation was increased in diabetics with hip fractures (OR = 1.825 [95%CI: 1.373–2.425) [90]. Geriatric care needs to intensify preventive measures in these patients. Pressure ulcers are also associated with surgical delay: a meta-analysis showed an increase in complications including pressure ulcers among patients with higher surgical delay [91].

Approximately 12% of patients suffered category II or higher pressure ulcers in a prospective cohort study that identified five risk factors associated with developing sores: higher preoperative Braden score, surgical procedure with internal fixation, a higher percentage of days with the presence of foam valves before surgery, use of a urinary catheter, and use of a diaper in the postoperative period [92]. Another prospective cohort study also found an incidence of 12% and linked this geriatric syndrome to low albumin levels, history of atrial fibrillation, coronary artery disease and diabetes. Pressure ulcers were also associated with 6-month mortality (RR = 2.38, 95%CI = 1.31–4.32, p = 0.044) [93].

In another cohort study of 8871 geriatric hip fracture patients, 457 (5.15%) developed pressure ulcers. Risk factors of developing pressure ulcers were preoperative sepsis, elevated platelet count, insulin-dependent diabetes, pre-existing pressure ulcers, postoperative pneumonia, urinary tract infection, and delirium [94]. Pressure sores appeared in 22.7% of 1083 older adult patients with fragility hip fractures included in a prospective multicentric prognostic cohort study; risk factors identified were: age over 80 years, the length of time an indwelling urinary catheter was used, duration of pain, the absence of side rails on the bed, and the use of a foam position valve [95]. The incidence of pressure ulcers was 25.7% in a cohort study of 462 patients with hip fracture. The incidence was higher in weaker subjects, and baseline Barthel index, and MNA scores were lower among those developing ulcers. However, only low handgrip strength remained associated with the development of pressure ulcers upon multivariate adjustment [96].

The effects of multidisciplinary co-management of older hip fracture patients were evaluated in a retrospective study that included 3540 patients. Half of the patients who received co-management received surgery within 48 h of ward admission, compared to 6.4% before the intervention, 0.3% (vs 1.4%) developed pressure ulcers, and 76% (vs 19%) were assessed for osteoporosis [97].

In a prospective prognostic cohort study of patients admitted with fragility hip fractures and monitored over a 12-month period, 27% developed pressure sores. Multivariate analysis identified the following risk factors: age older than 81 years, type of surgery, and placement of the limb in a foam rubber splint. Pressure ulcers are a relatively common complication in older adults with hip fractures, especially high-risk patients or with certain treatments. Pre-emptively identifying patients at highest risk of pressure injury taking these factors into account could help provide and targeted care [98].

5. Polypharmacy

Polypharmacy, fall-risk increasing drugs and inadequate prescription are very common in older adults. A retrospective cohort study analysed polypharmacy and fall-risk increasing drugs (FRIDS) in 228 patients older than 80 years discharged from an Orthogeriatric Unit who were able to walk before surgery. The mean number of drugs and FRIDS prescribed at discharge was 11.6 (SD 3.0) and 2.9 (SD 1.6), respectively. Polypharmacy was very prevalent: 23.3% (5–9 drugs) and 75.9% (≥10 drugs); only three patients did not meet the definition of polypharmacy. In addition, only 11 patients had no FRIDS and 35.5% were on <3 FRIDS. The most prevalent FRIDS were: agents acting on the renin-angiotensin system (43.9%) and anxiolytics (39.9%). The number of FRIDS was higher in patients with extreme polypharmacy. Those independent in instrumental activities had lower risk of extreme polypharmacy (≥10 drugs), while patients living in a nursing home had higher risk of >3FRIDS [99].

Orthogeriatric co-management with CGA based care could help stop inappropriate prescriptions. The differences in drugs prescribed at admission and discharge were analysed in a randomized clinical trial that compared comprehensive geriatric care (CGC) in a geriatric ward with traditional orthopaedic care (OC). The mean number of drugs prescribed at discharge in the CGC group was lower compared with OC (7.1 (SD 2.8) versus 6.2 (SD 3.0)) and the total number of withdrawals and of starts was higher in the CGC group. The number of drug changes during hospitalisation was negatively associated with mobility and function at 4-month follow-up in both groups, but this association disappeared in multivariate analysis using baseline function and comorbidities as a confounders [100]. CGA interventions including assessment of drugs prescription at hospital discharge could have a potential impact on adverse events and the incidence of falls in older patients. Table 1 summarizes the most important papers on geriatric syndromes included in this review. The studies were included in this selection according to the level of evidence and the authors' consideration of their clinical relevance.

Table 1. Summary of the some most relevant studies on geriatric syndromes and functional recovery included in this review.

Authors	Year	Country	Sample Size	Inclusion Criteria	Exclusion Criteria	Study Design	Conclusion Summary	Level of Evidence
Zusman [61]	2017	Canada	53	Hip fracture aged 65 years or older with a recent hip fracture (3–12 months).	older adults who, prior to the fracture, were unable to walk 10 m, dementia, and/or older adults moved to a residential care facility.	RCT	44% of study participants self-reported UI.	Ib
Morri [65]	2018	Italy	840	65 years of age or older hospitalized	The absence of a legal guardian to sign the consent form in cases of cognitive deficit, and a diagnosis of periprosthetic or pathological fracture	Prospective cohort study	50% sample studied unable to recover their prefracture autonomy levels. Risk factors: increased number of days with diapers ($B = 0.003$; $p < 0.001$), urinary catheter ($B = 0.03$; $p < 0.001$)	IIb
Díaz de Bustamante [71]	2017	Spain	509	Patients aged ≥ 65 yo admitted due to hip fracture		Cohort study	81.2% protein malnutrition. 17.1% energy and protein malnutrition. 93% Low vitamin D levels. Sarcopenia prevalence 17.1%	IIb
Inoue [73]	2019	Japan	205	Patients aged ≥ 65 yo, fractures caused by falling and surgical treatment.	Terminal malignant disease, uncontrolled chronic liver disease and/or pre-fracture ambulation difficulty	Longitudinal cohort study	MNA-SF had a significant association with discharge motor-FIM, efficiency on the motor-FIM and 10-m walking speed. GNRI significantly associated with 10-m walking speed.	IIb
Inoue [77]	2017	Japan	204	Age ≥ 65 yo, fractures incurred as a result of falls and required surgery.	Terminal malignant disease, uncontrolled chronic liver disease, and/or pre-fracture ambulation difficulty, partial or no weight-bearing indications during postoperative rehabilitation	Multicentre cohort study	MNA-SF was a significant independent predictor for FIM at discharge (well-nourished vs. malnourished, $\beta = 0.86$, $p < 0.01$).	IIb
Beauchamp-Chalifour [78]	2020	Canada	209	Geriatric patients (>65 yo) admitted for a hip fracture.	Subtrochanteric fracture, pathologic hip fracture and polytrauma patients	Cohort study	Deceased patients had lower MNA scores (mean 19.9 (SD 5.2); $p < 0.001$) and lower MMSE scores (mean 16.0 (SD 10.9, $p < 0.001$).	IIb
Torbergsen [79]	2019	Norway	71 patients (31 in the intervention group and 40 controls)	Fracture resulted of a low energy trauma.	Moribund at admittance.	RCT	Intervention group: Vitamin K1 K1: 1.0 (SD 1.2) vs 0.6 (SD 0.6) ng/mL, $p = 0.09$; 25(OH)D: 60 (SD 29) vs 43 (SD 22) nmol/L, $p = 0.01$	Ib
Landi [83]	2017	Italy	127	Age ≥ 70 yo admitted to in-hospital Geriatric Rehabilitation Unit with hip fracture.		Longitudinal cohort study	Sarcopenia 33.9%. Sarcopenia increased risk of incomplete functional recovery: OR 3.07, 95%CI 1.07–8.75. Sarcopenia showed lower Barthel index scores at discharge: 69.2 versus 58.9; $p < 0.001$); and after 3 months of follow-up (90.9 versus 80.5; $p = 0.02$).	IIb
van de Ree [84]	2019	Netherlands	696	Patients ≥ 65 yo with hip fracture	Pathological hip fractures.	Multicentre longitudinal cohort study	53.3% were frail. Frailty was negatively associated with HS (β −0.333; 95%CI −0.366 to −0.299), self-rated health (β −21.9; 95%CI −24.2 to −19.6) and capability well-being (β −0.296; 95%CI −0.322 to −0.270) in elderly patients 1 year after hip fracture. After adjusting for confounders, associations were weakened but remained significant.	IIb

Table 1. Cont.

Authors	Year	Country	Sample Size	Inclusion Criteria	Exclusion Criteria	Study Design	Conclusion Summary	Level of Evidence
Wei [89]	2017	China	8 studies (22,180 patients)	Types of studies: observational studies; Types of participants: patients with hip fracture; Comorbidity: compared patients with diabetes with those without diabetes		Meta-analysis	Mean PU incidence: 15.1% in group with diabetes compared to 7.5% without diabetes group. Diabetes PU OR 1.825 (95%CI: 1.373–2.425; $p < 0.001$). Subgroup analysis by PU stage: OR 1.474 [95%CI 0.984–2.207] for $\geq$category II PU, and 2.814 [95%CI: 2.115–3.742] for $\geq$category I PU.	Ia
Klestil [90]	2018	Austria	28 prospective studies (31,242 patients).	Randomised controlled trials, non-randomised controlled trials, and prospective controlled cohort studies. Adults aged 60 years or older undergoing surgery for acute intra- and extracapsular hip fracture.		Meta-analysis	48 h surgery: RR dying within 12 months (RR) 0.80, 95%CI 0.66–0.97. Adjusted data: fewer complications (8% vs. 17%) in patients who had early surgery.	Ia
Ganizeo [91]	2019	Italy	761	Fragility hip fracture patients aged $\geq$65 years.	Patients with periprosthetic or pathological fractures.	Prospective cohort study	The incidence of category II or higher PUs was 12%. Five factors independently associated with category $\geq$II PU development: Higher preoperative Braden score (Hazard Ratio [HR]: 0.884; 95% confidence interval [CI]: 0.806–0.969), surgical procedure with internal fixation (HR 1.876; 95%CI: 1.183–2.975), a higher percentage of days with the presence of foam valve before surgery (HR: 1.010; 95%CI: 1.010–1.023) and a urinary catheter (HR: 1.013; 95%CI: 1.006–1.019) and diaper (HR: 1.007; 95%CI 1.001–1.013) in the postoperative period.	IIb
Chiari [94]	2017	Italy	1083	Patients $\geq$ 65 years of age with fragility hip fracture.	Patients with periprosthetic or pathological fractures, and patients who presented with pressure ulcers.	Prospective cohort study	Pressure ulcers incidence: 22.7%. Two risk factors: age > 80 years (odds ratio (OR) 1.03; 95%IC 1.006; 1.054, $p = 0.015$), the length of time a urinary catheter was used (OR 1.013; 95%IC 1.008; 1.018, $p < 0.001$.	IIb
Forni [97]	2018	Italy	467			Prospective cohort study	Of these, 27% ($n = 127$) developed a pressure injury. Multivariate analysis identified the following predictive factors: age older than 81 years, type of surgery, and placing the limb in a foam rubber splint.	IIb

6. Perioperative Care

6.1. Renal Function

Low glomerular filtration rates have been associated with increased comorbidity, lower haemoglobin concentrations at admission, longer surgical delay, and greater incidence of delirium. Of 1425 consecutive hip fracture patients included in a population-based prospective study, 40% had renal dysfunction on admission using the Chronic Kidney Disease Epidemiology equation (eGFRCDK-EPI) [101]. In the multivariate analyses, eGFRCDK-EPI values of 30–44 mL/min/1.73 m^2 (HR = 1.91; 95%CI = 1.44–2.52) and <30 mL/min/1.73 m^2 (HR = 1.95; 95%CI = 1.36–2.78) were associated with increased mortality. In summary, moderate to severe renal dysfunction measured by eGFRCDK-EPI and polypharmacy increased mortality after hip fracture. Frequent assessment of renal function and medications are essential in the care of geriatric hip fracture patients.

6.2. Anemia and Patients Blood Management

Approximately 40% of all hip fracture patients have haemoglobin (Hb) values below 12 g/dL upon admission to hospital. Anaemia progresses significantly during the days before surgery, more so in extracapsular fractures. In hip fracture patients, anaemia has been associated with increased risk of blood transfusion, poorer functional outcomes and increased mortality [102]. Hip fracture surgery is additionally associated with perioperative blood loss frequently requiring transfusion. Patient blood management (PBM) involves multidisciplinary strategies to optimize outcomes. The management of anaemic patients includes preoperative fluid resuscitation, the administration of iron alone or combined with vitamin B12, folic acid, and on occasion erythropoietin, as well as blood products; it also includes the minimization of further intraoperative and perioperative losses.

Some risk factors for increased hidden blood loss after a hip fracture are higher ASA score, perioperative gastrointestinal bleeding/ulcer and use of general anaesthesia compared to spinal anaesthesia. Patients with higher hidden blood loss were more likely to receive transfusions [103]. Advanced age, preoperative anaemia, female sex, lower BMI, higher ASA scores, chronic obstructive pulmonary disease (COPD), hypertension, increased surgical delay, and having intertrochanteric and subtrochanteric femur fractures were perioperative independent risk factors associated with receiving postoperative blood transfusions in older patients with hip fractures included in the American College of Surgeons National Surgical Quality Improvement Program (ACS NSQIP) [104]. Patients receiving postoperative transfusions had a significantly higher risk-adjusted 30-day mortality, total hospital length of stay and readmission rates. Survival at 90 days, 180 days, and one year after surgery was significantly lower among patients with a Hb level below 12 g/dL at admission [105].

The 2018 PBM International Consensus Conference defined the current status of the PBM evidence base for clinical practice in major orthopaedic surgery. It recommended using intravenous (IV) iron for patients with iron deficiency anaemia to reduce red blood cell (RBC) transfusion rates; erythropoietin therapy in addition to IV iron in patients with Hb levels < 13 g/dL; and it also established a conditional recommendation in favour of using a RBC transfusion threshold of Hb < 8 g/dL in adults with hip fractures and cardiovascular disease or risk factors [106].

PBM-based strategies for the prevention and treatment of anaemia and transfusion have demonstrated an improvement of outcomes after hip fracture. A meta-analysis comparing restrictive versus liberal transfusion strategies in patients undergoing hip fracture surgery found no differences in the rates of delirium, mortality, the overall incidence of infections, the incidence of pneumonia, wound infection, cardiovascular events, congestive heart failure, thromboembolic events or length of hospital stay between restrictive (haemoglobin level threshold $\leq$ 8 g/dL or symptoms) and liberal (Hb level threshold $\leq$ 10 g/dL) RBC transfusion strategies ($p > 0.05$). However, the authors found that restrictive transfusion thresholds were associated with higher rates of acute coronary syndrome and a 40% decrease in the risk of cerebrovascular accidents. The authors concluded that that clinicians should individualise treatment based on patient condition before adopting a transfusion strategy, rather than using haemoglobin level thresholds [107]. In a retrospective study, a restrictive transfusion strategy was associated with fewer acute cardiovascular complications and a reduction in packed RBC units used per participant, but also with a greater frequency of transfusion in the rehabilitation setting [108]. Another retrospective cohort study compared a restrictive (transfusion threshold of haemoglobin < 8 g/dL) with a very restrictive transfusion protocol (threshold of <7 g/dL Hb in hemodynamically stable patients and <8 g/dL in patients with symptomatic anaemia or a history of coronary artery disease); the very restrictive protocol decreased transfusion rates, a lower likelihood of transfusion of more than 1 unit of RBCs, and lower inpatient cardiac morbidity without differences in morbidity, in-hospital mortality and readmission and survival at one month follow-up [109].

Intravenous iron is an alternative to avoid RBC transfusion. A meta-analysis comparing iron supplementation with placebo in 1201 patients undergoing hip fracture surgery, found that administering 200–300 mg iron IV preoperatively was associated with a reduction in transfusion volume and length of stay, but was not found to reduce infections or mortality [110]. Preoperative iron supplementation combined with restrictive transfusion strategy (Hb level threshold ≤ 8 g/dL or symptoms) was compared with a liberal transfusion strategy (Hb level threshold ≤ 10 g/dL) without iron supplementation during hospitalization for hip fracture in a retrospective cohort study. The restrictive transfusion strategy was associated with a reduction in packed RBC units used per patient, but more transfusions in rehabilitation settings [111].

The combined use of IV iron and erythropoietin (EPO) did not reduce the percentage of transfused patients in two cohort studies [112,113] but it did reduce the number of RBC units required. Patients in the intervention group showed improved functional recovery at 3 and 6 months after the fracture, measured with the Barthel index and the Functional Ambulation Categories (FAC scale) [112]. A retrospective study compared RBC transfusion with a patients treated with iron and EPO [114]. The transfusion group had higher haemoglobin levels on the first postoperative day without differences in mortality; haemoglobin levels were completely recovered within 2 weeks in both groups. Treatment with EPO could improve functional recovery as well, as suggested by a randomized clinical trial [115] that used EPO in sarcopenic patients with femoral intertrochanteric fractures and reported a higher handgrip strength in sarcopenic women in the intervention group, but not in men. The appendicular skeletal muscle increment of the intervention group was markedly increased regardless of sex. The postoperative infection rate and length of stay were lower in the intervention group. In summary, EPO could improve the muscle strength of female patients with sarcopenia during the perioperative period-but not revert sarcopenia itself. EPO could also increase muscle mass in both sexes. Postoperative administration of EPO could therefore potentially accelerate postoperative rehabilitation.

Intravenous tranexamic acid (TXA) is another option in PBM. It possesses great potential in reducing blood loss and allogeneic blood transfusion safely in patients with hip fractures undergoing surgery. Five meta-analyses [116–120] of RCTs comparing intraoperative administration of TXA with placebo in patients undergoing hip fracture surgery showed significant differences between groups regarding transfusion rates of allogeneic blood, total blood loss, intraoperative blood loss, postoperative blood loss and postoperative haemoglobin, without affecting the rates of thromboembolic events, deep venous thrombosis, acute coronary syndrome, cerebrovascular events, wound complications or mortality.

6.3. Pain Management

Insufficient control of pain during hospitalisation for hip fracture has been associated with an increased incidence of delirium and poorer outcomes. A review published in 2016 warned of the importance of pain associated with hip fracture due to its severe consequences and delayed recovery. However, the prevailing opioid-dependent model of analgesia, presents multiple disadvantages and risks that can compromise outcomes in the hip fracture population. The pain management process includes fundamental preoperative, intraoperative, and postoperative interventions and lacks sufficient well-designed studies to unequivocally show which pain management approaches work best after hip fracture surgery [121].

A study used the initial pain evaluation by emergency medical services using the Numeric Rating Scale (NRS) and reported that 28% of patients received analgesics, with their score dropping from 7.0 (SD, 2.6) to 2.8 (SD, 1.4) upon hospital arrival [122]. The authors of this study highlighted that only a minority of patients received pre-hospital analgesia and this treatment was linked to significant pain relief. Treatment of pain during transfer to hospital could be implemented in hip fracture treatment guidelines.

Pain was measured with the Western Ontario and McMaster Universities Osteoarthritis Index questionnaire's short form (WOMAC-SF) in a prospective study [123]. Predictors of worse pain at six or eighteen months after the fracture were: living in a home care situation or nursing home before the fracture and low pre-fracture pain. Predictors of functional deterioration at six months were: age ≥ 85 years, lower income, high pre-fracture hip function, referral to rehabilitation upon discharge, and longer surgical delay. In summary, prefracture frailty is a predictor of greater post-fracture pain and functional decline. Prevention of frailty by promoting exercise in older adults could improve the prognosis following hip fracture.

The application of femoral nerve blocks in the Emergency Department among older adults with acute hip fracture has been evaluated in a systematic review that included seven randomized controlled trials [124]. All reported reductions in pain intensity with femoral nerve blocks, and all studies but one reported a decrease in the requirements of rescue analgesia. No adverse effects were found to be associated with the femoral block procedure; in fact, two studies reported a decreased risk of adverse events such as respiratory and cardiac complications. Femoral nerve blocks are beneficial both in terms of decreasing the pain experienced by older patients, as well as limiting the amount of systemic opioids administered. A Cochrane systematic review and meta-analysis on peripheral nerve blocks (PNBs) for hip fractures in adults included 49 trials (3061 participants; 1553 randomized to PNBs and 1508 to no nerve block (or sham block)) published from 1981 to 2020 [125]. The average age of participants ranged from 59 to 89 years. People with dementia were often excluded from the included trials. The results of 11 trials with 503 participants showed that PNBs reduced pain on movement within 30 min of block placement (standardized mean difference (SMD) -1.05, 95% confidence interval (CI) -1.25 to -0.86; equivalent to -2.5 on a scale from 0 to 10; high-certainty evidence). The effect size was proportional to the concentration of local anaesthetic used ($p = 0.0003$). Based on 13 trials with 1072 participants, PNBs decreased the risk of acute confusional state (RR = 0.67; 95%CI = 0.50–0.90; number needed to treat for an additional beneficial outcome (NNTB) = 12, 95%CI 7–47; high-certainty evidence). PNBs are likely to reduce the risk for chest infection (RR = 0.41 95%CI = 0.19–0.89; NNTB = 7, 95%CI 5–72; moderate-certainty evidence). The effects of PNBs on six-month mortality are uncertain, due to very serious imprecision (RR = 0.87, 95%CI = 0.47–1.60; low-certainty evidence). PNBs are likely to reduce time to first mobilization (mean difference (MD) -10.80 h, 95%CI: -12.83 to -8.77 h; moderate-certainty evidence). In summary, PNBs reduce pain on movement within 30 min after block placement, risk of acute confusional state, and probably also reduce the risk of chest infection and time to first mobilization.

A randomized clinical trial examined the effect on pain intensity and mobility of incorporating transcutaneous electrical nerve stimulation (TENS) treatment added to standard rehabilitation care during the acute post-operative phase following Gamma-nail surgical fixation of extracapsular hip fractures. The authors reported a significantly greater pain reduction during walking in the active TENS group compared to sham TENS group. Additional improvements in the active TENS group were a greater increase in walking distance on the fifth postoperative day and a higher level of mobility compared to the sham

TENS group. The authors concluded that adding TENS to the standard care of elderly patients in the early postoperative period following surgical fixation of extracapsular hip fracture with a Gamma nail could be recommended for pain management during walking and functional gait recovery [126].

Functional Recovery

Orthogeriatric units can be defined as a transversal and multidisciplinary care model, with the main objective of recovering of previous function in older patients with hip fracture.

Several aspects play a relevant role in the functional recovery after hip surgery in older people. Awareness of the expected recovery following hip fracture is essential for setting of realistic goals. An observational study of 733 patients aged ≥65 years with hip fracture found a low rate of return to previous function, regardless of prefracture functional capacity. Return to independence in activities of daily living (ADLs) was less likely for those >85 years old (20% vs. 44%), with dementia (8% vs. 39%) and with a Charlson comorbidity index greater than 2 (23% vs 44%) [52]

Functional outcomes after a hip fragility fracture seem to depend more on patient characteristics than treatment-related factors [127] In a retrospective cohort study of 519 patients with hip fracture admitted to rehabilitation settings, it has been reported that both delirium and clinical adverse events (infections, respiratory failure, pulmonary embolism, falls) affected functional outcome. A clinical orthogeriatric approach is necessary in order to minimize the impact of these adverse events on the rehabilitation program [128].

A correlation between grip strength measured early after hip fracture and subsequent short and long-term functional recovery was found in a prospective cohort study that included 190 patients. Hand grip weakness was an independent predictor of worse functional outcome 3 and 6 months after hip fracture [129].

Early mobilization after surgery for hip fracture reduces medical complications and mortality. A higher time upright at discharge, measured in the first week after surgery, was associated with less fear of falling, a higher gait speed and a faster Timed Up and Go test time [130].

A single-blind controlled trial reported that a motivational interview conducted with hip fracture patients after being discharged from rehabilitation was related to an increase in physical activity and ambulation capacity [131].

The relationship between specific aspects of the rehabilitation program and functional outcome has been examined in several studies. A randomized controlled trial showed that a hospital rehabilitation program based on the training of specific balance tasks was useful to improve physical function, pain, ADL and quality of life in older patients with hip fracture [132]. Muscle quality (muscle mass and muscle strength) after a hip fracture improved with high-intensity resistance training with the knee in extension in a case series, possibly leading to significant gains in physical function [133].

A systematic review concluded that progressive resistance exercise after hip fracture surgery improved mobility, ADLs, balance, lower extremity strength, and performance task outcomes [134].

7. Prognostic Factors and Mortality

Of 2443 patients included in a prospective cohort study included, 36.8% were receiving treatment with β-blocker therapy before surgery. The group treated with beta-blockers was significantly older, had more comorbidities, and was less fit for surgery based on their ASA score; despite these risk factors, 90-day mortality was significantly lower in patients receiving beta-blockers (adjusted incidence rate ratio = 0.82, 95%CI: 0.68 to 0.98, $p = 0.03$) [135].

Preoperative CGA with shared decision-making was compared in a before-after, single-centre, retrospective study. Significantly more patients (or representatives) in the CGA group chose non-surgical management after hip fracture (9.1% vs. 2.7%, $p = 0.008$). Patient characteristics were comparable. Reasons not to undergo surgery included aversion to be more dependent on others and severe dementia [136].

Several studies have researched mortality after hip fracture and its risk factors. Baseline characteristics explained less than two-thirds of the six-month mortality after hip fracture in a retrospective observational study including 1010 individuals (mean age 86 (SD 6) years). The six-month mortality rate was 14.8%. The six-month attributable mortality estimates were as follows: baseline characteristics (including age, gender, comorbidities, autonomy, type of fracture) accounted for 62.4%; perioperative factors (including blood transfusion and delayed surgery) for 12.3%; and severe postoperative complications for 11.9% of attributable mortality [137].

One-year mortality in hip fracture patients from the Nan Province (Thailand) was 19%, or 6.21 times higher than expected compared with the age-matched population. Mortality among hip fracture patients was also significantly higher among those aged older than 80 years, non-ambulatory before the fracture and at hospital discharge, or suffering end-stage renal disease, delirium, and pneumonia [138].

In a retrospective study of 254 patients (mean age, 78.74 years), one-year mortality was 22.8% (58 patients). Univariate analysis identified age >85 years, male gender, ASA score ≥ 3, having ≥ 3 comorbidities, and a C Reactive Protein to albumin ratio (CAR) ≥ 2.49 were identified as mortality risk factors. The ASA score, CAR and number of comorbidities were included in the binary logistic regression analysis to determine the major predictors of 1-year mortality. The presence of a CAR ≥ 2.49 was found to be a strong indicator for 1-year mortality in patients operated due to hip fracture in the elderly population, while an ASA score ≥ 3 and the presence of ≥ 3 comorbidities were also related to mortality [139].

A retrospective French cohort study of 309 patients studied risk factors for 1-tear mortality, which was 23.9%. Over half had a surgical delay greater than 48 h (181 patients, 58.6%). Factors independently associated with 1-year mortality were: advanced age (HR = 1.06, 95%CI: 1.01–1.12; p =0.032), comorbidities as defined by the revised cardiac index or Lee score ≥ 3 (HR = 1,52, 95%CI: 1,05–2,20; p = 0.026) and surgical delay over 48 h (HR = 1.06, 95%CI = 1.01–1.11; p = 0.024) [140].

Mortality at one year was 35% and was associated with low IADL day −15 ($p < 0.01$), elevated CIRS-G ($p < 0.01$), severity ($p = 0.05$) and malnutrition ($p = 0.05$) in a prospective study of 113 patients (mean age 87 years (range 76–100). Of those who survived, 45% had a functional decline one year after the fracture and 11% were admitted in a nursing home [141].

The HULP-HF score was designed to predict one-year mortality after hip fractures, using a prospective study of 509 patients with a 1-year mortality of 23.2%. The eight independent mortality risk factors included in the score were age >85 years, baseline functional and cognitive impairment, low body mass index, heart disease, low hand-grip strength, anaemia on admission, and secondary hyperparathyroidism associated with vitamin D deficiency. The AUC was 0.79 for the HULP-HF score, greater than other tools such as the Nottingham Hip Fracture Score (NHFS), ASA classification or Charlson Comorbidity index [142].

Another study evaluated the usefulness of the Hip-MFS (Multidimensional Frailty Score) to predict 6-month all-cause mortality. Secondary outcomes were 1-year all-cause mortality, postoperative complications prolonged hospital stay, and institutionalization. 6-month mortality was 7.3% (35 patients), after a median of 2.9 months (interquartile range 1.4–3.9 months). The fully adjusted hazard ratio per 1-point increase in Hip-MFS was 1.46 (95%CI: 1.21–1.76) for 6-month mortality. The odds ratios for postoperative complications and prolonged total hospital stay were 1.24 (95%CI: 1.12–1.38) and 1.16 (95%CI: 1.03–1.30), respectively. After adjustment, high-risk patients (Hip-MFS > 8) had a higher risk of 6-month mortality (HR: 3.55, 95%CI: 1.47–8.57) than low-risk patients. The Hip-MFS successfully predicted 6-month mortality better than age or other existing tools (p-values of comparisons of ROC curves: 0.002, 0.004, and 0.044 for the ASA classification, age and

NHFS, respectively). It also predicted postoperative complications and prolonged hospital stay in older hip fracture patients after surgery [143].

8. Costs

The acute and post-acute care of patients with an osteoporotic hip fracture pose a significant burden for health care resources all over the world, involving up to 1.5% of total health care budgets [144]. The cost of acute inpatient care of this type of fracture is estimated globally at $13,331 according to a recent systematic review [145]. Costs were significantly associated with prefracture comorbidities prior to fracture and developing a medical or surgical complication during hospitalisation, due to an increase in the length of stay.

The mean cost of hospitalisation of an osteoporotic hip fracture patient was Singapore dollars (SGD) 13,313.81 (€8280,00 at current rates) in a retrospective analysis of patients admitted under a mature orthogeriatric co-management care service in Singapore. The presence of complications significantly increased average cost (SGD 2,689.99 [€1672,93] more than if there were no complications). Each additional day between admission and time of surgery led to an increased cost of SGD 575.89 (€358,15), with surgery after more than 48 h costing an average of SGD 2,716.63 (€1689,50) more than surgery within 48 h. The authors concluded that a standardised co-management model of care could accelerate surgical treatment and help reduce peri- and postoperative complications, reducing overall costs of these fractures [146].

A prospective, 12-month observational study from Spain calculated the mean total cost in the first year after an osteoporotic hip fracture at €9690 (95%CI: 9184–10,197) in women and €9019 (95%CI: 8079–9958) in men. Initial hospitalization was the main determinant of cost, followed by ambulatory care and home care. The cost per day of hospital stay has been estimated at €1,000, so a delay of 1 day for hip surgery would cost approximately 1800 € [144,147].

In addition to the direct costs derived from inpatient acute care, most of the costs for osteoporotic hip fractures are associated with post-acute care, including the direct costs for rehabilitation, medium and long-term care, and the indirect costs related with absence from work of family caregivers [148,149]. All these contribute to total costs reaching $43,669 per patient in the first year after a hip fracture, higher than those estimated for acute coronary syndrome ($32,345) and ischaemic stroke ($34,772) [145].

Many initiatives have been created in order to improve outcomes and reduce costs in an attempt to alleviate this overall burden of health care systems. The implementation of the orthogeriatric co-management model of care, integrated in specific functional units, has been a vital tool to improve outcomes [150].

The implementation of orthogeriatric programs has been shown by several studies to offer greater cost-effectiveness than usual care, decreasing surgical delay, length of stay and improving physical function, with a decrease in one-year morbidity and mortality, while using fewer resources per patient and saving money [151,152], as has also been shown in systematic reviews and meta-analysis that associated orthogeriatric programs with decreases in time to surgery, LOS, complication rates and costs [32,153].

Another recent study evaluated the cost-effectiveness of orthogeriatric models and nurse-led fracture liaison services (FLS), compared with usual care. Orthogeriatric models of care were the most effective and cost-effective models, at a threshold of £30,000 per quality-adjusted life years gained (QALY). The authors concluded that introducing an orthogeriatric model of care and a FLS was cost-effective when compared with usual care, regardless of how patients were stratified in terms of age, sex, and Charlson comorbidity score at the moment of index hip fracture [154].

A systematic review of eight studies (two high-quality and six moderate or low-quality studies) showed that the implementation of Comprehensive Geriatric Assessment (CGA) improved return of function and mortality, with reduced cost. The authors concluded that CGA was the most cost-effective care model for orthogeriatric patients [155].

The effect of orthogeriatric clinical care pathways (OG-CCPs) on physical function and health-related quality of life (HRQoL) following hip fracture was evaluated in a systematic review and meta-analysis that included 22 studies (21 included hip fracture patients, and one included wrist fracture patients; the majority were assessed as high quality). Compared with usual care, the OG-CCP group showed moderate improvements in physical function and HRQoL. Inpatient OG-CCPs that extended to the outpatient setting showed greater improvements compared to those that only included inpatient or outpatient management. OG-CCPs that incorporated a care coordinator, geriatric assessment, nutritional advice, prevention of inpatient complications, rehabilitation, and discharge planning also demonstrated greater improvements in outcomes [32].

Though certain questions remain open regarding which model of care should be considered ideal, implementation of an orthogeriatric co-management model of care, integrated in specific functional units, benefits older patients with hip fractures, improving standards of care in a cost-effective manner. Because of that we undoubtedly recommend developing orthogeriatric units as a standard of care of older patients with this type of fracture [156].

9. Future Perspectives and Lines of Research

Some recent publications should be mentioned that evaluate the role of advanced practice nurses in the management of hip fracture patients in reducing length of stay and mortality, as in a systematic review by Allsop et al. that included 19 papers [157]. Nurses could play an important role in the multidisciplinary team, for example as coordinator or case manager, improving bone health assessment and falls prevention programs in Fracture Liaison Services (FLS).

The effect of different models of orthogeriatric care for older hip fracture patients was compared to usual orthopaedic care in a meta-analysis and showed that orthogeriatric care was associated with higher odds of diagnosing osteoporosis, initiation of calcium and vitamin D supplements and discharge on anti-osteoporosis medication, but evidence on fall prevention and subsequent fractures was scarce and inconclusive [158]. Future studies could assess combination of orthogeriatric care and FLS with orthogeriatric care alone. Another area of interest is reducing inequity in research regarding rehabilitation interventions in hip fracture patients. In over half of the trials included in a systematic review, potential participants were excluded based on residency in a nursing home, cognitive impairment, mobility/functional impairment, minimum age and/or non-surgical candidacy [159]. These sources of bias should be avoided in future studies.

An emergent topic for study is the race and sex-related differences in hip fracture outcomes. A review published ten years ago, including an important number of papers from USA [160] showed that men were younger and sicker than women with hip fractures, but mortality in men was twice that of women. African-Americans, as well as Hispanics and Native Americans had higher mortality than Whites. Another recent study from the USA reported a significant disparity in surgical delay and perioperative complication rates between races, with African-Americans having a longer time to surgery than Whites [161]. While sex-related differences in some outcomes have been studied more extensively, race-related differences in outcomes are an interesting line of research especially in countries and regions where socioeconomic factors or other factors related to ethnicity could change the access of individuals to healthcare services.

10. Conclusions

The efficiency and benefits of orthogeriatric care in a co-management pathway should be generalized globally. Over the past 70 years, orthogeriatric units have enabled major improvements in the standards of care provided to geriatric patients admitted at hospital due to hip fracture. Increased survival and functional recovery rates have been reported across these years, as well as decreased complications and adverse events during hospitalisation, such as the incidence of infections and geriatric syndromes. All these points have led to a decrease in the length of stay and health and social costs. A large number of clinical trials and meta-analyses published over the last 5 years support this evidence.

Nevertheless, there are still knowledge gaps regarding specific clinical issues. Furthermore, lack of continuity of care after hospital discharge is still common nowadays. Gender- and sex-related differences should be further studies, particularly in regions where they entail differences in access to care. While future studies are needed to help answer these open questions but we could ask ourselves if we should apply the strong evidence available in our routine in the meantime, as well.

Author Contributions: Conceptualization, F.J.T.-S. and J.R.C.; methodology, F.J.T.-S.; software, C.O.-T.; validation, J.F.R., C.C.-O. and J.R.C.; formal analysis, F.J.T.-S., J.R.C.; investigation, F.J.T.-S., J.R.C.; resources, C.O.-T., J.F.R., C.C.-O.; data curation, J.F.R., C.C.-O.; writing—original draft preparation, F.J.T.-S., C.O.-T., J.R.C.; writing—review and editing, all authors.; visualization, all authors.; supervision, C.O.-T., J.R.C.; project administration, all authors.; funding acquisition, J.R.C. All authors have read and agreed to the published version of the manuscript.

Funding: This research received no external funding.

Institutional Review Board Statement: This is a review manuscript. We did not ask for a institutional review statement.

Informed Consent Statement: This a review manuscript, we did not need an informed consent statement.

Data Availability Statement: This a review manuscript, we did not need a data availability statement.

Acknowledgments: The authors who thank Amgen-UCB Pharma for sponsoring the expenses derived from the publication of this manuscript.

Conflicts of Interest: The authors received financial support from Amgen-UCB.

References

1. Johnell, O.; Kanis, J.A. An Estimate of the Worldwide Prevalence, Mortality and Disability Associated with Hip Fracture. *Osteoporos. Int.* **2004**, *15*, 897–902. [CrossRef]
2. Cooper, C.; Campion, G.; Melton, L.J. Hip Fractures in the Elderly: A World-Wide Projection. *Osteoporos. Int.* **1992**, *2*, 285–289. [CrossRef]
3. Lauritzen, J.B.; Schwarz, P.; Lund, B.; McNair, P.; Transbøl, I. Changing Incidence and Residual Lifetime Risk of Common Osteoporosis-Related Fractures. *Osteoporos. Int.* **1993**, *3*, 127–132. [CrossRef]
4. Aschkenasy, M.T.; Rothenhaus, T.C. Trauma and Falls in the Elderly. *Emerg. Med. Clin. N. Am.* **2006**, *24*, 413–432. [CrossRef] [PubMed]
5. Roche, J.J.W.; Wenn, R.T.; Sahota, O.; Moran, C.G. Effect of Comorbidities and Postoperative Complications on Mortality after Hip Fracture in Elderly People: Prospective Observational Cohort Study. *BMJ* **2005**, *331*, 1374. [CrossRef] [PubMed]
6. Morris, A.H.; Zuckerman, J.D.; AAOS Council of Health Policy and Practice, USA. American Academy of Orthopaedic Surgeons National Consensus Conference on Improving the Continuum of Care for Patients with Hip Fracture. *J. Bone Jt. Surg. Am.* **2002**, *84*, 670–674. [CrossRef]
7. Hawley, S.; Javaid, M.K.; Prieto-Alhambra, D.; Lippett, J.; Sheard, S.; Arden, N.K.; Cooper, C.; Judge, A.; REFReSH Study Group. Clinical Effectiveness of Orthogeriatric and Fracture Liaison Service Models of Care for Hip Fracture Patients: Population-Based Longitudinal Study. *Age Ageing* **2016**, *45*, 236–242. [CrossRef] [PubMed]
8. Grigoryan, K.V.; Javedan, H.; Rudolph, J.L. Orthogeriatric Care Models and Outcomes in Hip Fracture Patients: A Systematic Review and Meta-Analysis. *J. Orthop. Trauma* **2014**, *28*, e49–e55. [CrossRef] [PubMed]
9. Bertram, M.; Norman, R.; Kemp, L.; Vos, T. Review of the Long-Term Disability Associated with Hip Fractures. *Inj. Prev.* **2011**, *17*, 365–370. [CrossRef]
10. Braithwaite, R.S.; Col, N.F.; Wong, J.B. Estimating Hip Fracture Morbidity, Mortality and Costs. *J. Am. Geriatr. Soc.* **2003**, *51*, 364–370. [CrossRef] [PubMed]
11. Magaziner, J.; Hawkes, W.; Hebel, J.R.; Zimmerman, S.I.; Fox, K.M.; Dolan, M.; Felsenthal, G.; Kenzora, J. Recovery from Hip Fracture in Eight Areas of Function. *J. Gerontol. A Biol. Sci. Med. Sci.* **2000**, *55*, M498–M507. [CrossRef]
12. Leibson, C.L.; Tosteson, A.N.A.; Gabriel, S.E.; Ransom, J.E.; Melton, L.J. Mortality, Disability, and Nursing Home Use for Persons with and without Hip Fracture: A Population-Based Study. *J. Am. Geriatr. Soc.* **2002**, *50*, 1644–1650. [CrossRef] [PubMed]
13. Devas, M. *Geriatric Orthopaedics*; Academic Press: London, UK, 1977.
14. Sabharwal, S.; Wilson, H. Orthogeriatrics in the Management of Frail Older Patients with a Fragility Fracture. *Osteoporos. Int.* **2015**, *26*, 2387–2399. [CrossRef] [PubMed]

15. Khasraghi, F.A.; Christmas, C.; Lee, E.J.; Mears, S.C.; Wenz, J.F. Effectiveness of a Multidisciplinary Team Approach to Hip Fracture Management. *J. Surg. Orthop. Adv.* **2005**, *14*, 27–31.
16. Vidán, M.; Serra, J.A.; Moreno, C.; Riquelme, G.; Ortiz, J. Efficacy of a Comprehensive Geriatric Intervention in Older Patients Hospitalized for Hip Fracture: A Randomized, Controlled Trial. *J. Am. Geriatr. Soc.* **2005**, *53*, 1476–1482. [CrossRef]
17. Friedman, S.M.; Mendelson, D.A.; Bingham, K.W.; Kates, S.L. Impact of a Comanaged Geriatric Fracture Center on Short-Term Hip Fracture Outcomes. *Arch. Intern. Med.* **2009**, *169*, 1712–1717. [CrossRef]
18. Tarazona-Santabalbina, F.J.; Belenguer-Varea, Á.; Rovira, E.; Cuesta-Peredó, D. Orthogeriatric Care: Improving Patient Outcomes. *Clin. Interv. Aging* **2016**, *11*, 843–856. [CrossRef]
19. De Rui, M.; Veronese, N.; Manzato, E.; Sergi, G. Role of Comprehensive Geriatric Assessment in the Management of Osteoporotic Hip Fracture in the Elderly: An Overview. *Disabil. Rehabil.* **2013**, *35*, 758–765. [CrossRef]
20. Pillai, A.; Eranki, V.; Shenoy, R.; Hadidi, M. Age Related Incidence and Early Outcomes of Hip Fractures: A Prospective Cohort Study of 1177 Patients. *J. Orthop. Surg. Res.* **2011**, *6*, 5. [CrossRef] [PubMed]
21. Wilson, H.; Harding, K.; Sahota, O. Best Practice Tariff for Hip Fracture-Making Ends Meet. *British Geriatrics Society Newsletter*. June 2010. Available online: https://www.bgs.org.uk/?option=com_content&view=article&id=700%3Atariffhipfracture&catid=47%3Afallsandbones&Itemid=307 (accessed on 12 October 2020).
22. Payment by Results Guidance for 2013–2014. Available online: https://www.gov.uk/government/publications/payment-by-results-pbr-operational-guidance-and-tariffs (accessed on 12 October 2020).
23. National Institute for Health and Care Excellence Quality Standards for Hip Fracture 2012. Available online: https://www.nice.org.uk/guidance/qs16 (accessed on 9 November 2020).
24. Fernandez, M.A.; Griffin, X.L.; Costa, M.L. Management of Hip Fracture. *Br. Med. Bull.* **2015**, *115*, 165–172. [CrossRef]
25. Komadina, R.; Wendt, K.W.; Holzer, G.; Kocjan, T. Outcome Parameters in Orthogeriatric Co-management—A Mini-Review. *Wien. Klin. Wochenschr.* **2016**, *128*, 492–496. [CrossRef] [PubMed]
26. Liem, I.S.; Kammerlander, C.; Suhm, N.; Blauth, M.; Roth, T.; Gosch, M.; Hoang-Kim, A.; Mendelson, D.; Zuckerman, J.; Leung, F.; et al. Identifying a Standard Set of Outcome Parameters for the Evaluation of Orthogeriatric Co-Management for Hip Fractures. *Injury* **2013**, *44*, 1403–1412. [CrossRef] [PubMed]
27. Baroni, M.; Serra, R.; Boccardi, V.; Ercolani, S.; Zengarini, E.; Casucci, P.; Valecchi, R.; Rinonapoli, G.; Caraffa, A.; Mecocci, P.; et al. The Orthogeriatric Comanagement Improves Clinical Outcomes of Hip Fracture in Older Adults. *Osteoporos. Int.* **2019**, *30*, 907–916. [CrossRef]
28. Ojeda-Thies, C.; Sáez-López, P.; Currie, C.T.; Tarazona-Santalbina, F.J.; Alarcón, T.; Muñoz-Pascual, A.; Pareja, T.; Gómez-Campelo, P.; Montero-Fernández, N.; Mora-Fernández, J.; et al. Spanish National Hip Fracture Registry (RNFC): Analysis of Its First Annual Report and International Comparison with Other Established Registries. *Osteoporos. Int.* **2019**, *30*, 1243–1254. [CrossRef] [PubMed]
29. Pincus, D.; Ravi, B.; Wasserstein, D.; Huang, A.; Paterson, J.M.; Nathens, A.B.; Kreder, H.J.; Jenkinson, R.J.; Wodchis, W.P. Association Between Wait Time and 30-Day Mortality in Adults Undergoing Hip Fracture Surgery. *JAMA* **2017**, *318*, 1994–2003. [CrossRef]
30. Aletto, C.; Aicale, R.; Pezzuti, G.; Bruno, F.; Maffulli, N. Impact of an Orthogeriatrician on Length of Stay of Elderly Patient with Hip Fracture. *Osteoporos. Int.* **2020**, *31*, 2161–2166. [CrossRef] [PubMed]
31. Lin, S.-N.; Su, S.-F.; Yeh, W.-T. Meta-Analysis: Effectiveness of Comprehensive Geriatric Care for Elderly Following Hip Fracture Surgery. *West. J. Nurs. Res.* **2020**, *42*, 293–305. [CrossRef]
32. Talevski, J.; Sanders, K.M.; Duque, G.; Connaughton, C.; Beauchamp, A.; Green, D.; Millar, L.; Brennan-Olsen, S.L. Effect of Clinical Care Pathways on Quality of Life and Physical Function After Fragility Fracture: A Meta-Analysis. *J. Am. Med. Dir. Assoc.* **2019**, *20*, 926.e1–926.e11. [CrossRef]
33. Yang, Y.; Zhao, X.; Gao, L.; Wang, Y.; Wang, J. Incidence and Associated Factors of Delirium after Orthopedic Surgery in Elderly Patients: A Systematic Review and Meta-Analysis. *Aging Clin. Exp. Res.* **2020**. [CrossRef] [PubMed]
34. Poeran, J.; Cozowicz, C.; Zubizarreta, N.; Weinstein, S.M.; Deiner, S.G.; Leipzig, R.M.; Friedman, J.I.; Liu, J.; Mazumdar, M.; Memtsoudis, S.G. Modifiable Factors Associated with Postoperative Delirium after Hip Fracture Repair: An Age-Stratified Retrospective Cohort Study. *Eur. J. Anaesthesiol.* **2020**, *37*, 649–658. [CrossRef]
35. Tao, L.; Xiaodong, X.; Qiang, M.; Jiao, L.; Xu, Z. Prediction of Postoperative Delirium by Comprehensive Geriatric Assessment among Elderly Patients with Hip Fracture. *Ir. J. Med. Sci.* **2019**, *188*, 1311–1315. [CrossRef]
36. Aldwikat, R.K.; Manias, E.; Nicholson, P. Incidence and Risk Factors for Acute Delirium in Older Patients with a Hip Fracture: A Retrospective Cohort Study. *Nurs. Health Sci.* **2020**, *22*, 958–966. [CrossRef]
37. Pioli, G.; Bendini, C.; Giusti, A.; Pignedoli, P.; Cappa, M.; Iotti, E.; Ferri, M.A.; Bergonzini, E.; Sabetta, E. Surgical Delay Is a Risk Factor of Delirium in Hip Fracture Patients with Mild-Moderate Cognitive Impairment. *Aging Clin. Exp. Res.* **2019**, *31*, 41–47. [CrossRef]
38. Yang, Y.; Zhao, X.; Dong, T.; Yang, Z.; Zhang, Q.; Zhang, Y. Risk Factors for Postoperative Delirium Following Hip Fracture Repair in Elderly Patients: A Systematic Review and Meta-Analysis. *Aging Clin. Exp. Res.* **2017**, *29*, 115–126. [CrossRef] [PubMed]
39. Smith, T.O.; Cooper, A.; Peryer, G.; Griffiths, R.; Fox, C.; Cross, J. Factors Predicting Incidence of Post-Operative Delirium in Older People Following Hip Fracture Surgery: A Systematic Review and Meta-Analysis. *Int. J. Geriatr. Psychiatry* **2017**, *32*, 386–396. [CrossRef] [PubMed]

40. Hamilton, G.M.; Wheeler, K.; Di Michele, J.; Lalu, M.M.; McIsaac, D.I. A Systematic Review and Meta-Analysis Examining the Impact of Incident Postoperative Delirium on Mortality. *Anesthesiology* **2017**, *127*, 78–88. [CrossRef]
41. Mazzola, P.; Ward, L.; Zazzetta, S.; Broggini, V.; Anzuini, A.; Valcarcel, B.; Brathwaite, J.S.; Pasinetti, G.M.; Bellelli, G.; Annoni, G. Association Between Preoperative Malnutrition and Postoperative Delirium After Hip Fracture Surgery in Older Adults. *J. Am. Geriatr. Soc.* **2017**, *65*, 1222–1228. [CrossRef] [PubMed]
42. Monacelli, F.; Pizzonia, M.; Signori, A.; Nencioni, A.; Giannotti, C.; Minaglia, C.; Granello di Casaleto, T.; Podestà, S.; Santolini, F.; Odetti, P. The In-Hospital Length of Stay after Hip Fracture in Octogenarians: Do Delirium and Dementia Shape a New Care Process? *J. Alzheimers Dis.* **2018**, *66*, 281–288. [CrossRef] [PubMed]
43. Radinovic, K.S.; Markovic-Denic, L.; Dubljanin-Raspopovic, E.; Marinkovic, J.; Jovanovic, L.B.; Bumbasirevic, V. Effect of the Overlap Syndrome of Depressive Symptoms and Delirium on Outcomes in Elderly Adults with Hip Fracture: A Prospective Cohort Study. *J. Am. Geriatr. Soc.* **2014**, *62*, 1640–1648. [CrossRef] [PubMed]
44. Shields, L.; Henderson, V.; Caslake, R. Comprehensive Geriatric Assessment for Prevention of Delirium after Hip Fracture: A Systematic Review of Randomized Controlled Trials. *J. Am. Geriatr. Soc.* **2017**, *65*, 1559–1565. [CrossRef] [PubMed]
45. Wang, Y.; Tang, J.; Zhou, F.; Yang, L.; Wu, J. Comprehensive Geriatric Care Reduces Acute Perioperative Delirium in Elderly Patients with Hip Fractures: A Meta-Analysis. *Medicine (Baltimore)* **2017**, *96*, e7361. [CrossRef]
46. Ravi, B.; Pincus, D.; Choi, S.; Jenkinson, R.; Wasserstein, D.N.; Redelmeier, D.A. Association of Duration of Surgery With Postoperative Delirium Among Patients Receiving Hip Fracture Repair. *JAMA Netw. Open* **2019**, *2*, e190111. [CrossRef]
47. Hack, J.; Eschbach, D.; Aigner, R.; Oberkircher, L.; Ruchholtz, S.; Bliemel, C.; Buecking, B. Medical Complications Predict Cognitive Decline in Nondemented Hip Fracture Patients-Results of a Prospective Observational Study. *J. Geriatr. Psychiatry Neurol.* **2018**, *31*, 84–89. [CrossRef] [PubMed]
48. Seitz, D.P.; Adunuri, N.; Gill, S.S.; Rochon, P.A. Prevalence of Dementia and Cognitive Impairment among Older Adults with Hip Fractures. *J. Am. Med. Dir. Assoc.* **2011**, *12*, 556–564. [CrossRef] [PubMed]
49. Yiannopoulou, K.G.; Anastasiou, I.P.; Ganetsos, T.K.; Efthimiopoulos, P.; Papageorgiou, S.G. Prevalence of Dementia in Elderly Patients with Hip Fracture. *Hip. Int.* **2012**, *22*, 209–213. [CrossRef]
50. Delgado, A.; Cordero, G.-G.E.; Marcos, S.; Cordero-Ampuero, J. Influence of Cognitive Impairment on Mortality, Complications and Functional Outcome after Hip Fracture: Dementia as a Risk Factor for Sepsis and Urinary Infection. *Injury* **2020**, *51* (Suppl. 1), S19–S24. [CrossRef] [PubMed]
51. Tarazona-Santabalbina, F.J.; Belenguer-Varea, Á.; Rovira Daudi, E.; Salcedo Mahiques, E.; Cuesta Peredó, D.; Doménech-Pascual, J.R.; Gac Espínola, H.; Avellana Zaragoza, J.A. Severity of Cognitive Impairment as a Prognostic Factor for Mortality and Functional Recovery of Geriatric Patients with Hip Fracture. *Geriatr. Gerontol. Int.* **2015**, *15*, 289–295. [CrossRef]
52. Tang, V.L.; Sudore, R.; Cenzer, I.S.; Boscardin, W.J.; Smith, A.; Ritchie, C.; Wallhagen, M.; Finlayson, E.; Petrillo, L.; Covinsky, K. Rates of Recovery to Pre-Fracture Function in Older Persons with Hip Fracture: An Observational Study. *J. Gen. Intern. Med.* **2017**, *32*, 153–158. [CrossRef] [PubMed]
53. Yoshii, I.; Satake, Y.; Kitaoka, K.; Komatsu, M.; Hashimoto, K. Relationship between Dementia Degree and Gait Ability after Surgery of Proximal Femoral Fracture: Review from Clinical Pathway with Regional Alliance Data of Rural Region in Japan. *J. Orthop. Sci.* **2016**, *21*, 481–486. [CrossRef] [PubMed]
54. Zerah, L.; Cohen-Bittan, J.; Raux, M.; Meziere, A.; Tourette, C.; Neri, C.; Verny, M.; Riou, B.; Khiami, F.; Boddaert, J. Association between Cognitive Status before Surgery and Outcomes in Elderly Patients with Hip Fracture in a Dedicated Orthogeriatric Care Pathway. *J. Alzheimers Dis.* **2017**, *56*, 145–156. [CrossRef] [PubMed]
55. Shibasaki, K.; Asahi, T.; Mizobuchi, K.; Akishita, M.; Ogawa, S. Rehabilitation Strategy for Hip Fracture, Focused on Behavioral Psychological Symptoms of Dementia for Older People with Cognitive Impairment: A Nationwide Japan Rehabilitation Database. *PLoS ONE* **2018**, *13*, e0200143. [CrossRef] [PubMed]
56. Romero Pisonero, E.; Mora Fernández, J. Multidisciplinary geriatric rehabilitation in the patient with hip fracture and dementia. *Rev. Esp. Geriatr. Gerontol.* **2019**, *54*, 220–229. [CrossRef] [PubMed]
57. Ogunwale, A.N.; Colon-Emeric, C.S.; Sloane, R.; Adler, R.A.; Lyles, K.W.; Lee, R.H. Acetylcholinesterase Inhibitors Are Associated with Reduced Fracture Risk among Older Veterans with Dementia. *J. Bone Miner. Res.* **2020**, *35*, 440–445. [CrossRef]
58. Wu, Q.; Liu, J.; Gallegos-Orozco, J.F.; Hentz, J.G. Depression, Fracture Risk, and Bone Loss: A Meta-Analysis of Cohort Studies. *Osteoporos. Int.* **2010**, *21*, 1627–1635. [CrossRef] [PubMed]
59. van de Ree, C.L.P.; de Munter, L.; Biesbroeck, B.H.H.; Kruithof, N.; Gosens, T.; de Jongh, M.A.C. The Prevalence and Prognostic Factors of Psychological Distress in Older Patients with a Hip Fracture: A Longitudinal Cohort Study. *Injury* **2020**, *51*, 2668–2675. [CrossRef] [PubMed]
60. Charles-Lozoya, S.; Cobos-Aguilar, H.; Barba-Gutiérrez, E.; Brizuela-Ventura, J.M.; Chávez-Valenzuela, S.; García-Hernández, A.; Tamez-Montes, J.C. Depression and Geriatric Assessment in Older People Admitted for Hip Fracture. *Rev. Med. Chil.* **2019**, *147*, 1005–1012. [CrossRef]
61. Tseng, M.-Y.; Shyu, Y.-I.L.; Liang, J.; Tsai, W.-C. Interdisciplinary Intervention Reduced the Risk of Being Persistently Depressive among Older Patients with Hip Fracture. *Geriatr. Gerontol. Int.* **2016**, *16*, 1145–1152. [CrossRef]
62. Zusman, E.Z.; McAllister, M.M.; Chen, P.; Guy, P.; Hanson, H.M.; Merali, K.; Brasher, P.M.A.; Cook, W.L.; Ashe, M.C. Incontinence and Nocturia in Older Adults After Hip Fracture: Analysis of a Secondary Outcome for a Parallel Group, Randomized Controlled Trial. *Gerontol. Geriatr. Med.* **2017**, *3*. [CrossRef]

63. Schluter, P.J.; Askew, D.A.; Jamieson, H.A.; Arnold, E.P. Urinary and Fecal Incontinence Are Independently Associated with Falls Risk among Older Women and Men with Complex Needs: A National Population Study. *Neurourol. Urodyn.* **2020**, *39*, 945–953. [CrossRef]
64. Nuotio, M.S.; Luukkaala, T.; Tammela, T. Elevated Post-Void Residual Volume in a Geriatric Post-Hip Fracture Assessment in Women-Associated Factors and Risk of Mortality. *Aging Clin. Exp. Res.* **2019**, *31*, 75–83. [CrossRef] [PubMed]
65. Cialic, R.; Shvedov, V.; Lerman, Y. Risk Factors for Urinary Retention Following Surgical Repair of Hip Fracture in Female Patients. *Geriatr. Orthop. Surg. Rehabil.* **2017**, *8*, 39–43. [CrossRef]
66. Morri, M.; Chiari, P.; Forni, C.; Orlandi Magli, A.; Gazineo, D.; Franchini, N.; Marconato, L.; Giamboi, T.; Cotti, A. What Factors Are Associated With the Recovery of Autonomy After a Hip Fracture? A Prospective, Multicentric Cohort Study. *Arch. Phys. Med. Rehabil.* **2018**, *99*, 893–899. [CrossRef]
67. Trads, M.; Pedersen, P.U. Constipation and Defecation Pattern the First 30 Days after Hip Fracture. *Int. J. Nurs. Pract.* **2015**, *21*, 598–604. [CrossRef] [PubMed]
68. Trads, M.; Deutch, S.R.; Pedersen, P.U. Supporting Patients in Reducing Postoperative Constipation: Fundamental Nursing Care—A Quasi-Experimental Study. *Scand. J. Caring Sci.* **2018**, *32*, 824–832. [CrossRef] [PubMed]
69. Bohl, D.D.; Shen, M.R.; Hannon, C.P.; Fillingham, Y.A.; Darrith, B.; Della Valle, C.J. Serum Albumin Predicts Survival and Postoperative Course Following Surgery for Geriatric Hip Fracture. *J. Bone Jt. Surg. Am.* **2017**, *99*, 2110–2118. [CrossRef] [PubMed]
70. Malafarina, V.; Reginster, J.-Y.; Cabrerizo, S.; Bruyère, O.; Kanis, J.A.; Martinez, J.A.; Zulet, M.A. Nutritional Status and Nutritional Treatment Are Related to Outcomes and Mortality in Older Adults with Hip Fracture. *Nutrients* **2018**, *10*, 555. [CrossRef]
71. Nuotio, M.; Tuominen, P.; Luukkaala, T. Association of Nutritional Status as Measured by the Mini-Nutritional Assessment Short Form with Changes in Mobility, Institutionalization and Death after Hip Fracture. *Eur. J. Clin. Nutr.* **2016**, *70*, 393–398. [CrossRef]
72. Díaz de Bustamante, M.; Alarcón, T.; Menéndez-Colino, R.; Ramírez-Martín, R.; Otero, Á.; González-Montalvo, J.I. Prevalence of Malnutrition in a Cohort of 509 Patients with Acute Hip Fracture: The Importance of a Comprehensive Assessment. *Eur. J. Clin. Nutr.* **2018**, *72*, 77–81. [CrossRef]
73. Helminen, H.; Luukkaala, T.; Saarnio, J.; Nuotio, M.S. Predictive Value of the Mini-Nutritional Assessment Short Form (MNA-SF) and Nutritional Risk Screening (NRS2002) in Hip Fracture. *Eur. J. Clin. Nutr.* **2019**, *73*, 112–120. [CrossRef]
74. Inoue, T.; Misu, S.; Tanaka, T.; Kakehi, T.; Ono, R. Acute Phase Nutritional Screening Tool Associated with Functional Outcomes of Hip Fracture Patients: A Longitudinal Study to Compare MNA-SF, MUST, NRS-2002 and GNRI. *Clin. Nutr.* **2019**, *38*, 220–226. [CrossRef]
75. Koren-Hakim, T.; Weiss, A.; Hershkovitz, A.; Otzrateni, I.; Anbar, R.; Gross Nevo, R.F.; Schlesinger, A.; Frishman, S.; Salai, M.; Beloosesky, Y. Comparing the Adequacy of the MNA-SF, NRS-2002 and MUST Nutritional Tools in Assessing Malnutrition in Hip Fracture Operated Elderly Patients. *Clin. Nutr.* **2016**, *35*, 1053–1058. [CrossRef] [PubMed]
76. Nishioka, S.; Wakabayashi, H.; Momosaki, R. Nutritional Status Changes and Activities of Daily Living after Hip Fracture in Convalescent Rehabilitation Units: A Retrospective Observational Cohort Study from the Japan Rehabilitation Nutrition Database. *J. Acad. Nutr. Diet* **2018**, *118*, 1270–1276. [CrossRef] [PubMed]
77. Mendelson, G.; Katz, Y.; Shahar, D.R.; Bar, O.; Lehman, Y.; Spiegel, D.; Ochayon, Y.; Shavit, N.; Mimran Nahon, D.; Radinski, Y.; et al. Nutritional Status and Osteoporotic Fracture Rehabilitation Outcomes in Older Adults. *J. Nutr. Gerontol. Geriatr.* **2018**, *37*, 231–240. [CrossRef]
78. Inoue, T.; Misu, S.; Tanaka, T.; Sakamoto, H.; Iwata, K.; Chuman, Y.; Ono, R. Pre-Fracture Nutritional Status Is Predictive of Functional Status at Discharge during the Acute Phase with Hip Fracture Patients: A Multicenter Prospective Cohort Study. *Clin. Nutr.* **2017**, *36*, 1320–1325. [CrossRef] [PubMed]
79. Beauchamp-Chalifour, P.; Belzile, E.L.; Racine, L.-C.; Nolet, M.-P.; Lemire, S.; Jean, S.; Pelet, S. The Long-Term Postoperative Trajectory of Geriatric Patients Admitted for a Hip Fracture: A Prospective Observational Cohort Study. *Orthop. Traumatol. Surg. Res.* **2020**, *106*, 621–625. [CrossRef] [PubMed]
80. Torbergsen, A.C.; Watne, L.O.; Frihagen, F.; Wyller, T.B.; Mowè, M. Effects of Nutritional Intervention upon Bone Turnover in Elderly Hip Fracture Patients. Randomized Controlled Trial. *Clin. Nutr. ESPEN* **2019**, *29*, 52–58. [CrossRef]
81. Malafarina, V.; Malafarina, C.; Biain Ugarte, A.; Martinez, J.A.; Abete Goñi, I.; Zulet, M.A. Factors Associated with Sarcopenia and 7-Year Mortality in Very Old Patients with Hip Fracture Admitted to Rehabilitation Units: A Pragmatic Study. *Nutrients* **2019**, *11*, 2243. [CrossRef] [PubMed]
82. González-Montalvo, J.I.; Alarcón, T.; Gotor, P.; Queipo, R.; Velasco, R.; Hoyos, R.; Pardo, A.; Otero, A. Prevalence of Sarcopenia in Acute Hip Fracture Patients and Its Influence on Short-Term Clinical Outcome. *Geriatr. Gerontol. Int.* **2016**, *16*, 1021–1027. [CrossRef]
83. Ha, Y.-C.; Won Won, C.; Kim, M.; Chun, K.-J.; Yoo, J.-I. SARC-F as a Useful Tool for Screening Sarcopenia in Elderly Patients with Hip Fractures. *J. Nutr. Health Aging* **2020**, *24*, 78–82. [CrossRef]
84. Landi, F.; Calvani, R.; Ortolani, E.; Salini, S.; Martone, A.M.; Santoro, L.; Santoliquido, A.; Sisto, A.; Picca, A.; Marzetti, E. The Association between Sarcopenia and Functional Outcomes among Older Patients with Hip Fracture Undergoing In-Hospital Rehabilitation. *Osteoporos. Int.* **2017**, *28*, 1569–1576. [CrossRef]
85. van de Ree, C.L.P.; Landers, M.J.F.; Kruithof, N.; de Munter, L.; Slaets, J.P.J.; Gosens, T.; de Jongh, M.A.C. Effect of Frailty on Quality of Life in Elderly Patients after Hip Fracture: A Longitudinal Study. *BMJ Open* **2019**, *9*, e025941. [CrossRef]

86. Rajeev, A.; Anto, J. The Role of Edmonton Frailty Scale and Asa Grade in the Assessment of Morbidity and Mortality after Fracture Neck of Femur in Elderly. *Acta Orthop. Belg.* **2019**, *85*, 346–351.
87. Winters, A.M.; Hartog, L.C.; Roijen, H.; Brohet, R.M.; Kamper, A.M. Relationship between Clinical Outcomes and Dutch Frailty Score among Elderly Patients Who Underwent Surgery for Hip Fracture. *Clin. Interv. Aging* **2018**, *13*, 2481–2486. [CrossRef] [PubMed]
88. McGuckin, D.G.; Mufti, S.; Turner, D.J.; Bond, C.; Moonesinghe, S.R. The Association of Peri-Operative Scores, Including Frailty, with Outcomes after Unscheduled Surgery. *Anaesthesia* **2018**, *73*, 819–824. [CrossRef] [PubMed]
89. Kua, J.; Ramason, R.; Rajamoney, G.; Chong, M.S. Which Frailty Measure Is a Good Predictor of Early Post-Operative Complications in Elderly Hip Fracture Patients? *Arch. Orthop. Trauma Surg.* **2016**, *136*, 639–647. [CrossRef] [PubMed]
90. Wei, R.; Chen, H.-L.; Zha, M.-L.; Zhou, Z.-Y. Diabetes and Pressure Ulcer Risk in Hip Fracture Patients: A Meta-Analysis. *J. Wound Care* **2017**, *26*, 519–527. [CrossRef]
91. Klestil, T.; Röder, C.; Stotter, C.; Winkler, B.; Nehrer, S.; Lutz, M.; Klerings, I.; Wagner, G.; Gartlehner, G.; Nussbaumer-Streit, B. Impact of Timing of Surgery in Elderly Hip Fracture Patients: A Systematic Review and Meta-Analysis. *Sci. Rep.* **2018**, *8*, 13933. [CrossRef]
92. Gazineo, D.; Chiari, P.; Chiarabelli, M.; Morri, M.; D'Alessandro, F.; Sabattini, T.; Ambrosi, E.; Forni, C. Predictive Factors for Category II Pressure Ulcers in Older Patients with Hip Fractures: A Prospective Study. *J. Wound Care* **2019**, *28*, 593–599. [CrossRef]
93. Magny, E.; Vallet, H.; Cohen-Bittan, J.; Raux, M.; Meziere, A.; Verny, M.; Riou, B.; Khiami, F.; Boddaert, J. Pressure Ulcers Are Associated with 6-Month Mortality in Elderly Patients with Hip Fracture Managed in Orthogeriatric Care Pathway. *Arch. Osteoporos.* **2017**, *12*, 77. [CrossRef]
94. Galivanche, A.R.; Kebaish, K.J.; Adrados, M.; Ottesen, T.D.; Varthi, A.G.; Rubin, L.E.; Grauer, J.N. Postoperative Pressure Ulcers After Geriatric Hip Fracture Surgery Are Predicted by Defined Preoperative Comorbidities and Postoperative Complications. *J. Am. Acad. Orthop. Surg.* **2020**, *28*, 342–351. [CrossRef]
95. Chiari, P.; Forni, C.; Guberti, M.; Gazineo, D.; Ronzoni, S.; D'Alessandro, F. Predictive Factors for Pressure Ulcers in an Older Adult Population Hospitalized for Hip Fractures: A Prognostic Cohort Study. *PLoS ONE* **2017**, *12*, e0169909. [CrossRef]
96. Gonzalez, E.D.D.L.; Mendivil, L.L.L.; Garza, D.P.S.; Hermosillo, H.G.; Chavez, J.H.M.; Corona, R.P. Low Handgrip Strength Is Associated with a Higher Incidence of Pressure Ulcers in Hip Fractured Patients. *Acta Orthop. Belg.* **2018**, *84*, 284–291. [PubMed]
97. Wu, X.; Tian, M.; Zhang, J.; Yang, M.; Gong, X.; Liu, Y.; Li, X.; Lindley, R.I.; Anderson, M.; Peng, K.; et al. The Effect of a Multidisciplinary Co-Management Program for the Older Hip Fracture Patients in Beijing: A "Pre- and Post-" Retrospective Study. *Arch. Osteoporos.* **2019**, *14*, 43. [CrossRef]
98. Forni, C.; D'Alessandro, F.; Genco, R.; Mini, S.; Notarnicola, T.; Vitulli, A.; Capezzali, D.; Morri, M. Prospective Prognostic Cohort Study of Pressure Injuries in Older Adult Patients with Hip Fractures. *Adv. Skin Wound Care* **2018**, *31*, 218–224. [CrossRef] [PubMed]
99. Correa-Pérez, A.; Delgado-Silveira, E.; Martín-Aragón, S.; Rojo-Sanchís, A.M.; Cruz-Jentoft, A.J. Fall-Risk Increasing Drugs and Prevalence of Polypharmacy in Older Patients Discharged from an Orthogeriatric Unit after a Hip Fracture. *Aging Clin. Exp. Res.* **2019**, *31*, 969–975. [CrossRef] [PubMed]
100. Heltne, M.; Saltvedt, I.; Lydersen, S.; Prestmo, A.; Sletvold, O.; Spigset, O. Patterns of Drug Prescriptions in an Orthogeriatric Ward as Compared to Orthopaedic Ward: Results from the Trondheim Hip Fracture Trial—A Randomised Clinical Trial. *Eur. J. Clin. Pharmacol.* **2017**, *73*, 937–947. [CrossRef] [PubMed]
101. Pajulammi, H.M.; Luukkaala, T.H.; Pihlajamäki, H.K.; Nuotio, M.S. Decreased Glomerular Filtration Rate Estimated by 2009 CKD-EPI Equation Predicts Mortality in Older Hip Fracture Population. *Injury* **2016**, *47*, 1536–1542. [CrossRef] [PubMed]
102. Ryan, G.; Nowak, L.; Melo, L.; Ward, S.; Atrey, A.; Schemitsch, E.H.; Nauth, A.; Khoshbin, A. Anemia at Presentation Predicts Acute Mortality and Need for Readmission Following Geriatric Hip Fracture. *JB JS Open Access* **2020**, *5*. [CrossRef] [PubMed]
103. Guo, W.-J.; Wang, J.-Q.; Zhang, W.-J.; Wang, W.-K.; Xu, D.; Luo, P. Hidden Blood Loss and Its Risk Factors after Hip Hemiarthroplasty for Displaced Femoral Neck Fractures: A Cross-Sectional Study. *Clin. Interv. Aging* **2018**, *13*, 1639–1645. [CrossRef] [PubMed]
104. Arshi, A.; Lai, W.C.; Iglesias, B.C.; McPherson, E.J.; Zeegen, E.N.; Stavrakis, A.I.; Sassoon, A.A. Blood Transfusion Rates and Predictors Following Geriatric Hip Fracture Surgery. *Hip. Int.* **2020**. [CrossRef]
105. Yombi, J.C.; Putineanu, D.C.; Cornu, O.; Lavand'homme, P.; Cornette, P.; Castanares-Zapatero, D. Low Haemoglobin at Admission Is Associated with Mortality after Hip Fractures in Elderly Patients. *Bone Jt. J.* **2019**, *101-B*, 1122–1128. [CrossRef]
106. Mueller, M.M.; Van Remoortel, H.; Meybohm, P.; Aranko, K.; Aubron, C.; Burger, R.; Carson, J.L.; Cichutek, K.; De Buck, E.; Devine, D.; et al. Patient Blood Management: Recommendations From the 2018 Frankfurt Consensus Conference. *JAMA* **2019**, *321*, 983–997. [CrossRef] [PubMed]
107. Zhu, C.; Yin, J.; Wang, B.; Xue, Q.; Gao, S.; Xing, L.; Wang, H.; Liu, W.; Liu, X. Restrictive versus Liberal Strategy for Red Blood-Cell Transfusion in Hip Fracture Patients: A Systematic Review and Meta-Analysis. *Medicine (Baltimore)* **2019**, *98*, e16795. [CrossRef] [PubMed]
108. Zerah, L.; Dourthe, L.; Cohen-Bittan, J.; Verny, M.; Raux, M.; Mézière, A.; Khiami, F.; Tourette, C.; Neri, C.; Le Manach, Y.; et al. Retrospective Evaluation of a Restrictive Transfusion Strategy in Older Adults with Hip Fracture. *J. Am. Geriatr. Soc.* **2018**, *66*, 1151–1157. [CrossRef] [PubMed]

109. Amin, R.M.; DeMario, V.M.; Best, M.J.; Shafiq, B.; Hasenboehler, E.A.; Sterling, R.S.; Frank, S.M.; Khanuja, H.S. A Restrictive Hemoglobin Transfusion Threshold of Less Than 7 g/DL Decreases Blood Utilization without Compromising Outcomes in Patients With Hip Fractures. *J. Am. Acad. Orthop. Surg.* **2019**, *27*, 887–894. [CrossRef] [PubMed]
110. Chen, R.; Li, L.; Xiang, Z.; Li, H.; Hou, X.-L. Association of Iron Supplementation with Risk of Transfusion, Hospital Length of Stay, and Mortality in Geriatric Patients Undergoing Hip Fracture Surgeries: A Meta-Analysis. *Eur. Geriatr. Med.* **2020**. [CrossRef]
111. Yoon, B.-H.; Lee, B.S.; Won, H.; Kim, H.-K.; Lee, Y.-K.; Koo, K.-H. Preoperative Iron Supplementation and Restrictive Transfusion Strategy in Hip Fracture Surgery. *Clin. Orthop. Surg.* **2019**, *11*, 265–269. [CrossRef] [PubMed]
112. Pareja Sierra, T.; Bartolome Martín, I.; Rodríguez Solis, J.; Morales Sanz, M.D.; Torralba Gonzalez de Suso, M.; Barcena Goitiandia, L.Á.; Hornillos Calvo, M. Results of an Anaemia Treatment Protocol Complementary to Blood Transfusion in Elderly Patients with Hip Fracture. *Rev. Esp. Geriatr. Gerontol.* **2019**, *54*, 272–279. [CrossRef] [PubMed]
113. Long, Y.; Wang, T.; Liu, J.; Duan, X.; Xiang, Z. Clinical study of recombinant human erythropoietin combined with iron to correct perioperative anemia in elderly patients with intertrochanteric fractures. *Zhongguo Xiu Fu Chong Jian Wai Ke Za Zhi* **2019**, *33*, 662–665. [CrossRef] [PubMed]
114. Yoon, B.-H.; Ko, Y.S.; Jang, S.-H.; Ha, J.K. Feasibility of Hip Fracture Surgery Using a No Transfusion Protocol in Elderly Patients: A Propensity Score-Matched Cohort Study. *J. Orthop. Trauma* **2017**, *31*, 414–419. [CrossRef]
115. Zhang, Y.; Chen, L.; Wu, P.; Lang, J.; Chen, L. Intervention with Erythropoietin in Sarcopenic Patients with Femoral Intertrochanteric Fracture and Its Potential Effects on Postoperative Rehabilitation. *Geriatr. Gerontol. Int.* **2020**, *20*, 150–155. [CrossRef]
116. Xiao, C.; Zhang, S.; Long, N.; Yu, W.; Jiang, Y. Is Intravenous Tranexamic Acid Effective and Safe during Hip Fracture Surgery? An Updated Meta-Analysis of Randomized Controlled Trials. *Arch. Orthop. Trauma Surg.* **2019**, *139*, 893–902. [CrossRef] [PubMed]
117. Baskaran, D.; Rahman, S.; Salmasi, Y.; Froghi, S.; Berber, O.; George, M. Effect of Tranexamic Acid Use on Blood Loss and Thromboembolic Risk in Hip Fracture Surgery: Systematic Review and Meta-Analysis. *Hip. Int.* **2018**, *28*, 3–10. [CrossRef] [PubMed]
118. Qi, Y.-M.; Wang, H.-P.; Li, Y.-J.; Ma, B.-B.; Xie, T.; Wang, C.; Chen, H.; Rui, Y.-F. The Efficacy and Safety of Intravenous Tranexamic Acid in Hip Fracture Surgery: A Systematic Review and Meta-Analysis. *J. Orthop. Translat.* **2019**, *19*, 1–11. [CrossRef] [PubMed]
119. Haj-Younes, B.; Sivakumar, B.S.; Wang, M.; An, V.V.; Lorentzos, P.; Adie, S. Tranexamic Acid in Hip Fracture Surgery: A Systematic Review and Meta-Analysis. *J. Orthop. Surg. (Hong Kong)* **2020**, *28*. [CrossRef]
120. Luo, X.; Huang, H.; Tang, X. Efficacy and Safety of Tranexamic Acid for Reducing Blood Loss in Elderly Patients with Intertrochanteric Fracture Treated with Intramedullary Fixation Surgery: A Meta-Analysis of Randomized Controlled Trials. *Acta Orthop. Traumatol. Turc.* **2020**, *54*, 4–14. [CrossRef] [PubMed]
121. Sanzone, A.G. Current Challenges in Pain Management in Hip Fracture Patients. *J. Orthop. Trauma* **2016**, *30* (Suppl. 1), S1–S5. [CrossRef]
122. Oberkircher, L.; Schubert, N.; Eschbach, D.-A.; Bliemel, C.; Krueger, A.; Ruchholtz, S.; Buecking, B. Prehospital Pain and Analgesic Therapy in Elderly Patients with Hip Fractures. *Pain Pract.* **2016**, *16*, 545–551. [CrossRef] [PubMed]
123. Orive, M.; Anton-Ladislao, A.; García-Gutiérrez, S.; Las Hayas, C.; González, N.; Zabala, J.; Quintana, J.M. Prospective Study of Predictive Factors of Changes in Pain and Hip Function after Hip Fracture among the Elderly. *Osteoporos. Int.* **2016**, *27*, 527–536. [CrossRef]
124. Riddell, M.; Ospina, M.; Holroyd-Leduc, J.M. Use of Femoral Nerve Blocks to Manage Hip Fracture Pain among Older Adults in the Emergency Department: A Systematic Review. *CJEM* **2016**, *18*, 245–252. [CrossRef] [PubMed]
125. Guay, J.; Kopp, S. Peripheral Nerve Blocks for Hip Fractures in Adults. *Cochrane Database Syst. Rev.* **2020**, *11*, CD001159. [CrossRef]
126. Elboim-Gabyzon, M.; Andrawus Najjar, S.; Shtarker, H. Effects of Transcutaneous Electrical Nerve Stimulation (TENS) on Acute Postoperative Pain Intensity and Mobility after Hip Fracture: A Double-Blinded, Randomized Trial. *Clin. Interv. Aging* **2019**, *14*, 1841–1850. [CrossRef] [PubMed]
127. Ganczak, M.; Chrobrowski, K.; Korzeń, M. Predictors of a Change and Correlation in Activities of Daily Living after Hip Fracture in Elderly Patients in a Community Hospital in Poland: A Six-Month Prospective Cohort Study. *Int. J. Environ. Res. Public Health* **2018**, *15*, 95. [CrossRef]
128. Morandi, A.; Mazzone, A.; Bernardini, B.; Suardi, T.; Prina, R.; Pozzi, C.; Gentile, S.; Trabucchi, M.; Bellelli, G. Association between Delirium, Adverse Clinical Events and Functional Outcomes in Older Patients Admitted to Rehabilitation Settings after a Hip Fracture: A Multicenter Retrospective Cohort Study. *Geriatr. Gerontol. Int.* **2019**, *19*, 404–408. [CrossRef]
129. Selakovic, I.; Dubljanin-Raspopovic, E.; Markovic-Denic, L.; Marusic, V.; Cirkovic, A.; Kadija, M.; Tomanovic-Vujadinovic, S.; Tulic, G. Can Early Assessment of Hand Grip Strength in Older Hip Fracture Patients Predict Functional Outcome? *PLoS ONE* **2019**, *14*, e0213223. [CrossRef]
130. Kronborg, L.; Bandholm, T.; Palm, H.; Kehlet, H.; Kristensen, M.T. Physical Activity in the Acute Ward Following Hip Fracture Surgery Is Associated with Less Fear of Falling. *J. Aging Phys. Act.* **2016**, *24*, 525–532. [CrossRef] [PubMed]
131. O'Halloran, P.D.; Shields, N.; Blackstock, F.; Wintle, E.; Taylor, N.F. Motivational Interviewing Increases Physical Activity and Self-Efficacy in People Living in the Community after Hip Fracture: A Randomized Controlled Trial. *Clin. Rehabil.* **2016**, *30*, 1108–1119. [CrossRef] [PubMed]

132. Monticone, M.; Ambrosini, E.; Brunati, R.; Capone, A.; Pagliari, G.; Secci, C.; Zatti, G.; Ferrante, S. How Balance Task-Specific Training Contributes to Improving Physical Function in Older Subjects Undergoing Rehabilitation Following Hip Fracture: A Randomized Controlled Trial. *Clin. Rehabil.* **2018**, *32*, 340–351. [CrossRef]
133. Briggs, R.A.; Houck, J.R.; Drummond, M.J.; Fritz, J.M.; LaStayo, P.C.; Marcus, R.L. Muscle Quality Improves with Extended High-Intensity Resistance Training after Hip Fracture. *J. Frailty Aging* **2018**, *7*, 51–56. [CrossRef]
134. Lee, S.Y.; Yoon, B.-H.; Beom, J.; Ha, Y.-C.; Lim, J.-Y. Effect of Lower-Limb Progressive Resistance Exercise after Hip Fracture Surgery: A Systematic Review and Meta-Analysis of Randomized Controlled Studies. *J. Am. Med. Dir. Assoc.* **2017**, *18*, 1096.e19–1096.e26. [CrossRef] [PubMed]
135. Mohammad Ismail, A.; Borg, T.; Sjolin, G.; Pourlotfi, A.; Holm, S.; Cao, Y.; Wretenberg, P.; Ahl, R.; Mohseni, S. β-Adrenergic Blockade Is Associated with a Reduced Risk of 90-Day Mortality after Surgery for Hip Fractures. *Trauma Surg. Acute Care Open* **2020**, *5*, e000533. [CrossRef]
136. van der Zwaard, B.C.; Stein, C.E.; Bootsma, J.E.M.; van Geffen, H.J.A.A.; Douw, C.M.; Keijsers, C.J.P.W. Fewer Patients Undergo Surgery When Adding a Comprehensive Geriatric Assessment in Older Patients with a Hip Fracture. *Arch. Orthop. Trauma Surg.* **2020**, *140*, 487–492. [CrossRef] [PubMed]
137. Zerah, L.; Hajage, D.; Raux, M.; Cohen-Bittan, J.; Mézière, A.; Khiami, F.; Le Manach, Y.; Riou, B.; Boddaert, J. Attributable Mortality of Hip Fracture in Older Patients: A Retrospective Observational Study. *J. Clin. Med.* **2020**, *9*, 2370. [CrossRef] [PubMed]
138. Daraphongsataporn, N.; Saloa, S.; Sriruanthong, K.; Philawuth, N.; Waiwattana, K.; Chonyuen, P.; Pimolbutr, K.; Sucharitpongpan, W. One-Year Mortality Rate after Fragility Hip Fractures and Associated Risk in Nan, Thailand. *Osteoporos. Sarcopenia* **2020**, *6*, 65–70. [CrossRef]
139. Capkin, S.; Guler, S.; Ozmanevra, R. C-Reactive Protein to Albumin Ratio May Predict Mortality for Elderly Population Who Undergo Hemiarthroplasty Due to Hip Fracture. *J. Investig. Surg.* **2020**, 1–6. [CrossRef]
140. Huette, P.; Abou-Arab, O.; Djebara, A.-E.; Terrasi, B.; Beyls, C.; Guinot, P.-G.; Havet, E.; Dupont, H.; Lorne, E.; Ntouba, A.; et al. Risk Factors and Mortality of Patients Undergoing Hip Fracture Surgery: A One-Year Follow-up Study. *Sci. Rep.* **2020**, *10*, 9607. [CrossRef]
141. Drevet, S.; Bornu, B.-J.C.; Boudissa, M.; Bioteau, C.; Mazière, S.; Merloz, P.; Couturier, P.; Tonetti, J.; Gavazzi, G. One-year mortality after a hip fracture: Prospective study of a cohort of patients aged over 75 years old. *Geriatr. Psychol. Neuropsychiatr. Vieil.* **2019**, *17*, 369–376. [CrossRef]
142. Menéndez-Colino, R.; Gutiérrez Misis, A.; Alarcon, T.; Díez-Sebastián, J.; Díaz de Bustamante, M.; Queipo, R.; Otero, A.; González-Montalvo, J.I. Development of a New Comprehensive Preoperative Risk Score for Predicting 1-Year Mortality in Patients with Hip Fracture: The HULP-HF Score. Comparison with 3 Other Risk Prediction Models. *Hip. Int.* **2020**. [CrossRef] [PubMed]
143. Choi, J.-Y.; Cho, K.-J.; Kim, S.-W.; Yoon, S.-J.; Kang, M.-G.; Kim, K.-I.; Lee, Y.-K.; Koo, K.-H.; Kim, C.-H. Prediction of Mortality and Postoperative Complications Using the Hip-Multidimensional Frailty Score in Elderly Patients with Hip Fracture. *Sci. Rep.* **2017**, *7*, 42966. [CrossRef]
144. Chesser, T.J.S.; Inman, D.; Johansen, A.; Belluati, A.; Pari, C.; Contini, A.; Voeten, S.C.; Hegeman, J.H.; Ponsen, K.J.; Montero-Fernández, N.; et al. Hip Fracture Systems—European Experience. *OTA Int.* **2020**, *3*, e050. [CrossRef]
145. Williamson, S.; Landeiro, F.; McConnell, T.; Fulford-Smith, L.; Javaid, M.K.; Judge, A.; Leal, J. Costs of Fragility Hip Fractures Globally: A Systematic Review and Meta-Regression Analysis. *Osteoporos. Int.* **2017**, *28*, 2791–2800. [CrossRef]
146. Tan, L.T.J.; Wong, S.J.; Kwek, E.B.K. Inpatient Cost for Hip Fracture Patients Managed with an Orthogeriatric Care Model in Singapore. *Singap. Med. J.* **2017**, *58*, 139–144. [CrossRef]
147. Bartra, A.; Caeiro, J.-R.; Mesa-Ramos, M.; Etxebarría-Foronda, I.; Montejo, J.; Carpintero, P.; Sorio-Vilela, F.; Gatell, S.; Canals, L.; en representación de los investigadores del estudio PROA. Cost of Osteoporotic Hip Fracture in Spain per Autonomous Region. *Rev. Esp. Cir. Ortop. Traumatol.* **2019**, *63*, 56–68. [CrossRef] [PubMed]
148. Adeyemi, A.; Delhougne, G. Incidence and Economic Burden of Intertrochanteric Fracture: A Medicare Claims Database Analysis. *JB JS Open Access* **2019**, *4*, e0045. [CrossRef] [PubMed]
149. Arshi, A.; Rezzadeh, K.; Stavrakis, A.I.; Bukata, S.V.; Zeegen, E.N. Standardized Hospital-Based Care Programs Improve Geriatric Hip Fracture Outcomes: An Analysis of the ACS NSQIP Targeted Hip Fracture Series. *J. Orthop. Trauma* **2019**, *33*, e223–e228. [CrossRef] [PubMed]
150. Reyes, B.J.; Mendelson, D.A.; Mujahid, N.; Mears, S.C.; Gleason, L.; Mangione, K.K.; Nana, A.; Mijares, M.; Ouslander, J.G. Postacute Management of Older Adults Suffering an Osteoporotic Hip Fracture: A Consensus Statement From the International Geriatric Fracture Society. *Geriatr. Orthop. Surg. Rehabil.* **2020**, *11*. [CrossRef]
151. González Montalvo, J.I.; Gotor Pérez, P.; Martín Vega, A.; Alarcón Alarcón, T.; Mauleón Álvarez de Linera, J.L.; Gil Garay, E.; García Cimbrelo, E.; Alonso Biarge, J. La Unidad de Ortogeriatría de Agudos. Evaluación de Su Efecto En El Curso Clínico de Los Pacientes Con Fractura de Cadera y Estimación de Su Impacto Económico. *Rev. Esp. Geriatr. Gerontol.* **2011**, *46*, 193–199. [CrossRef]
152. Ginsberg, G.; Adunsky, A.; Rasooly, I. A Cost-Utility Analysis of a Comprehensive Orthogeriatric Care for Hip Fracture Patients, Compared with Standard of Care Treatment. *Hip. Int.* **2013**, *23*, 570–575. [CrossRef]
153. Eamer, G.; Taheri, A.; Chen, S.S.; Daviduck, Q.; Chambers, T.; Shi, X.; Khadaroo, R.G. Comprehensive Geriatric Assessment for Older People Admitted to a Surgical Service. *Cochrane Database Syst. Rev.* **2018**, *1*, CD012485. [CrossRef]

154. Leal, J.; Gray, A.M.; Hawley, S.; Prieto-Alhambra, D.; Delmestri, A.; Arden, N.K.; Cooper, C.; Javaid, M.K.; Judge, A.; REFReSH Study Group. Cost-Effectiveness of Orthogeriatric and Fracture Liaison Service Models of Care for Hip Fracture Patients: A Population-Based Study. *J. Bone Miner. Res.* **2017**, *32*, 203–211. [CrossRef]
155. Eamer, G.; Saravana-Bawan, B.; van der Westhuizen, B.; Chambers, T.; Ohinmaa, A.; Khadaroo, R.G. Economic Evaluations of Comprehensive Geriatric Assessment in Surgical Patients: A Systematic Review. *J. Surg. Res.* **2017**, *218*, 9–17. [CrossRef] [PubMed]
156. Mesa Ramos, M.; Caeiro-Rey, J.R. Orthogeriatric Units. They Are Really Necessary. *Glob. J. Ortho. Res.* **2020**, *2*, 4.
157. Allsop, S.; Morphet, J.; Lee, S.; Cook, O. Exploring the Roles of Advanced Practice Nurses in the Care of Patients Following Fragility Hip Fracture: A Systematic Review. *J. Adv. Nurs.* **2020**. [CrossRef]
158. Van Camp, L.; Dejaeger, M.; Tournoy, J.; Gielen, E.; Laurent, M.R. Association of Orthogeriatric Care Models with Evaluation and Treatment of Osteoporosis: A Systematic Review and Meta-Analysis. *Osteoporos. Int.* **2020**, *31*, 2083–2092. [CrossRef] [PubMed]
159. Sheehan, K.J.; Fitzgerald, L.; Hatherley, S.; Potter, C.; Ayis, S.; Martin, F.C.; Gregson, C.L.; Cameron, I.D.; Beaupre, L.A.; Wyatt, D.; et al. Inequity in Rehabilitation Interventions after Hip Fracture: A Systematic Review. *Age Ageing* **2019**, *48*, 489–497. [CrossRef] [PubMed]
160. Sterling, R.S. Gender and Race/Ethnicity Differences in Hip Fracture Incidence, Morbidity, Mortality, and Function. *Clin. Orthop. Relat. Res.* **2011**, *469*, 1913–1918. [CrossRef]
161. Nayar, S.K.; Marrache, M.; Ali, I.; Bressner, J.; Raad, M.; Shafiq, B.; Srikumaran, U. Racial Disparity in Time to Surgery and Complications for Hip Fracture Patients. *Clin. Orthop. Surg.* **2020**, *12*, 430–434. [CrossRef]

Article

Predictive Model of Gait Recovery at One Month after Hip Fracture from a National Cohort of 25,607 Patients: The Hip Fracture Prognosis (HF-Prognosis) Tool

Cristina González de Villaumbrosia [1,*], Pilar Sáez López [2], Isaac Martín de Diego [3], Carmen Lancho Martín [3], Marina Cuesta Santa Teresa [3], Teresa Alarcón [4], Cristina Ojeda Thies [5], Rocío Queipo Matas [6], Juan Ignacio González-Montalvo [4] and on behalf of the Participants in the Spanish National Hip Fracture Registry [†]

1. Hospital Universitario Rey Juan Carlos, Universidad Rey Juan Carlos, 28933 Móstoles, Spain
2. Hospital Universitario Fundación Alcorcón, Instituto de Investigación Hospital Universitario La Paz, 28046 Madrid, Spain; pisalop@gmail.com
3. Data Science Lab, Universidad Rey Juan Carlos, 28933 Móstoles, Spain; isaac.martin@urjc.es (I.M.d.D.); carmen.lancho@urjc.es (C.L.M.); marina.cuesta@urjc.es (M.C.S.T.)
4. Hospital Universitario La Paz, Instituto de Investigación Hospital Universitario La Paz, 28046 Madrid, Spain; mteresa.alarcon@salud.madrid.org (T.A.); juanignacio.gonzalez@salud.madrid.org (J.I.G.-M.)
5. Hospital Universitario 12 De Octubre, 28041 Madrid, Spain; cristina.ojeda@salud.madrid.org
6. Data Science Lab, Universidad Europea de Madrid, 28005 Madrid, Spain; rocio.queipo@universidadeuropea.es
* Correspondence: cristina.gonzalez@hospitalreyjuancarlos.es
† SNHFR are listed in acknowledgments.

Abstract: The aim of this study was to develop a predictive model of gait recovery after hip fracture. Data was obtained from a sample of 25,607 patients included in the Spanish National Hip Fracture Registry from 2017 to 2019. The primary outcome was recovery of the baseline level of ambulatory capacity. A logistic regression model was developed using 40% of the sample and the model was validated in the remaining 60% of the sample. The predictors introduced in the model were: age, prefracture gait independence, cognitive impairment, anesthetic risk, fracture type, operative delay, early postoperative mobilization, weight bearing, presence of pressure ulcers and destination at discharge. Five groups of patients or clusters were identified by their predicted probability of recovery, including the most common features of each. A probability threshold of 0.706 in the training set led to an accuracy of the model of 0.64 in the validation set. We present an acceptably accurate predictive model of gait recovery after hip fracture based on the patients' individual characteristics. This model could aid clinicians to better target programs and interventions in this population.

Keywords: predictive model; hip fracture; gait recovery

1. Introduction

Hip fractures are highly prevalent in aging societies, with an incidence of over 150 cases annually per 100,000 inhabitants in the general population [1], increasing to 511 cases per year per 100,000 inhabitants over 65 years old [2]. This incidence is expected to rise due to the demographic changes foreseen in the coming decades [3]. These fractures entail high mortality rates (9% the first month after the fracture, 15.5% at 3 months, 26.5% at one year and 36.2% at two years [4,5]), high morbidity and readmission rates (9.3% in the first month [6]). They also affect the patients' functional status. Even one year after the fracture, approximately 50% of patients have been reported to newly require walking aids, and 90% need help climbing stairs, compared to 21–26% of controls matched for age, sex, comorbidity, and baseline functional status. Functional impairment and increased dependency often become chronic and increase the likelihood of other adverse outcomes such as institutionalization, cognitive impairment, risk of new falls and mortality, worsening the patient's quality of life and increasing healthcare costs [7–9].

The main component of functional recovery is regaining the ability to walk, so a better understanding of the probability that each individual has of recovering baseline ambulatory capacity following a hip fracture could potentially be useful for several reasons: first, clinicians would be able to counsel patients and caregivers on what degree of recovery of the ability to walk can be expected, allowing for better planning of their needs and improved clinical decision making. Second, awareness of the modifiable factors associated with greater deterioration of ambulation could guide clinicians and researchers on interventions to optimize the functional recovery of patients. Advances in surgical techniques, anesthesia, perioperative care, early rehabilitation and multidisciplinary teamwork have improved clinical outcomes in recent years. However, the functional impairment associated with hip fracture remains in need of improvement.

National hip fracture registries have been launched in several countries, allowing for audit of the care process, identification of the appropriateness or deviation from established quality standards and introduction of corrective measures to improve quality of care and efficiency. Often, however, there is insufficient clear data on the functional recovery following hip fracture. While previous studies have analyzed the prevalence of functional impairment and identified several predictive factors, they are generally single-center studies focusing on predictors of functional impairment or cluster analysis [10–12]. To our knowledge, no predictive model has been established to estimate the specific probability of each individual's functional recovery in our setting.

The objective of this study is to develop a predictive model serving as a tool to estimate the individual probability of recovering the previous level of gait independency one month after hip fracture and to build a practical tool applicable in the clinical setting.

2. Materials and Methods

2.1. Study Sample

We included patients aged 75 years old or older hospitalized for fragility hip fracture between January 2017 and December 2019 at any of the 61 participating hospitals in the Spanish National Hip Fracture Registry (SNHFR). This registry is a previously described initiative carried out voluntarily by a group of clinicians throughout Spain [13]. It is a prospective audit including the variables proposed by the Fragility Fracture Network, endorsed by over 20 regional and national scientific societies. Data is collected during acute hospitalization and one month after the fracture. The SNHFR has established and monitors several standards of quality of care, with the final goal of progressively improving care for patients suffering hip fractures [14].

Patients were included if: they were aged 75 years old or more and admitted to hospital for a fragility hip fracture, included in the SNHFR and provided written informed consent to data collection and analysis (by patients or their legally authorized representatives).

Exclusion criteria were: patients who were non-ambulatory before the fracture or whose walking ability was unknown, and those lost to one-month follow-up due to death, or unknown vital status or walking ability one month after the fracture.

The SNHFR recorded 31,882 cases between 1 January 2017 and 31 December 2019. After excluding 6275 cases, a final sample of 25,607 patients (80.3% of the initial sample) was used, as shown in Figure 1. Another 244 samples were omitted (0.95%) after the missing values analysis.

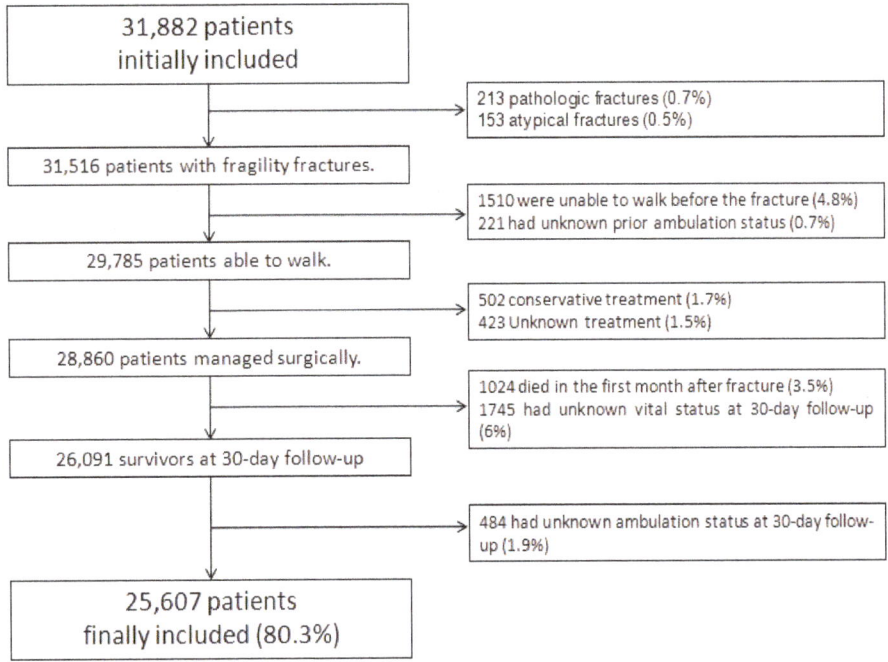

Figure 1. Inclusion and exclusion criteria.

2.2. Data Collection

Study data was collected by over 200 volunteer research clinicians or nurses from hospitals participating in the SNHFR. Baseline data on demographic and clinical variables and self-reported measures of their prefracture functional status was obtained during acute admission from interviewing the individuals or their representatives and through the patients' medical records. These included age, gender, place of residence (home, nursing home or acute hospitalization), date of arrival to the emergency room, date of surgery (if applicable) and date of discharge to calculate operative delay and total length of stay. Prefracture mobility was collected using the Functional Ambulation Classification Scale (FAC) [15], which scores between 0 (worst) and 5 (best): 0 (no gait at all, or needing the aid of two people), 1 (gait with great assistance of one person), 2 (gait with little help of one person), 3 (gait with supervision of one person), 4 (independent gait on flat surfaces, but needing help to climb stairs) and 5 (independent gait both on flat surfaces and climbing stairs). The target variable was recoded into three categories to facilitate understanding: unable to walk (FAC 0), dependent gait (FAC 1,2,3) and independent gait (FAC 4,5). It is summarized in Table 1. This classification emphasizes the need of another person's assistance to walk, regardless of the technical aids used. Cognitive status during admission was collected using the Pfeiffer Short Portable Mental State Questionnaire [16] (SPMSQ), defining cognitive impairment as 4 errors or more according to the validated Spanish version [17]. Other data collected was: Fracture type (intracapsular, intertrochanteric or subtrochanteric), anesthetic risk according to the American Society of Anesthesiologists' (ASA [18]) Physical Status Classification, type of anesthesia (general or spinal), early postoperative mobilization (in the first 24 h after surgery), development of pressure ulcers (grade II or more), involvement of a clinician in addition to the surgical specialist, applying a peripheral nerve block, destination at discharge (private home, nursing home, geriatric rehabilitation unit or other locations such as acute hospitalization or a long stay units), and vital status at discharge. Authorization of weight bearing on the operated limb started to be recorded mid-2018.

Table 1. Functional ambulation classification scale.

Functional Ambulation Category	Description
5	Independent, all surfaces
4	Independent, level surfaces only
3	Dependent for supervision
2	Dependent for physical assistance—level I (light touch)
1	Dependent for physical assistance—level II (support body weight)
0	Nonambulator

Follow-up data was obtained one month after the fracture by contacting the patients by telephone or in person during the follow-up visit. Information regarding vital status and level of ambulation (again using the Functional Ambulation Classification Scale [19]) was collected.

Study protocols were approved by the local institutional review boards of each of the 61 participating centers. A representative in each participating hospital is in charge of data custody and submission in an encrypted format at defined intervals to the registry's data manager, who is responsible for data cleaning, analysis, and database maintenance.

2.3. Outcome Definition

The primary outcome of this study is the recovery of the previous level of walking ability, defined as one of two possible outcomes: for previously independent patients (FAC 4,5), if they were again independent at follow-up (FAC 4,5). For previously dependent patients (FAC 1,2,3), if they were still able to walk at follow-up (FAC > 0). Patients meeting these criteria were defined as "patients recovering ambulation" and those who did not, "patients not recovering ambulation".

2.4. Statistical Analysis

An exploratory analysis was performed first to study variable distributions, the relationship of each variable with the outcome variable, and the presence of missing values. Missing values were treated in the following manner: if the percentage of the missing values was greater than 1%, a new category was created. That applies to the following variables; cognitive impairment (15.9% missing values), ASA (3.7%), weight bearing not allowed (61.2%) and pressure ulcers (1.6%). Regarding weight bearing, the high number of missing data can be explained by the fact that it was a variable that started to be collected after initiating the study. When the percentage of missing values was under 1%, as was the case for the rest of variables, that missing data was deleted. As a consequence, 0.95% of the observations from the entire dataset were eliminated.

Afterwards, in order to reduce overfitting, we split our sample into a training set (20% of the sample), test set (20%) and validation set (60%) [20]. Training and test sets were used in the first phase of the study to develop the predictive model. To assess the model's accuracy, the developed model was then tested to correctly predict the outcome in a different group of patients (the validation sample).

2.4.1. Training Phase

A descriptive analysis of the variables included in the SNHFR and relationship of each regressive variable with the target variable was carried out as follows: qualitative variables were expressed as counts and percentages, while continuous variables (age, presurgical length of stay, and total length of stay) were described using the median and interquartile range, after observing they did not conform to normal distribution using the Kolmogorov Smirnov test. Baseline characteristics of patients who recovered ambulation were compared with patients not recovering ambulation using the Chi-squared test for categorical variables and the Kruskal-Wallis test for continuous variables. Significance was set with an alpha error of $p = 0.05$. Univariate analysis allowed detecting which variables showed significant differences between groups.

The relationship between the explanatory variables and the target variable "recovery of ambulation" was studied using a logistic regression model, that allowed the likelihood of recovering ambulation to be estimated based on the values observed in the explanatory variables. All variables significantly associated with recovery of ambulation in the univariate analysis were selected and subjected to logistic regression. To select the best logistic regression model, cross-validation and a step-by-step selection of variables in the training set was applied.

Variables with several categories were recoded defining the most frequent category as the reference in the logistic regression model, shown in first place. This was the case for anesthetic risk (ASA III being the most common category), destination at discharge (home) and operative delay (more than 24 h). Some categories were grouped with the reference category, as a significant relation with the target variable was not found in the logistic regression. This was the case for the missing categories regarding pressure ulcers and weight bearing. Intracapsular and intertrochanteric fractures were similarly grouped together.

The probability of recovering ambulation for each individual of the training set through the adjusted regression model was calculated. A calculator using this model called the Hip Fracture Prognosis (HF-prognosis) tool will be included on the SNHFR website (http://rnfc.es/, accessed on 20 March 2021) and/or in a smartphone app.

The optimal threshold for the classification as presence or absence of recovery of ambulation was calculated with the probabilities obtained, optimizing the F1 score 21. This way, a trade-off between precision and recall is achieved [21].

Several cut-off points were defined for the probability of recovering ambulation, creating 5 groups: "very low" (probability less than 0.2), "low" (0.2–0.4), "medium" (0.4–0.6), "high" (0.6–0.8), and "very high" (probability greater than 0.8), allowing us to study the relationship between the predicted probabilities and the observed response variable.

2.4.2. Test Phase

The test set was used to ensure an adequate generalization of the results obtained in the training phase.

2.4.3. Validation Phase

The performance of the adjusted model that is presented in the next section as well as in the probability plot has been obtained using the validation set. All statistical analysis was performed with IBM SPSS Statistics version 27.0 software (IBM, Armonk, NY, USA).

3. Results

The baseline characteristics of the overall population and in the groups of patients who do and do not recover ambulation are shown in Table 2. All baseline characteristics had statistically significant differences between the group of patients with and without gait recovery, except gender (p value = 0.278), and the evaluation of a clinical doctor in addition to the Traumatology surgeon (p value = 0.167).

Table 2. Baseline characteristics of the global sample and according to the presence or absence of gait recovery. Univariate analysis.

		All Patients $n = 25{,}607$	Patients Recovering Ambulation $n = 16{,}839\ (65.8)$	Patients Not Recovering Ambulation $n = 8768\ (34.2)$	p Value
Age (years) Median ± IQR		87 (83–90)	86 (82–90)	88 (84–91)	<0.001
Gender (Female) n (%)		19,753 (77.1)	13,024 (77.4)	6729 (76.8)	0.278
Place of residence: nursing home n (%)		5404 (21.1)	2585 (15.4)	2819 (32.2)	<0.001
Prefracture ambulation n (%)	FAC 1	1073 (4.2)	514 (3.1)	559 (6.4)	<0.001
	FAC 2	1072 (4.2)	659 (3.9)	6413 (4.7)	
	FAC 3	908 (3.5)	616 (3.7)	292 (3.3)	
	FAC 4	7588 (29.6)	3662 (21.7)	3926 (44.8)	
	FAC 5	14,966 (58.4)	11,388 (67.6)	3578 (40.8)	
Cognitive impairment n (%)		8701 (40.4)	4589 (32.1)	4112 (57.0)	<0.001
ASA n (%)	I	295 (1.2)	253 (1.6)	42 (0.5)	<0.001
	II	7063 (28.6)	5224 (32.2)	1839 (21.8)	
	III	15,032 (61)	9481 (58.4)	5551 (65.9)	
	IV–V	2266 (9.2)	1275 (7.9)	991 (11.8)	
Fracture type n (%)	Intracapsular	10,005 (39.3)	7266 (43.4)	2739 (31.5)	<0.001
	Intertrochanteric	13,496 (53.1)	8490 (50.8)	5006 (57.5)	
	Subtrochanteric	1925 (7.6)	968 (5.8)	957 (11.0)	
Spinal anesthesia n (%)		23,948 (93.9)	15,805 (94.2)	8143 (93.5)	0.036
Peripheral nerve block n (%)		3534 (16.5)	2472 (18.0)	1062 (13.8)	<0.001
Time to surgery (hours) Median ± IQR		50.8 (26.1–90)	49.4 (25.1–89)	54,5 (28.2–91.6)	<0.001
Surgery in the first 24 h n (%)		5788 (22.6)	3966 (23.6)	1822 (20.8)	<0.001
Mobilization on the first postoperative day n (%)		17,685 (69.1)	12,354 (73.4)	5331 (60.9)	<0.001
Weight bearing not permitted n (%)		789 (7.9)	230 (3.6)	559 (15.8)	<0.001
Pressure ulcers n (%)		1233 (4.9)	592 (3.6)	641 (7.5)	<0.001
Clinician in addition to surgeon. n (%)		24,615 (96.2)	16,206 (96.3)	8409 (95.9)	0.167
Discharge destination n (%)	Home	11,345 (44.3)	8743 (51.9)	2602 (29.7)	<0.001
	Nursing home	7910 (30.9)	3928 (23.3)	3982 (45.4)	
	Geriatric rehabilitation unit	5893 (23.0)	3985 (23.7)	1908 (21.8)	
	Other	450 (1.8)	178 (1.1)	272 (3.1)	
Length of stay (days) Median ± IQR		8.9 (6.6–12.1)	8.7 (6.5–11.8)	9.2 (6.8–12.9)	<0.001

Abbreviations: IQR = interquartile range. FAC = Functional Ambulation Clasification. ASA = American Society of Anesthesiologists' Physical Status Classification.

3.1. Training Set; Logistic Regression Model

Figure 2 summarizes the adjusted logistic regression model explaining the target variable "recovery of ambulation" through the explanatory variables. The odds ratios [22] resulting from that model are shown in Table 3.

$$logit(P(Y = 1)) = \beta\_0 + \beta\_1 \; [\cdot x] \_1 + \ldots + \beta\_n \cdot x\_n =$$

+5.823
−0.048 · Age
+0.246 · Prefracture ambulation (FAC 1, 2, 3)
−0.768 · Cognitive impairment (present)
−0.384 · Cognitive impairment (unknown)
+0.194 · ASA (II)
+1.062 · ASA (I)
−0.335 · ASA (IV, V)
−0.284 · ASA (Unknown)
+0.148 · Surgical delay (≤ 24h)
−0.440 · No early postoperative mobilization
−0.985 · Discharge destination (Nursing home)
−0.358 · Discharge destination (Rehab facility)
−1.306 · Discharge destination (Others)
−0.631 · Fracture type (Subtrochanteric)
−1.906 · Weight bearing not allowed
−0.546 · Pressure ulcers (present)

Figure 2. Equation of the logistic regression model. Note that in the model some variables appear several times; this is because each time it refers to one of the variable's categories. Thus, for example, the ASA variable has 5 categories: reference (ASA III), I, II, IV-V and unknown. ASA III level does not appear in the formula because this is the reference level. If a patient has ASA I, in the model it will be translated as ASA I = 1 and the rest of ASA levels = 0. If a patient has ASA II, it will be ASA II = 1 and the rest of the ASA levels will be = 0.

Table 3. Results of the logistic regression model. Odds ratios of the explanatory variables, with the target variable "recovery of ambulation".

		Odds Ratio	95% Confidence Interval	
			Lower Margin	Higher Margin
	Age	0.953	0.942	0.964
Prefracture ambulation	Dependent (FAC 1–3)	1.279	1.055	1.550
Cognitive impairment	Present	0.464	0.401	0.537
	Unknown	0.681	0.566	0.820
ASA	I	2.891	1.273	6.565
	II	1.214	1.043	1.413
	IV–V	0.715	0.573	0.892
	Unknown	0.753	0.539	1.052
Type of fracture; Subtrochanteric fracture		0.532	0.422	0.671
Surgical delay ≤24 h.		1.159	0.993	1.352
Postoperative mobilization >24 h		0.644	0.562	0.737
Weight bearing Not allowed		0.149	0.098	0.224
Pressure ulcers Present		0.579	0.443	0.758
Discharge destination	Nursing home	0.373	0.321	0.434
	Geriatric rehabilitation unit	0.699	0.592	0.826
	Other	0.271	0.173	0.425

Abbreviations: FAC = Functional Ambulation Clasification. ASA = American Society of Anesthesiologists' Physical Status Classification. Reference categories are: Prefracture ambulation; Independent (FAC 4–5). Cognitive impairment; absent. Anaesthetic risk; ASA III. Type of fracture; intracapsular or intertrochanteric. Surgical delay; >24 h. Postoperative mobilization; ≤24 h. Weight bearing; allowed or unknown. Development of pressure ulcers; absent or unknown. Discharge destination; home.

3.2. Performance Measures in Validation

The optimum threshold for the prediction of the presence or absence of recovery of ambulation in patients included in the training set was 0.706. This threshold led to an accuracy of 0.64, a precision of 0.48, a recall of 0.74, a specificity of 0.58 and a F1 score of 0.59 in the validation set.

3.3. Groups by Predicted Probability of Recovery

Figure 3 shows the percentage of patients in each of the five groups of predicted probability of recovery, being the most common group the one with high probability of recovery. Figure 4 shows the observed percentages of recovered patients in each of the groups in the validation set. For example, 27.3% of the patients had a very high predicted probability of recovery. Of these, 86.8% recovered. Meanwhile, only 1.8% of the validation sample was classified as patients with a very low probability of recovery, of which only 22.1% managed to recover.

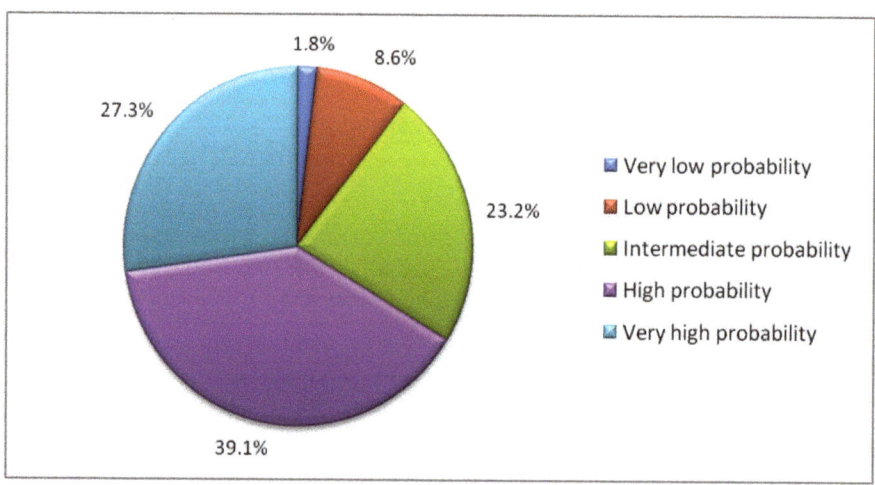

Figure 3. Distribution of the sample according to the groups of predicted probability of recovery.

The most common features of each group are summarized in Figure 5, and were the following:

- "Very low" group (less than 0.2 probability). This group represented 1.8% of the sample. With a mean age of 89.6 years, was characterized by patients admitted for subtrochanteric fractures, in whom postoperative weight bearing was not allowed, who develop pressure ulcers and who are discharged to locations other than their home, nursing homes or geriatric rehabilitation units, such as acute hospitalization or long-stay units.
- "Low" group (probability 0.2–0.4). This group represented 8.6% of the sample. Patients discharged to nursing homes, suffering subtrochanteric fractures, developing pressure ulcers, and not mobilized on the first postoperative day, characterized this group, that had an average age of 90.2 years. The scarcity of mild systemic disease (ASA = I–II) also stand out.
- "Medium" group (probability 0.4–0.6). This group represented 23.2% of the sample. With an average age of 88.7 years, was characterized by patients who walked with assistance (FAC 1–3) before the fracture, discharged to nursing homes, and who had cognitive impairment. The scarcity of mild systemic disease (ASA = I–II) was also noteworthy.

- "High" group (probability 0.6–0.8): This group represented 39.1% of the sample. With an average age of 86.6 years, was characterized by the scarcity of patients discharged to nursing homes and by the predominance of patients in whom weight bearing was allowed and who were sent to geriatric rehabilitation units at discharge.
- "Very high" group (probability greater than 0.8): This group represented 27.3% of the sample. The mean age of this group was 83 years. It was characterized by the scarcity of patients dependent for walking at baseline, as well as the scarcity of cognitive impairment, subtrochanteric fractures and pressure ulcers. ASA levels = I and II stand out as well as mobilization on the first postoperative day. There is also a predominance of short operative delay (less than 24 h) and discharge back home.

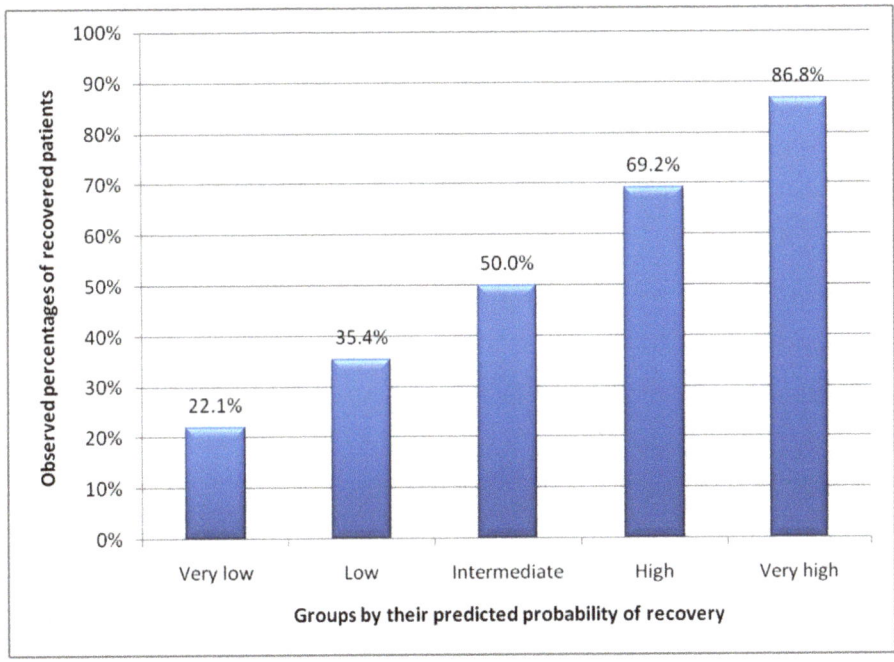

Figure 4. Rate of recovered patients within each group by their predicted probability of recovery.

3.4. Examples of Hypothetical Patients with Different Probabilities of Recovery

Here we show how the predicted probability of patients' recovery of ambulation is affected in the validation database when its explanatory variables are modified.

A 79-year-old patient who walks with little assistance (FAC = 2), is cognitively impaired, has mild systemic disease (ASA = II), suffered an intracapsular fracture. Surgery was delayed more than 24 h, the patient was not mobilized on the first postoperative day, but weight bearing was authorized; no pressure ulcers were developed, and the patient was discharged home. The estimated probability of recovery is 0.778. For this same patient:

- If weight bearing had not been authorized, probability of recovery would drop to 0.343.
- If weight bearing had not been authorized in addition to discharge to a nursing home, the probability of recovery would fall to 0.163.

A 96-year-old patient without cognitive impairment, but requiring continuous support of another person to walk (FAC = 1), who has suffered an intertrochanteric fracture, with an anesthetic risk score of ASA = III, has surgery delayed more than 24 h after admission, and was not mobilized on the first postoperative day. The patient did not develop pressure ulcers and was discharged to a nursing home. The probability of recovering ambulation is 0.506. If this patient:

- Had undergone surgery within 24 h after admission, the probability of recovery would be 0.543.
- Had been mobilized the first day after surgery, the probability of recovery would be 0.614.
- If both situations had occurred, the probability would reach 0.649.
- If weight bearing had not been authorized then the probability of recovery would fall to 0.132.

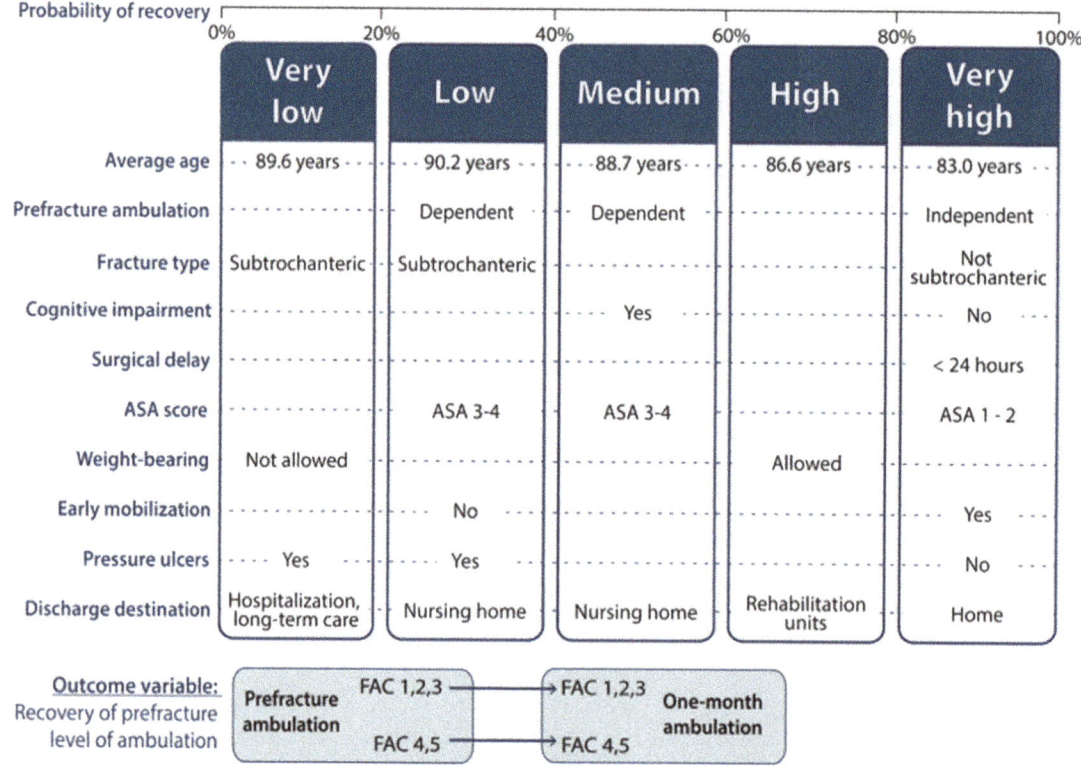

Figure 5. Clusters predicting the probability of functional recovery (very low; 0–20%; low, 20–40%; medium, 40–60%; high, 60–80%; very high, 80–100%), The boxes show the average age of the patients include in each cluster, as well as the most relevant features for the variables included in the model. Dashed lines represent transitions in which the difference between one cluster and the next were not relevant for the variable. Below: definition of the outcome variable as recovery of prefracture ambulation at one month, depending on FAC categories (1,2,3 vs. 4,5).

4. Discussion

This study proposes a method to estimate the probability of recovering previous ambulation one month after hip fracture. It allows us to stratify hip fracture patients into five risk groups (very low, low, medium, high, and very high probability of recovering ambulation).

We have identified several predictors of recovering ambulation after hip fracture, consistent with most studies. Age is one of the most cited factors, with older patients taking longer to regain their baseline walking ability or at greater risk of not achieving it [23–28]. Gender did not significantly affect ambulatory recovery in our study, nor in previous ones [29–31]. Our results, however differed from others regarding previous ambulatory dependence; while in other studies it seems to be a risk factor for not recovering ambulation [23,26,27] as also observed in the univariate analysis in our study, it proved to be a factor in favor of recovery in our regression model. This could be explained by the wide definition we have made of recovery of ambulation, despite it being similar to that of other authors. For example, in our study, a patient who walked regularly with supervision (FAC 3), may be more likely to recover as the margin up to the category of FAC 1 is wider, while for a patient with a baseline FAC 4 ambulation level, deteriorating to FAC 3 at one month was considered "not recovered".

Other risk factors of not recovering ambulation identified in our study, as well as in previous ones, are comorbidity [25,27,32], cognitive impairment [24–26], subtrochanteric fractures [24,26], not permitting weight-bearing [33,34], and late postoperative mobilization [35]. Operative delay has widely been studied as a risk factor for mortality, but there are few studies focusing on its relation with functional recovery [36,37]. In our study, an operative delay of more than 24 h was related to a higher risk of not recovering ambulation in the univariate analysis, but lost its significance in the multivariate analysis. This could be due to the relatively low proportion of patients treated in less than 24 h, inferior to that reported by other audits [13]. Analysis of other thresholds for delay and the combined effect of early surgery and early postoperative mobilization would be of interest. Pressure ulcers have been associated with longer surgical delay and increased mortality and morbidity [38] but their relation with recovery of ambulation has been studied less. We observed that they were associated with a lower probability of recovering ambulation, perhaps acting as an effect as well as a cause of reduced mobilization during hospitalization. The discharge destination showing the greatest likelihood of ambulatory recovery was home, followed by geriatric rehabilitation units; nursing homes and other locations such as acute hospitalization were associated with the lowest probability of recovering ambulation. The lack of recovery of walking ability could be a cause rather than consequence of the discharge destination. For example, a patient who recovers quickly and adequately during acute admission is more likely to return home, while a patient who does not regain ambulation—perhaps due to numerous intercurrent medical complications—is more likely to be transferred to a geriatric rehabilitation unit, and has still not recovered after a month. Finally, a patient who does not regain ambulation during acute admission and has little chance of doing so even in a rehabilitation facility is more likely to be sent to a nursing home. The appearance of medical complications, which could explain the worse functional results observed compared to those expected in some patients, is not included in the SNHFR and could therefore not be controlled for in the multivariate analysis.

Several factors such as the anesthetic risk are non-modifiable. Others, however, are modifiable and have an even greater impact on the likelihood of recovery, such as the permission to bear weight. With an Odds Ratio of 0.149, the risk of recovery is $1/0.149 = 6.71$ times higher in patients in whom weight bearing is permitted versus patients who are not allowed to bear weight. The modifiable factors found were time to surgery, early mobilization, weight-bearing status, and the development of pressure ulcers. Although the best discharge destination in our study was home, it is important to have the possibility to discharge patients to geriatric rehabilitation units in order to minimize the loss of ambulatory independency in complex patients. It is likely that a longer follow-up is needed to fully appreciate their effect.

Predictors of ambulatory recovery were similar to other studies focusing on tools that calculate the individual probability of recovering ambulation. Other factors not included in our model are gender, body mass index, polypharmacy, type of surgery performed, pre-fracture Barthel Index, and postoperative complications [32,39–41]. One of the studies cited has the advantage of using a longer (one year) follow-up [41]. Some developed a regression model similar to the one presented here [32,41], while others have reported a score instead [32,39]. All of them have been validated using less than 500 patients, and none of them have been validated in our setting. The most similar predictive model is the one developed by Kim et al., who retrospectively reviewed patients aged 60 and older with hip fractures and developed a predictive model of ambulation at one month postoperatively, which included age, gender, prefracture ambulation and the generic term of "combined medical diseases", defined as diseases which could affect ambulatory capacity. Their model showed an accuracy of 0.704 but did not include any modifiable variables on which to act [32].

One of the strengths of our study is the large number of patients included, offering enough statistical power to be able to study multiple predictive factors of gait recovery. The casemix reported by the SNHFR is similar to that in other studies from Spain [42–47], and it can be inferred it is representative of the population of hip fractures. The possibility of calculating the individual probability of recovering ambulation using a simple web based calculator makes this study particularly interesting.

We are aware our study has several weaknesses. First, comorbidity was adjusted using to the ASA score instead of a specific score for comorbidity. The ASA score is however collected universally through hospitals and recommended in the Fragility Fracture Network dataset for hip fracture audit. Second, possible confounding factors like the presence of medical complications during admission was not recorded, as previously mentioned. Data on the rehabilitation and mobilization carried out during admission—not only on the first postoperative day—would also be interesting to take into account. Third, this is an observational study; the theoretical contribution of each factor to ambulatory recovery can be examined, and hypotheses can be formulated, but the effect of individual interventions on each of the prognostic factors cannot be quantified, nor can causality be determined. We are limited to showing statistically significant associations. Fourth, ambulatory capacity was measured using the FAC scale, which relies mainly on the responses given by the patient and/or family during admission. This is less accurate than measures such as the Timed up and go [48], SPPB [49] tests. In the setting of an acute hip fracture, it would be impossible to obtain preoperative baseline measurements for these tests. Fifth, more than 200 professionals are involved in data collection, which may increase the risk of classification errors and variability, especially if the one-month follow-up information was obtained by telephone instead of in person. Finally, follow-up is carried out at one month. Thirty days is a very short period for recovery compared with other studies and registries with longer follow-up periods (usually 3 or 6 months), which more accurately determine the level of long-term functional recovery. Again, our registry follows the Fragility Fracture Network's Minimum Common Dataset, which recommends 30-day follow-up. In our opinion, predicting short-term recovery is also interesting. Few studies that provide information on the ability to walk at one month, and the ability to walk at 30 days is an important factor in planning short-term patient care. It also could potentially be a predictor of recovery at 3 or 6 months or even 1 year.

In summary, hip fracture commonly leads to dependence in older patients that frequently persists one month after the fracture. The ambulatory capacity of patients with a lower functional reserve is more likely compared to those who do not deteriorate. The former group is more likely to be older, be admitted from nursing homes, have dementia or significant comorbidity, and therefore has a more unfavorable baseline situation. They are less likely to receive peripheral nerve blocks, to be operated on in less than 24 h or be mobilized on the first postoperative day, and they are referred to rehabilitation units less frequently. In order to maximize the likelihood of recovering the ability to walk, our resources should be focused on optimizing these modifiable factors.

A tool that identifies the probability of each patient to recover pre-fracture walking independence following hip fracture surgery is useful for aiding clinicians and health care administrators to develop targeted programs and interventions. Healthcare administrators could also use it to estimate the need of post-acute care facilities adapted to patients' needs. This aid is also useful to counsel patients and caregivers on the functional prognosis following hip fracture, so they can plan the social support they may need.

Further studies are, of course, needed to validate this tool for different populations and settings. More complex machine learning models rather than logistic regression models could help us to improve this model in the near future.

5. Conclusions

The aim of this study was the development of a predictive model that aid clinicians to calculate the probability for patient of recovering the baseline level of independent or assisted ambulation one month after hip fracture. This is important, as the ability to walk is the main component of functional recovery after a hip fracture.

In this study of 25,607 Spanish hip fracture patients, 16,839 (65.8%) recovered prefracture ambulatory capacity at one month. Non-modifiable risk factors independently associated with worse recovery were cognitive impairment, elevated anesthetic risk, and a suffering subtrochanteric fractures. The modifiable factors affecting the probability of regaining prefracture ambulation were performing surgery in less than 24 h, early mobilization, allowance of weight-bearing, avoiding pressure ulcers and discharging the patient home.

We have successfully developed a predictive model that included all these factors, based on logistic regression. Our model has shown similar accuracy to prior studies by other authors. This predictive model estimates the individual probability of recovery (ranging from 0 to 100%), and we have defined 5 groups or clusters of patients depending on this probability. Patients with a very low and low probability of recovery are usually older, have suffered subtrochanteric fractures, are not allowed to bear weight, and are commonly discharged to nursing homes. On the other hand, patients with high and very high probabilities of recovery are younger, without cognitive impairment, present with intracapsular or intertrochanteric fractures, and walked independently before the fracture; they also have a shorter surgical delay and are likely to be sent home at discharge. In other words, those with the least probability of recovery start off from a worse baseline situation, but also managed more poorly, with worse performance indicators during admission, such as greater surgical delay or not allowing weight bearing. On the opposite end of the spectrum, patients most likely to recover have a better prefracture status and are better managed, fulfilling key performance indicators.

These findings can be used to aid risk stratification in this population to support informed treatment decisions and to aid conversations regarding goals of care. Future work on this topic could refine the precision of the model using more complex machine learning models, and longer follow-up time.

Author Contributions: Conceptualization: P.S.L., I.M.d.D. and C.G.d.V. Methodology, software, validation, formal analysis: C.G.d.V., I.M.d.D., C.L.M., M.C.S.T., R.Q.M. Writing (Original Draft Preparation): C.G.d.V. and I.M.d.D. Writing (Review & Editing): P.S.L., J.I.G.-M., T.A., C.O.T. Visualization, supervision, project Administration, funding acquisition: P.S.L., J.I.G.-M., T.A. All authors have read and agreed to the published version of the manuscript.

Funding: This project was funded by AMGEN SA, UCB PharmaSA, Abbott Laboratories SA and FAES Farma, as well as a research grant awarded by the Fundación Mutua Madrileña (grant number AP169672018) and Fundación Mapfre. The sponsors had no role in the design, execution, interpretation, or writing of the study.

Institutional Review Board Statement: The study was conducted according to the guidelines of the Declaration of Helsinki, and approved by the Ethics Committee of each participating hospital, headed by "Instituto de Investigación Hospital Universitario La Paz, Madrid, Comunidad de Madrid, Spain".

Informed Consent Statement: Written informed consent was obtained from all subjects involved in the study.

Data Availability Statement: The data obtained from the SNHFR is anonymized and guarded by the data manager. They are available to the participants in the registry for the preparation of reports with the intention of anonymously comparing the results between centers, and for the development of studies, under the supervision of the organizing board of the Registry. The data is not accessible on any freely accessible web page.

Acknowledgments: The authors wish to thank Jesús Martín García from BSJ Marketing for his administrative help, Laura Navarro Castellanos for her work as data manager, and Raquel Barba Martín for her contribution in the revision of the manuscript and proposals of improvement. We want to give special thanks to each participant of the SNHFR. Thanks to their collaboration and perseverance during these years, it has been possible to continue improving the results of our clinical practice and to develop studies like this. The list of participants is: Iñigo Etxebarría, Amaia Santxez, Uxue Barrena. Natalia Sánchez Hernández, Flavia Lorena Hünicken Torrez. Leonor Cuadra Llopart, Laura de Haro García, Georgina Cerdà Mas, Pedro Zubeldia Centeno. Anabel Llopis, Gustavo Adolfo Lucar López, Adrián Oller Bonache, Montserrat Méndez Brich. Macarena Morales Yáñez, Estela Mañana Vázquez, Marcela Camps Ferrer. Abelardo Montero Sáez. José Manuel Cancio, Jose Luis Rodríguez García. José Salvador Barreda Puchades, Anca Dragoi Dragoi. Noelia Míguez Alonso. Raquel Ortés Gómez, Guadalupe Lozano Pino, Estela Villalba Lancho, Jean Carlos Heredia Pons. Nuria Fernández Martínez, Francisco Manuel García Navas, Javier Gil Moreno y Virginia Mazoteras Muños. José Ramón Caeiro, Eduardo del Río Pombo y Aurora Freire Romero. Regina Feijoo. Elena Ubis Diez, Isabel Peralta y Amparo Fontestad, Caterina Soler. Sonia Jiménez Mola, Javier Idoate Gil, Isabel Porras Guerra. Mariano de Miguel Artal, Ana Scott-Tennet de Rivas, Amer Mustafa Gondolbeu, Olga Roca Chacón. Nuria Montero Fernández, Virginia Mendoza Moreno. Fátima Brañas Baztan y María Alcantud Ibáñez. María Isabel Pérez Millán, Concepción Fernández Mejía y María Jesús López Ramos. Ana Isabel Hormigo, Teresa de la Huerga Fernandez Boffil, Javier Sánchez Martín, Myriam Rodríguez Couso, María Almudena Milán Vegas, Manuel Vicente Mejía Ramírez De Arellano, Virginia Ruiz Almarza. Jesús Mora Fernández, Ana Mª Moreno Morillo, Mijail Méndez Hinojosa, Diana K Villacrés Estrada, Ana Garrido, Marta Echevarría, Ana Broughton Díez. Raquel Vállez Romero. Elisa Martín de Francisco. Verónica García Cárdenas, Nuria El Kadaooui Calvo, Verónica Martín. Miriam Rosa Ramos Cortés. Marta Neira Álvarez, Ana Mª Hurtado Ortega, Ruben Herreros Ruiz Valdepeñas, Guillermo Carretero Cristobal, Lorena Vicente Díaz. María Auxiliadora Julia Illán Moyano, Fernando Garcia Navarrete. María Jesús Molina Hernández, Rosario García Martín, Jaime Rodríguez Salazar. Teresa Pareja Sierra, Juan Rodríguez Solis, Irene Bartolomé Martín. Cristina González de Villaumbrosia, Javier Martínez Peromingo, Carlos Oñoro Algar, Sonia Torras Cortada, Yanira Suárez Sánchez. Inmaculada Boyano, Agustín Prieto Sánchez, Francisco Javier Cid Abasalo, Sonia Nieto Colino. María Gonzalo Lázaro, Bernardo Abel Cedeño Veloz. María Elvira Salgado. Mónica Suárez, Carmen Fidalgo, Francisco Jiménez Muela, Laura Pellitero Blanco. Laura Pellitero. Mª Luisa Taboada Martínez. Marta Alonso Álvarez, David Bonilla Diez. Ana Andrés Marta Pérez García, Lucía Ferradás García, Patricia María Balvís, Diego Matías Domínguez Prado, Alejandro García Reza, Alberto Carpintero Vara, Constantino Iglesias Núñez. Jesús Pérez del Molino Martín, Mª Jesús Sanz-Aranguez Avila, Zoilo Yusta Escudero, Marta Madariaga Canoura, Mª Begoña Busta Vallina, Mª Isabel Pérez Nuñez. María Teresa Guerrero, Elena Ridruejo, Ángelica Muñoz, Ma Cruz Macias, Pilar del Pozo Tagarro. Mª Carmen Barrero Raya, Romeo Enrique Rivas Espinoza, Miguel Antonio Araujo Ordóñez. Paula Santos Patiño, Samuel Díaz Gómez, José Carlos Armada Pérez, Alonso Sepúlveda Martínez, María Alonso Seco, Clara Pedro Monfort, Leonel Porta González. Mariano Barres Carsi, María José Pérez Dura, Adrián Alonso Caravaca, Miguel Ángel CastilloSoriano, Miguel de Pedro Abascal, Amparo Ortega Yago. Mª Carmen Cervera, Virginia García Virto, María Bragado González, Juan Berrocal Cuadrado, Ricardo León Fernández, Hector J. Aguado Hernández. María Pilar Mesa Lampré, Sofía Solsona Fernández, Jorge Corrales Cardenal, Claudia Murillo Erazo, Nora Molina Torres, Elisa Lasala Hernández. Concepción Casinnello Ogea. Ángel Castro Sauras, María Teresa Espallargas Donate, María Pilar Muniesa Herrro, Miguel Ranera García, José Adolfo Blanco Llorca, Alejandro Urgel Granados, María Royo Agustín, Agustín Rillo Lázaro, Jorge García Fuente, Alberto Planas Gil, Vicente Sánchez Ramos, SilviaAldabas Soriano. Raquel Bachiller. Eugenia Sonia Sopnea. Carmen Benítez González, Belén Cámara Marín, María Adela Delgado Álvarez de Sotomayor, Ines Gil Broceño. Laura Alexandra Ivanov, Alfred Dealbert Andres, Oscar Macho Perez. Amparo Cerón González. Pablo Díaz de Rada Lorente, María Rosa González Panisello, José Ramón Mora Martínez. Manuel Mesa Ramos, Pilar Márquez de Torres, María del Mar Higuera Álvarez de los Corrales. Silvia Comas Herrero. José Luis Navarro López, Miguel Fernández Sánchez, Teresa Flores Ruano, Gema Paterna Mellinas. Cristina Bermejo Boixareu, Jesús Campo Loarte, Gema Piña Delgado, Macarena Díaz de Bustamante de Ussía, Samuel González González, Fernando Segismundo Jañez Moral, Armando Pardo Gómez, Ainhoa Guijarro Valtueña, María Iluminada Martín García, Juan Martínez Candial. Silvia Lozoya Moreno, Sergio Salmerón

Ríos, Esther Martínez Sánchez, Isabel María Soler Moratalla, María Isabel Azabarte Cano, Lucia Sánchez Cózar, María Luisa Sánchez Galletero. Laura Puertas, Pablo Castillón, Cristina Estrada, Verónica Gil, Olga Gómez, Irene Omiste. Verónica Pérez del Rio. Sonia Bartolomé Blanco. Javier Sainz Reig, Jesús Más Martínez. María Cinta Escuder Capafons, Verónica Rico Ramírez, Adriana Soria Franch, Cristina Corral Martínez, Daniel Salamanca Rodríguez, Alejandro Pastor Zaplana, Petra Llull Riera. Amalia Navarro Martínez, Lourdes Sáez, Sergio Losa Palacios, MaríaEsther Ladrón de Guevara Córcoles, Ainara Achaerandio de Nova, Joaquín Alfaro mico, Maía del Carmen Viejobueno Mayordomo, Leticia García Sánchez, Virginia Parra Ramos, Cristina Rosa Felipe, María Cortés Avilés Martínez. Javier Pérez-Jara Carrera, María Ángeles Helguera de la Cruz. Regina Feijoo. Jordi Robert. Paloma Muñoz Mingarro, Pedro Gray, Oscar Perez Simanca, Carlos Prato, Jose Juárez, Jose Miguel Guijarro. Jose Eduardo Salinas, Elena Blay, Silvia Correoso, Beatriz Muela, Eva Veracruz, Francisco Navarro, Miguel Palazón, Vicente Mira, Antonio Ortín, Alberto Garcia, Javier Ricon, Ana Corraliza, David Coves, Mari Luz Aguilar, Jesus Jimenez, Carmen Rosa, Juan Antonio Lozano María Aritizta Arreta. Josu Lauzirika Uranga, Unai García De Cortázar Antolín, Mirentxu Arrieta Salinas, Daniel Escobar Sánchez, Estibaliz Castrillo Carrera, Mar Abeal López, Javier Hoyos Cillero, Lara Fernández Gutiérrez, Ainara Izaguirre Zurinaga, César García Puertas, Arkaitz Lara Quintana, Borja Cuevas Martínez, David García Marinas, Ivan Arrizabalaga Legorburu, Andrea Domínguez Ibarrola, Julia Isabel Martino Quintela, Idoia Villamor García, Ander Moso Bilbao. Esther Lueje Alonso, Lucía Fernández Arana, Elisa Martín de Francisci, Guillermo Sánchez Inchaust, Jaime Mateos Delgado, Carlos Zorzo Godes. Pilar Sáez López, Beatriz Perdomo Ramírez, Miguel Ángel Marín Aguado, Álvaro López Hualda, José Luis Patiño Contreras, Irene Blanca Moreno Fenol, María Angeles Pizarro Jaraiz, Pilar Martínez Velasco, Leandro Valdez Disla, Sara Aya Rodriguez, Mally Veras Basora, Isabel González Anglada, Javier Martínez Martín. Magali González-Colaço Harmand. María Victoria Farré Mercadé, Nuria Pérez Muñoz, Georgina Codina Frutos. Gregorio Jiménez Díaz, Natalia González García, María Madrigal López. Carmen Deza Pérez, Raquel Rodríguez Herrero. Ignacio Maestre. Juan Manuel Fernandez Domínguez, Antoine Nicolas Najem Rizk. María Cristina Rodríguez González.

Conflicts of Interest: Cristina González de Villaumbrosia has received honoraria for speaking at symposia and financial support for attending symposia from Abbott and Nutricia, none of them related to the present work. Pilar Sáez López has received financial aid for attendance to scientific events from Nutricia Advanced Medical Nutrition and Nestlé and has received speakers' honoraria from Abbott Laboratories SA and AMGEN SA, none of them related to the present work. Cristina Ojeda Thies has received financial aid for attendance to scientific events from AMGEN SA and UCB Pharma, and has received speakers' honoraria from AMGEN SA, Grünenthal Pharma and MBA Iberica, none of them related to the present work. Juan Ignacio González Montalvo has received speakers' honoraria from AMGEN SA, Nutricia Advanced Medical Nutrition and Nestlé and has coordinated educational activities financed by Nutricia Advanced Medical Nutrition, AMGEN SA and GSK, none of them related to the present work. Isaac Martín de Diego, Carmen Lancho Martín, Marina Cuesta Santa Teresa, Rocío Queipo Matas and Teresa Alarcón have no conflict of interest to declare.

References

1. Kanis, J.A.; on behalf of the IOF Working Group on Epidemiology and Quality of Life; Odén, A.; McCloskey, E.V.; Johansson, H.; Wahl, D.A.; Cooper, C. A systematic review of hip fracture incidence and probability of fracture worldwide. *Osteoporos. Int.* **2012**, *23*, 2239–2256. [CrossRef] [PubMed]
2. Alvarez-Nebreda, M.L.; Jiménez, A.B.; Rodríguez, P.; Serra, J.A. Epidemiology of hip fracture in the elderly in Spain. *Bone* **2008**, *42*, 278–285. [CrossRef] [PubMed]
3. Azagra, R.; López-Expósito, F.; Martin-Sánchez, J.C.; Aguyé, A.; Moreno, N.; Cooper, C.; Díez-Pérez, A.; Dennison, E.M. Changing trends in the epidemiology of hip fracture in Spain. *Osteoporos. Int.* **2014**, *25*, 1267–1274. [CrossRef]
4. Haleem, S.; Lutchman, L.; Mayahi, R.; Grice, J.; Parker, M. Mortality following hip fracture: Trends and geographical variations over the last 40 years. *Injury* **2008**, *39*, 1157–1163. [CrossRef]
5. Giversen, I.M. Time trends of mortality after first hip fractures. *Osteoporos. Int.* **2007**, *18*, 721–732. [CrossRef] [PubMed]
6. Pollock, F.H.; Bethea, A.; Samanta, D.; Modak, A.; Maurer, J.P.; Chumbe, J.T. Readmission within 30 days of discharge after hip fracture care. *Orthopedics* **2015**, *38*, e7–e13. [CrossRef]
7. Alarcón, T.A.; González-Montalvo, J.I. Fractura osteoporótica de cadera: Factores predictivos de recuperación funcional a corto y largo plazo. *An. Med. Interna* **2004**, *21*, 49–58. [CrossRef]
8. Liem, I.S.L.; Kammerlander, C.; Suhm, N.; Kates, S.L.; Blauth, M. Literature review of outcome parameters used in studies of geriatric fracture centers. *Arch. Orthop. Trauma Surg.* **2012**, *134*, 181–187. [CrossRef]

9. Liem, I.; Kammerlander, C.; Suhm, N.; Blauth, M.; Roth, T.; Gosch, M.; Hoang-Kim, A.; Mendelson, D.; Zuckerman, J.; Leung, F.; et al. Identifying a standard set of outcome parameters for the evaluation of orthogeriatric co-management for hip fractures. *Injury* **2013**, *44*, 1403–1412. [CrossRef]
10. Eastwood, E.A.; Magaziner, J.; Wang, J.; Silberzweig, S.B.; Hannan, E.L.; Strauss, E.; Siu, A.L. Patients with hip fracture: Subgroups and their outcomes. *J. Am. Geriatr. Soc.* **2002**, *50*, 1240–1249. [CrossRef]
11. Colón-Emeric, C.; Whitson, H.E.; Pieper, C.F.; Sloane, R.; Orwig, D.; Huffman, K.M.; Bettger, J.P.; Parker, D.; Crabtree, D.M.; Gruber-Baldini, A.; et al. Resiliency Groups Following Hip Fracture in Older Adults. *J. Am. Geriatr. Soc.* **2019**, *67*, 2519–2527. [CrossRef]
12. Michel, J.-P.; Hoffmeyer, P.; Klopfenstein, C.; Bruchez, M.; Grab, B.; D'Epinay, C.L. Prognosis of Functional Recovery 1 Year after Hip Fracture: Typical Patient Profiles Through Cluster Analysis. *J. Gerontol. Ser. A Boil. Sci. Med. Sci.* **2000**, *55*, M508–M515. [CrossRef]
13. Ojeda-Thies, C.; Rnfc, O.B.O.T.P.I.T.; Sáez-López, P.; Currie, C.; Tarazona-Santalbina, F.; Alarcón, T.; Muñoz-Pascual, A.; Pareja, T.; Gómez-Campelo, P.; Montero-Fernández, N.; et al. Spanish National Hip Fracture Registry (RNFC): Analysis of its first annual report and international comparison with other established registries. *Osteoporos. Int.* **2019**, *30*, 1243–1254. [CrossRef] [PubMed]
14. Condorhuamán-Alvarado, P.Y.; Pareja-Sierra, T.; Muñoz-Pascual, A.; Sáez-López, P.; Ojeda-Thies, C.; Alarcón-Alarcón, T.; Cassinello-Ogea, M.C.; Pérez-Castrillón, J.L.; Gómez-Campelo, P.; Navarro-Castellanos, L.; et al. First proposal of quality indicators and standards and recommendations to improve the healthcare in the Spanish National Registry of Hip Fracture. *Rev. Española Geriatría Gerontol.* **2019**, *54*, 257–264. [CrossRef]
15. Holden, M.K.; Gill, K.M.; Magliozzi, M.R.; Nathan, J.; Piehl-Baker, L. Clinical Gait Assessment in the Neurologically Impaired. *Phys. Ther.* **1984**, *64*, 35–40. [CrossRef]
16. Pfeiffer, E. A Short Portable Mental Status Questionnaire for the Assessment of Organic Brain Deficit in Elderly Patients. *J. Am. Geriatr. Soc.* **1975**, *23*, 433–441. [CrossRef]
17. De La Iglesiaa, J.M.; Dueñasherrerob, R.; Vilchesa, M.C.O.; Tabernéa, C.A.; Colomerc, C.A.; Luquec, R.L. Adaptación y validación al castellano del cuestionario de Pfeiffer (SPMSQ) para detectar la existencia de deterioro cognitivo en personas mayores e 65 años. *Med. Clínica* **2001**, *117*, 129–134. [CrossRef]
18. Owens, W.D.; Felts, J.A.; Spitznagel, E.L. ASA physical status classifications: A study of consistency of ratings. *Anesthe-Siology* **1978**, *49*, 239–243. [CrossRef]
19. Viosca, E.; Martínez, J.L.; Almagro, P.L.; Gracia, A.; González, C. Proposal and Validation of a New Functional Ambulation Classification Scale for Clinical Use. *Arch. Phys. Med. Rehabil.* **2005**, *86*, 1234–1238. [CrossRef]
20. Efron, B. The Jackknife, the Bootstrap and Other Resampling Plans. *Soc. Ind. Appl. Math.* **1982**. [CrossRef]
21. James, G.; Witten, D.; Hastie, T.; Tibshirani, R. *An Introduction to Statistical Learning: With Applications in R*; Springer: New York, NY, USA, 2013; Volume 112, p. 18.
22. *Applied Logistic Regression*, 3rd ed.; Wiley: Hoboken, NJ, USA; Available online: https://www.wiley.com/en-us/Applied+Logistic+Regression%2C+3rd+Edition-p-9780470582473 (accessed on 26 December 2020).
23. Hannan, E.L.; Magaziner, J.; Wang, J.J.; Eastwood, E.A.; Silberzweig, S.B.; Gilbert, J.; Morrison, R.S.; McLaughlin, M.A.; Orosz, G.M.; Siu, A.L. Mortality and Locomotion 6 Months After Hospitalization for Hip Fracture: Risk factors and risk-adjusted hospital outcomes. *JAMA* **2001**, *285*, 2736–2742. [CrossRef]
24. Kim, S.-M.; Moon, Y.-W.; Lim, S.-J.; Yoon, B.-K.; Min, Y.-K.; Lee, D.-Y.; Park, Y.-S. Prediction of survival, second fracture, and functional recovery following the first hip fracture surgery in elderly patients. *Bone* **2012**, *50*, 1343–1350. [CrossRef]
25. Tang, V.L.; Sudore, R.; Cenzer, I.S.; Boscardin, W.J.; Smith, A.; Ritchie, C.; Wallhagen, M.; Finlayson, E.; Petrillo, L.; Covinsky, K. Rates of Recovery to Pre-Fracture Function in Older Persons with Hip Fracture: An Observational Study. *J. Gen. Intern. Med.* **2017**, *32*, 153–158. [CrossRef]
26. Pajulammi, H.M.; Pihlajamäki, H.K.; Luukkaala, T.H.; Nuotio, M.S. Pre- and perioperative predictors of changes in mobility and living arrangements after hip fracture—A population-based study. *Arch. Gerontol. Geriatr.* **2015**, *61*, 182–189. [CrossRef]
27. Pioli, G.; Lauretani, F.; Pellicciotti, F.; Pignedoli, P.; Bendini, C.; Davoli, M.L.; Martini, E.; Zagatti, A.; Giordano, A.; Nardelli, A.; et al. Modifiable and non-modifiable risk factors affecting walking recovery after hip fracture. *Osteoporos. Int.* **2016**, *27*, 2009–2016. [CrossRef]
28. Ouellet, J.A.; Ouellet, G.M.; Romegialli, A.M.; Hirsch, M.; Berardi, L.; Ramsey, C.M., Jr.; Walke, L.M. Functional Outcomes after Hip Fracture in Independent Community-Dwelling Patients. *J. Am. Geriatr. Soc.* **2019**, *67*, 1386–1392. [CrossRef]
29. Sterling, R.S. Gender and Race/Ethnicity Differences in Hip Fracture Incidence, Morbidity, Mortality, and Function. *Clin. Orthop. Relat. Res.* **2011**, *469*, 1913–1918. [CrossRef]
30. Endo, Y.; Aharonoff, G.B.; Zuckerman, J.D.; Egol, K.A.; Koval, K.J. Gender Differences in Patients With Hip Fracture: A Greater Risk of Morbidity and Mortality in Men. *J. Orthop. Trauma* **2005**, *19*, 29–35. [CrossRef]
31. Woodward, L.M.; Clemson, L.; Moseley, A.M.; Lord, S.R.; Cameron, I.D.; Sherrington, C. Most functional outcomes are similar for men and women after hip fracture: A secondary analysis of the enhancing mobility after hip fracture trial. *BMC Geriatr.* **2014**, *14*, 140. [CrossRef]
32. Kim, J.L.; Jung, J.S.; Kim, S.J. Prediction of Ambulatory Status after Hip Fracture Surgery in Patients Over 60 Years Old. *Ann. Rehabil. Med.* **2016**, *40*, 666–674. [CrossRef]

33. Ariza-Vega, P.; Jiménez-Moleón, J.J.; Kristensen, M.T. Non-Weight-Bearing Status Compromises the Functional Level Up to 1 yr after Hip Fracture Surgery. *Am. J. Phys. Med. Rehabil.* **2014**, *93*, 641–648. [CrossRef] [PubMed]
34. Baer, M.; Neuhaus, V.; Pape, H.C.; Ciritsis, B. Influence of mobilization and weight bearing on in-hospital outcome in geriatric patients with hip fractures. *SICOT-J* **2019**, *5*, 4. [CrossRef]
35. Siu, A.L.; Penrod, J.D.; Boockvar, K.S.; Koval, K.; Strauss, E.; Morrison, R.S. Early Ambulation after Hip Fracture. *Arch. Intern. Med.* **2006**, *166*, 766–771. [CrossRef]
36. Cohn, M.R.; Cong, G.-T.; Nwachukwu, B.U.; Patt, M.L.; Desai, P.; Zambrana, L.; Lane, J.M. Factors Associated With Early Functional Outcome after Hip Fracture Surgery. *Geriatr. Orthop. Surg. Rehabil.* **2016**, *7*, 3–8. [CrossRef] [PubMed]
37. Al-Ani, A.N.; Samuelsson, B.; Tidermark, J.; Norling, Å.; Ekström, W.; Cederholm, T.; Hedström, M. Early Operation on Patients with a Hip Fracture Improved the Ability to Return to Independent Living. *J. Bone Jt. Surg. Am.* **2008**, *90*, 1436–1442. [CrossRef] [PubMed]
38. Magny, E.; Vallet, H.; Cohen-Bittan, J.; Raux, M.; Meziere, A.; Verny, M.; Riou, B.; Khiami, F.; Boddaert, J. Pressure ulcers are associated with 6-month mortality in elderly patients with hip fracture managed in orthogeriatric care pathway. *Arch. Osteoporos.* **2017**, *12*, 77. [CrossRef]
39. Belelli, G.; Noale, M.; Guerini, F.; Turco, R.; Maggi, S.; Crepaldi, G.; Trabucchi, M. A prognostic model predicting recovery of walking independence of elderly patients after hip-fracture surgery. An experiment in a rehabilitation unit in Northern Italy. *Osteoporos. Int.* **2012**, *23*, 2189–2200. [CrossRef]
40. Zuckerman, J.D.; Koval, K.J.; Aharonoff, G.B.; Hiebert, R.; Skovron, M.L. A Functional Recovery Score for Elderly Hip Fracture Patients: I. Development. *J. Orthop. Trauma* **2000**, *14*, 20–25. [CrossRef]
41. Hirose, J.; Ide, J.; Yakushiji, T.; Abe, Y.; Nishida, K.; Maeda, S.; Anraku, Y.; Usuku, K.; Mizuta, H. Prediction of Postoperative Ambulatory Status 1 Year after Hip Fracture Surgery. *Arch. Phys. Med. Rehabil.* **2010**, *91*, 67–72. [CrossRef]
42. Cancio, J.M.; Vela, E.; Santaeugènia, S.; Clèries, M.; Inzitari, M.; Ruiz, D. Long-term Impact of Hip Fracture on the Use of Healthcare Resources: A Population-Based Study. *J. Am. Med Dir. Assoc.* **2019**, *20*, 456–461. [CrossRef]
43. Hernández, M.J.M.; De Villaumbrosia, C.G.; Murga, E.M.D.F.D.; Alarcón, T.A.; Montero-Fernández, N.; Illán, J.; Bielza, R.; Mora-Fernández, J. Registro de fracturas de cadera multicéntrico de unidades de Ortogeriatría de la Comunidad Autónoma de Madrid. *Rev. Española Geriatría Gerontol.* **2019**, *54*, 5–11. [CrossRef]
44. Muñoz-Pascual, A.; Sáez-López, P.; Jiménez-Mola, S.; Sánchez-Hernández, N.; Alonso-García, N.; Andrés-Sainz, A.I.; Macias-Montero, M.C.; Vázquez-Pedrezuela, C.; Juez, N.P.D.C.; Del Pozo-Tagarro, P.; et al. Ortogeriatría: Primer registro multicéntrico autonómico de fracturas de cadera en Castilla y León (España). *Rev. Española Geriatría Gerontol.* **2017**, *52*, 242–248. [CrossRef] [PubMed]
45. Prieto-Alhambra, D.; Reyes, C.; Sainz, M.S.; González-Macías, J.; Delgado, L.G.; Bouzón, C.A.; Gañan, S.M.; Miedes, D.M.; Vaquero-Cervino, E.; Bardaji, M.F.B.; et al. In-hospital care, complications, and 4-month mortality following a hip or proximal femur fracture: The Spanish registry of osteoporotic femur fractures prospective cohort study. *Arch. Osteoporos.* **2018**, *13*, 1–11. [CrossRef]
46. Caeiro, J.R.; Bartra, A.; Mesa-Ramos, M.; Etxebarría, Í.; Montejo, J.; Carpintero, P.; Sorio, F.; Gatell, S.; Farré, A.; Canals, L.; et al. Burden of First Osteoporotic Hip Fracture in Spain: A Prospective, 12-Month, Observational Study. *Calcif. Tissue Int.* **2016**, *100*, 29–39. [CrossRef] [PubMed]
47. Sáez-López, P.; Ojeda-Thies, C.; Alarcón, T.; Pascual, A.M.; Mora-Fernández, J.; De Villaumbrosia, C.G.; Hernández, M.J.M.; Montero-Fernández, N.; Trujillo, J.M.C.; Pérez, A.D.; et al. Spanish National Hip Fracture Registry (RNFC): First-year results and comparison with other registries and prospective multi-centric studies from Spain. *Rev. Esp. Salud. Publica.* **2019**, *93*, 201910072.
48. Podsiadlo, D.; Richardson, S. The Timed "Up & Go": A Test of Basic Functional Mobility for Frail Elderly Persons. *J. Am. Geriatr. Soc.* **1991**, *39*, 142–148. [CrossRef] [PubMed]
49. Guralnik, J.M.; Simonsick, E.M.; Ferrucci, L.; Glynn, R.J.; Berkman, L.F.; Blazer, D.G.; Scherr, P.A.; Wallace, R.B. A Short Physical Performance Battery Assessing Lower Extremity Function: Association with Self-Reported Disability and Prediction of Mortality and Nursing Home Admission. *J. Gerontol.* **1994**, *49*, M85–M94. [CrossRef]

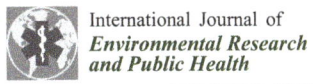

Article

Reliability, Validity, and Feasibility of the Frail-VIG Index

Anna Torné [1,2], Emma Puigoriol [3,4], Edurne Zabaleta-del-Olmo [5,6,7], Juan-José Zamora-Sánchez [6], Sebastià Santaeugènia [1,8] and Jordi Amblàs-Novellas [1,2,8,*]

1. Central Catalonia Chronicity Research Group (C3RG), Centre for Health and Social Care Research (CESS), Faculty of Medicine, University of Vic-Central University of Catalonia (UVIC-UCC), 08500 Barcelona, Spain; atorneco@gmail.com (A.T.); sebastia.santaeugenia@gencat.cat (S.S.)
2. Geriatric and Palliative Care Department, Hospital Universitari de la Santa Creu and Hospital Universitari de Vic, 08500 Barcelona, Spain
3. Clinical Epidemiology Unit, Consorci Hospitalari de Vic, 08500 Barcelona, Spain; epuigoriol@chv.cat
4. Tissue Repair and Regeneration Laboratory (TR2Lab), Faculty of Sciences and Technology, Faculty of Medicine, University of Vic-Central University of Catalonia, 08500 Barcelona, Spain
5. Fundació Institut Universitari per a la Recerca a L'atenció Primària de Salut Jordi Gol I Gurina (IDIAPJGol), 08500 Barcelona, Spain; ezabaleta@idiapjgol.org
6. Gerència Territorial de Barcelona, Institut Català de la Salut, 08500 Barcelona, Spain; juanjozamora72@gmail.com
7. Nursing Department, Faculty of Nursing, Universitat de Girona, 17005 Girona, Spain
8. Chronic Care Program, Ministry of Health, Generalitat de Catalunya, 08830 Catalonia, Spain
* Correspondence: jordiamblas@gmail.com

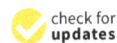

Citation: Torné, A.; Puigoriol, E.; Zabaleta-del-Olmo, E.; Zamora-Sánchez, J.-J.; Santaeugènia, S.; Amblàs-Novellas, J. Reliability, Validity, and Feasibility of the Frail-VIG Index. *IJERPH* **2021**, *18*, 5187. https://doi.org/10.3390/ijerph18105187

Academic Editor: Graziano Onder

Received: 31 March 2021
Accepted: 9 May 2021
Published: 13 May 2021

Publisher's Note: MDPI stays neutral with regard to jurisdictional claims in published maps and institutional affiliations.

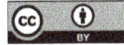

Copyright: © 2021 by the authors. Licensee MDPI, Basel, Switzerland. This article is an open access article distributed under the terms and conditions of the Creative Commons Attribution (CC BY) license (https://creativecommons.org/licenses/by/4.0/).

Abstract: The study aimed to assess the reliability of the scores, evidence of validity, and feasibility of the Frail-VIG index. A validation study mixing hospitalized and community-dwelling older people was designed. Intraclass correlation coefficient (ICC) was used to assess the inter-rater agreement and the reliability. The construct validity of the Frail-VIG index with respect to the Frailty Phenotype (FP) was evaluated by calculating the area under the receiver operating characteristic curve (AUC-ROC). Convergent validity with the Clinical Frailty Scale (CFS) was assessed using Pearson's correlation coefficients. The feasibility was evaluated by calculating the average time required to administer the Frail-VIG index and the percentage of unanswered responses. A sample of 527 older people (mean age of 81.61, 56.2% female) was included. The inter-rater agreement and test–retest reliability were very strong: 0.941 (95% CI, 0.890 to 0.969) and 0.976 (95% CI, 0.958 to 0.986), respectively. Results indicated adequate convergent validity of the Frail-VIG index with respect to the FP, AUC-ROC 0.704 (95% CI, 0.622 to 0.786), and a moderate to strong positive correlation between the Frail-VIG index and CFS ($r = 0.635$, 95% CI, 0.54 to 0.71). The Frail-VIG index administration required an average of 5.01 min, with only 0.34% of unanswered responses. The Frail-VIG index is a reliable, feasible, and valid instrument to assess the degree of frailty in hospitalized and community-dwelling older people.

Keywords: feasibility; frailty; frailty index; psychometrics; reliability; validity

1. Introduction

1.1. Background

Over the last few decades, developed countries have undergone a demographic and epidemiological shift that has led to progressive aging of the population and to an increased prevalence of people with chronic diseases [1,2]. While the two most prevalent chronic health problems are multimorbidity and frailty [3], frailty is the chronic condition most frequently associated with poor health outcomes, such as mortality or disability [4,5], as has become apparent during the COVID-19 pandemic [6,7]. In this scenario, the concept of frailty—understood as a vulnerability state against stressing factors due to limited compensatory mechanisms [8]—seems to emerge as a sound line of argument for health systems and their professionals, which require understandable narratives and pragmatic instruments [9,10]. However, despite the widespread consensus regarding the usefulness of the concept of frailty [11] and the need for its routine assessment in the clinical practice [12], there is still some controversy over the operational approach to address it [8].

These difficulties may be explained by two facts. On the one hand, the broadness of the concept of frailty (which ranges from the syndromic view to the accumulation of deficits approach) [13], in addition to the enriching academic debate, may have determined difficulties in its applicability to the healthcare practice. In summary, it can be said that frailty may be presented as a syndromic/dichotomous reality (*"Is this person frail or not?"*) [14], which becomes especially useful for screening for the population that can potentially benefit from preventive actions; the Frailty Phenotype (FP) [14] criteria, the Fatigue, Resistance, Ambulation, Illnesses, and Loss of Weight (FRAIL) [15] questionnaire, the Gérontopôle Frailty Screening Tool [16], or functional performance tests (such as the gait speed test [17] or the Short Physical Performance Battery [18]) are examples of useful instruments for this approach. However, frailty can also be seen as a continuous reality based on the accumulation of different deficits (*"How frail is this person?"*) [19], which is particularly useful to assess a person's situational diagnosis or degree of reserve [20]. Both the Clinical Frailty Scale (CFS) [21] and the frailty indices (FIs) [22] may be effective instruments in this approach to frailty.

On the other hand, there are many frailty assessment tools available [12], which are not always sufficiently pragmatic or feasible in the daily clinical practice, or which are not valid or reliable enough [23]. In this sense, the psychometric assessment of frailty instruments should be a research priority, in order to produce even stronger evidence on the practical usefulness of the concept of frailty [24,25]. This need becomes especially relevant in the case of FIs [26], for which there are limited studies on reliability of its scores, construct validity, and feasibility [27].

One of the FIs that has shown better mortality predictive capacity is the Frail-VIG index, with an area under the receiver operating characteristic curve (AUC-ROC) of 0.90 and 0.85 at 1 and 2 years, respectively [28,29]. Published in 2017 by Amblàs-Novellas et al., this FI, based on the Comprehensive Geriatric Assessment, consists of 22 trigger questions that are used to assess 25 deficits from eight different dimensions, with a final score that can range from 0 to 1 (with the submaximal limit in the clinical practice being close to 0.7). There is an excel calculator available at https://en.c3rg.com/index-fragil-vig (31 March 2021).

1.2. Objective/Rationale

Although previous papers have shown an excellent mortality predictive capacity, as well as good content validity and interpretability, there are no conclusive data on its reliability, construct validity, and feasibility. Therefore, this article aims to analyze the reliability of the scores, evidence of validity, and feasibility of the Frail-VIG index.

2. Methods

This article follows the guidelines established by the Consensus-Based Standards for the Selection of Health Measurement Instruments (COSMIN) on the design of studies to assess the measurement properties of instruments [30]. The study protocol was approved by the Ethics Committee of the University Hospital of Vic (2018958/PR189).

2.1. Study Design and Participants

This is an observational study, based on the classical test theory [31] and conducted in the prospective FIS/VIG cohort designed for the validation of the Frail-VIG index and the dynamic assessment of frailty over time. Participant recruitment was performed at an intermediate care hospital, with a home-based follow-up of 12 months and quarterly assessments of the degree of frailty by means of the Frail-VIG index.

The inclusion criteria for the study were individuals ≥75 years of age and/or identified as people with complex care needs (PCC, in Catalan) or with palliative care needs (MACA, in Catalan), based on the criteria developed by the Health Department of Catalonia [32,33], who were admitted to the Santa Creu de Vic University Hospital (Barcelona, Spain) during the study enrolment period (July 2018–July 2019). This intermediate care hospital was equipped with 100 beds, as well as subacute care, functional rehabilitation, palliative care, and psychogeriatric units. Patients were admitted from primary care or acute care hospitals, generally in the context of an acute intercurrent process. Those individuals for whom the in-person home follow-up was deemed difficult due to geographical reasons (more than 30 km away from the hospital) were excluded from the study.

2.2. Variables and Data Sources

In terms of epidemiological variables, these included age, gender, and usual place of residence. At the clinical level, all the variables included in the Frail-VIG index (Table 1) were collected, as well as the degree of frailty according to the classification into four categories commonly used in our clinical practice: non-frailty (Frail-VIG index score < 0.2), mild frailty (Frail-VIG index score 0.2–0.35), moderate frailty (Frail-VIG index score 0.36–0.5), and severe frailty (Frail-VIG index score > 0.5).

Table 1. Epidemiological and clinical characteristics of the cohort at baseline and at the 6 and 12 month follow-ups. At the 6 month follow-up (when the different frailty measurement instruments were compared), the characteristics of the group of non-frail (Frail-VIG index 0–0.19) vs. frail individuals (Frail-VIG index 0.20–1.00) are also shown.

	Baseline Total N = 527	Month 6 Follow-Up			Month 12 Follow-Up n = 176
		Total n = 200	No Frailty n = 20 (10.0%)	Frailty n = 180 (90.0%)	
		Demographic characteristics			
Age (years), mean ± SD	81.61 ± 9.9	80.9 ± 10.6	82.6 ± 7.2	80.7 ± 10.9	81.7 ± 9.6
Sex (women), N (%)	296 (56.2)	114 (57.0)	11 (55.0)	103 (57.2)	98 (55.7)
		Usual habitat, No (%)			
Nursing home	68 (12.9)	63 (31.5)	0 (0.0)	63 (35.0)	48 (27.3)
Home	440 (83.5)	129 (64.5)	20 (100.0)	109 (60.5)	111 (63.1)
Others	2 (0.4)	1 (0.5)	0 (0.0)	1 (0.6)	0 (0.0)
Missing information	17 (3.2)	7 (3.5)	0 (0.0)	7 (3.9)	17 (9.6)
		Living arrangement [1], No (%)			
With family	303 (68.5)	93 (71.6)	15 (75.0)	78 (70.9)	76 (68.5)
With caregiver	22 (5.0)	6 (4.6)	0 (0.0)	6 (5.5)	5 (4.5)
Alone	105 (23.8)	25 (19.2)	4 (20.0)	21 (19.1)	18 (16.2)
Others	4 (0.9)	0 (0.0)	0 (0.0)	0 (0.0)	0 (0.0)
Missing information	8 (1.8)	6 (4.6)	1 (5.0)	5 (4.5)	12 (10.8)
		Frail-VIG variables			
Functional IADLs (0–3), mean ± SD	1.48 ± 1.3	1.81 ± 1.2	0.15 ± 0.3	1.99 ± 1.1	1.80 ± 1.3
Barthel index (0–100), mean ± SD	73.87 ± 27.5	57.5 ± 32.4	90.5 ± 22.5	53.9 ± 31.3	62.2 ± 31.1
Malnutrition, N (%)	144 (27.3)	34 (17.1)	2 (10.0)	32 (17.9)	15 (9.1)
Cognitive impairment, N (%)	198 (37.6)	83 (41.7)	0 (0.0)	83 (46.3)	62 (37.8)
Depressive syndrome, N (%)	165 (31.3)	78 (39.6)	2 (10.0)	76 (42.9)	75 (44.9)
Insomnia/anxiety, N (%)	255 (48.4)	119 (59.8)	4 (20.0)	115 (64.2)	96 (56.8)
Social vulnerability, N (%)	74 (14.0)	4 (2.0)	0 (0.0)	4 (2.0)	8 (4.8)
Delirium, N (%)	85 (16.1)	59 (29.5)	1 (5.0)	58 (32.2)	45 (26.8)
Falls, N (%)	111 (21.1)	35 (17.7)	1 (5.0)	34 (19.1)	23 (13.9)
Ulcers, N (%)	56 (10.6)	27 (13.5)	0 (0.0)	27 (15.0)	17 (10.4)
Polypharmacy, N (%)	425 (80.6)	176 (88.0)	357 (86.7)	176 (88.0)	141 (83.9)
Dysphagia, N (%)	88 (16.7)	41 (20.6)	0 (0.0)	41 (22.9)	28 (17.2)
Pain, N (%)	131 (24.9)	62 (31.0)	2 (10.0)	60 (33.3)	36 (21.7)
Dyspnoea, N (%)	47 (8.9)	34 (17.1)	1 (5.0)	33 (18.4)	21 (12.8)
Cancer, N (%)	128 (24.3)	43 (21.8)	2 (10.0)	41 (23.2)	25 (15.3)
Chronic respiratory disease, N (%)	147 (27.9)	78 (39.4)	3 (15.0)	75 (42.1)	63 (37.3)
Chronic cardiac disease, N (%)	232 (44.1)	111 (55.5)	6 (30.0)	105 (58.3)	89 (53.9)
Chronic neurological disease, N (%)	74 (14.1)	47 (23.5)	2 (10.0)	45 (25.0)	34 (20.5)
Chronic digestive disease, N (%)	40 (7.6)	39 (20.1)	2 (10.0)	37 (21.2)	28 (17.2)
Chronic renal disease, N (%)	210 (39.8)	91 (46.4)	3 (15.8)	88 (49.8)	68 (40.7)

Table 1. Cont.

	Baseline Total N = 527	Month 6 Follow-Up			Month 12 Follow-Up n = 176
		Total n = 200	No Frailty n = 20 (10.0%)	Frailty n = 180 (90.0%)	
		Frailty degree [2]			
Total cohort average, mean ± SD	0.31 ± 0.15	0.39 ± 0.16	0.11 ± 0.05	0.42 ± 0.14	0.35 ± 0.16
No frailty, N (%)	115 (21.8)	20 (10.0)	20 (100.0)	-	35 (20.5)
Mild frailty, N (%)	190 (36.1)	52 (26.0)	-	52 (28.9)	43 (25.1)
Intermediate frailty, N (%)	147 (27.9)	77 (38.5)	-	77 (42.8)	59 (34.5)
Severe frailty, N (%)	75 (14.2)	51 (25.5)	-	51 (28.3)	34 (19.9)

[1] Refers to patients not living in a nursing home. [2] The frailty degree was calculated using the categorization of the Frail-VIG index into no frailty (Frail-VIG index score <0.2), mild frailty (Frail-VIG index score 0.2–0.35), moderate frailty (Frail-VIG index score 0.36–0.5), and advanced frailty (Frail-VIG index score >0.5). IADLs, Instrumental Activities of Daily Living; SD, standard deviation.

The collection of data at the time of hospitalization was conducted by the hospital's healthcare professionals (physicians and nurses), with the Frail-VIG index being an instrument used in the regular clinical practice at the Geriatrics and Palliative Care units. Home follow-up upon discharge was performed by four research nurses combining face-to-face visits (months 1, 6, and 12) and telephone visits (months 3 and 9).

2.3. Psychometric Assessment of the Frail-VIG Index

This study evaluated the following psychometric parameters: reliability of the scores, evidence of construct validity, and feasibility. The evaluation was performed at different time points (Figure 1).

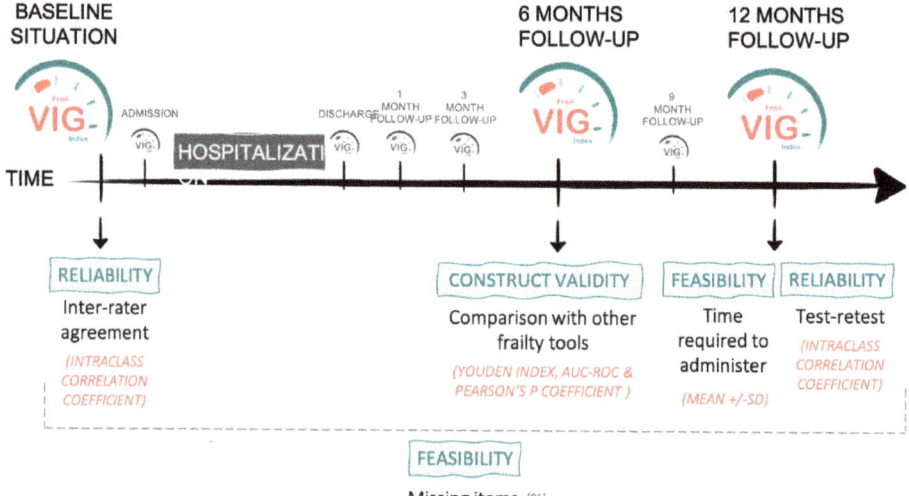

Figure 1. Cohort follow-up timeline, showing the psychometric characteristics assessed at the different moments of the follow-up (as well as the statistical methodology used to assess it).

2.3.1. Reliability

Reliability is the extent to which scores for people who have not changed are the same for repeated measurement under several conditions [34]. Following COSMIN recommendations, the following measures were assessed: (A) inter-rater reliability, by different persons on the same occasion, evaluated by administering the Frail-VIG index with respect to the individual's baseline situation by two different teams: the geriatrics professionals (physicians and/or nurses) responsible for admission, and by the team responsible for hospitalization of that individual, which was performed blindly (without having the result of the test performed by the other team); (B) test–retest reliability, over time: in this case, the four nurses administered the Frail-VIG index on two separate occasions for about a week in a blind manner (without having the results of the previous test), ensuring similar conditions to the baseline measurement (assessing, in particular, the absence of any added concurrent processes). For the assessment of frailty, the calculation of the internal consistency of the Frail-VIG index was dismissed upon considering it not relevant, given that it was developed as a formative model (in which the items together form the construct) and not as a reflective model (in which all items are a manifestation of the same underlying construct) [35].

2.3.2. Validity

Since previous studies published on the Frail-VIG index have already demonstrated evidence of its content validity and its criterion validity related to mortality [28,29], as well as its convergent discriminative validity related to the EQ-5D-3L index, this study focused on evidence of construct validity between the Frail-VIG index and other frailty measurement tools. To this end, the Frail-VIG index was administered at the same time and in the same subjects at the cohort's 6 month follow-up, together with the following tools:

- As a categorical instrument for the assessment of frailty (frail vs. not frail), the five original FP criteria based on the physical characteristics as reported in the original Cardiovascular Health Study by Fried were used: weight loss, exhaustion, low energy, expenditure, slow walking speed, and weak grip strength [36]. The JAMAR PLUS+ Hand Dynamometer was used to assess grip strength, assessing the average score of two grips of the grip strength of the dominant hand. Those with no characteristics were identified as fit, those with one or two characteristics were identified as pre-frail, and those with three to five characteristics were identified as frail.
- CFS [21], a validated ordinal measure of frailty based on nine category clinical descriptors and pictographs ranging from one (fit) to nine (terminally ill), was used as a tool to assess continuous frailty.

Although frailty indices assess frailty as a continuous variable, different cutoffs have been proposed in the literature to distinguish between non-frail and frail individuals (≥ 0.2 [37] vs. ≥ 0.25 [12]); in some cases, a distinction has also been proposed for non-frail individuals (≤ 0.08), pre-frail individuals (0.09–0.24), and frail individuals (≥ 0.25), even weighing the FI result according to the individual's chronological age [38].

2.3.3. Feasibility

Feasibility measures whether a questionnaire is affordable for use in the environment in which it is intended to be used, and it should be a usual feature in frailty measurements, while also being simple to apply [39]. The two most frequently used measurements are the calculation of percentage of unanswered responses and the time required to administer the measure. To assess the percentage of unanswered responses, the total number of tests performed since the start of the study to the 12 month follow-up was analyzed. To assess the time of administration of the Frail-VIG, the duration of the 12 month home follow-up was timed. Other aspects to consider when assessing feasibility based on COSMIN recommendations that have been incorporated into this study are the education or training required to administer each test, the need for special equipment/devices, and the physical space required [40].

2.4. Statistical Methods

Categorical variables are described as frequencies. Quantitative variables are shown as the mean and standard deviation (SD) when the distribution was normal, and as medians with 25th and 75th percentiles when the distribution was asymmetric. We considered a

p-value <0.05 as statistically significant. The data were analyzed using the latest available version of the IBM SPSS Statistics 27 software.

2.4.1. Reliability

Reliability was assessed using the intraclass correlation coefficients (ICCs) (two-way random) for the inter-rater agreement and test–retest reliability, as well as Bland–Altman plots for their graphical representation. We calculated a minimum requirement of 40 subjects [41], who were randomly selected. ICCs greater than or equal to 0.70 were interpreted as optimal [34].

2.4.2. Validity

In accordance with COSMIN recommendations, we used the AUC-ROC as the method of choice for the assessment of the convergent validity of the Frail-VIG index (continuous score) with respect to the FP (noncontinuous score). AUC-ROCs of <0.70, 0.70–0.89, and $\geq$0.90 were considered poor, adequate, and excellent, respectively [42]. While there is no gold-standard tool for the assessment of frailty [34], most frailty tools have ended up conducting comparative studies with FP, since it was the first published tool and represented a benchmark for the other initiatives. Thus, for the calibration of the Frail-VIG index with respect to FP, the prevalence of frail individuals was assessed using both instruments, as well as the sensitivity, specificity, positive and negative predictive value, and Youden index for different cutoffs for the identification of a condition of frailty ($\geq$0.20, $\geq$0.23 and $\geq$0.25). We also analyzed the discriminative validity of the Frail-VIG index by comparing it between people classified as frail and non-frail using the FP. We hypothesized that people classified as frail would have a substantially higher average index than non-frail people.

On the other hand, the convergent validity between the two continuous score instruments (CFS and Frail-VIG index) was evaluated using Pearson's correlation coefficients. We expected moderate to strong positive correlations ($r \geq 0.50$) between the measurement instruments.

2.4.3. Feasibility

Feasibility was evaluated by calculating the average and SD of time required to administer Frail-VIG, as well as the percentage of unanswered responses. To evaluate the time of administration of the Frail-VIG index, a minimum requirement of 40 subjects [41] was estimated, which were randomly selected.

3. Results

3.1. General Characteristics

A total of 527 individuals were enrolled: 296 (56.2%) women and 231 (43.8%) men, with a mean (SD) age of 81.6 (9.9) years. Table 1 shows the demographic and clinical characteristics of the cohort at the time of enrolment in the study (corresponding to the baseline Frail-VIG index, administered by the team responsible for hospitalization of the subjects), and at the 6 and 12 month follow-ups (administered by the nurses conducting follow-up).

3.2. Psychometric Results of the Frail-VIG Index

3.2.1. Reliability

The inter-rater reliability by the two professionals corresponding to the baseline Frail-VIG of the 41 individuals assessed was ICC 0.941 (95% IC, 0.890 to 0.969)—Figure 2A. The test–retest reliability for the 51 individuals assessed was ICC 0.976 (95% CI, 0.958 to 0.986)—Figure 2B. Both results suggest excellent reliability.

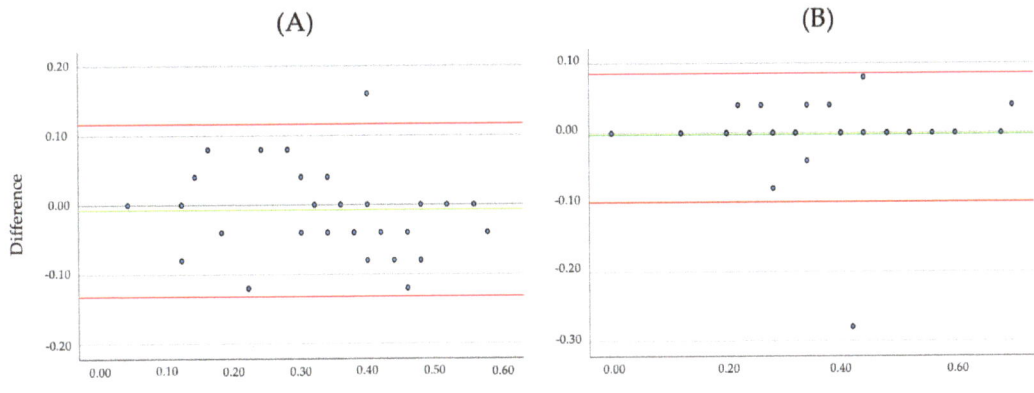

Mean Frail-VIG index score

Figure 2. Bland–Altman correlation for the inter-rater reliability (**A**) and test–retest reliability (**B**).

3.2.2. Validity

All of the 6 month follow-up subjects were included ($n = 200$). Losses to follow-up with respect to the initial cohort ($n = 527$) corresponded to (1) deaths (227), of which 136 died during hospitalization, mainly (65.4%) in the palliative care unit, (2) definitive losses to follow-up ($n = 39$), (3) and occasional losses to follow-up (n = 62), who were later followed up at 9 months.

Table 2 shows the prevalence of frail individuals in the 6 month follow-up cohort using the FP and the Frail-VIG index for the different cutoffs proposed in the literature (between 0.2 [37] and 0.25 [12]).

Table 2. Prevalence of frail people in the cohort using Frailty Phenotype (FP), as well as different cutoffs of the Frail-VIG index.

		Non-Frailty/Pre-Frailty	Frailty
FP	No (%)	52 (26.0)	148 (74.0)
	Frail-VIG, mean ± SD	0.30 (0.16)	0.42 (0.15)
IF-VIG (Frailty cutoff ≥0.20)	No (%)	20 (10)	180 (90)
	Frail-VIG, mean ± SD	0.11 (0.05)	0.42 (0.14)
IF-VIG (Frailty cutoff ≥0.23)	No (%)	32 (16)	168 (84)
	Frail-VIG, mean ± SD	0.14 (0.06)	0.44 (0.13)
IF-VIG (Frailty cutoff ≥0.25)	mean ± SD	45 (22.5)	155 (77.5)
	Frail-VIG, mean (DS)	0.17 (0.07)	0.45 (0.12)

When assessing the construct validity of the Frail-VIG index with respect to FP, the AUC-ROC was 0.704 (95% CI, 0.622 to 0.786) (Figure 3), consistently with an adequate convergent validity. Table 3 shows the sensitivity, specificity, positive and negative predictive value, and Youden index for different cutoffs. The Youden index presented its best score (0.43) for the cutoff of the Frail-VIG index at a ≥0.20.

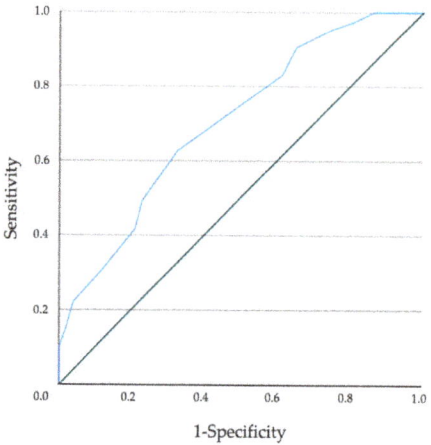

Figure 3. Graphical representation of the ROC plot of the Frail-VIG index, for the people identified as frail according to the Frailty Phenotype criteria.

Table 3. Sensitivity, specificity, and positive and negative predictive value between the Frail-VIG index and the Frailty Phenotype (FP).

	Sensitivity	Specificity	PPV	NPV	Youden Index	Frail-VIG Index (Frailty Value Cutoff)
	78.3%	65.0%	95.3%	25.0%	0.43	≥0.20
FP	79.8%	56.3%	90.5%	34.6%	0.36	≥0.23
	79.4%	44.4%	83.1%	38.5%	0.24	≥0.25

NPV, negative predictive value; PPV, positive predictive value.

The correlation coefficient between the two continuous score instruments (Frail-VIG index and CFS) for the calculation of their convergent validity showed moderate to strong positive correlation between the Frail-VIG index and CFS ($r = 0.64$, 95% CI, 0.54 to 0.71) (Figure 4).

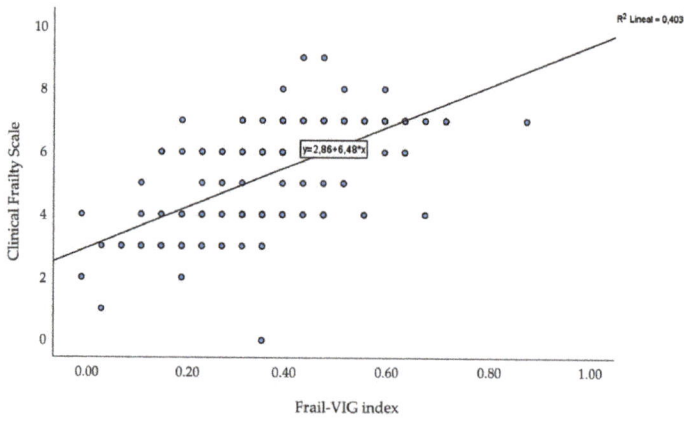

Figure 4. Scatter plots of the correlation between the Frail-VIG index and Clinical Frailty Scale.

3.2.3. Feasibility

Of the 2273 tests performed during the first year of follow-up (equivalent to 50,006 variables; 22 variables for each test), the number of missing variables was 170. This is equivalent to 0.34%. Supplementary File 1 includes the number of losses of variables in the Frail-VIG index administered in a hospital setting (baseline situation, admission, and discharge) and in the follow-up at community level (1, 3, 6, 9, and 12 months). Losses in this follow-up period at 6 and 12 months correspond to deaths (n = 55) or losses to follow-up (n = 19). The administration time of 68 individuals was evaluated, with an average of 5.01 min (SD 2.86).

With respect to the more qualitative aspects, a two-session training was conducted for the interviewers, who also had an instruction manual available. For the administration of the Frail-VIG index, no special equipment or physical space was required. In the context of this study, a dynamometer (for grip strength assessment) was only required for the evaluation of convergent validity, as well as a 4 m space and a chronometer to calculate gait speed.

4. Discussion

The results obtained support the Frail-VIG index as a reliable, feasible, and valid tool to assess the degree of frailty in hospitalized and community-dwelling older people.

4.1. Psychometric Assessment of the Frail-VIG Index

There are limited high-quality reliability, validity, and feasibility data for many of the FI tools. A recent systematic review of the psychometric characteristics of multicomponent tools designed to assess frailty in older adults found that, for example, there were reliability and validity data available for only 21% of the tools [27]. This could be explained by the fact that, as opposed to the Frail-VIG index, many of the frailty assessment tools were developed and tested retrospectively using data available from large-scale longitudinal studies or were developed in conjunction with a larger trial whose main aim was not the development of a frailty assessment tool [27].

4.1.1. Reliability

The reliability of the Frail-VIG index scores can be classified as very strong. There are virtually no previous studies on the reliability of FI [43], which makes it difficult to compare the results obtained. With respect to other frailty instruments, the Frail-VIG index showed better inter-rater reliability (0.94) than, for example, the Edmonton Frail Scale (0.77) [44] or the CFS (from 0.97 [21] to 0.68 [45]).

Test–retest was also excellent (0.97), indicating that if frail elderly people are stable and the Frail-VIG index is administered under similar conditions, their scores remain stable over time. These results are as good as or better than those published for other assessment instruments, such as the CFS (0.87), the Tilburg Frailty Indicator (0.79) [46], or the FRAIL questionnaire (0.71) [47].

4.1.2. Validity

Convergent validity between Frail-VIG index and FP was substantial (0.70), similar to the results previously published by other FIs (0.65) [26]. When the dichotomized Frail-VIG index for the different cutoffs proposed by the literature was compared with the FP, better results of the Youden index were obtained for values ≥ 0.20, which would endorse it as a cutoff for considering someone frail when using the Frail-VIG index. For this cutoff, the Frail-VIG index showed an overall higher sensitivity (78.3%) than other FIs (45.9 to 60.7%), but a lower specificity (65.0% vs. 83.5 to 90.0%) [26]. However, this assessment of the FIs from a dichotomic perspective is likely to have academic importance rather than clinical implications; clearly, the two measures (FI vs. FP) cannot be considered equivalent, since they are different instruments with different objectives, and the combined/sequential use of both instruments is advisable, as they provide different and complementary clinical information on the individual's condition [13,48].

Lastly, the degree of correlation between the two instruments that assess frailty as a continuous reality, Frail-VIG index and CFS ($r = 0.66$), was similar to previous studies for these two instruments ($r = 0.71$) [49]. This is consistent with published evidence on convergent validity between CFS and other FIs, ranging from 0.59 of the electronic frailty index [50] to 0.91 of the FI used by Chong et al. [51].

4.1.3. Feasibility

In terms of feasibility, most published studies used administration time as the most common measure, ranging from 44 s for the CFS to 5 to 20 min for the Fried Phenotype [4,52]. In the case of the FI, in the FI-CGA [53], the administration time ranges from 10 [54] or 12.5 min [55] to 25 min [56]. The CSHA-FI [21] requires about 20–30 min [12]. In fact, the time required for the administration of the FIs has been mentioned by some authors as one of the main limitations to their implementation in routine clinical practice [57]. Thus, the Frail-VIG index would fall in the low range of time of administration of the frailty indices, probably as a result of the lower number of variables involved (22), compared, for example, with the more than 30 items of the different versions of the CSHA-FI [21]. There are not many studies either on the completion rate of FI forms. In the study conducted by Lin et al. [55], a completion rate of 45% was found for the FI-CGA, with the majority (91%) of the incomplete forms having minimal amount of data missing—fewer than four items. In this sense, the low number of missing data in our study is remarkable. Lastly, the Frail-VIG index does not require any additional equipment or space, which has sometimes proven an obstacle to the use of CP, GSFT, and some other versions of the FI [55].

4.2. Limitations of the Study

The main limitations of the study are probably related to the generalizability of its results; on the one hand, the inclusion criteria determined a relatively large sample of individuals, with a significant degree of frailty. On the other hand, even though this is an instrument designed to be used by both physicians and nurses in all settings, in this study, it was used by geriatrics specialists, who are very familiar with the use of the Frail-VIG index (commonly used in clinical practice in our environment). Thus, for instance, in the assessment of feasibility, both the time of administration of the Frail-VIG index and the low number of missing data could also be explained by the expertise of the professionals involved (there is probably a learning curve in its use by professionals), as well as the thoroughness inherent to the context of a research study.

Another limitation to bear in mind is that not all psychometric properties were assessed in all settings and by all professional profiles. Therefore, for example, reliability and inter-rater reliability were assessed in hospital settings by physicians and nurses, while the test–retest has been performed in a community setting by the follow-up nurses. Thus, more studies are needed to evaluate the psychometric properties in daily clinical practice by other professionals in different settings and populations.

4.3. Healthcare Implications and Future Research

It is essential to have reliable, valid, and feasible tools to take advantage of the multiple opportunities offered by the assessment of frailty as a central element of clinical practice, research, and planning in the care of the elderly [9,12,58], ranging from the prevention of disability to the care of individuals with complex and palliative care needs [20,39]. Unfortunately, only 5% of the frailty assessment tools have shown evidence of reliability and validity that was within statistically significant parameters and of fair methodological quality [27].

There are two areas of special interest for future research, which are related to the multidimensional nature of the IF and the assessment of the dynamic behavior of frailty. In the first place, the validity of the content of the instruments should be enhanced with respect to physical, cognitive-psychological, and social frailty [59,60]. In the second place, the serial administration of the Frail-VIG index in a prospective cohort is likely to provide knowledge on the different courses of frailty [61], as well as on the ability of this FI to assess sensitivity to change and responsiveness, understood as the ability of an instrument to distinguish clinically important changes as the result of an intervention [34]. Further studies are also needed to continue to advance in the validation process of the Frail-VIG index, especially with respect to its cross-cultural validity and generalizability.

5. Conclusions

According to the COSMIN guidelines, the results obtained endorse the Frail-VIG index as a reliable, feasible, and valid instrument. Firstly, a very strong reliability of the scores was found in its administration among different professionals (inter-rater reliability), as well as in test–retest reliability. Secondly, the Frail-VIG showed a moderate to strong positive correlation with CFS, as well as adequate convergent validity with respect to the FP. This also allowed calibrating the Frail-VIG index for the identification of frail individuals, establishing a frailty threshold at a score of ≥ 0.20. Lastly, excellent feasibility has been observed in relation to the time of administration, with respect to the few items missed, and due to the lack of specific space or equipment requirements.

All these characteristics, together with their good correlation, with the mortality demonstrated in previous studies, and with the discriminating capacity between the different degrees of frailty, make the Frail-VIG index a particularly interesting tool to assess frail elderly people in hospitalized and community-dwelling settings.

Supplementary Materials: The following are available online at https://www.mdpi.com/article/10.3390/ijerph18105187/s1: Table S1. Missing variables for the different follow-up cutoffs.

Author Contributions: Conceptualization, A.T., E.P., and J.A.-N.; methodology, A.T., E.P., E.Z.-d.-O., J.-J.Z.-S., and J.A.-N.; software, E.P.; validation, A.T., E.P., E.Z.-d.-O., J.-J.Z.-S., S.S., and J.A.-N.; formal analysis, E.P.; investigation, A.T. and E.P.; resources, E.P.; data curation, A.T. and E.P.; writing—original draft preparation, J.A.-N.; writing—review and editing, A.T., E.P., E.Z.-d.-O., J.-J.Z.-S., S.S., and J.A.-N.; visualization, J.A.-N.; supervision, J.A.-N.; project administration, A.T. and E.P.; funding acquisition, J.A.-N. All authors have read and agreed to the published version of the manuscript.

Funding: This study was funded by the Instituto de Salud Carlos III (ISCIII) 17/02240 grant.

Institutional Review Board Statement: The study protocol was approved by the Ethics Committee of the University Hospital of Vic (2018958/PR189). This study was conducted in accordance with the Helsinki Declaration and the local Personal Data Protection Law (LOPD 15/1999).

Informed Consent Statement: All patients and family relatives of patients with advanced dementia situation (GDS ≥ 6) signed the written informed consent for participation before any data were recorded.

Data Availability Statement: The data presented in this study are available on request from the corresponding author.

Acknowledgments: The authors would like to acknowledge all the professionals who contributed to the collection of the data, especially the nurses who conducted the fieldwork (Rut Cabestany, Esther Fontserè, Alba Márquez, and Ramona Sandu), for their extraordinary work in the field and their strong commitment to the project. We would also like to thank the professionalism of i2e3 Biomedical Research Institute for providing medical writing assistance.

Conflicts of Interest: The authors declare no conflict of interest.

References

1. World Health Organization. *Global Strategy on Integrated People-Centered Health Services 2016–2026*; World Health Organization: Geneva, Switzerland, 2017.
2. Busse, R.; Blümel, M.; Scheller-Kreinsen, D.; Zentner, A. *Tackling Chronic Disease in Europe: Strategies, Interventions and Challenges*; WHO Regional Office for Europe: Copenhagen, Denmark, 2010.

3. Harrison, J.K.; Clegg, A.; Conroy, S.P.; Young, J. Managing frailty as a long-term condition. *Age Ageing* **2015**, *44*, 732–735. [CrossRef] [PubMed]
4. Kojima, G.; Iliffe, S.; Walters, K. Frailty index as a predictor of mortality: A systematic review and meta-analysis. *Age Ageing* **2018**, *47*, 193–200. [CrossRef]
5. Rivera-Almaraz, A.; Manrique-Espinoza, B.; Ávila-Funes, J.A.; Chatterji, S.; Naidoo, N.; Kowal, P.; Salinas-Rodríguez, A. Disability, quality of life and all-cause mortality in older Mexican adults: Association with multimorbidity and frailty. *BMC Geriatr.* **2018**, *18*, 236. [CrossRef]
6. Marengoni, A.; Zucchelli, A.; Vetrano, D.L.; Armellini, A.; Botteri, E.; Nicosia, F.; Romanelli, G.; Beindorf, E.A.; Giansiracusa, P.; Garrafa, E.; et al. Beyond Chronological Age: Frailty and Multimorbidity Predict In-Hospital Mortality in Patients With Coronavirus Disease 2019. *J. Gerontol. A Biol. Sci. Med. Sci.* **2021**, *76*, e38–e45. [CrossRef]
7. Hewitt, J.; Carter, B.; Vilches-Moraga, A.; Quinn, T.J.; Braude, P.; Verduri, A.; Pearce, L.; Stechman, M.; Short, R.; Price, A.; et al. The effect of frailty on survival in patients with COVID-19 (COPE): A multicentre, European, observational cohort study. *Lancet Public Health* **2020**, *5*, e444–e451. [CrossRef]
8. Rodríguez-Mañas, L.; Féart, C.; Mann, G.; Viña, J.; Chatterji, S.; Chodzko-Zajko, W.; Harmand, M.G.-C.; Bergman, H.; Carcaillon, L.; Nicholson, C.; et al. Searching for an operational definition of frailty: A delphi method based consensus statement. the frailty operative definition-consensus conference project. *J. Gerontol. A Biol. Sci. Med. Sci.* **2013**, *68*, 62–67. [CrossRef] [PubMed]
9. Cesari, M.; Marzetti, E.; Thiem, U.; Pérez-Zepeda, M.U.; Abellan Van Kan, G.; Landi, F.; Petrovic, M.; Cherubini, A.; Bernabei, R. The geriatric management of frailty as paradigm of "The end of the disease era". *Eur. J. Intern. Med.* **2016**, *31*, 11–14. [CrossRef]
10. Turner, G.; Clegg, A. Best practice guidelines for the management of frailty: A British Geriatrics Society, Age UK and Royal College of General Practitioners report. *Age Ageing* **2014**, *43*, 744–747. [CrossRef] [PubMed]
11. Hoogendijk, E.O.; Afilalo, J.; Ensrud, K.E.; Kowal, P.; Onder, G.; Fried, L.P. Series Frailty 1 Frailty: Implications for clinical practice and public health. *Lancet* **2019**, *394*, 1365–1375. [CrossRef]
12. Dent, E.; Kowal, P.; Hoogendijk, E.O. Frailty measurement in research and clinical practice: A review. *Eur. J. Intern. Med.* **2016**, *31*, 3–10. [CrossRef]
13. Cesari, M.; Gambassi, G.; van Kan, G.A.; Vellas, B. The frailty phenotype and the frailty index: Different instruments for different purposes. *Age Ageing* **2014**, *43*, 10–12. [CrossRef] [PubMed]
14. Fried, L.P.; Tangen, C.M.; Walston, J.; Newman, A.B.; Hirsch, C.; Gottdiener, J.; Seeman, R.; Tracy, R.; Kop, W.J.; Burke, G.; et al. Frailty in older adults: Evidence for a phenotype. *J. Gerontol. A Biol. Sci. Med. Sci.* **2001**, *56*, M146–M156. [CrossRef]
15. Morley, J.E.; Malmstrom, T.K.; Miller, D.K. A simple frailty questionnaire (FRAIL) predicts outcomes in middle aged african americans. *J. Nutr. Health Aging* **2012**, *16*, 601–608. [CrossRef] [PubMed]
16. Vellas, B.; Balardy, L.; Gillette-Guyonnet, S.; Abellan Van Kan, G.; Ghisolfi-Marque, A.; Subra, J.; Bismuth, S.; Oustric, S.; Cesari, M. Looking for Frailty in Community-Dwelling Older Persons: The Gérontopôle Frailty Screening Tool (GFST). *J. Nutr. Health Aging* **2013**, *17*, 629–631. [CrossRef] [PubMed]
17. Abellan Van Kan, G.; Rolland, Y.; Andrieu, S.; Bauer, J.; Beauchet, O.; Bonnefoy, M.; Cesari, M.; Donini, L.M.; Gillette-Guyonnet, S.; Inzitari, M.; et al. Gait speed at usual pace as a predictor of adverse outcomes in community-dwelling older people an International Academy on Nutrition and Aging (IANA) task force. *J. Nutr. Health Aging* **2009**, *13*, 881–889. [CrossRef]
18. Guralnik, J.M.; Simonsick, E.M.; Ferrucci, L.; Glynn, R.J.; Berkman, L.F.; Blazer, D.G.; Scherr, P.A.; Wallace, R.B. A short physical performance battery assessing lower extremity function: Association with self-reported disability and prediction of mortality and nursing home admission. *J. Gerontol.* **1994**, *49*, M85–M94. [CrossRef]
19. Mitnitski, A.B.; Mogilner, A.J.; Rockwood, K. Accumulation of deficits as a proxy measure of aging. *Sci. World J.* **2001**, *1*, 323–336. [CrossRef]
20. Amblàs-Novellas, J.; Espaulella, J.; Rexach, L.; Fontecha, B.; Inzitari, M.; Blay, C.; Gómez-Batiste, X. Frailty, severity, progression and shared decision-making: A pragmatic framework for the challenge of clinical complexity at the end of life. *Eur. Geriatr. Med.* **2015**, *6*, 189–194. [CrossRef]
21. Rockwood, K.; Song, X.; MacKnight, C.; Bergman, H.; Hogan, D.B.; McDowell, I.; Mitnitski, A. A global clinical measure of fitness and frailty in elderly people. *CMAJ* **2005**, *173*, 9–13. [CrossRef]
22. Rockwood, K.; Mitnitski, A. Frailty in relation to the accumulation of deficits. *J. Gerontol. A Biol. Sci. Med. Sci.* **2007**, *62*, 722–727. [CrossRef]
23. Abbasi, M.; Rolfson, D.; Khera, A.S.; Dabravolskaj, J.; Dent, E.; Xia, L. Identification and management of frailty in the primary care setting. *CMAJ* **2018**, *191*, E54. [CrossRef] [PubMed]
24. Huisingh-Scheetz, M.; Martinchek, M.; Becker, Y.; Ferguson, M.K.; Thompson, K. Translating Frailty Research Into Clinical Practice: Insights From the Successful Aging and Frailty Evaluation Clinic. *J. Am. Med. Dir. Assoc.* **2019**, *20*, 672–678. [CrossRef] [PubMed]
25. Warnier, R.M.J.; van Rossum, E.; van Velthuijsen, E.; Mulder, W.J.; Schols, J.M.G.A.; Kempen, G.I.J.M. Validity, reliability and feasibility of tools to identify frail older patients in inpatient hospital care: A systematic review. *J. Nutr. Health Aging* **2016**, *20*, 218–230. [CrossRef] [PubMed]
26. Drubbel, I.; Numans, M.E.; Kranenburg, G.; Bleijenberg, N.; De Wit, N.J.; Schuurmans, M.J. Screening for frailty in primary care: A systematic review of the psychometric properties of the frailty index in community-dwelling older people. *BMC Geriatr.* **2014**, *14*, 27. [CrossRef]

27. Sutton, J.L.; Gould, R.L.; Daley, S.; Coulson, M.C.; Ward, E.V.; Butler, A.M.; Nunn, S.P.; Howard, R.J. Psychometric properties of multicomponent tools designed to assess frailty in older adults: A systematic review. *BMC Geriatr.* **2016**, *16*, 55. [CrossRef]
28. Amblàs-Novellas, J.; Martori, J.; Molist Brunet, N.; Oller, R.; Gomez-Batiste, X.; Espaulella, J. Índice Frágil-VIG: diseño y evaluación de un Índice de Fragilidad basado en la Valoración Integral Geriátrica. *Rev. Esp. Geriatr. Gerontol.* **2016**, *52*, 119–123. [CrossRef]
29. Amblàs-Novellas, J.; Martori, J.C.; Espaulella, J.; Oller, R.; Molist-Brunet, N.; Inzitari, M.; Romero-Ortuno, R. Frail-VIG index: A concise frailty evaluation tool for rapid geriatric assessment. *BMC Geriatr.* **2018**, *18*, 29. [CrossRef] [PubMed]
30. Mokkink, L.B.; Prinsen, C.A.C.; Patrick, D.L.; Alonso, J.; Bouter, L.M.; de Vet, H.C.W.; Terwee, C.B. *COSMIN Study Design Checklist for Patient-Reported Outcome Measurement Instruments*; Amsterdam University Medical Centers: Amsterdam, The Netherlands, 2019.
31. DeVellis, R.F. Classical test theory. *Med. Care* **2006**, *33*, S50–S59. [CrossRef]
32. Contel, J.C.; Ledesma, A.; Blay, C.; González Mestre, A.; Cabezas, C.; Puigdollers, M.; Zara, C.; Amil, P.; Sarquella, E.; Constante, C. Chronic and integrated care in Catalonia. *Int. J. Integr. Care* **2015**, *15*, e025. [CrossRef]
33. Gómez-Batiste, X.; Martínez-Muñoz, M.; Blay, C.; Amblàs-Novellas, J.; Vila, L.; Costa, X.; Espaulella, J.; Espinosa, J.; Constante, C.; Mitchell, G.K. Prevalence and characteristics of patients with advanced chronic conditions in need of palliative care in the general population: A cross-sectional study. *Palliat. Med.* **2014**, *28*, 302–311. [CrossRef]
34. Mokkink, L.B.; Terwee, C.B.; Knol, D.L.; Stratford, P.W.; Alonso, J.; Patrick, D.L.; Bouter, L.M.; De Vet, H.C. The COSMIN checklist for evaluating the methodological quality of studies on measurement properties: A clarification of its content. *BMC Med. Res. Methodol.* **2010**, *10*, 22. [CrossRef]
35. Streiner, D.L. Being inconsistent about consistency: When coefficient alpha does and doesn't matter. *J. Pers. Assess.* **2003**, *80*, 217–222. [CrossRef]
36. Alonso Bouzón, C.; Rodríguez-Mañas, L.; Carnicero, J.A.; García-García, F.J.; Turín, J.G.; Rodríguez-Mañas, L.; Turín, J.G. The Standardization of Frailty Phenotype Criteria Improves Its Predictive Ability: The Toledo Study for Healthy Aging. *J. Am. Med. Dir. Assoc.* **2017**, *18*, 402–408. [CrossRef]
37. Searle, S.; Mitnitski, A.; Gahbauer, E. A standard procedure for creating a frailty index. *BMC Geriatr.* **2008**, *8*, 24. [CrossRef] [PubMed]
38. Romero-Ortuno, R. An alternative method for Frailty Index cut-off points to define frailty categories. *Eur. Ger. Med.* **2013**, *4*. [CrossRef] [PubMed]
39. Clegg, A.; Young, J.; Iliffe, S.; Rikkert, M.O.; Rockwood, K. Frailty in elderly people. *Lancet* **2013**, *381*, 752–762. [CrossRef]
40. Ambagtsheer, R.; Visvanathan, R.; Cesari, M.; Yu, S.; Archibald, M.; Schultz, T.; Karnon, J.; Kitson, A.; Beilby, J. Feasibility, acceptability and diagnostic test accuracy of frailty screening instruments in community-dwelling older people within the Australian general practice setting: A study protocol for a cross-sectional study. *BMJ Open* **2017**, *7*, e016663. [CrossRef]
41. Giraudeau, B.; Mary, J.Y. Planning a reproducibility study: How many subjects and how many replicates per subject for an expected width of the 95 per cent confidence interval of the intraclass correlation coefficient. *Stat. Med.* **2001**, *20*, 3205–3214. [CrossRef]
42. McDowell, I. *Measuring Health: A Guide to Rating Scales and Questionnaires*; Oxford University Press: Oxford, UK, 2009.
43. Bouillon, K.; Kivimaki, M.; Hamer, M.; Sabia, S.; Fransson, E.I.; Singh-Manoux, A.; Gale, C.R.; Batty, G.D. Measures of frailty in population-based studies: An overview. *BMC Geriatr.* **2013**, *13*, 64. [CrossRef] [PubMed]
44. Rolfson, D.B.; Majumdar, S.R.; Tsuyuki, R.T.; Tahir, A.; Rockwood, K. Validity and reliability of the Edmonton Frail Scale. *Age Ageing* **2006**, *35*, 526–529. [CrossRef]
45. Chan, D.C.; Tsou, H.H.; Chen, C.Y.; Chen, C.Y. Validation of the Chinese-Canadian study of health and aging clinical frailty scale (CSHA-CFS) telephone version. *Arch. Gerontol. Geriatr.* **2010**, *50*, e74–e80. [CrossRef]
46. Gobbens, R.J.J.; van Assen, M.A.L.M.; Luijkx, K.G.; Wijnen-Sponselee, M.T.; Schols, J.M.G.A. The tilburg frailty indicator: Psychometric properties. *J. Am. Med. Dir. Assoc.* **2010**, *11*, 344–355. [CrossRef] [PubMed]
47. Dong, L.; Qiao, X.; Tian, X.; Liu, N.; Jin, Y.; Si, H.; Gale, C.R.; Batty, G.D. Cross-Cultural Adaptation and Validation of the FRAIL Scale in Chinese Community-Dwelling Older Adults. *J. Am. Med. Dir. Assoc.* **2018**, *19*, 12–17. [CrossRef]
48. Clegg, A.; Rogers, L.; Young, J. Diagnostic test accuracy of simple instruments for identifying frailty in community-dwelling older people: A systematic review. *Age Ageing* **2015**, *44*, 148–152. [CrossRef]
49. Moreno-Ariño, M.; Torrente Jiménez, I.; Cartanyà Gutiérrez, A.; Oliva Morera, J.C.; Comet, R. Assessing the strengths and weaknesses of the Clinical Frailty Scale through correlation with a frailty index. *Aging Clin. Exp. Res.* **2020**, *32*, 2225–2232. [CrossRef] [PubMed]
50. Brundle, C.; Heaven, A.; Brown, L.; Teale, E.; Young, J.; West, R.; Clegg, A. Convergent validity of the electronic frailty index. *Age Ageing* **2019**, *48*, 152–156. [CrossRef] [PubMed]
51. Chong, E.; Chia, J.Q.; Law, F.; Chew, J.; Chan, M.; Lim, W.S. Validating a Standardised Approach in Administration of the Clinical Frailty Scale in Hospitalised Older Adults. *Ann. Acad. Med. Singap.* **2019**, *48*, 115–124.
52. Kim, D.H.; Kim, C.A.; Placide, S.; Lipsitz, L.A.; Marcantonio, E.R. Preoperative frailty assessment and outcomes at 6 months or later in older adults undergoing cardiac surgical procedures: A systematic review. *Ann. Intern. Med.* **2016**, *165*, 650–660. [CrossRef] [PubMed]

53. Jones, D.; Song, X.; Mitnitski, A.; Rockwood, K. Evaluation of a frailty index based on a comprehensive geriatric assessment in a population based study of elderly Canadians. *Aging Clin. Exp. Res.* **2005**, *17*, 465–471. [CrossRef]
54. Hubbard, R.E.; Peel, N.M.; Smith, M.; Dawson, B.; Lambat, Z.; Bak, M.; Best, J.; Johnson, D.W. Feasibility and construct validity of a Frailty index for patients with chronic kidney disease. *Australas. J. Ageing* **2015**, *34*, E9–E12. [CrossRef]
55. Lin, H.; Peel, N.M.; Scott, I.A.; Vardesh, D.L.; Sivalingam, P.; McBride, R.L.; Morong, J.J.; Nelson, M.J.; Hubbard, R.E. Perioperative assessment of older surgical patients using a frailty index-feasibility and association with adverse post-operative outcomes. *Anaesth. Intensive Care* **2017**, *45*, 676–682. [CrossRef] [PubMed]
56. Evans, S.J.; Sayers, M.; Mitnitski, A.; Rockwood, K. The risk of adverse outcomes in hospitalized older patients in relation to a frailty index based on a comprehensive geriatric assessment. *Age Ageing* **2014**, *43*, 127–132. [CrossRef] [PubMed]
57. Hubbard, R.E.; O'mahony, M.S.; Woodhouse, K.W. Characterising frailty in the clinical setting—A comparison of different approaches. *Age Ageing* **2009**, *38*, 115–119. [CrossRef]
58. Cesari, M.; Prince, M.; Thiyagarajan, J.A.; De Carvalho, I.A.; Bernabei, R.; Chan, P.; Gutierrez-Robledo, L.M.; Michel, J.-P.; Morley, J.E.; Ong, P.; et al. Frailty: An Emerging Public Health Priority. *J. Am. Med. Dir. Assoc.* **2016**, *17*, 188–192. [CrossRef] [PubMed]
59. Gobbens, R.J.J.; van Assen, M.A.L.M.; Luijkx, K.G.; Wijnen-Sponselee, M.T.; Schols, J.M.G.A. Determinants of frailty. *J. Am. Med. Dir. Assoc.* **2010**, *11*, 356–364. [CrossRef]
60. Bunt, S.; Steverink, N.; Olthof, J.; van der Schans, C.P.; Hobbelen, J.S.M. Social frailty in older adults: A scoping review. *Eur. J. Ageing* **2017**, *14*, 323–334. [CrossRef] [PubMed]
61. Chamberlain, A.M.; Finney Rutten, L.J.; Manemann, S.M.; Yawn, B.P.; Jacobson, D.J.; Fan, C.; Ms, B.R.G.; Roger, V.L.; Sauver, J.L.S. Frailty Trajectories in an Elderly Population-Based Cohort. *J. Am. Geriatr. Soc.* **2016**, *64*, 285–292. [CrossRef] [PubMed]

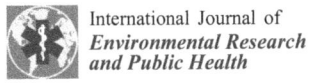

Article

"Not Alone in Loneliness": A Qualitative Evaluation of a Program Promoting Social Capital among Lonely Older People in Primary Health Care

Laura Coll-Planas [1,2,*], Dolors Rodríguez-Arjona [1], Mariona Pons-Vigués [3,4], Fredrica Nyqvist [5], Teresa Puig [2,6,7] and Rosa Monteserín [2,8]

1. Fundació Salut i Envelliment (Foundation on Health and Ageing), Universitat Autònoma de Barcelona, 08041 Barcelona, Spain; lrodriguez79@hotmail.com
2. Institute of Biomedical Research (IIB Sant Pau), 08041 Barcelona, Spain; tpuig@santpau.cat (T.P.); rmonteserin@eapsardenya.cat (R.M.)
3. Servei Català de la Salut (CatSalut), Planning and Assessment Area, 08028 Barcelona, Spain; mariona.pons@catsalut.cat
4. Nursing Department at the Faculty of Nursing, Universitat de Girona, 17003 Girona, Spain
5. Faculty of Education and Welfare Studies, Social Policy, Åbo Akademi University, 65101 Vaasa, Finland; fredrica.nyqvist@abo.fi
6. Universitat Autònoma de Barcelona, 08193 Bellaterra (Cerdanyola del Vallès), Spain
7. Epidemiology and Public Health Department, Hospital de la Santa Creu i Sant Pau, 08041 Barcelona, Spain
8. Equip d'Atenció Primària Sardenya, EAP Sardenya, 08025 Barcelona, Spain
* Correspondence: laura.coll@uab.cat

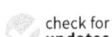

Citation: Coll-Planas, L.; Rodríguez-Arjona, D.; Pons-Vigués, M.; Nyqvist, F.; Puig, T.; Monteserín, R. "Not Alone in Loneliness": A Qualitative Evaluation of a Program Promoting Social Capital among Lonely Older People in Primary Health Care. *IJERPH* **2021**, *18*, 5580. https://doi.org/10.3390/ijerph18115580

Academic Editors: Francisco José Tarazona Santabalbina, José Augusto García Navarro and José Viña

Received: 18 March 2021
Accepted: 17 May 2021
Published: 23 May 2021

Publisher's Note: MDPI stays neutral with regard to jurisdictional claims in published maps and institutional affiliations.

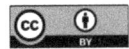

Copyright: © 2021 by the authors. Licensee MDPI, Basel, Switzerland. This article is an open access article distributed under the terms and conditions of the Creative Commons Attribution (CC BY) license (https://creativecommons.org/licenses/by/4.0/).

Abstract: The weekly group-based program "Paths: from loneliness to participation" was conducted face-to-face over 15 sessions by nurses, social workers and volunteers in primary care in Catalonia (Spain) to alleviate loneliness among older people by promoting peer support and participation in community assets. We aimed at exploring participants' experiences of loneliness and participation prior to the program and its perceived benefits. The qualitative design was descriptive-interpretative. Data were collected through three focus groups and 41 interviews applying a semistructured topic guide involving 26 older participants, six professionals and nine volunteers. Participant-observation of all sessions involved the 38 older people who started the program. A thematic content analysis was applied. Older persons with diverse profiles of loneliness and participation explained different degrees of decrease in loneliness, an increase in participation in local community assets, companionship, peer support and friendship, and an empowerment process. Successful cases reported improvements in mental wellbeing and recovering the sense that life was worth living. Loneliness persisted among some widowed participants and vulnerabilities hampered some benefits. Participants, professionals and volunteers reported different degrees of success in older people to alleviate loneliness by enhancing social relationships and activities through complex processes interrelated with health and socioeconomic factors.

Keywords: ageing; qualitative research; primary health care; loneliness; social capital

1. Introduction

Loneliness is defined as a negative feeling due to the perception that the social needs of the person are not corresponded, neither in quantity nor in quality, by the social relationships that the person has [1]. In the last years, the public awareness and the scientific concern about the phenomenon of loneliness has increased [2]. Furthermore, the current SARS-COV2 pandemic has accentuated the value of social interactions and social support and the need to alleviate loneliness among older people [3]. Older people undergo major changes in their social environment mainly due to retirement, widowhood, loss of peers, and age-related disability [4]. Likewise, three ageing crises are related to loneliness: the identity (no longer feeling like who they used to be), autonomy (not being able to do what they used to do) and belonging crises (not belonging to the places and groups of persons to which they used to belong) [5].

At a personal level, several risk factors related with sociodemographic characteristics and health status are associated with loneliness: being female, living alone, limited education, small social network, low self-efficacy, poor self-rated health, depression and recent bereavement (often due to widowhood) [6,7]. Geographically, loneliness differs across Europe being higher in Southern countries such as Spain [8]. In Southern Europe, the cultural emphasis on family and social relationships generates high expectations and social needs that might be more challenging to fulfil. Moreover, active participation in social organizations is seen as vital to build relationships while ageing, but it is lower among older people in Spain in a European comparative perspective [9–12]. From a policy perspective, the WHO Active Ageing and Healthy Ageing paradigms have encouraged for the last 20 years to enhance social participation and social networks for ageing people [13,14]. In this vein, Putnam's definition of social capital has been adapted to older age placing more relevance on the interaction between individuals at the micro level. Accordingly, social capital is an umbrella concept that involves individual (family and friends) and collective social resources (e.g., neighborhoods), their structural (e.g., social networks, social contacts and participation) and cognitive aspects (e.g., social support and sense of belonging) [15–17]. However, the processes involved in the promotion of social capital in ageing, including social relationships and participation, remain unclear [4].

Certain intervention characteristics are related to a higher efficiency at reducing loneliness, such as theory-driven interventions [18–20]. However, it is not yet clear which theory supports more effective interventions. The loneliness model supports cognitive behavioral therapy to correct deficits in social skills and address maladaptive social cognition [21]. On the contrary, the empowerment theory considers that loneliness is potentially alleviated through empowering lonely older people to increase their self-esteem and feeling of mastery over their own life [22–24]. Moreover, theories of behavior change might be used to better understand how to promote social relations and social participation [25,26]. Finally, the most widely applied strategy among older people to tackle loneliness is increasing social support. However, controlled trials evaluating this intervention strategy are scarce [21].

Regarding intervention effectiveness, a systematic review on interventions based on social capital targeting older people showed few and diverse trials assessing the impact on loneliness and they were generally ineffective [27]. However, some successful studies targeted complex cases of loneliness, and social capital interventions successfully increased quality of life, well-being and self-perceived health among lonely older people. In this vein, the intervention Circle of Friends in Finland, which focused on empowering lonely older people, achieved successful improvements in a wide range of health outcomes including mortality, but not in loneliness [24]. Their qualitative analysis showed how lonely participants built trust and encouragement and continued to meet [28]. A program based on facilitating community knowledge and networking among older migrants in Japan through volunteers as gatekeepers, decreased loneliness and increased social support [29].

In Spain, the program "Paths: from loneliness to participation" was designed, conducted and evaluated to alleviate loneliness among older people attending primary health care [30]. The intervention promoted peer support and social participation by enhancing engagement in activities in community assets. The intervention was evaluated with mixed methods. According to the quantitative evaluation, loneliness decreased and social participation and support significantly increased [30].

In summary, despite a diversity of programs in place around the world and isolated successful results, evidence and detailed understanding on whether and how programs decrease loneliness is lacking, as well as how the characteristics of the target population influence the impact. Likewise, while previous literature clearly suggests health beneficial effects of social capital, less is known about social capital interventions and how social capital can be built for health promoting purposes. Qualitative evaluation of interventions to explore participants and professionals' perspective on the experiences and perceived benefits is a complementary approach to the quantitative evaluation of objective impacts that can help understand the processes and interpret the effects of the programs.

Therefore, this paper reports the qualitative evaluation of the program "Paths: from loneliness to participation" aimed at exploring participants' experiences of loneliness and social participation prior to the program; and describing its perceived benefits on loneliness, social participation, and support and health according to participants' experience, volunteers and professionals' observations.

2. Materials and Methods

The study was conducted adhering to the rigor and quality criteria for qualitative research: description of context, of participants and of the research process, methodological adequacy, triangulation of data and reflexivity of the research team [31]. Moreover, it is reported according to the Standards for Reporting Qualitative Research [32].

Throughout the paper, "participants" refers to older people participating in the program and "informants" comprises all agents involved: participants, volunteers, and professionals.

2.1. Design

Following a constructivist research paradigm, a qualitative study with a phenomenological approach was chosen, in order to explore the lived experiences of the involved agents applying a descriptive-interpretative design.

The perceived benefits of the program were identified among participants according to their experiences and then triangulated with the perceptions of volunteers and health and social care professionals and with the researchers' observations.

This research applies the social capital theory adapted to ageing by Nyqvist and Forsman [33].

2.2. Description of the Program

The "Paths: from loneliness to participation" program is theory-driven and was designed around the mentioned operationalization of the social capital theory applied to ageing with the goal to alleviate loneliness among older people by promoting peer support and participation in local community assets [15,30,34]. It was conducted from December 2011 to July 2012 in primary health and social care centers in Catalonia (Spain). Sessions were one and half hours long and took place once a week during 15 weeks. The program has been previously described in detail, as well as its overall intervention framework [30]. In summary, older people with low or no participation in social activities and suffering from loneliness at least sometimes were referred by primary health and social care professionals to the group. The group met face-to-face and was led by social workers or nurses from the primary health or social care center. The group dynamic was grounded on active participation in line with the empowerment theory. Along the 15 sessions, peer support was promoted through sharing opinions and experiences around loneliness and participation prompted by a diversity of pictures. Furthermore, older people active in the same neighborhood were involved as volunteers to connect participants with the local community assets. As a group, they visited and experienced activities in five local community assets to promote their engagement in these settings. An intervention guide specified all activities with its purposes and professionals and volunteers were specifically trained for their roles.

One intervention group was conducted in a semirural area (Cardedeu, zone A), and two in an urban area, Barcelona: one in a low socioeconomic level neighborhood (zone B) and one in a medium level one (zone C). Settings were selected by convenience to evaluate the viability of the intervention in different contexts.

2.3. Study Participants

The study population reached through the focus groups and interviews comprised 26 older people who participated in the program, nine older volunteers and six health and social care professionals. All 38 participants (37 women, 1 man) who started the program were involved in the participant-observation. Participants of the program were invited in person to the interviews and focus groups by the researcher (LCP) to take part in this qualitative study and agreed to participate. All volunteers and professionals directly involved in the program were invited to participate. The characteristics of all 38 participants have been previously described in detail. [30] Table 1 details the main characteristics of the 41 informants of the interviews and focus groups.

Table 1. Characteristics of participants, volunteers, and professionals interviewed.

Context	Technique	Number of Informants	Age	Gender	Educational Level/Occupation **
		Participants *			
Zone A: Semirural context with a medium socioeconomic level.	One focus group	Five participants	65–74 y.: 1 75–80 y.: 2 over 80 y.: 2	Five women	One with medium education and four with low education
	Eight individual semistructured interviews	Eight participants	65–74 y.: 1 75–80 y.: 5 over 80 y.: 2	Eight women	One with medium education and seven with low education
		Volunteers			
	One interview in small group	Four volunteers	65–74 y.: 1 75–80 y.: 2 over 80 y.: 1	Four women	Low education
	Professionals				
	Two individual semistructured interviews	Two professionals from primary health care and social services	30–50 y.: 1 51–65 y.: 1	Two women	One nurse One social worker
		Participants *			
Zone B: Urban context with a low socioeconomic level.	Focus groups	Nine participants	65–74 y.: 2 75–80 y.: 4 over 80 y.: 3	Nine women	Low education
	Individual semistructured interviews	Eleven participants	65–74 y.: 2 75–80 y.: 6 over 80 y.: 3	Eleven women	Low education
		Volunteers			
	One interview in small group	Two volunteers	63 and 80 years old	Two women	Medium and low education
	Individual semistructured interview	One volunteer	63 years old	One woman	High education
		Professionals			
	Two individual semistructured interviews	Two professionals from primary health care	30–50 y.: 1 51–65 y.: 1	Two women	Two social workers

Table 1. Cont.

Context	Technique	Number of Informants	Age	Gender	Educational Level/Occupation **
		Participants *			
Zone C: Urban context with medium socioeconomic level.	One focus group	Seven participants	65–74 y.: 1	Six women and one man	One with high education, six with low education
	Seven individual semistructured interviews		75–80 y.: 2		
			over 80 y.: 4		
		Volunteers			
	One interview in small group	Two volunteers	65–74 y.: 1	Two women	Medium education
			75–80 y.: 1		
		Professionals			
	Two individual semistructured interviews	Two professionals from primary health care	30–50 y.: 2	Two women	One social worker and one nurse
			51–65 y.: 0		

* Note: All participants who were individually interviewed had previously participated in the focus groups, except three from zone A and two from zone B, who were only individually interviewed. ** "Educational level" applies to older participants and volunteers and "occupation" refers to professionals.

We intended to interview all 26 participants who finished the program out of 38 older people who started, but only 23 were available. None of the participants were excluded for any other reason. Moreover, one participant who had dropped out of each intervention group was selected taking into account their gender and the heterogeneous reasons for leaving the program: two women, one of whom dropped out to care for a family member and the other had an injurious fall, and one man who started a social activity. Furthermore, nine older volunteers who accompanied the three intervention groups were interviewed. One man and one woman initially involved as volunteers were not available. All six professionals involved as facilitators or observers were interviewed.

2.4. Data Collection Techniques

Focus groups and interviews were semistructured and followed a topic guide with open-end questions. The topic guide had been previously planned and prepared based on a review of the literature and the objectives of the study. The guide included adaptation according to the type of informant and had been agreed by the research team (Appendix A: "Topic guides of the semistructured interviews and focus groups with participants, volunteers and professionals"). The topic guide was pilot tested with the first two informants of each profile. Despite the structured script, the interviewer had the possibility to adapt the topics, add and change questions according to the progress of the group discussion. Focus groups with participants explored the perceived benefits on participants regarding loneliness, social support and participation, and health, accounting for contextual factors. In the interviews, participants were asked about their loneliness and participation prior to the program and the perceived benefits. Volunteers and professionals were asked about their perceptions of the process and benefits observed on participants.

Three focus groups with older participants and 41 semistructured interviews were conducted: 26 with older participants, six with professionals and nine with volunteers (one individual interview and three with small groups). Interviews and focus groups were conducted at the end of the intervention, in June–July 2012. Twenty-six older people were interviewed twice: in the focus groups conducted in their natural group during the last session of the program, and in an individual interview, in order to gain more personal information about their situation prior to the program, the process carried out and the perceived benefits.

Interviews with participants were partly conducted at participants' homes and partly in a local senior club. Focus groups and interviews with professionals and volunteers were conducted in each primary health care center. Interviews lasted approximately one hour and focus groups around 1.5 h.

Moreover, participant-observation was conducted in all 15 sessions of the program in the three zones by one or two members of the research team. Field notes included any positive and negative information on the implementation of the intervention and the attitudes and reactions of participants, volunteers and professionals along the sessions. Notes were rigorously collected differentiating observed facts from subjective interpretations. A total of 58 field notes from observations were taken. All techniques were conducted by two female researchers (LCP, medical doctor, and GV, sociologist), both with experience in ageing research. As a consequence of the observation period, researchers established a rapport with participants during the 4.5 months. Participants were aware of the researchers' involvement in the program.

2.5. Data Analysis

All conversational techniques were digitally recorded and transcribed (by DR, sociologist). A thematic content analysis was conducted. The analysis involved a triangulation of techniques, researchers, and informants. Two female researchers (DRA, sociologist, and LCP, medical doctor) independently analyzed the transcripts. DRA is an expert on qualitative research and was not involved in the program. The analysis was conducted according to following steps: (1) formulation of pre-analytical intuitions after successive readings of the transcriptions and the notes from documentary techniques; (2) creation of an initial analytical framework and text codification; (3) creation of categories by grouping the codes according to the analogy criterion based on predefined themes (experiences prior to the program, processes undergone during the intervention, influences of health, and context and perceived benefits according to the social capital theory) and new emerging elements from the discourses, with a continuous cross-checking between the categorization and the source of the data that combined a deductive and inductive approach; (4) analysis of each category and relationship with the others; (5) elaboration of the new text with the main results.

The loneliness model, the theories of behavior change, such as the social cognitive theory and the stages of change of the trans-theoretical model, and the three ageing crises were used to interpret the findings once data had been coded and categorized.

The results were structured to build an explanatory framework of the processes that participants underwent during the program, their perceived benefits and the main influencing factors. The results and the framework were discussed with the entire research team and verified with the corpus when needed. Informants verified results by providing their feedback on preliminary results. Informative richness for a deeper understanding of the phenomenon studied around the program was achieved according to the study aims and research questions. Data saturation was reached at the end of the analysis in the main categories for women, since participants were not contributing with new information.

2.6. Ethical Considerations

The ethics committees from IDIAP Jordi Gol and Universitat Autònoma de Barcelona approved the protocol (Ref number 1403). The informants participated voluntarily after signing informed consent forms. Anonymity, confidentiality and protection of stored data were guaranteed. No financial or material compensation was offered to informants.

3. Results

As recommended in the Standards for Reporting Qualitative Research [32] the results section comprises the synthesis and interpretation of the main findings with interpretations, inferences, and themes. Those are illustrated with quotes and field notes gathered in the qualitative procedures as evidence linking the results to the empirical data to substantiate the analytic findings and illustrate the process of interpretation based on these data. The verbatim quotations selected are the most representative of each theme, according to the richness of the idea or result they illustrate. Quotations from participants' discussions included were translated by a professional scientific bilingual translator.

3.1. Participants' Experiences of Participation and Loneliness prior to the Program

Two profiles of participants were identified regarding previous experiences of participation. The first profile was composed of participants with no previous experience of formal participation. They were women with a low educational level and mainly widowed. Their life had been focused on family and house care, and caring had been a barrier for participation. They shared trajectories of disempowerment, lack of courage to participate alone and renouncing to make decisions that they considered would be unfaithful towards others. Some women had no friends, had participated in social activities only with their husbands and stopped participating when they passed away. Some of them had no previous knowledge on community assets, or had prejudices, especially about senior clubs.

> "He didn't want to go, because I sometimes said "let's go and see". We live beside the senior club ... (...) but I didn't have the strength to say "if you don't come, then I'll go on my own"". Participant 5, Woman, 78 years old, Zone C.

The second profile had previous experience of social participation. They were mainly single, divorced or widowed, including the only widower. Widows who had participated together with their husbands in community assets had ended participation when their husbands passed away. Those who had participated on their own had conducted activities for other people (e.g., sewing), with others (e.g., social activities) or to help others (e.g., volunteering) and it had been a source of mental wellbeing. They had stopped mainly due to age-related health problems (e.g., chronic pain), economic problems, or translocation. Stopping them had contributed to their loneliness. Nevertheless, some participants reported having found ways of coping with limitations to maintain some informal activities, like overcoming pain to go for a walk.

> "For a long time I used to go there every day (to a center for disabled children) ... look at my knee, I've needed an operation for 18 years but I decided not to have it, and I can't feed them from sitting, because sometimes you have to hold their head and I can't." Participant 1, Woman, 83 years old, Zone C.

Three main profiles of participants were identified regarding experiences of loneliness. In the first profile, participants expressed their loneliness as a consequence of widowhood. Their husbands' absence had left a void that was impossible to fill and finding a new partner was disregarded to avoid being a "servant" again or because their husband was irreplaceable. They were living alone, suffered from loneliness mainly at home and coped with it by talking with their deceased husband, going out for a walk or having a pet.

> "I'm missing the most important thing, I'm missing my husband." Participant 29, Woman, 78 years old, Zone B.

In contrast, a recently widowed man who dropped out had joined the program to find a new partner.

Many of them had cared for family members and started to feel lonely after or while caring. They explained feeling lonely despite the support perceived and received from their family and neighbors. In some cases, widows suffered depressive symptoms and anxiety or had a pharmacologically treated depression. Nevertheless, it is to be mentioned that a minority of them expressed widowhood as a relief from a constrictive marriage.

The second profile comprised some long-term widowed, divorced or single participants who expressed that they were solitary. They expressed having a fear of relating with others, a lack of social relationships and that they received pressure from their family to interact more.

> "I've done it (joining the program) mainly because I had a problem relating with others, isn't that right?" Participant, N. 18, Woman, 65 years old, Zone A.

In the third profile, participants were suffering from loneliness in company. They had moved to live with their children due to health problems, or their children and grandchildren had moved to live with them due to economic problems. Older women expressed missing having their own space and a lack of communication with their children, who had little time for them.

"My daughter and I have a good relationship, but I can't have any conversations with her . . . She takes care of me if I am ill . . . but I can't tell her stories about older people; they are very tedious, because she has no time. It's true, she works long hours and has no time. She would like to listen to me and so on, but she says "Ah Mum, not today, I have no time, maybe on Sunday . . . ". "Participant 28, woman, 71 years old, Zone B.

In addition, providing economic support to their children was a strong source of worry that intensified their loneliness.

"And now I'm turning 74 years old. I thought than when I was old, I would have my retirement prepared, I thought I could live my life a bit. But I see it is the other way round, that now I have to be there for the others, instead of them being there for me; I am the one who has to be there for everyone." Participant 2, Woman, 73 years old, Zone C.

Table 2 summarizes the previous results regarding participants' experiences when entering the program showing the identified profiles on loneliness and participation.

Table 2. Summary of results regarding participants' experiences prior to the program.

	Participants' Experiences Prior to the Program		
Experiences of participation	No previous experience of formal participation	Knowledge about local community assets: no knowledge, perceived barriers or prejudices	
		Life focused on family and house care	
	Previous experience of social participation but stopped	Participation linked to husband (stopped when widowhood)	
		Due to health-related limitations	
		Due to changing neighborhood	
		Due to economic constraints	
Experiences of loneliness	Loneliness attributed to widowhood		
	Participants who expressed that they were solitary but wishing more social relationships		
	Suffering from loneliness in company	Lack of communication	
		Lack of own space	
	Factors worsening loneliness	Economic constraints, e.g., providing economic support to family	
		Urban–rural translocation with insufficiently built social network	

3.2. Perceived Benefits on Participants during and after the Program

Professionals and volunteers observed changes in participants that they attributed to the intervention. The benefits were more intensive among those participants who adhered more, suggesting a dose–response effect.

3.2.1. Perceived Benefits on Social Support

Professionals and participants expressed that the program was especially successful at promoting mutual support. Living in the same area gave them a feeling of familiarity, and participants often met each other on the street, and sometimes walked back to their homes together.

According to participants, the group provided companionship, a feeling of social integration and sense of belonging to the group. The group was perceived as a space of attention, respect and affection to give and receive emotional support. When a participant suffered an injurious fall, was in low mood or had a new illness, support relationships could be observed.

Many participants were part of a group for the first time and for some participants, the group was the only place they had to socialize.

Participants discovered that peer relationships, as opposed to relationships within the family, provided a way of communicating shared worries and interests by sharing a similar age.

"We are the same age, you can talk about the same things ... youth, depending on the topic ... you talk but ... , I don't know, youth is very different. (...) For me, the company of one or the other is different. With the group companions there ... , I don't know, maybe it's another freedom, another thing because since we all speak about the same thing, pretty much, about what happens to us and about what we do not have ... " Participant 29, Woman, 78 years old, Zone B.

Participants identified others as a model to follow or, on the contrary, as a model to avoid, evoking positive changes.

Some participants became friends and started visiting and calling each other. While some people were previously aware of missing having friends, others made friends for the first time.

"(...) because I don't tend to go out with friends here and there. But now it's different, since I've been coming here (...) Look, I get on very well with Maria, she's a lovely and good woman and we get on great together. For her it's the same; she says "I've found a shoe for my foot, because I don't trust anybody but you"." Participant 37, Woman, 77 years old, Zone B.

In some cases, new friends generated subgroups that integrated other participants, including those who were more socially isolated. In other cases, friendships were closed, and some participants felt excluded.

"... and they seem to have become very united to go out on walks together (...), but I go by and they are sitting there and never say "do you want to come with us", so I go home...." Participant 2, Woman, 74 years old, Zone C.

The group comprised different profiles regarding educational levels, age-related disability and health problems, which unified but also divided the group. Some participants expressed having felt united and treated without differences. In some cases, participants and volunteers developed support relationships with more vulnerable participants, moved by compassion. Telephone contact was especially relevant between participants with mobility limitations or living apart, and also for volunteers to support participants.

"The one I see who needs to cheer up is Margalida, she is very down... (...) For me it's no effort because it's something I've done all my life, listen to people and be at their side and support them. Let them tell you things, especially that ... I'll go and see her this week, because she called me the other day and I went to her house and now I want her to come to my house". Volunteer 2, Woman, 77 years old, Zone A.

However, those participants with mobility limitations and hearing impairment were at higher risk of not establishing friendships and dropping out, thus losing the opportunity to benefit of the program at any level.

The few participants with a higher educational level expressed not sharing interests with the rest. For them, feeling valued and helpful for more vulnerable participants was key to remain in the program. In one group, there was a conflict with one participant. She felt more skillful and was jealous of those who participated more in the group.

"You can see that she doesn't stop talking, she always wants to speak . . . and from the first day there has been a conflict, and everybody saw there was a conflict. Even Jose said he didn't feel comfortable because of her. And of course, this has restricted the dynamic a bit, hasn't it? It hasn't been easy . . . " Social care professional 1, Woman, Zone C.

3.2.2. Perceived Benefits on Loneliness

Most of the participants reported that their loneliness decreased after the program by feeling accompanied by peers and professionals, and thanks to the bonds established and to having become aware of and engaged in local activities of their interest. While some people said they no longer felt lonely because of new friendships, others continued to suffer from loneliness, but with less intensity. The awareness that loneliness was a common matter helped them to cope with it by realizing they were not alone in their loneliness.

"I don't feel lonely, now I have friends". Participant 28, Woman, 71 years old, Zone B.

"Like bread and butter: loneliness is easier to digest when in company". Participant 4, Woman, 78 years old, Zone C.

Some participants expressed a transitory benefit on loneliness. For them, home was the space of loneliness, while the group and the street were relational spaces. Likewise, some participants said that the improvement would vanish once the group finished. Nevertheless, thinking and talking about the program with others also helped them to feel less lonely.

"I am happy to join the group, but then, when I get back home, I fall apart, I need to be on the street with someone . . . at home, alone, is bad . . . " Participant 35, Woman, 81 years old, Zone B.

Some widows who attributed loneliness to widowhood reported no decrease in loneliness after the program. Accordingly, in these cases the main effect desired of the intervention was not achieved. However, these participants reported other benefits such as an increase in social relationships, well-being and empowerment.

"Since my loneliness is due to missing my husband, it cannot be replaced, at the moment, or ever." Participant 13, Woman, 75 years old, Zone A.

3.2.3. Perceived Benefits on Social Participation

According to all types of informants, the program was generally successful at helping participants to discover and sometimes engage in local activities.

Visiting community assets allowed participants to get a sense of what was available and to remove prejudices. Moreover, some people returned to community resources where they used to go with their husbands.

"The satisfaction of seeing things I had never seen before, although you imagine them, you've seen them on TV, but being there inside, you see it, you touch it, it is a big satisfaction . . . " Participant 5, Woman, 78 years old, Zone C.

The visits included testing local activities and triggered participation in a wide range of activities. Some participants started participating in activities immediately and others started later during the program. They became engaged in activities that suited their interests, abilities or worries (e.g., memory training). Belonging to the group facilitated becoming engaged with other peers. Thus, new friends easily did new activities together, accompanying each other and reinforcing their friendship.

"Carme and Teresa meet up to go to the cinema, since they live near each other, and Carme does not like going out on the street on her own at night. They meet up to see the film that the parish puts on in the cinema and has been recommended to them, but it's not a planned activity; it's an extra outing." Field note, researcher LCP, referring to participants 10 and 13, Women, 75 and 80 years old, Zone A.

Other participants made specific plans to start activities the following year and some exclusively connected with their wish to participate. For some participants, socializing was very important but participating in activities was not. Some participants, especially those who had been caregivers over the past years, discovered the value of doing activities with other people.

> "Everything we did there was new to me. Everything . . . " Participant 12, Woman, 79 years old, Zone A

Low self-confidence and low communication ability, often related with low education, limited the benefits on participation to the extent of feeling they were not up to join community assets.

> "She tells me she's odd and that she thinks everything is very nice and would like to get involved but she doesn't feel capable because she is silly, she doesn't express herself well, she talks poorly..." Field note, researcher LCP, referring to the participant 30, Woman, 84 years old, Zone B.

3.2.4. Perceived Benefits on Health

Participants, professionals, and volunteers agreed on the improvement in mental health. The program was seen as a strategy to prevent or alleviate depressive symptoms. Many participants took antidepressive drugs and/or tranquillizers and explained feeling better after the program. Some women expressed that the program was a salvation to them. One participant explained having solved her sleep problems.

> "For me, beforehand, I wasn't able to go anywhere on my own. Now, I've changed! If I had to go for an X-ray, I had to be accompanied, and, since I have claustrophobia, in a lift and things like that . . . but now, I go alone wherever it may be, an X-ray, Sant Pau (Hospital) . . . I'm a different woman!" Participant 5, Woman, 78 years old, Zone C.

According to the professionals, some participants were initially trapped in a loop linked to loneliness with an obsessive focus on illnesses and woes, but the intervention successfully broke it by connecting them with others, awakening the wish to remain connected and helping them to forget about their worries.

Sharing their woes and coping strategies among peers during the sessions was generally relieving and helped them to deal with them, although specific people needed to feel their suffering was greater.

> "By participating, you don't feel lonely, with everything you are experiencing." Participant 18, Woman, 65 years old, Zone A.

Specifically, sharing the way in which they talked with their deceased husbands to overcome loneliness helped them to feel better instead of "crazy", as they said.

In terms of positive mental health, participants reported an improved subjective well-being, becoming aware of worse circumstances and valuing their situation more. They reported being more understanding and empathic, and having more trust in other people; particularly those who were more closed and socially isolated. Others explained being more compassionate, respectful and having learned not to judge others. Likewise, they also reported feeling less worried and more able to deal with economic, family and health problems. Those living with family members expressed having learned to be more tolerant in cohabitation with other household members.

An empowerment process was observed that contributed to alleviating their loneliness. According to the three groups of informants, the program contributed to the development of personal potential and autonomy to participate and to live their life as they wanted, with less dependency on their children. They had a feeling of strength and of power to decide.

> "My daughter wanted me to spend every Sunday with them, but I didn't like it and I used to say: "but why do I have to be here every Sunday?" and she'd say "so that you're not on your own" (. . .) And now, if one day I don't want to go for lunch I say "today, I won't come for lunch, don't wait for me because I'll be with Maria", now it's different." Participant 37, Woman, 77 years old, Zone B.

Participants attributed their empowerment to the attention and value received. Additionally, realizing they had helped peers was very satisfying and increased their self-esteem, since it gave value to their life experience. Accordingly, feeling useful and able instead of useless meant that their life was not ending and was worth living.

> *"(With the program) you have another stimulus, you feel like living, you feel like someone needs you for something. You feel that you, life, or God or whatever, needs you for something. Do you know what that feels like?"* Participant 29, Woman, 78 years old, Zone C.

In particular, those participants with a life trajectory that was family-oriented, said that they reached a new sense of freedom in their lives. Those participants with severe physical conditions felt connected with their wish to live by becoming aware that others do care about them. They were aware of their own empowerment process and participants mutually reinforced each other. It was strange for them having lived until then without these satisfying aspects of life. However, participants did not see themselves able to lead the continuity of the group and wanted someone as a leader to tell them where to go.

Empowerment was also enhanced by discovering new interests. Becoming engaged in local activities like physical activity and memory training especially promoted healthy ageing, but their physical activity also increased by starting to participate.

The program had some benefits on self-care and healthy lifestyles. Participants were motivated to dress smartly, some of them rediscovering the desire to get dressed up after widowhood by identifying some participants as a model to follow.

Two participants with hearing impairment felt motivated to wear the hearing aid that they had not used before because they wanted to feel connected to others in the group.

Through the program, they became aware of the relevance of taking care of their own health, especially those who had cared for a spouse and whose own health and self-care had not been a priority before.

Nevertheless, participants reported limited benefits on physical health, since many participants reported suffering from chronic conditions with aches that were difficult to alleviate.

Table 3 summarizes the results on the benefits of the program attributed to the intervention on social support, loneliness, participation and health. In each category, no effect, adverse effects, facilitators and mediators are specified when identified. Mediators are factors interpreted to be necessary in the pathway to reach benefits, while facilitators are factors considered as enhancing that area.

Table 3. Summary of results regarding perceived benefits of the program.

	Perceived Benefits of the Program
Perceived benefits on social support	Company Social integration Sense of belonging Support relationships: ○ Friendship: participants with affinity becoming friends, including or excluding others *(adverse effects)* ○ Compassion: Relationship with more vulnerable participants moved by compassion Conflicts *(adverse effects)*
Mediator	Social network among peers from the same neighborhood
Facilitators	Previous knowledge among participants
Perceived benefits on loneliness	Loneliness decreased Transitory improvement in loneliness: during the program or during the group sessions No improvement in loneliness (in case of loneliness attributed to widowhood)

Table 3. *Cont.*

	Perceived Benefits of the Program
Perceived benefits on participation	Do not want to participate (*no effect on participation*) Connecting with the wish to participate Plans for participating Started participation
Mediator	Knowledge on local community assets
Facilitator	Local activities that meet interests, abilities and worries
Perceived benefits on health	Disconnect from worries and discomfort Self-reported improvement of mood and decrease depressive symptoms Better strategies to affront health and personal problems Increase trust in others Better self-care and healthier lifestyles Feeling useful, able and strong; life is not ending, life is worth living
Mediator	Empowerment process, autonomy to participate, feeling of strength and of the power to decide
Barriers	Vulnerabilities: • Age-related health limitations: acoustic limitations, chronic diseases and mobility disability • Low education: poor communication ability • Personal resources: low self-efficacy and poor coping strategies

3.3. The Role of Urban, Semirural and Socioeconomic Context

Some differences and communalities could be identified between the three zones considering their semirural and urban contexts and the different socioeconomic levels in the urban neighborhoods.

As mentioned in Table 2, loneliness was worsened by a recent or prolonged translocation when the older person had not built a sufficiently fulfilling social life. This phenomenon was observed in all three zones, with translocations from urban to the semirural area, from rural areas to the city or when moving within the same city.

"I say: so, you (meaning the husband who had died) were the one who wanted to live here (in the semirural area), you go, you leave me alone and I remain here". Participant 13, Woman, 75 years old, Zone A.

Only in the urban context, participants mentioned that the program contributed to a less hostile neighborhood. In the semirural area, many of the participants knew each other before, but the previous dynamics greatly influenced future relationships that could be built. Otherwise, in both urban areas, it was uncommon that participants knew each other and in these few cases, a previous relationship facilitated developing supportive friendships. Community assets were also already known in the semirural area but not their full range of offers. Whereas in the urban areas, many participants expressed surprise when discovering the opportunities for participation that they had near their homes.

Although the urban zones were different in terms of socioeconomic levels, observed processes and perceived impacts were more influenced by the socioeconomic characteristics of the participants than the contextual ones. Indeed, both zones were similar regarding some features that were relevant to enhance the effects of the program by promoting social interactions beyond the sessions. For instance, at that time, in both urban zones several community assets offered a diversity of activities and older people were present and relevant in the community life, e.g., participants easily met in their daily errands, sitting in benches or walking in pedestrian zones.

4. Discussion

4.1. Interpretation of Findings

The results of the qualitative evaluation of the program were convergent with the already published quantitative effects on loneliness, social support, and participation [30]. However, regarding reported health benefits at post-intervention, qualitative findings suggested changes that validated scales in the quantitative study could not detect at post-intervention. Nevertheless, at two years follow-up, the quantitative evaluation did detect a decrease in depressive symptoms in line with the qualitative findings. Accordingly, the main benefits of the program on mental health are in line with the protective effect of social capital on mental well-being among older adults [34].

Our results are consistent with research reflecting that handling loss is key in the attitude towards participation and social relationships [35]. Our study adds that interventions might encourage lonely people overwhelmed by loss to connect with meaningful activities and establish positive social relationships.

Our findings are consistent with the qualitative results of other programs in the same area like the Circle of Friends [28]. In both studies, participants felt alleviated sharing their diverse experiences of loneliness, although particular cases competed to be the worst case. Additionally, in both programs mutual support was observed, subgroups developed, and participants especially helped those who were more vulnerable. Meetings outside the groups were self-organized. Similarly, mild conflicts in relation with power games were rare but present and affected the group dynamic. Both studies showed that participants increasingly paid more attention to their appearance. Equally, the heterogeneity in age-related limitations influenced the group dynamics, limiting the participation of those more vulnerable participants.

The loneliness model could partly correspond to the type of loneliness observed by professionals prior to the program. The loneliness model proposes that chronic loneliness entails a cognitive bias consisting of a self-reinforcing loop associated with negative social expectations that cause social distance [36]. In this case, the self-reinforcing loop would be centered on illnesses and woes. However, participants were released from it at least during the program. Indeed, social relationships and participation seemed to create a positive self-reinforcing loop; opening participants up to others and to new experiences, relativizing their situations and encouraging them to get out of an introspective state, and thus involving more social relationships, and more participation that brought more meaning to their life. Accordingly, the observed empowerment process confirms the suitability of the empowerment model informing a successful design of the intervention.

The program helped participants to overcome, at least in part, the three ageing crises of autonomy, identity and belonging and consequently brought the feeling that life was worth living to participants and alleviated their loneliness [5]. It helped them to take care of their image and health, to take up their interests again, and provided them with the feeling of belonging to the group and their neighborhood. Mutual support helped them to overcome or cope better with their limitations and they felt more capable and useful.

The role of modeling, and the reported increased self-efficacy are in line with social cognitive theory [25]. Moreover, the stages of change of the trans-theoretical model supports the different levels of change described among participants: some participants started the action during the program (participation), others were in the preparation stage (were ready and made concrete plans), while others were in the contemplation stage (getting ready, connecting with their wish to participate) [26].

In line with the salutogenic approach, benefits were mainly reported on well-being, the social aspects of health and positive mental health, and there was also a decrease in ill mental health [4].

However, some participants did not report benefits from the program in certain spheres of their lives. Poor physical function and low socioeconomic level, especially when linked to low education, low self-confidence and low communication abilities, hindered engaging in the program and limited the process of change among participants. This is in line with previous research that shows that socioeconomic factors are key factors linking social relationships with health [4]. Nevertheless, it is to be remarked that this group of women had difficulties to access and continue formal education in their childhood and youth, which explains their low educational level. However, those with certain personal capabilities and social abilities could further develop and grow with the program. Moreover, some widowed participants who attributed loneliness to their widowhood continuously felt lonely although expressing an increase in social relationships. The distinction between social and emotional loneliness could partly explain why these cases remained emotionally but not socially lonely. While social loneliness occurs when the number of relationships with family, friends and colleagues is smaller than desired, emotional loneliness refers to situations where the wished intimacy in confidant relationships is not realized [37].

Lastly, the historical and cultural context seems to configure a generation of older women who had grown up assuming traditional roles of dependence on their husbands. Some of them remained powerless in widowhood, while others were relieved, and others managed widowhood well alone over time. In addition, the 2008–2009 financial crisis seems to have worsened the experience of the ageing process and enhanced loneliness by stressing family dynamics.

4.2. Strengths and Limitations

The rapport built between researchers and participants during the program generated a trust that facilitated the observation of the sessions and sharing personal experiences in the interviews, although it might also have influenced their answers, consciously or unconsciously wanting to please researchers. Nevertheless, the assumptions we had as researchers regarding how and why the program should have reduced their loneliness were challenged from the first group session to the last interview.

Among informants, men were rare, since women were a clear majority among participants and the only gender among volunteers, professionals and researchers. This fact has as consequences that the men's discourse is underrepresented in the results. However, community-based programs targeting older people in Spain are frequently dominated by women [38]. Accordingly, our study contributes to the understanding of the experiences of women, who are the majority of users of this type of program. Moreover, older people who adhered to the intervention were the majority among informants. Nevertheless, three people who dropped out for different reasons were interviewed, and the participant observation technique involved all participants since all sessions were observed.

Benefits reported by older people at the end of the program were triangulated with those perceived by volunteers and professionals and with the observations of researchers during the process. Accordingly, the richness and complementarity of the information generated with the different techniques and the three types of informants are a strength of the study, since triangulation of informants and techniques is a criteria for rigor and quality in qualitative research to enhance trustworthiness and credibility of data analysis [31]. Nevertheless, the constructivist research paradigm framing qualitative research does not aim to study a representative sample and generalize the results, but to study in depth a phenomenon in a given context that can be transferred to similar contexts [39]. Moreover, qualitative results can guide further quantitative research to objectify, quantify and generalize the magnitude of effects.

Qualitative findings are limited to the post-intervention timepoint with no further data on whether and how the perceived effects lasted and what was the trajectory of participants not experiencing certain effects. However, the quantitative evaluation was repeated at two years follow-up and significant long-term effects on loneliness, social participation and depressive symptoms were detected [30]. Moreover, almost half of the participants maintained long-term contact with at least one person from the group and 40% continued participating in activities [30].

Lastly, primary care professionals involved in the program were especially motivated to work on loneliness, and the implementation of the program might face barriers in primary health care contexts with a strong biomedical focus. Accordingly, caution is required before transferring these results to other settings. Nevertheless, similar community-based programs in different contexts, such as Circle of Friends, have shown their applicability.

4.3. Implications for Research, Practice and Policy

This program supports the WHO Active and Healthy Ageing policies and provides insight into how to enhance social networks and participation while ageing to enhance well-being.

In addition, our findings should support current practices and policies of social prescribing programs, which link primary care patients with community resources with the aim of strengthening participation and social support, and promoting health, particularly mental health, and well-being [40].

Nevertheless, the role of primary health care in loneliness interventions may differ according to the cultural context and the characteristics of the health and social care system and the available community resources [41]. In any case, attention must be placed on not medicalizing loneliness when interventions are developed in primary health care.

Regarding the intervention design, guaranteeing the continuity of the group remains a challenge, as well as an appropriate follow-up to enhance, if needed, participants' engagement in the social activities in community assets. Strategies are needed to focus on those persons with social and health vulnerabilities and, consequently, at risk of dropping out or of being socially excluded during or after the program.

4.4. Future Research Directions

Future research should include more qualitative evaluations of interventions for a better understanding of personal processes and perceived intervention benefits on loneliness and unintended effects, addressing its complexity, including context specificities [42].

Programs addressing loneliness tend to reach and work well with certain profiles of people (e.g., widow women), while they might be missing some others [43]. Indeed, loneliness is crossed by inequality axes such as gender, age, social class, disability and ethnicity [44]. Some of these profiles might be "hard-to-reach" if they are not specifically targeted by programs. In this vein, a deeper understanding of the perspective of men and participants dropping out of programs tackling loneliness is fundamental to rethink interventions to reach them, identify profiles at risk of dropping out and address their potential reasons. Therefore, there is an urgent need to move towards personalizing interventions with and for older people with an equity perspective. Moreover, future studies should assess the long-term effects of such interventions, also from a qualitative perspective, especially when the ageing process might further affect their abilities and opportunities to participate and socialize.

Finally, with the expectation of an increasing number of vulnerable older people vaccinated against COVID-19 in Europe, research should guide post-pandemic times on how to rebuild social capital, especially in older people with aggravated loneliness during the pandemic.

5. Conclusions

The qualitative evaluation of the Paths program has contributed to understanding the complex processes that are involved when promoting social capital in older people with low participation and loneliness. The intervention tried to promote social capital to make it a social resource available to all group members. Different degrees of success were observed among participants on their reported alleviation of loneliness, increase in social relationships and engagement in social activities. In the most successful cases, the program enabled their empowerment and enhanced processes of change. Those participants reported an improvement in mental well-being, experienced new freedoms and became reconnected with the sense that life was worth living. However, some widowed participants remained emotionally lonely and other participants were not interested in joining social activities. Moreover, vulnerabilities related to health, socioeconomic factors and age-related disability limited the adherence to the program and the perceived benefits of the intervention.

These findings should support further designs, and the implementation and evaluation of interventions. The cultural context of the study is a familistic society with a primary health and social care system with a community-based approach in Catalonia, Spain. However, our results can inspire other programs that should be flexible to adapt intervention components to the specific contexts and to participants' characteristics.

Our results might guide post-pandemic programs on how to resume face-to-face social interactions and social activities among older people suffering from loneliness.

Author Contributions: Conceptualization, L.C.-P. and R.M.; methodology, D.R.-A. and M.P.-V.; data analysis, L.C.-P. and D.R.-A.; writing—original draft preparation, L.C.-P.; writing—review and editing, M.P.-V., F.N., D.R.-A., R.M. and T.P.; supervision, R.M. and T.P.; funding acquisition, L.C.-P. and R.M. All authors have read and agreed to the published version of the manuscript.

Funding: This research received no external funding.

Institutional Review Board Statement: The study was conducted according to the guidelines of the Declaration of Helsinki, and approved by the ethics committees from IDIAP Jordi Gol and Universitat Autònoma de Barcelona (Ref number 1403, October 2011).

Informed Consent Statement: Informed consent was obtained from all subjects involved in the study.

Data Availability Statement: The data presented in this study are available on request from the corresponding author.

Acknowledgments: We gratefully acknowledge the contribution of the participants sharing their experiences with us. We would like to thank Àlex Domingo for the proofreading.

Conflicts of Interest: The authors declare no conflict of interest. The funders had no role in the design of the study; in the collection, analyses, or interpretation of data; in the writing of the manuscript, or in the decision to publish the results.

Appendix A

Topic guides of the semistructured interviews and focus groups with participants, volunteers and professionals.

References

1. Peplau, L.; Perlman, D. *Loneliness: A Sourcebook of Current Theory, Research, and Therapy*; Wiley-Interscience: New York, NY, USA, 1982; ISBN 0471080284.
2. Prohaska, T.; Burholt, V.; Burns, A.; Golden, J.; Hawkley, L.; Lawlor, B.; Leavey, G.; Lubben, J.; O'Sullivan, R.; Perissinotto, C.; et al. Consensus statement: Loneliness in older adults, the 21st century social determinant of health? *BMJ Open* **2020**, *10*, e034967. [CrossRef] [PubMed]
3. Dahlberg, L. Loneliness during the COVID-19 pandemic. *Aging Ment. Health* **2021**, 1–4. [CrossRef]
4. *The Handbook of Salutogenesis*, 1st ed.; Mittlemark, M.B., Sagy, S., Eriksson, M., Bauer, G.F., Pelikan, J.M., Lindström, B., Espnes, G.A., Eds.; Springer: Berlin, Germany, 2017; ISBN 9783319045993.
5. Rey Calero, J. Epidemiología y sociología de la vejez. In *Anales de Academia Nazionale dei Lincei*; Università di Roma Tor Vergata: Roma, Italy, 1995.
6. Victor, C.R.; Scambler, S.J.; Bowling, A.N.N.; Bond, J. The prevalence of, and risk factors for, loneliness in later life: A survey of older people in Great Britain. *Ageing Soc.* **2005**, *25*, 357–375. [CrossRef]
7. Cattan, M.; Kime, N.; Bagnall, A.-M. The use of telephone befriending in low level support for socially isolated older people-an evaluation. *Health Soc. Care Community* **2010**, *19*, 198–206. [CrossRef] [PubMed]
8. Sundström, G.; Fransson, E.; Malmberg, B.; Davey, A. Loneliness among older Europeans. *Eur. J. Ageing* **2009**, *6*, 267–275. [CrossRef] [PubMed]
9. Dykstra, P.A. Older adult loneliness: Myths and realities. *Eur. J. Ageing* **2009**, *6*, 91–100. [CrossRef]
10. Litwin, H. Social Networks and Well-being: A Comparison of Older People in Mediterranean and Non-Mediterranean Countries. *J. Gerontol. Ser. B* **2009**, *65*, 599–608. [CrossRef]
11. Van Tilburg, T.; Gierveld, J.D.J.; Lecchini, L.; Marsiglia, D. Social Integration and Loneliness: A Comparative Study among Older Adults in the Netherlands and Tuscany, Italy. *J. Soc. Pers. Relationsh.* **1998**, *15*, 740–754. [CrossRef]

12. Sirven, N.; Debrand, T. Social participation and healthy ageing: An international comparison using SHARE data. *Soc. Sci. Med.* **2008**, *67*, 2017–2026. [CrossRef]
13. World Health Organization Active Ageing: A Policy Framework. 2002. Available online: http://www.who.int/ageing/publications/active_ageing/en/ (accessed on 19 May 2021).
14. *International Longevity Centre Brazil (ILC-BR) Active Ageing: A Policy Framework in Response to the Longevity Revolution*, 1st ed.; Faber, P., Ed.; Centro Internacional de Longevidade Brasil: Rio de Janeiro, RJ, Brazil, 2015; Volume 9, ISBN 9788569483007.
15. Islam, M.K.; Merlo, J.; Kawachi, I.; Lindström, M.; Gerdtham, U.-G. Social capital and health: Does egalitarianism matter? A literature review. *Int. J. Equity Health* **2006**, *5*, 3. [CrossRef]
16. Forsman, A.K.; Nyqvist, F.; Wahlbeck, K. Cognitive components of social capital and mental health status among older adults: A population-based cross-sectional study. *Scand. J. Public Health* **2011**, *39*, 757–765. [CrossRef] [PubMed]
17. Nyqvist, F.; Pape, B.; Pellfolk, T.; Forsman, A.K.; Wahlbeck, K. Structural and Cognitive Aspects of Social Capital and All-Cause Mortality: A Meta-Analysis of Cohort Studies. *Soc. Indic. Res.* **2014**, *116*, 545–566. [CrossRef]
18. Cattan, M.; White, M.; Bond, J.; Learmouth, A. Preventing social isolation and loneliness among older people: A systematic review of health promotion interventions. *Ageing Soc.* **2005**, *25*, 41–67. [CrossRef]
19. Dickens, A.; Richards, S.H.; Greaves, C.J.; Campbell, J.L. Interventions targeting social isolation in older people: A systematic review. *BMC Public Health* **2011**, *11*, 647. [CrossRef] [PubMed]
20. Findlay, R.A. Interventions to reduce social isolation amongst older people: Where is the evidence? *Ageing Soc.* **2003**, *23*, 647–658. [CrossRef]
21. Masi, C.M.; Chen, H.-Y.; Hawkley, L.C.; Cacioppo, J.T. A Meta-Analysis of Interventions to Reduce Loneliness. *Pers. Soc. Psychol. Rev.* **2010**, *15*, 219–266. [CrossRef] [PubMed]
22. Victor, C.; Scambler, S.; Bond, J.; Bowling, A. Being alone in later life: Loneliness, social isolation and living alone. *Rev. Clin. Gerontol.* **2000**, *10*, 407–417. [CrossRef]
23. Stevens, N. Combating loneliness: A friendship enrichment programme for older women. *Ageing Soc.* **2001**, *21*, 183–202. [CrossRef]
24. Routasalo, P.E.; Tilvis, R.S.; Kautiainen, H.; Pitkala, K.H. Effects of psychosocial group rehabilitation on social functioning, loneliness and well-being of lonely, older people: Randomized controlled trial. *J. Adv. Nurs.* **2009**, *65*, 297–305. [CrossRef]
25. Bandura, A. *Social Learning Theory*; Prentice Hall: Englewood Cliffs, NJ, USA, 1977; Volume 28, ISBN 0138167516.
26. Prochaska, J.O.D.C. Stages and Processes of Self-Change in Smoking. Towards an Integrative Model of Change. *J. Consult. Clin. Psych.* **1983**, *59*, 259–304. [CrossRef]
27. Coll-Planas, L.; Nyqvist, F.; Puig, T.; Urrútia, G.; Solà, I.; Monteserín, R. Social capital interventions targeting older people and their impact on health: A systematic review. *J. Epidemiol. Community Health* **2017**, *71*, 663–672. [CrossRef]
28. Pitkälä, K.H.; Savikko, N.; Routasalo, P. Group dynamics in older people's closed groups: Findings from finnish psychosocial group rehabilitation. In *Group Therapy*; Derrickson, H., Ed.; Nova Science Publishers, Inc.: New York, NY, USA, 2015; ISBN 9781634631730.
29. Saito, T.; Kai, I.; Takizawa, A. Effects of a program to prevent social isolation on loneliness, depression, and subjective well-being of older adults: A randomized trial among older migrants in Japan. *Arch. Gerontol. Geriatr.* **2012**, *55*, 539–547. [CrossRef]
30. Coll-Planas, L.; Gómez, G.D.V.; Bonilla, P.; Masat, T.; Puig, T.; Monteserín, R. Promoting social capital to alleviate loneliness and improve health among older people in Spain. *Health Soc. Care Community* **2015**, *25*, 145–157. [CrossRef] [PubMed]
31. Guba, E.; Lincoln, Y. Establishing Trustworthiness. In *Naturalistic Inquiry*; SAGE Publications: Sauzend Oaks, CA, USA, 1985.
32. O'Brien, B.C.; Harris, I.B.; Beckman, T.J.; Reed, D.A.; Cook, D.A. Standards for reporting qualitative research: A synthesis of recommendations. *Acad. Med.* **2014**, *89*, 1245–1251. [CrossRef]
33. *Social Capital as a Health Resource in Later Life: The Relevance of Context*, 1st ed.; Nyqvist, F.; Forsman, A.K., Eds.; Springer: Berlin/Heidelberg, Germany, 2015.
34. Nyqvist, F.; Forsman, A.K.; Giuntoli, G.; Cattan, M. Social capital as a resource for mental well-being in older people: A systematic review. *Aging Ment. Health* **2013**, *17*, 394–410. [CrossRef] [PubMed]
35. Kirkevold, M.; Moyle, W.; Wilkinson, C.; Meyer, J.; Hauge, S. Facing the challenge of adapting to a life 'alone' in old age: The influence of losses. *J. Adv. Nurs.* **2013**, *69*, 394–403. [CrossRef]
36. Hawkley, L.C.; Cacioppo, J.T. Loneliness Matters: A Theoretical and Empirical Review of Consequences and Mechanisms. *Ann. Behav. Med.* **2010**, *40*, 218–227. [CrossRef] [PubMed]
37. Gierveld, J.D.J.; Van Tilburg, T. The De Jong Gierveld short scales for emotional and social loneliness: Tested on data from 7 countries in the UN generations and gender surveys. *Eur. J. Ageing* **2010**, *7*, 121–130. [CrossRef]
38. Alias, S.B.; Nadal, R.M.; Moral, I.; Fígols, M.R.; i Luque, X.R.; Coll-Planas, L. Promoting social capital, self-management and health literacy in older adults through a group-based intervention delivered in low-income urban areas: Results of the randomized trial AEQUALIS. *BMC Public Health* **2021**, *21*, 1–12. [CrossRef]
39. Guba, E.; Lincoln, Y. Paradigmas en pugna en la investigación cualitativa (Denzin, N. and Lincoln, I.). In *Handbook of Qualitative Research*; SAGE Publications Inc.: London, UK, 1994; pp. 105–117.
40. Wilson, P.; Booth, A. University of York Centre for Reviews & Dissemination Evidence to Inform the Commissioning of Social Prescribing. 2015. Available online: https://www.york.ac.uk/media/crd/Ev%20briefing_social_prescribing.pdf (accessed on 19 May 2021).

41. Kharicha, K.; Iliffe, S.; Ma, J.M.; Chew-Graham, C.A.; Cattan, M.; Goodman, C.; Kirby-Barr, M.; Bsc, J.H.W.; Walters, K. What do older people experiencing loneliness think about primary care or community based interventions to reduce loneliness? A qualitative study in England. *Health Soc. Care Community* **2017**, *25*, 1733–1742. [CrossRef]
42. Power, J.E.M.; Dolezal, L.; Kee, F.; Lawlor, B.A. Conceptualizing loneliness in health research: Philosophical and psychological ways forward. *J. Theor. Philos. Psychol.* **2018**, *38*, 219–234. [CrossRef]
43. Liljas, A.E.M.; Walters, K.; Jovicic, A.; Iliffe, S.; Manthorpe, J.; Goodman, C.; Kharicha, K. Strategies to improve engagement of 'hard to reach' older people in research on health promotion: A systematic review. *BMC Public Health* **2017**, *17*, 349. [CrossRef] [PubMed]
44. Gierveld, J.D.J.; Van Tilburg, T.G.; Dykstra, P.A.; Vangelisti, A.L.; Perlman, D. New Ways of Theorizing and Conducting Research in the Field of Loneliness and Social Isolation. *Camb. Handb. Pers. Relatsh.* **2018**, 391–404. [CrossRef]

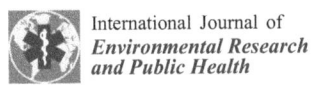

Review

Colorectal Cancer in Elderly Patients with Surgical Indication: State of the Art, Current Management, Role of Frailty and Benefits of a Geriatric Liaison

Nicolás M. González-Senac [1,†], Jennifer Mayordomo-Cava [1,2,3,†], Angela Macías-Valle [4], Paula Aldama-Marín [1], Sara Majuelos González [1,5,‡], María Luisa Cruz Arnés [1], Luis M. Jiménez-Gómez [6], María T. Vidán-Astiz [1,2,3,7,*] and José Antonio Serra-Rexach [1,2,3,7]

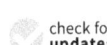

Citation: González-Senac, N.M.; Mayordomo-Cava, J.; Macías-Valle, A.; Aldama-Marín, P.; Majuelos González, S.; Cruz Arnés, M.L.; Jiménez-Gómez, L.M.; Vidán-Astiz, M.T.; Serra-Rexach, J.A. Colorectal Cancer in Elderly Patients with Surgical Indication: State of the Art, Current Management, Role of Frailty and Benefits of a Geriatric Liaison. IJERPH 2021, 18, 6072. https://doi.org/10.3390/ijerph18116072

Academic Editors: Francisco José Tarazona Santabalbina, Sebastià Josep Santaeugènia Gonzàlez, José Augusto García Navarro and José Viña

Received: 29 April 2021
Accepted: 29 May 2021
Published: 4 June 2021

Publisher's Note: MDPI stays neutral with regard to jurisdictional claims in published maps and institutional affiliations.

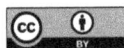

Copyright: © 2021 by the authors. Licensee MDPI, Basel, Switzerland. This article is an open access article distributed under the terms and conditions of the Creative Commons Attribution (CC BY) license (https://creativecommons.org/licenses/by/4.0/).

1. Geriatric Department, Hospital General Universitario Gregorio Marañón, 28007 Madrid, Spain; nic.gsenac@gmail.com (N.M.G.-S.); jennifer.mayordomo@gmail.com (J.M.-C.); paula.aldama.marin@gmail.com (P.A.-M.); saramajuelos@gmail.com (S.M.G.); mcarnes@salud.madrid.org (M.L.C.A.); joseantonio.serra@salud.madrid.org (J.A.S.-R.)
2. Instituto de Investigación Sanitaria Gregorio Marañón, 28007 Madrid, Spain
3. Biomedical Research Networking Center on Frailty and Healthy Aging, CIBERFES, 28029 Madrid, Spain
4. School of Physical Activity and Sport Sciences, Universidad Politécnica de Madrid, 28040 Madrid, Spain; angela.macias.valle@alumnos.upm.es
5. Centro Asistencial San Camilo de Tres Cantos, 28760 Madrid, Spain
6. General Surgery Department, Hospital General Universitario Gregorio Marañón, 28007 Madrid, Spain; luismiguel.jimenez@salud.madrid.org
7. School of Medicine, Universidad Complutense, 28040 Madrid, Spain
* Correspondence: maite.vidan@salud.madrid.org
† These authors contributed equally to this work.
‡ Majuelos González is in collaboration with Fundación La Caixa.

Abstract: Six out of every 10 new colorectal cancer (CRC) diagnoses are in people over 65 years of age. Current standardized surgical approaches have proved to be tolerable on the elderly population, although post-operative complications are more frequent than in the younger CRC population. Frailty is common in elderly CRC patients with surgical indication, and it appears to be also associated with an increase of post-operative complications. Fast-track pathways have been developed to assure and adequate post-operative recovery, but comprehensive geriatric assessments (CGA) are still rare among the preoperative evaluation of elderly CRC patients. This review provides a thorough study of the effects that a CGA assessment and a geriatric intervention have in the prognosis of CRC elderly patients with surgical indication.

Keywords: colorectal cancer; elderly; frailty; geriatric syndromes; comprehensive geriatric assessment; geriatric liaison; multicomponent programs; functional capacity

Highlights

(1) Individualizing interventions in the colorectal cancer elderly population undergoing elective surgery could boost the benefits of fast-track pathways (as ERAS program), which may be gained by CGA-guided care and a geriatric liaison or co-management.

(2) CGA should be the first step towards a multidisciplinary network which would give the patient access to a personalized pre-habilitation and rehabilitation program.

1. Background

1.1. Epidemiology

Colorectal cancer (CRC) is the third most common cancer in the world. In 2019, the worldwide number of new CRC cases was 1,931,590, which accounts for 10% of new cancer diagnosis. The median age of CRC diagnosis is 67 years, with 56% of the cases newly diagnosed corresponding to patients ≥65 years, and 31% to patients ≥75 years [1]. The median age at death is 72 years, and 45% of the deaths occur in patients ≥75 years old, with 21% of them in the oldest (≥85 years) [1]. The incidence of CRC has increased in countries with a medium-high human development index (HDI), whilst it has stabilized—or even declined—in some of the highest HDI, such as the United States [2] or certain European countries, possibly linked to the effect of screening CRC programs [3], changes in lifestyle and dietary habits [4,5]. Although more than 90% of colorectal carcinomas are adenocarcinomas, other rare types include neuroendocrine, squamous cell, adenosquamous, spindle cell and undifferentiated carcinomas [6].

1.2. Risk Factors

Main risk factors for the development of CRC are positive family history [7], male sex and advanced age, although lifestyle-related factors such as smoking, processed/red meat and alcohol intake, low-fruit and vegetable diets and increased bodyweight are also of importance [5,8].

1.3. Screening for Colorectal Cancer

The lack of specificity in CRC symptoms makes screening highly relevant, and many tests have been developed over the years (e.g., stool test, colonoscopy). It is generally recommended to give patients the opportunity to choose the test of their preference, as that may increase adherence to the screening program [9]. It appears that the early detection by screening may have contributed to the reduction of mortality by decreasing incidence (removing precancerous polyps) and increasing survival (detecting the disease at an early stage) [8,10]. Since the early 2000s a decrease in the elective and emergency admission rates for CRC resection (8% and 6%, respectively) has been observed in the U.S. aging population (≥65 years) [11].

Screening is carried out mainly in patients between 60 and 70 years of age [12], although it is recommended for subjects of 50 years and older [13]. A large proportion of patients 80 years and older still require urgent admissions, which could be related to the possible lack of screening in elderly patients. Moreno et al. described how only 4% of CRC diagnosis in elderly patients (>75 years) of a medical institution in the U.S. were determined through screening colonoscopy, whereas in younger patients (range: 50–75 years) this percentage rose to 14% [14]. Both the U.S. Preventive Services Task Force and the American Cancer Society recommend CRC screening until the age of 75 years (when life expectancy is greater than 10 years) and individualization in patients between 76 to 85 years, as in this age group screening benefits decrease while the risk of suffering associated complications increases [9,15]. The U.S. Multi-Society Task Force of Colorectal Cancer suggests continuing screening up to 85 years only if no previous screening has been done, and stopping it at 75 years if prior screening tests have been negative [16]. Interestingly, Van Hees et al. carried out a microsimulation modeling study to try to determine at what age CRC screening should still be considered and they concluded that in unscreened elderly without comorbidity colonoscopy screening was cost-effective up to age 85 years, decreasing to 82 and 79 years in the case of elderly patients with moderate to severe comorbidities, respectively [17].

1.4. Colorectal Cancer Management

Endoscopic management is achievable in early malignant lesions, but surgery remains the main foundation of CRC treatment. According to the U.S. Healthcare Cost and Utilization Project Nationwide Inpatient Sample, comprised by 1,043,108 patients over 45 years of age that had undergone CRC resection, most of them (64%) were 65 years or older, including 29% septuagenarians and 23% octogenarians and nonagenarians [11]. Even though a mean decrease in mortality after CRC surgery was described in the early 2000s (being this improvement most notable in patients 85 years and older) [11], and that long-term survival is achieved in the surgical CRC elderly population [10], it has been stated in the literature that differences of CRC management exist between age groups. Elderly patients are less likely to undergo CRC surgery in comparison to younger individuals [18]. Simmonds et al. showed how, in a population of 34,194 patients with CRC from various studies, 21% of those aged over 85 years did not undergo operation, while the rates of no surgical intervention were 11% in the 75–84 years age group, 6% in the 65–74 group and 4% in those aged 64 years or younger. Additionally, 33% of the surgeries performed in patients over 85 years had a palliative intent [19].

Also, elderly patients with a more advanced tumor stage were less often offered adjuvant therapy [18]. These differences have been sustained by other groups. Sell et al. recently described, in a retrospective analysis of patients with colon adenocarcinoma who underwent surgical resection in an American hospital, how younger patients (aged 79 years or less) were more likely to receive adjuvant chemotherapy when compared to octogenarians, with rates of 48% vs. 9%, respectively. Although they found phenotypic tumor differences between groups (octogenarians presented with larger tumors but less extra-colonic spread) the difference in adjuvant therapy remained when analyzing patients of all stages and when excluding those with American Joint Committee on Cancer Stage IV disease. Interestingly, they also described how in younger patients the use of chemotherapy increased with tumor size, while in the elderly it decreased [20]. Serra–Rexach et al. conducted a retrospective cohort study in a Spanish university hospital in which it was found that age was the main reason for different therapeutic approaches in elderly ($\geq$75 years) and younger (<75 years) CRC patients. Although no differences were observed between groups in tumor degree of differentiation, extension or stage at diagnosis, those individuals aged over 75 years were less likely to receive surgery, radiotherapy, and chemotherapy [21]. Older population is frequently underrepresented in randomized clinical trials (RCTs) [22] and, consequently, it is difficult to reach evidence-based clinical recommendations that apply to the treatment of the elderly CRC population [23].

Laparoscopic surgery (LS) has gained importance over the years due to its short-term beneficial results compared to open colectomy (e.g., decreased post-operative morbidity, faster recovery of bowel function, reduction on length hospital of stay (LOS)) with a low rate of conversion to open surgery (OS) [24–26]. It has proven to be an effective and safe procedure for treating elderly CRC patients [27]. A matched case-control study by Hinoi et al. which only included elderly patients with a diagnosis of colon or rectum adenocarcinoma (median age: 83 years) pointed out how the outcomes of LS in this population are not inferior to those of OS [28]. Regarding the surgical act, they showed how the LS approach—for both colon and rectal cancer—was longer in duration, but had lower blood loss. In the post-operative period, patients who had undergone LS for colon cancer had a faster return of bowel function, a shorter hospital stay and were able to initiate fluid and solid diet in less time than OS patients. Those who had undergone rectum LS also had a faster return of bowel function and initiated fluid diet in less time than OS patients, but no differences were found regarding time to solid intake and hospital stay. Post-operative morbidity rates in colon cancer cases were 36% in the OS group and 25% in the LS group, at the expense of a reduction in the occurrence of delirium, organ/space surgical site infection and pneumonia. Although the post-operative morbidity rates in rectum patients were also lower (40% vs. 47%), the difference was not statistically significant [28]. Kannan et al. also observed how post-operative complications on elderly patients who had undergone laparoscopic partial colectomy were significantly fewer than in those that had undergone open partial colectomy, including every subcategory (cardiac, pulmonary, renal, and infectious). Additionally, the LS group had lower rates of unplanned return to the operating room, their LOS was shorter and 30-day mortality was also significantly lower [29].

Adjuvant therapy can be considered in high-risk Stage II patients (e.g., poorly differentiated tumor, vascular or perineural invasion, lymph nodes sampling <12, tumor presentation with obstruction or perforation) and is recommended in Stage III patients, as it improves survival [5,10]. As rectal cancer surgery is more complex, its approach tends to be different, and neoadjuvant radiotherapy is common [5].

2. Characteristics of Elderly Colorectal Cancer Population That Undergo Surgery

2.1. General Colorectal Cancer Characteristics

2.1.1. Disease Presentation

Patients over 75 years old are more likely to present with later-stage disease and to undergo emergency surgery [19]. Bircan et al. retrospectively analyzed the characteristics of 265 patients that had undergone a programmed colorectal surgery at two Turkish institutions and found that the most common causes of admission differed between age groups: blood stool for patients aged 60–69 years, bowel obstruction for those aged between 70–79 years and anemia for the oldest (>80 years) [30]. Although these last findings could be due to the inclusion of non-malignant colon surgeries in the study, differences like these can also be attributed as stated by the Colorectal Cancer Collaborative Group [19] to age-related variances in recognizing symptoms or seeking medical advice, as well as to primary-care referral patterns.

2.1.2. Complications and Post-Surgical Survival

Although intraoperative complications do not seem to be more frequent among elderly CRC patients [30–32], no clear consensus exists regarding surgical post-operative complications. Some authors have described that elderly patients suffer more ileus, peritonitis/septic shock, pelvic abscess, incisional/post-herniation and have significant longer time to first flatus, bowel motion or to resume normal diet compared to younger patients [31]. Others have not reported differences regarding post-operative surgical complications between age groups [30]. These last findings were also found in a prospective multicenter study conducted by the Colon/Rectum Cancer Working Group that included 19,080 surgical CRC patients: the rate of surgical post-operative complications was not higher in the elderly group (≥80 years) compared to the younger one [32].

Regarding systemic post-operative complications, all studies agree on how they tend to be more frequent in the elderly when compared to younger CRC patients. This type of complications includes respiratory [11,31,32], cardiovascular [11,31,32], renal [31,32], and infectious [11,31,32], among others. There is also certain consensus on how elderly CRC patients have longer LOS which may be attributed to, precisely, the higher rates of post-operative complications [11,30–33]. Kunitake et al. described an increase of 90-day post-discharge readmission rates in the elderly of a large CRC population (83,897 with colon cancer, 26,794 with rectal cancer). These readmissions were mainly justified by non-surgical complications and associated with higher comorbidity and male gender [33].

Although mortality after CRC surgery in the elderly has decreased in the past few years [11], age is an independent predictor of post-operative mortality following CRC resection [34,35]. Excess mortality is sustained throughout the whole year after CRC surgery, and most patients seem to die after the 30-day post-operative period, especially those aged 75 years or more [36]. Interestingly, older CRC patients who survive the first year after surgery may have the same overall cancer-related survival as younger patients [37].

2.2. Geriatric Syndromes

Geriatric syndromes (GS), such as cognitive impairment, functional dependency, falls or urinary incontinence, are clinical conditions more commonly detected on elderly patients. Its cause is believed to be multifactorial, and their presentation is the result of the accumulation of impairments in different systems and the inability of the individual to compensate for them. In the elderly population, GS are associated with higher risk of hospitalization and mortality. Both cancer and oncologic treatments can behave as potential stressors that may overwhelm the patient's reserve capacity and, consequently, favor the development of GS. Therefore, the assessment of GS in the elderly cancer population is of interest when designing care plans or interventions [38].

2.2.1. Functional Dependency

Functional dependency, understood as a person's inability to live independently and perform basic activities of daily living, has proved to be a predictor of morbidity and mortality in the elderly population [39]. It has also been independently associated with shorter survival time in cancer patients [40].

In a systematic review by Hamaker et al. that gathered 23 studies which assessed long-term physical and role functioning changes in CRC patients after treatment, it was discovered that both physical and role functioning were significantly limited at three months after treatment [41]. Ronning et al. in an observational prospective cohort that evaluated predictors of postoperative complications in older patients with CRC, found a significant decline in both basic activities of daily living (ADLs) and instrumental activities of daily living (IADLs) in the 16–28 months that followed surgery, measuring ADLs and IADLs with Barthel Index and the Nottingham Extended Activities of Daily Living Scale, respectively [42].

2.2.2. Frailty

Frailty is a dynamic clinical state characterized by an increased vulnerability to stressors that leads to a loss of homeostasis and a subsequent increase in the risk of developing adverse outcomes (such as disability, falls, delirium or death) [43,44]. Traditionally, it has been defined by two different models: the phenotype model [45] and the deficit accumulation model [46], both of which have showed overlap in their identification of frailty and statistical convergence [43]. The prevalence of frailty among community-dwelling older adults is variable, between 11% in subjects over 65 years of age (ascending to 16% in those aged 80–84 years and 26% in those aged ≥85 years) [47]. Regarding cancer patients, in a sample of 2349 Medicare beneficiaries with 65 years or more and a history of cancer the prevalence of frailty ranged from 46% to 80% [48]. It has been described in the literature how cancer patients and those who are undergoing surgery are more likely to be frail and have more adverse outcomes than those who are not frail [49]. As a result of this, oncologic scientific societies like the International Society of Geriatric Oncology (SIOG) recommend the screening of frailty in older cancer patients [50]. However, there is no standard evaluation and several tools to identify frail cancer patients have been developed, such as the Balducci criteria [51], the Vulnerable Elders Survey-13 [52] and the G8 Geriatric Screening Tool [53], among others. Many of these tools consider comorbidities, cognition, nutritional status, functionality, and physical performance as components of frailty, and others like the Fried criteria [45] only focus on a physical phenotype. Consequently, the prevalence of frailty in older individuals with CRC and surgical indication ranges between 25% and 46%, a variability that depends on both the population studied and the tools used to measure it [54]. It has been proposed that, regarding CRC treatment in the elderly, standard approaches may be offered to robust CRC patients while a need for an individualized therapeutic plan must be considered on frail CRC patients [55].

Using frailty as a risk-stratification tool in surgical elderly patients is a relatively new concept that could change their pre-operative assessment paradigm, as a growing body of scientific evidence has emerged over the past few years. Robinson et al., in a prospective cohort study that included patients ≥65 years undergoing elective colorectal or cardiac surgeries, described how those classified as frail had a higher risk of developing post-operative complications. The definition of frailty they used was based in a deficit accumulation model in which frailty was detected when at least 4 of 7 frailty-related characteristics (regarding function, cognition, chronic disease burden, walking speed, nutrition and geriatric syndromes) were met [56]. Independently of the way frailty is assessed, studies in CRC are concordant in the association of frailty and an increased risk of postoperative complications and mortality. Table 1 shows a detailed description of the main studies that have assessed the influence of frailty (defined by different criteria, such as the Groningen Frailty Indicator (GFI), the Fried Criteria and a modified version of the Balducci criteria) on post-operative outcomes in CRC patients, with similar results.

2.2.3. Cognitive Impairment and Mental Health

The prevalence of dementia in patients with CRC is not clear. Gupta et al. in a population-level cohort study that included 17,507 patients of 67 years or more of the SEER-Medicare file diagnosed with colon cancer, found that the prevalence of dementia in newly-diagnosed patients was 7%. Also, they described how dementia patients were not only twice as likely to be diagnosed with non-invasive methods (without biopsy) but also twice as likely to have their cancer diagnosed after death [57].

The most frequently described psychological alterations in oncologic patients are reactive conditions, mainly adjustment disorder, followed by depressed mood and anxiety [58]. It has been described how depression prevalence in cancer patients can range from 0% to 58%, with this variability attributed to factors such as tumor type, stage of the disease, assessment instruments or diagnostic criteria employed [59]. Few data regarding mental illness in CRC patients have been published, but both depression and anxiety are common in this population, with published prevalence rates that range between 2–57% and 1–47%, respectively [60]. In a recent cohort study, Lloyd et al. described an increase in any mental illness (including depression, anxiety, and adjustment disorders, among others) in CRC survivors since diagnosis. They also found that risk factors for mental illness among CRC survivors include colostomy, female gender (for depression), radiation therapy, chemotherapy, older age, advanced disease, and comorbid conditions. CRC survivors who developed mental illness had increased mortality [61]. Regarding age, some studies have observed higher rates of depression in elderly CRC patients, but no difference on anxiety levels [62,63].

2.2.4. Malnutrition and Social Support

Malnutrition prevalence in cancer population ranges from 20–70%, with differences attributed to patient's age, cancer type and stage [64,65]. In the elderly cancer subpopulation, malnutrition has been described as a risk factor for mortality, functional decline and, among others, poor treatment response [66]. In a prospective multi-center study whose primary objective was to evaluate the impact of a geriatric screening and assessment in elderly patients with cancer (n = 1967, median age 76 years, 22% with CRC) it was found that, according to the Mini Nutritional Assessment, 68% of the patients were at risk of malnutrition and 15% had malnutrition. It was also found how, following the assessment, the most frequently planned geriatric intervention was related to nutrition (57%) [67].

Haviland et al. in a multicenter prospective cohort study that included 857 adult patients with CRC, found how—in a 2-year follow-up after surgery—levels of social support decreased over time and how health-related quality of life outcomes were associated with levels of social support. Also, their findings suggest that those patients with lower and declining social support were more likely to be older [68].

Table 1. Summary of studies in which the influence of frailty on post-operative outcomes in colorectal cancer populations was assessed.

Author, yr.	Sample (n)	Age (yr.)	Setting	Frailty Measure	Frailty Prevalence	Outcomes & Results
Kristjansson el al. (2010) [69]	178	Mean: 80 SD: 6 Range: 70–94	Hospitalization Elective surgery	CGA (Frail: ≥1 domain affected) − Barthel < 19 − NEADL: NR − CIRS: any grade 4/>2 comorbidity grade 3 − MNA < 17 − MMSE < 24 − Polypharmacy > 7 − GDS > 13	F: 76 (43%) NF: 102 (57%)	30-Day Postoperative Complications Any complication (Clav. I–IV) RR 1.59, 95% CI (1.25–2.01) F: 58 (76%), NF: 59 (48%) Severe Complications (Clav. ≥II) RR 1.75, 95% CI (1.28, 2.41) F: 47 (62%), NF: 36 (35%)
Ommundsen et al. (2014) [70]	178	Age Groups: 70–79 (50%) 80–89 (44%) ≥90 (6%)	Hospitalization Elective surgery	CGA (Frail: ≥1 domain affected) − Barthel < 19 − NEADL: NR − CIRS: any grade 4/>2 co-morbidity grade 3 − MNA < 17 − MMSE < 24 − Polypharmacy > 7 − GDS > 13	F: 76 (43%) NF: 102 (57%)	5-Year Survival F: 18 (24%), NF: 67 (66%) $p < 0.001$
Reisinger et al. (2015) [71]	153 *	>70	Hospitalization Elective surgery	GFI (Frail: ≥5/15) − Mobility − Cognition − Nutrition − Vision − Hearing − Co-morbidity − Physical fitness − Psychosocial	F: 39 (26%) NF: 114 (75%)	Postoperative Sepsis OR 3.96, 95% CI (1.14–13.83) F: 6 (15.4%), NF: 5 (4.4%) $p = 0.03$
Tan et al. (2012) [72]	83	Mean: 81 Range: 75–93	Hospitalization Elective surgery	Fried Criteria (Frail: ≥3/5) − Weigth loss (≥10 lb, >5%) − Physical exhaustion − Physical activity level − Grip strenght − Walking speed	F: 23 (28%) NF: 60 (72%)	Major Postoperative Complications (Clav. ≥ II) OR 4.083, 95% CI (1.433–11.638) F: 11 (47.8%), NF: 11 (18.3%) $p = 0.006$

* Reporting a subgroup of patients that had >70 years, a GFI performed preoperatively and outcomes in the post-operative period. Abbreviations: F: Frail; NF: Not Frail; CGA: Comprehensive Geriatric Assessment; GFI: Groningen Frailty Indicator; Clav.: Clavien-Dindo; OR: Odds Ratio; RR: Relative Risk; CI: Confidence Interval.

3. Multidisciplinary Team and Comprehensive Interventions in Colorectal Cancer Patients

To assure an adequate recovery after major abdominal surgery, fast-track pathways such as the Enhanced Recovery After Surgery (ERAS) program have been developed. Among other elements, ERAS programs include preoperative counselling, preferred laparoscopic approach, avoidance of nasogastric tubes or drains when not necessary, enforcement of postoperative early mobilization or feeding and detailed postoperative nursing-care programs [73,74]. It has been described how the implementation of at least four ERAS elements in the colorectal surgery pathway reduces LOS and the rate of post-operative complications without increasing readmission or mortality risk [75]. Its feasibility and benefits in elderly patients who undergo CRC surgery have already been described as well [76]. However, fast-track surgery programs do not discriminate between frail or robust elderly patients, which is of importance considering the higher rates of complications in the former collective.

3.1. Benefits of a Geriatrics Liaison

The Comprehensive Geriatric Assessment (CGA) has been defined as a "multidimensional interdisciplinary diagnostic process intended to determine a frail elderly's person's medical, psychosocial and functional capabilities and limitations in order to develop an overall plan for treatment and long-term follow-up" [77]. It encompasses many domains of an elderly's life to ensure the detection of a wide variety of problems (such as cognitive disorders, depression, social isolation, frailty, comorbidities, undernutrition, polypharmacy, and other geriatric syndromes) so that they can be properly managed to ensure the patient's well-being and independence.

To address the heterogeneity of elderly patients with cancer and guide oncologic treatment decisions, scientific societies such as the SIOG have recommended improving scientific research regarding CGA and cancer patients [78]. Although it has been described how CGA can contribute to the detection of problems and risks often unrecognized in regular oncologic assessments, or how CGA components have predictive risk of complications and toxicity related to treatment, a lack of standardized assessment tools and the heterogeneity regarding CGA models in geriatric oncology difficult its implementation [78]. Nevertheless, in the most recent American Society of Clinical Oncology Guideline for Geriatric Oncology, a CGA is recommended to all patients 65 years of age or older that are receiving chemotherapy [48], and many randomized controlled trials have shown that CGA-guided interventions improve key outcomes for older patients with cancer [79]. Unfortunately, its use in daily practice is complex and time-consuming.

There are studies which show how a geriatric co-management (including both preoperative and postoperative care) in older patients undergoing cancer-related surgery is associated with a reduction of LOS [80] and a lower 90-day postoperative mortality [81]. As a result of this, individualizing interventions in the CRC elderly population undergoing elective surgery could boost the benefits of ERAS programs, which may be gained by CGA-guided care and a geriatric liaison or co-management. Interestingly, few surgeons appear to collaborate on a regular basis with geriatricians [82].

CGA-guided assessments in CRC patients can function as a risk assessment or as a tool to design individualized patient-centered interventions. Many studies have been described with conflicting results. Lee et al. carried out a retrospective review of a prospective single-center database to assess whether a preoperative CGA in 240 elderly patients (aged 70 years or more) who had undergone elective CRC surgery was effective in predicting postoperative morbidity. This CGA included several domains (comorbidity, polypharmacy, physical function, cognitive, depression and nutrition), and a "high-risk" patient was defined as one who had deficits in at least two of those domains. A total of 95 high-risk patients (40%) were detected, and this condition was significantly and independently associated with postoperative complications. As well, they found how greater independence in ADLs and fewer comorbidities were predictive of a less eventful—and therefore better—recovery [83].

Shipway et al. evaluated the efficacy of an embedded geriatric liaison service for emergency and elective gastrointestinal surgery using a retrospective control and a preoperative, in-hospital and post-operative CGA and intervention. The primary aim of the study was the reduction in LOS. They included 682 patients (203 pre-intervention, 479 post-intervention). A total of 132 patients in the intervention group were referred to the preoperative CGA-based assessment (from which 60% had CRC) and 26% of them were considered unfit and did not proceed with surgery. Two hundred and thirty-three inpatient reviews were conducted, being some of the most frequent indications discharge planning, communication with family, high dependency unit interventions, fluid balance, cardiac assessment, and delirium. The implementation of this geriatric liaison service supposed a mean LOS reduction of 3 days considering all surgeries, and this reduction was maintained in patients aged 75 years or more. However, when considering patients admitted electively for cancer surgery, LOS reductions were not statistically significant, although a trend of greater reduction was observed with advancing age [84]. Ramirez et al. carried out a before–after study with the objective of assessing the effect that a geriatric co-management program had on the LOS of elderly patients admitted to a general surgery ward. The results of the study show how in both intervention subgroups (the emergency-admitted and the electively-admitted), LOS was lower when compared to the control, with the CRC group presenting a mean decrease of 9 days [85].

In-hospital geriatric co-management interventions have also been described. In a single-center retrospective cohort study that included 310 patients aged 70 years or older who were admitted for elective CRC surgery in a tertiary level hospital, it was found how a daily CGA-based hospital assistance was associated with a lower incidence of delirium and other geriatric syndromes (such as falls, pain, urinary incontinence, constipation, pressure ulcers, malnutrition, and immobility), as well as fewer blood transfusions. Nevertheless, they also found that the intervention group had higher rates of long hospitalizations, intensive care unit admissions, serious complications, and hospitalization within the year [86].

However, although these kinds of CGA interventions seem promising, there are studies that have not shown clear benefits. Indrakusuma et al. carried out a retrospective matched-controlled study with the main objective of assessing beneficial postoperative outcomes of a preoperative CGA in 443 elderly patients (aged 70 years or more) who underwent CRC surgery in two time periods. The most frequent preoperative interventions derived from the preoperative CGA assessment were detection of delirium risk (64%), vitamin supplementation (64%) and dietary supplementation (20%). Contrary to benefits showed in the previously mentioned studies, in this study no differences regarding mortality, postoperative delirium or LOS were found when the intervention group was compared to the control group [87]. Similarly, an RCT of frail older patients that were to undergo CRC surgery, failed to detect benefits of a preoperative and tailored geriatric intervention focused on nutritional advice (34%), increased medication (30%), other healthcare professional referral (30%) and exercise (23%). No differences between groups were found regarding the rate of postoperative severe complications, reoperations, readmission, or mortality. However, they found that the intervention group experienced fewer medical non severe complications [70]. A detailed description of all these findings has been summarized in Table 2.

Table 2. Summary of studies assessing the benefits of a geriatric liaison on the approach of colorectal cancer patients undergoing surgery.

Author, yr.	Sample (n; Groups)	Age (yr.) †	Design	Type of Program & Setting	Assessments & Interventions	Benefits ‡
Shipway et al., 2018 [84]	682 CG: 203 IG: 479	>60 CG: 73 (60–100) IG: 73 (60–94)	Single-center before-after study	Embedded Geriatric Liaison Hospitalization Elective & Emergency GI surgery	- Preoperative CGA - Comorbidity - Medication - Nutrition Status - Exercise Tolerance - Cognitive Function - Frailty - Depression Assessment - Functional Capacity - Social Circumstances - Screening, Investigations - Postoperative Follow-Up - Ward Rounds (selected patients) - Discharge Plan - Geriatrician-led rehabilitation ward (selected patients)	LOS (All Surgeries) All Patients Mean Reduction: 3.1 days 95% CI (0.7–5.5), $p = 0.007$ Patients ≥ 75 years Mean Reduction: 3 days 95% CI (0.2–5.8), $p = 0.045$ LOS (Elective Surgery) All Patients Mean Reduction: 1.3 days 95% CI (−1.4–4.03) Patients ≥ 75 years Mean Reduction: 5.2 days 95% CI (−1.7–12.1), $p = 0.099$
Tarazona-Santabalbina et al., 2019 [86]	310 CG: 107 IG: 203	≥ 70 CG: 75 ± 5 IG: 76 ± 5	Single-center retrospective cohort study	In-Hospital Program Elective CRC Surgery	8-Hour Ward Assessment/intervention - Pressure Ulcers - Pain - Urinary Continence - Constipation - Delirium Daily Ward Assessment - Endovenous Catheters - Medication - Infections - Thromboembolic Events - Anemia - Early Ambulation - Fall Risk - Hydration & Nutrition - Sleep Hygiene - Sensory Impairment	Delirium reduction CG: 31 (29.2), IG: 23 (11.3) $p < 0.001$ Geriatric Syndromes diagnosis * CG: 28 (26.2), IG: 21 (10.3) $p < 0.001$ Blood transfusions reduction CG: 24 (22.4); IG: 18 (8.9) $p = 0.001$

Table 2. Cont.

Author, yr.	Sample (n; Groups)	Age (yr.) †	Design	Type of Program & Setting	Assessments & Interventions	Benefits ‡
Ramirez-Martín et al., 2020 [85]	175 CG: 122 IG: 53	≥80	Single-center before-after cohort study	Emergency Surgery Inpatients - In-Hospital Collaborative Management Elective CRC Surgery - Preoperative CGA & Intervention - In-Hospital Collaborative Management	Preoperative CGA - Not Specified In-Hospital Management - Daily Ward Monitoring - Clinical Management Collaboration - Discharge Planning	LOS (days) Emergency Admissions CG: 27.2 (18.1), IG: 16.6 (10.7) $p < 0.01$ Elective Surgery (CRC) CG: 19.1 (13.4), IG: 10.6 (9.3) $p < 0.01$
Indrakusuma et al., 2015 [87]	100 ** CG: 50 IG: 50	≥70 CG: 75 (71–78) IG: 81 (79–85)	Single-center retrospective cohort and match-control study	Preoperative CGA & Intervention Elective CRC surgery	Preoperative CGA & Intervention - Full Medical Study - Social Circumstances - Review of Systems - Functional Capacity - Family History - Full Physical Examination - Laboratory Tests - Cognitive Function - Depression Assessment - Nutritional Status	Mortality No significant differences Postoperative Delirium No significant differences Postoperative Complications No significant differences Length of Stay No significant differences
Ommundsen et al., 2017 [70]	114 CG: 62 IG: 52	>65 CG: 79 ± 8 IG: 78 ± 7	Multi-center randomized controlled trial	Preoperative CGA & Intervention Elective CRC Surgery - Frail Subjects	Preoperative CGA - Activities of Daily Living - Use of Medication - Comorbidity - Nutritional Status - Cognitive Function - Depression Assessment	Mild Postop. Complications Mentioned. No specific data provided Postop. Complications (Clav. I–V) No significant differences Postop. Complications (Clav. II–V) No significant differences 30-Day Mortality No significant differences 3-Month Mortality No significant differences Length of Stay No significant differences

† Age: mean ± SD; median (interquartile ranges); ‡ Benefits: mean ± SD; absolute number (percentage); * 'Geriatric Syndromes & Events' include: falls, pain, urinary incontinence, constipation, pressure ulcers, malnutrition and immobility; ** From this study we only report a subgroup of patients (those in the intervention group that underwent the Geriatric Assessment and their matched controls). Abbreviations: CG: Control Group; IG: Intervention Group; GI: gastrointestinal; CGA: Comprehensive Geriatric Assessment; CRC: Colorectal Cancer; Postop: postoperative; Clav.: Clavien-Dindo.

3.2. Benefits of Exercise Programs

Observational studies have shown how the highest level of physical activity (PA), before and after CRC diagnosis, is associated with a lower risk of CRC mortality [88–90]. Therefore, CRC patients should avoid physical inactivity whenever possible [91]. Although PA is beneficial in several aspects [92,93] its benefits vary depending on factors such as the population included, the study design or the exercise programs themselves [94].

We found eleven RCTs assessing the effect of physical exercise in surgical CRC patients over the age of 60 years (mean age range: 60–81 years), with sample sizes from 42 to 185 patients (Table 3). The RCTs included multimodal programs with prehabilitation (before surgery) [95–98]. prehabilitation and rehabilitation (after surgery) [99–101] or comparing prehabilitation vs rehabilitation [102–105]. Prehabilitation's duration ranged between 2 and 4 weeks and rehabilitation from 4 to 8 weeks. Sessions were usually held one to three days per week for 30–60 min. Programs included exercise training alone [95,97,103], exercise training and psychological interventions with anxiety reduction strategies [98,99,102–105], adding in some of them a nutritional control [95,98,99,101–105]. Exercises included aerobic training [98], aerobic and resistance training [95,97,99–105], or only resistance training [96]. Aerobic training consisted of activities such as walking, treadmill walking or cycling, following the 150 min/week recommendations by the American College of Sport Medicine Guideline [88,91]. Resistance training consisted of exercises of the upper and lower limbs using elastic bands. Some of the RCTs did not report the exercise's intensity, but most of them opted for a moderate one [88,91] using the Borg Scale [97,99,102–104]. Home-based exercise sessions supervised weekly with phone calls were more prevalent [96,98,99,102–105], although some programs were carried out at the hospital or exercise center [97,100,101]. As shown in Table 3, the results were variable. Some of the studies demonstrate an increase in functional capacity [99,104,105], and others a decrease in postoperative complications [95,101] or LOS [100,101]. Only two RCTs studied mortality, but no decrease was found in 30-day [100] or 1-year mortality [101] with the intervention. No differences regarding quality of life were found [97,104].

Table 3. Description of interventions and results of randomized controlled trials in older than 60 years with CRC.

Author, yr.	Sample (n)	Age yr. (mean)	Duration	Features	Programs Analyzed	Principal and Other Outcomes and Results	Adherence
Prehabilitation Programs							
Dronkers et al., 2010 [97]	42	70	2–4 w.	Supervised vs unsupervised home-based exercise program.	Short-term intensive program Group: 2x/w. for 60 min per session. Resistance training, inspiratory muscle training, moderate aerobic training, and training functional activities. Daily 30 min walk and inspiratory muscle training. Home-based exercise group: Daily activation for minimally 30 min with a pedometer. Measurements: baseline and postsurgery.	Postoperative complications: NSD. LOS: NSD. Functional capacity (TUG): NSD; Strength (CRT): NSD; (Hand grip): NSD. Inspiratory muscle endurance (RMA): SD. Physical activity (LASA): NSD. Fatigue (AFQ): NSD. Quality of life (EORTC-QLQ-C30): NSD.	Supervised training: 97%; Unsupervised training: Non-reported.
Carli et al., 2010 [96]	112	60	4 w.	In-hospital supervised exercise program.	Bike/strengthening Group: 7x/w. 20–30 min of moderate intensity aerobic training and 3x/w. for 10–15 min of resistance training. Walk/breathing Group: 7x/w. training for 40–45 min per session. Measurements: baseline, 1-week presurgery, 2- and 4-month postsurgery.	Functional capacity (6MWT): NSD. Anxiety and Depression (HADS): NSD.	16%
Minnella et al., 2020 [98]	42	67	4 w.	Prehabilitation Unit-based supervised exercise program.	High-Intensity Interval Training (HIIT) Group: 3x/w. for 40 min per session. High intensity aerobic training on a bicycle and resistance training. Nutrition: Balanced macronutrient composition and protein. Anxiety: Relaxation techniques and breathing exercises. Moderate Intensity Continuous Training (MICT) group: 3x/w. for 50 min per session. Moderate intensity aerobic training on a bicycle and resistance training. Nutrition: Balanced macronutrient composition and protein. Anxiety: Relaxation techniques and breathing exercises. Measurements: baseline, presurgery, 1- and 2-month postsurgery	30-day complications (Clav.): NSD. LOS: NSD. Functional capacity (6MWT): NSD; (CPET): SD.	HIIT/MICT: Exercise: 89%/93%, Nutrition: 97%/99%, Loss of patients at follow-up: presurgery 19%/5% 1 month postsurgery 33%/38%, and 2 months postsurgery. 38%/48%.
Berkel et al., 2021 [95]	57	74	3 w.	Community-based supervised exercise program.	Intervention group: 3x/w. for 60 min per session. Moderate to high intensity aerobic training on a cycle ergometer and resistance training. Control group (usual care): ERAS protocol. Nutritional counseling and advice on smoking cessation. Measurements: 30-day postsurgery.	30-day postoperative complications (Clav.): SD. LOS: NSD. Readmissions: NSD. Functional capacity: Aerobic fitness (V02): NSD.	Non- reported.
Chia et al., 2015 [100]	117	80	PREHAB: 2w. and REHAB: 2–6 w.	Supervised exercise or unsupervised home-based exercise depending of patient situation.	Intervention group (STF): Cardiovascular strengthening, mobilizing and muscle strengthening. Nutrition: Individual attention. Control group (GSS): quality reviews and a patient-centered culture. Nutrition: Individual attention. Measurements: 30-day mortality and 6-week postsurgery.	Postoperative complications (Clav.): NSD. LOS: SD. 30-day mortality: NSD. Recovery functional capacity (Barthel): NSD.	80%

Table 3. *Cont.*

Author, yr.	Sample (n)	Age yr. (mean)	Duration	Features	Programs Analyzed	Principal and Other Outcomes and Results	Adherence
Prehabilitation Programs							
Awasthi et al., 2018 [99]	140	68	PREHAB: 4 w. and REHAB: 8 w.	Supervised exercise and unsupervised home-based exercise program.	Group 1: unsupervised exercise (Gillis et al. 2014) 3x/w. for 50 min per session: moderate intensity aerobic exercise and moderate intensity resistance training. Nutrition: Nutritional assessment and protein supplementation. Anxiety: Relaxation techniques. Group 2: supervised training (Bousquet-Dion et al., 2018) 1x/w. at hospital exercise laboratory for 65 min per session: moderate aerobic exercise and resistance exercise. 3 to 4x/w. at home for 30 min of moderate intensity aerobic training and resistance training. Nutrition: Nutritional assessment and protein supplementation. Anxiety: Relaxation techniques. Measurements: baseline, before surgery, 4- and 8-week postsurgery.	LOS: NSD Functional capacity (6MWT): SD. Muscle strength (Hand grip): SD. Anxiety and depression (HADS): NSD. Quality of life (SF36): SD.	Supervised exercise: 98%
Prehabilitation Programs							
Souwer et al., 2018 [101]	86	81	PREHAB: 4 w. and REHAB: 4–6 w.	In-hospital supervised exercise and home-based exercise program.	Intervention Group: 2x/w. for 30–45 min per session. PREHAB: Resistance and endurance training, and home exercise and breathing. REHAB: Physical training. Nutrition: Protein supplementation, dietary support. Anxiety: Cognitive and emotional guidance. Control group: usual care (previous cohort). Measurements: 30-day and 1-year postsurgery.	30-day postoperative complications. Only cardiac: SD. LOS: SD. 1-year mortality: NSD.	63%
Gillis et al., 2014 [104]	77	66	PREHAB: 4 w. vs REHAB: 8 w.	Unsupervised home-based exercise program.	PREHAB: 3x/w. for 50 min per session. Moderate intensity aerobic exercise and moderate resistance training. Nutrition: Protein intake. Anxiety: 60 min of relaxation techniques and breathing exercises. REHAB Group: 3x/w. for 50 min per session. Moderate intensity aerobic exercise and moderate resistance training. Nutrition: Protein intake. Anxiety: 60 min of relaxation techniques and breathing exercises. Measurements: baseline, presurgery, 4- and 8-week postsurgery.	30-day complications (Clav.): NSD. Functional capacity (6MWT): NSD. Health status (SF-36): NSD. Anxiety and depression (HADS): NSD.	PREHAB = 78%; 4 w.: 53%; 8w.: 53% REHAB = 4 w.: 31% 8w.: 40%

Table 3. Cont.

Author, yr.	Sample (n)	Age yr. (mean)	Duration	Features	Programs Analyzed	Principal and Other Outcomes and Results	Adherence
Prehabilitation Programs							
Minnella et al., 2017 [105]	185	68	PREHAB: 4 w. vs REHAB: 8 w.	Unsupervised home-based exercise and supervised exercise program.	PREHAB Group: 3x/w. for 20–30 min per session of endurance training and 2x/w. of resistance training. Nutrition: Dietary changes and protein supplementation. Anxiety: Relaxation techniques. Plus ERAS protocol. REHAB Group: 3x/w. for 20–30 min per session of endurance training and 2x/w. of resistance training. Nutrition: Dietary changes and protein supplementation. Anxiety: Relaxation techniques. Plus ERAS protocol. Measurements: baseline, presurgery, 4- and 8-week postsurgery.	Postoperative complications (Clav.): NDS. LOS: NDS. Functional capacity (6MWT): SD. Physical fitness (CHAMPS): SD.	PREHAB = 70–98% REHAB = 4 w.: 53–72% 8 w.: 53–82%
Prehabilitation Programs							
Bousquet-Dion et al., 2018 [102]	80	73	PREHAB: 4 w. vs REHAB: 8 w.	In-hospital supervised and unsupervised home-based exercise program.	PREHAB Group: At hospital: 1x/w. for 65 min per session. Moderate aerobic exercise and resistance exercise. At home: 3 to 4x/w. for 30 min of moderate intensity aerobic training and resistance training. Nutrition: Protein supplementation. Anxiety: 60 min of relaxation techniques and breathing exercises. Plus ERAS protocol. REHAB Group: At hospital: 1x/w. for 65 min per session. Moderate aerobic exercise and resistance exercise. At home: 3 to 4x/w. for 30 min of moderate intensity aerobic training and resistance training. Nutrition: Protein supplementation. Anxiety: 60 min of relaxation techniques and breathing exercises. Plus ERAS protocol. Measurements: baseline, presurgery, 4- and 8-week postsurgery.	LOS: NSD. Functional capacity (6MWT): NSD. Physical activity (CHAMPS): NSD.	Supervised exercise: PREHAB 98% REHAB = 4 w. 70% 8 w.: 75%
Carli et al., 2020 [103]	110	78	PREHAB: 4 w. vs REHAB: 4 w.	Unsupervised home-based multimodal program with 1 session/w. supervised at hospital (similar for PREHAB and REHAB).	PREHAB group: 1x/w. for 60 min per session. Supervised moderate aerobic exercises and resistance exercises at hospital and moderate intensity aerobic activities (walking) and resistance training at home. Anxiety: Relaxation techniques and breathing exercises. Nutrition: Protein intake. REHAB group: 3x/w. for 30 min per session. Supervised moderate aerobic exercises and resistance exercises at hospital and moderate-intensity aerobic activities (walking) and resistance training at home. Anxiety: Relaxation techniques and breathing exercises. Nutrition: Protein intake. Measurements: 4-week postsurgery.	30-day postoperative complications (CCI and Clav.): NSD. LOS: NSD. Functional capacity (6MWT): NSD. Readmissions: NSD.	PREHAB = 68% REHAB = 14%. General exercise and nutrition: PREHAB 80%, REHAB 30%.

Abbreviations: NSD = Non Significant Differences between groups; SD = Significant Differences between groups; LOS = Length of hospital Stay; TUG = Timed Up and Go; CRT = Chair Rise Time; RMA = Respiratory Muscle Analyzer; LASA = Physical Activity Questionnaire; AFQ = Abbreviated Fatigue Questionnaire; EORTC-QLQ C30 = The EORTC Quality of Life questionnaire QLQ-C30; 6MWT = 6-Minute Walking Test; HADS = Hospital Anxiety and Depression Scale; Clav. = Clavien-Dindo; CPET = Cardiopulmonary Exercise testing; VO2 = máx O$_2$ Volume; PREHAB = Prehabilitation; REHAB = Rehabilitation; SF36 = Short Form (36); STF = Trans-institutional transdisciplinary Start to Finish Programm; GGS = Geriatric Surgery Service; Health Survey; CHAMPS = Community Health Activities Model Program for Seniors; ERAS = Enhanced Recovery After Surgery; CCI = Comprehensive Complications Index; yr. = years; w. = weeks; min = minutes.

It is difficult to determine which is the most appropriate type of exercise program for elderly CRC population due to its heterogeneity [106]. The design of these programs must be adapted to the characteristics of the population studied (regarding functional capacity, frailty, comorbidity, etc.), the proposed outcomes (e.g., functional capacity recovery, change in functional state, reduction on complications or mortality, shortened LOS), the type of program (timing, duration, intensity ...) and patient´s preferences.

3.3. Benefits of Psychotherapeutic Interventions

Psychotherapeutic interventions have been described in CRC population, mainly in patients with newly-formed stomas, with generally satisfactory effects. Stoma patients, due to a distorted body image and the loss of an essential body function, face difficulties in everyday life in terms of physical, psychological, and social aspects [107]. One of the most common psychosocial intervention described in this population is preoperative education, which appears to satisfactorily reduce both LOS and days to stoma proficiency [108,109]. Moreover, cognitive therapy and emotional support interventions such a relaxation training has proven to be feasible (even with follow-up telephone calls) and appear to reduce anxiety levels [110]. However, a major limitation is the small sample sizes of the studies [111].

Beneficial effects on quality of life with psychosocial interventions (mainly face-to-face approaches) [112] have been described [113]. Also, interventions focused on enriching communication with CRC patients have also been carried out. Ohlen et al. designed a person-centered information and communication intervention to study its beneficial effects on the patients' preparedness for surgery, discharge, and their subsequent recovery, but no conclusive results were obtained [114].

A favorable trend on the effectiveness of a positive emotion-based psychological therapy and a cognitive-behavioral therapy on the quality of life of CRC patients receiving adjuvant chemotherapy has been suggested, although findings were not conclusive [115].

Ellis et al. in a report of a longitudinal study of psychological adjustment in 326 patients with advanced cancer (43% corresponding to CRC), found how elderly patients (aged 70 years or more) were less frequently referred for specialized psychosocial care in comparison to younger subjects with the same degree of depressive symptoms [116]. Whether this finding is related to the illness being less destabilizing to an older person when compared to a younger counterpart or to a possible ageist bias for which caregivers may assume the benefits of these therapies is greater in younger subjects, remains unknown.

The shortage of evidence regarding the effect of psychotherapeutic interventions in cancer patients is striking considering how receiving a cancer diagnosis is a complex and stressful experience that constitutes a vital crisis that can present itself with very diverse emotional reactions (e.g., sadness, anger, confusion) [117]. Future studies should focus on studying some of the mostly inconclusive findings mentioned above, adhere to standards of quality research, and try to, not only increase the number of individuals per study, but also focus on certain subpopulations, such as the elderly.

4. Conclusions

CRC is a frequent disease among the elderly. Although fast-track circuits such as the ERAS program include the assessment of relevant problems for the elderly CRC patient (e.g., malnutrition), other aspects that could influence therapeutic approaches are normally left out, such as functionality, frailty, cognitive impairment, depression/anxiety or social support. The adequate evaluation of these conditions could lead to its control or improvement, and therefore a change in the patient's prognosis.

CGA has proven to be a useful tool for the identification and assessment of these conditions. It allows the multidisciplinary team (conformed by surgeons, anesthesiologists, nutritionists, pharmacologists, physical therapists, nurses, etc.) to design a thorough care plan that comprises both the oncologic treatment (surgery and/or adjuvant therapy) and the approach of geriatric syndromes through a multicomponent program. A program of these characteristics would be individualized, adjusted to the patient's situation and preferences, and could include nutritional, psychotherapeutic, pharmacologic or exercise interventions, among others. Possible outcomes to be assessed would include not only length of stay, in-hospital mortality, or post-operative complications, but also improvement on the physical, functional, cognitive and mental health situation, quality of life and readmissions in both the medium and long term post-operative period.

The scarcity of randomized controlled trials that evaluate the benefits of preoperative geriatric assessments or the use of multicomponent interventions, methodological variability among studies already published and the use of standard outcomes mostly centered on surgical aspects, could be some of the reasons why the evidence regarding the benefits of these programs remains unclear. In the authors' opinion, CGA should be the first step towards the creation of a multidisciplinary network which would give the patient access to a personalized treatment plan conformed by integral interventions. Although the evaluation of multicomponent programs of these characteristics is difficult, research on this matter seems necessary, as the complexity of elderly patients needs to be confronted not in just one field separately (be it the surgical, clinical, physical, or psychological), but in all of them together.

Author Contributions: Conceptualization: N.M.G.-S., J.M.-C., M.T.V.-A., J.A.S.-R., Search: N.M.G.-S., J.M.-C., M.L.C.A., L.M.J.-G., S.M.G., A.M.-V.; Writing—original draft preparation, N.M.G.-S, J.M.-C., M.L.C.A., S.M.G., P.A.-M., A.M.-V.; writing—review and editing, N.M.G.-S., J.M.-C., L.M.J.-G., J.A.S.-R., M.T.V.-A., supervision, M.T.V.-A., J.A.S.-R.; funding acquisition, J.A.S.-R. All authors have read and agreed to the published version of the manuscript.

Funding: This study was supported by the Biomedical Research Networking Center on Frailty and Healthy Aging (CIBERFES, Spain); and FEDER funds from the European Union. The work of Jennifer Mayordomo-Cava is supported by a contract granted by Biomedical Research Networking Center on Frailty and Healthy Aging (CIBERFES, Spain).

Institutional Review Board Statement: Not applicable.

Informed Consent Statement: Not applicable.

Conflicts of Interest: The authors declare no conflict of interest.

References

1. Howlader, N.; Noone, A.; Krapcho, M.; Garshell, J.; Miller, D.; Altekruse, S.; Kosary, C.; Yu, M.; Ruhl, J.; Tatalovich, Z.; et al. *SEER Cancer Statistics Review, 1975–2018*; National Cancer Institute: Bethesda, MD, USA, 2020. Available online: https://seer.cancer.gov/csr/1975_2017/ (accessed on 30 January 2021).
2. Arnold, M.; Sierra, M.S.; Laversanne, M.; Soerjomataram, I.; Jemal, A.; Bray, F. Global patterns and trends in colorectal cancer incidence and mortality. *Gut* **2017**, *66*, 683–691. [CrossRef] [PubMed]
3. Ouakrim, D.A.; Pizot, C.; Boniol, M.; Malvezzi, M.; Boniol, M.; Negri, E.; Bota, M.; Jenkins, M.A.; Bleiberg, H.; Autier, P.J.B. Trends in colorectal cancer mortality in Europe: Retrospective analysis of the WHO mortality database. *BMJ* **2015**, *351:h4970*. [CrossRef] [PubMed]
4. Bray, F.; Ferlay, J.; Soerjomataram, I.; Siegel, R.L.; Torre, L.A.; Jemal, A. Global cancer statistics 2018: GLOBOCAN estimates of incidence and mortality worldwide for 36 cancers in 185 countries. *CA Cancer J. Clin.* **2018**, *68*, 394–424. [CrossRef] [PubMed]
5. Dekker, E.; Tanis, P.J.; Vleugels, J.L.A.; Kasi, P.M.; Wallace, M.B. Colorectal cancer. *Lancet* **2019**, *394*, 1467–1480. [CrossRef]
6. Bosman, F.T.; Carneiro, F.; Hruban, R.H.; Theise, N.D. *WHO Classification of Tumours of the Digestive System*, 4th ed.; World Health Organization, International Agency for Research on Cancer: Geneva, Switzerland, 2010.
7. Henrikson, N.B.; Webber, E.M.; Goddard, K.A.; Scrol, A.; Piper, M.; Williams, M.S.; Zallen, D.T.; Calonge, N.; Ganiats, T.G.; Janssens, A.C.; et al. Family history and the natural history of colorectal cancer: Systematic review. *Genet. Med. Off. J. Am. Coll. Med Genet.* **2015**, *17*, 702–712. [CrossRef]
8. Siegel, R.L.; Miller, K.D.; Goding Sauer, A.; Fedewa, S.A.; Butterly, L.F.; Anderson, J.C.; Cercek, A.; Smith, R.A.; Jemal, A. Colorectal cancer statistics, 2020. *CA Cancer J. Clin.* **2020**, *70*, 145–164. [CrossRef]
9. Wolf, A.M.D.; Fontham, E.T.H.; Church, T.R.; Flowers, C.R.; Guerra, C.E.; LaMonte, S.J.; Etzioni, R.; McKenna, M.T.; Oeffinger, K.C.; Shih, Y.T.; et al. Colorectal cancer screening for average-risk adults: 2018 guideline update from the American Cancer Society. *CA Cancer J. Clin.* **2018**, *68*, 250–281. [CrossRef]
10. Labianca, R.; Nordlinger, B.; Beretta, G.D.; Mosconi, S.; Mandala, M.; Cervantes, A.; Arnold, D.; Group, E.G.W. Early colon cancer: ESMO Clinical Practice Guidelines for diagnosis, treatment and follow-up. *Ann. Oncol.* **2013**, *24* (Suppl. 6), vi64–vi72. [CrossRef]

11. Jafari, M.D.; Jafari, F.; Halabi, W.J.; Nguyen, V.Q.; Pigazzi, A.; Carmichael, J.C.; Mills, S.D.; Stamos, M.J. Colorectal Cancer Resections in the Aging US Population: A Trend Toward Decreasing Rates and Improved Outcomes. *JAMA Surg.* **2014**, *149*, 557–564. [CrossRef]
12. Papamichael, D.; Audisio, R.A.; Glimelius, B.; de Gramont, A.; Glynne-Jones, R.; Haller, D.; Kohne, C.H.; Rostoft, S.; Lemmens, V.; Mitry, E.; et al. Treatment of colorectal cancer in older patients: International Society of Geriatric Oncology (SIOG) consensus recommendations 2013. *Ann. Oncol.* **2013**, *26*, 463–476. [CrossRef]
13. Simon, K. Colorectal cancer development and advances in screening. *Clin. Interv. Aging* **2016**, *11*, 967–976. [CrossRef]
14. Moreno, C.C.; Mittal, P.K.; Sullivan, P.S.; Rutherford, R.; Staley, C.A.; Cardona, K.; Hawk, N.N.; Dixon, W.T.; Kitajima, H.D.; Kang, J.; et al. Colorectal Cancer Initial Diagnosis: Screening Colonoscopy, Diagnostic Colonoscopy, or Emergent Surgery, and Tumor Stage and Size at Initial Presentation. *Clin. Colorectal Cancer* **2016**, *15*, 67–73. [CrossRef]
15. Force, U.P.S.T. Screening for Colorectal Cancer: US Preventive Services Task Force Recommendation Statement. *JAMA* **2016**, *315*, 2564–2575. [CrossRef]
16. Rex, D.K.; Boland, C.R.; Dominitz, J.A.; Giardiello, F.M.; Johnson, D.A.; Kaltenbach, T.; Levin, T.R.; Lieberman, D.; Robertson, D.J. Colorectal Cancer Screening: Recommendations for Physicians and Patients from the U.S. Multi-Society Task Force on Colorectal Cancer. *Am. J. Gastroenterol.* **2017**, *112*, 1016–1030. [CrossRef]
17. van Hees, F.; Habbema, J.D.; Meester, R.G.; Lansdorp-Vogelaar, I.; van Ballegooijen, M.; Zauber, A.G. Should colorectal cancer screening be considered in elderly persons without previous screening? A cost-effectiveness analysis. *Ann. Intern. Med.* **2014**, *160*, 750–759. [CrossRef]
18. van Leeuwen, B.L.; Pahlman, L.; Gunnarsson, U.; Sjovall, A.; Martling, A. The effect of age and gender on outcome after treatment for colon carcinoma. A population-based study in the Uppsala and Stockholm region. *Crit. Rev. Oncol. Hematol.* **2008**, *67*, 229–236. [CrossRef] [PubMed]
19. Colorectal Cancer Collaborative Group. Surgery for colorectal cancer in elderly patients: A systematic review. *Lancet* **2000**, *356*, 968–974. [CrossRef]
20. Sell, N.M.; Qwaider, Y.Z.; Goldstone, R.N.; Stafford, C.E.; Cauley, C.E.; Francone, T.D.; Ricciardi, R.; Bordeianou, L.G.; Berger, D.L.; Kunitake, H. Octogenarians present with a less aggressive phenotype of colon adenocarcinoma. *Surgery* **2020**, *168*, 1138–1143. [CrossRef]
21. Serra-Rexach, J.A.; Jimenez, A.B.; Garcia-Alhambra, M.A.; Pla, R.; Vidan, M.; Rodriguez, P.; Ortiz, J.; Garcia-Alfonso, P.; Martin, M. Differences in the therapeutic approach to colorectal cancer in young and elderly patients. *Oncologist* **2012**, *17*, 1277–1285. [CrossRef]
22. Townsley, C.A.; Selby, R.; Siu, L.L. Systematic review of barriers to the recruitment of older patients with cancer onto clinical trials. *J. Clin. Oncol. Off. J. Am. Soc. Clin. Oncol.* **2005**, *23*, 3112–3124. [CrossRef]
23. Pallis, A.G.; Papamichael, D.; Audisio, R.; Peeters, M.; Folprecht, G.; Lacombe, D.; Van Cutsem, E. EORTC Elderly Task Force experts' opinion for the treatment of colon cancer in older patients. *Cancer Treat. Rev.* **2010**, *36*, 83–90. [CrossRef] [PubMed]
24. Abraham, N.S.; Young, J.M.; Solomon, M.J. Meta-analysis of short-term outcomes after laparoscopic resection for colorectal cancer. *Br. J. Surg.* **2004**, *91*, 1111–1124. [CrossRef] [PubMed]
25. Braga, M.; Vignali, A.; Gianotti, L.; Zuliani, W.; Radaelli, G.; Gruarin, P.; Dellabona, P.; Di Carlo, V. Laparoscopic versus open colorectal surgery: A randomized trial on short-term outcome. *Ann. Surg.* **2002**, *236*, 759–766. [CrossRef]
26. Lacy, A.M.; Garcia-Valdecasas, J.C.; Delgado, S.; Castells, A.; Taura, P.; Pique, J.M.; Visa, J. Laparoscopy-assisted colectomy versus open colectomy for treatment of non-metastatic colon cancer: A randomised trial. *Lancet* **2002**, *359*, 2224–2229. [CrossRef]
27. Fujii, S.; Tsukamoto, M.; Fukushima, Y.; Shimada, R.; Okamoto, K.; Tsuchiya, T.; Nozawa, K.; Matsuda, K.; Hashiguchi, Y. Systematic review of laparoscopic vs open surgery for colorectal cancer in elderly patients. *World J. Gastrointest. Oncol.* **2016**, *8*, 573–582. [CrossRef]
28. Hinoi, T.; Kawaguchi, Y.; Hattori, M.; Okajima, M.; Ohdan, H.; Yamamoto, S.; Hasegawa, H.; Horie, H.; Murata, K.; Yamaguchi, S.; et al. Laparoscopic versus open surgery for colorectal cancer in elderly patients: A multicenter matched case-control study. *Ann. Surg. Oncol.* **2015**, *22*, 2040–2050. [CrossRef]
29. Kannan, U.; Reddy, V.S.; Mukerji, A.N.; Parithivel, V.S.; Shah, A.K.; Gilchrist, B.F.; Farkas, D.T. Laparoscopic vs open partial colectomy in elderly patients: Insights from the American College of Surgeons-National Surgical Quality Improvement Program database. *World J. Gastroenterol.* **2015**, *21*, 12843–12850. [CrossRef]
30. Bircan, H.Y.; Koc, B.; Ozcelik, U.; Adas, G.; Karahan, S.; Demirag, A. Are there any differences between age groups regarding colorectal surgery in elderly patients? *BMC Surg.* **2014**, *14*, 44. [CrossRef]
31. Grosso, G.; Biondi, A.; Marventano, S.; Mistretta, A.; Calabrese, G.; Basile, F. Major postoperative complications and survival for colon cancer elderly patients. *BMC Surg.* **2012**, *12* (Suppl. 1), S20. [CrossRef]
32. Marusch, F.; Koch, A.; Schmidt, U.; Steinert, R.; Ueberrueck, T.; Bittner, R.; Berg, E.; Engemann, R.; Gellert, K.; Arbogast, R.; et al. The impact of the risk factor "age" on the early postoperative results of surgery for colorectal carcinoma and its significance for perioperative management. *World J. Surg.* **2005**, *29*, 1013–1021; discussion 1021–1012. [CrossRef]
33. Kunitake, H.; Zingmond, D.S.; Ryoo, J.; Ko, C.Y. Caring for octogenarian and nonagenarian patients with colorectal cancer: What should our standards and expectations be? *Dis. Colon Rectum* **2010**, *53*, 735–743. [CrossRef]
34. Engel, A.F.; Oomen, J.L.; Knol, D.L.; Cuesta, M.A. Operative mortality after colorectal resection in the Netherlands. *Br. J. Surg.* **2005**, *92*, 1526–1532. [CrossRef]

35. Faiz, O.; Haji, A.; Bottle, A.; Clark, S.K.; Darzi, A.W.; Aylin, P. Elective colonic surgery for cancer in the elderly: An investigation into postoperative mortality in English NHS hospitals between 1996 and 2007. *Colorectal Dis. Off. J. Assoc. Coloproctol. Great Br. Irel.* **2011**, *13*, 779–785. [CrossRef]
36. Dekker, J.W.; Gooiker, G.A.; Bastiaannet, E.; van den Broek, C.B.; van der Geest, L.G.; van de Velde, C.J.; Tollenaar, R.A.; Liefers, G.J.; Steering Committee of the 'Quality Information System Colorectal Cancer' Project. Cause of death the first year after curative colorectal cancer surgery; a prolonged impact of the surgery in elderly colorectal cancer patients. *Eur. J. Surg. Oncol. J. Eur. Soc. Surg. Oncol. Br. Assoc. Surg. Oncol.* **2014**, *40*, 1481–1487. [CrossRef]
37. Dekker, J.W.; van den Broek, C.B.; Bastiaannet, E.; van de Geest, L.G.; Tollenaar, R.A.; Liefers, G.J. Importance of the first postoperative year in the prognosis of elderly colorectal cancer patients. *Ann. Surg. Oncol.* **2011**, *18*, 1533–1539. [CrossRef]
38. Magnuson, A.; Sattar, S.; Nightingale, G.; Saracino, R.; Skonecki, E.; Trevino, K.M. A Practical Guide to Geriatric Syndromes in Older Adults With Cancer: A Focus on Falls, Cognition, Polypharmacy, and Depression. *Am. Soc. Clin. Oncol. Educ. Book. Am. Soc. Clin. Oncology. Annu. Meet.* **2019**, *39*, e96–e109. [CrossRef]
39. Reuben, D.B.; Rubenstein, L.V.; Hirsch, S.H.; Hays, R.D. Value of functional status as a predictor of mortality: Results of a prospective study. *Am. J. Med.* **1992**, *93*, 663–669. [CrossRef]
40. Wedding, U.; Rohrig, B.; Klippstein, A.; Pientka, L.; Hoffken, K. Age, severe comorbidity and functional impairment independently contribute to poor survival in cancer patients. *J. Cancer Res. Clin. Oncol.* **2007**, *133*, 945–950. [CrossRef]
41. Hamaker, M.E.; Prins, M.C.; Schiphorst, A.H.; van Tuyl, S.A.; Pronk, A.; van den Bos, F. Long-term changes in physical capacity after colorectal cancer treatment. *J. Geriatr. Oncol.* **2015**, *6*, 153–164. [CrossRef]
42. Ronning, B.; Wyller, T.B.; Jordhoy, M.S.; Nesbakken, A.; Bakka, A.; Seljeflot, I.; Kristjansson, S.R. Frailty indicators and functional status in older patients after colorectal cancer surgery. *J. Geriatr. Oncol.* **2014**, *5*, 26–32. [CrossRef] [PubMed]
43. Clegg, A.; Young, J.; Iliffe, S.; Rikkert, M.O.; Rockwood, K. Frailty in elderly people. *Lancet* **2013**, *381*, 752–762. [CrossRef]
44. Hoogendijk, E.O.; Afilalo, J.; Ensrud, K.E.; Kowal, P.; Onder, G.; Fried, L.P. Frailty: Implications for clinical practice and public health. *Lancet* **2019**, *394*, 1365–1375. [CrossRef]
45. Fried, L.P.; Tangen, C.M.; Walston, J.; Newman, A.B.; Hirsch, C.; Gottdiener, J.; Seeman, T.; Tracy, R.; Kop, W.J.; Burke, G.; et al. Frailty in older adults: Evidence for a phenotype. *J. gerontology. Ser. A Biol. Sci. Med Sci.* **2001**, *56*, M146–M156. [CrossRef] [PubMed]
46. Rockwood, K.; Song, X.; MacKnight, C.; Bergman, H.; Hogan, D.B.; McDowell, I.; Mitnitski, A. A global clinical measure of fitness and frailty in elderly people. *CMAJ Can. Med Assoc. J.* **2005**, *173*, 489–495. [CrossRef]
47. Collard, R.M.; Boter, H.; Schoevers, R.A.; Oude Voshaar, R.C. Prevalence of frailty in community-dwelling older persons: A systematic review. *J. Am. Geriatr. Soc.* **2012**, *60*, 1487–1492. [CrossRef]
48. Mohile, S.G.; Dale, W.; Somerfield, M.R.; Schonberg, M.A.; Boyd, C.M.; Burhenn, P.S.; Canin, B.; Cohen, H.J.; Holmes, H.M.; Hopkins, J.O.; et al. Practical Assessment and Management of Vulnerabilities in Older Patients Receiving Chemotherapy: ASCO Guideline for Geriatric Oncology. *J. Clin. Oncol. Off. J. Am. Soc. Clin. Oncol.* **2018**, *36*, 2326–2347. [CrossRef]
49. Morley, J.E.; Vellas, B.; van Kan, G.A.; Anker, S.D.; Bauer, J.M.; Bernabei, R.; Cesari, M.; Chumlea, W.C.; Doehner, W.; Evans, J.; et al. Frailty consensus: A call to action. *J. Am. Med Dir. Assoc.* **2013**, *14*, 392–397. [CrossRef]
50. Extermann, M.; Aapro, M.; Bernabei, R.; Cohen, H.J.; Droz, J.P.; Lichtman, S.; Mor, V.; Monfardini, S.; Repetto, L.; Sorbye, L.; et al. Use of comprehensive geriatric assessment in older cancer patients: Recommendations from the task force on CGA of the International Society of Geriatric Oncology (SIOG). *Crit. Rev. Oncol. Hematol.* **2005**, *55*, 241–252. [CrossRef]
51. Balducci, L.; Extermann, M. Management of cancer in the older person: A practical approach. *Oncologist* **2000**, *5*, 224–237. [CrossRef]
52. Saliba, D.; Elliott, M.; Rubenstein, L.Z.; Solomon, D.H.; Young, R.T.; Kamberg, C.J.; Roth, C.; MacLean, C.H.; Shekelle, P.G.; Sloss, E.M.; et al. The Vulnerable Elders Survey: A tool for identifying vulnerable older people in the community. *J. Am. Geriatr. Soc.* **2001**, *49*, 1691–1699. [CrossRef]
53. Bellera, C.A.; Rainfray, M.; Mathoulin-Pelissier, S.; Mertens, C.; Delva, F.; Fonck, M.; Soubeyran, P.L. Screening older cancer patients: First evaluation of the G-8 geriatric screening tool. *Ann. Oncol.* **2012**, *23*, 2166–2172. [CrossRef]
54. Fagard, K.; Leonard, S.; Deschodt, M.; Devriendt, E.; Wolthuis, A.; Prenen, H.; Flamaing, J.; Milisen, K.; Wildiers, H.; Kenis, C. The impact of frailty on postoperative outcomes in individuals aged 65 and over undergoing elective surgery for colorectal cancer: A systematic review. *J. Geriatr. Oncol.* **2016**, *7*, 479–491. [CrossRef]
55. Sáez-López, P.; Filipovich Vegas, E.; Martinez Peromingo, J.; Jimenez Mola, S. Colorectal cancer in the elderly. Surgical treatment, chemotherapy, and contribution from geriatrics. *Rev. Esp. De Geriatr. Y Gerontol.* **2017**, *52*, 261–270. (In Spanish) [CrossRef]
56. Robinson, T.N.; Walston, J.D.; Brummel, N.E.; Deiner, S.; Brown, C.H., IV; Kennedy, M.; Hurria, A. Frailty for Surgeons: Review of a National Institute on Aging Conference on Frailty for Specialists. *J. Am. Coll. Surg.* **2015**, *221*, 1083–1092. [CrossRef]
57. Gupta, S.K.; Lamont, E.B. Patterns of presentation, diagnosis, and treatment in older patients with colon cancer and comorbid dementia. *J. Am. Geriatr. Soc.* **2004**, *52*, 1681–1687. [CrossRef]
58. Derogatis, L.R.; Morrow, G.R.; Fetting, J.; Penman, D.; Piasetsky, S.; Schmale, A.M.; Henrichs, M.; Carnicke, C.L., Jr. The prevalence of psychiatric disorders among cancer patients. *JAMA* **1983**, *249*, 751–757. [CrossRef]
59. Massie, M.J. Prevalence of depression in patients with cancer. *J. Natl. Cancer Inst. Monogr.* **2004**, *2004*, 57–71. [CrossRef]
60. Peng, Y.N.; Huang, M.L.; Kao, C.H. Prevalence of Depression and Anxiety in Colorectal Cancer Patients: A Literature Review. *Int. J. Environ. Res. Public Health* **2019**, *16*. [CrossRef]

61. Lloyd, S.; Baraghoshi, D.; Tao, R.; Garrido-Laguna, I.; Gilcrease, G.W., 3rd; Whisenant, J.; Weis, J.R.; Scaife, C.; Pickron, T.B.; Huang, L.C.; et al. Mental Health Disorders are More Common in Colorectal Cancer Survivors and Associated With Decreased Overall Survival. *Am. J. Clin. Oncol.* **2019**, *42*, 355–362. [CrossRef]
62. Mols, F.; Schoormans, D.; de Hingh, I.; Oerlemans, S.; Husson, O. Symptoms of anxiety and depression among colorectal cancer survivors from the population-based, longitudinal PROFILES Registry: Prevalence, predictors, and impact on quality of life. *Cancer* **2018**, *124*, 2621–2628. [CrossRef]
63. Zhang, A.Y.; Cooper, G.S. Recognition of Depression and Anxiety among Elderly Colorectal Cancer Patients. *Nurs. Res. Pract.* **2010**, *2010*, 693961. [CrossRef] [PubMed]
64. Arends, J.; Bachmann, P.; Baracos, V.; Barthelemy, N.; Bertz, H.; Bozzetti, F.; Fearon, K.; Hütterer, E.; Isenring, E.; Kaasa, S.; et al. ESPEN guidelines on nutrition in cancer patients. *Clin. Nutr.* **2017**, *36*, 11–48. [CrossRef] [PubMed]
65. Arends, J.; Baracos, V.; Bertz, H.; Bozzetti, F.; Calder, P.C.; Deutz, N.E.P.; Erickson, N.; Laviano, A.; Lisanti, M.P.; Lobo, D.N.; et al. ESPEN expert group recommendations for action against cancer-related malnutrition. *Clin. Nutr.* **2017**, *36*, 1187–1196. [CrossRef] [PubMed]
66. Zhang, X.; Edwards, B.J. Malnutrition in Older Adults with Cancer. *Curr. Oncol. Rep.* **2019**, *21*, 80. [CrossRef]
67. Kenis, C.; Bron, D.; Libert, Y.; Decoster, L.; Van Puyvelde, K.; Scalliet, P.; Cornette, P.; Pepersack, T.; Luce, S.; Langenaeken, C.; et al. Relevance of a systematic geriatric screening and assessment in older patients with cancer: Results of a prospective multicentric study. *Ann. Oncol.* **2013**, *24*, 1306–1312. [CrossRef]
68. Haviland, J.; Sodergren, S.; Calman, L.; Corner, J.; Din, A.; Fenlon, D.; Grimmett, C.; Richardson, A.; Smith, P.W.; Winter, J.; et al. Social support following diagnosis and treatment for colorectal cancer and associations with health-related quality of life: Results from the UK ColoREctal Wellbeing (CREW) cohort study. *Psycho-Oncology* **2017**, *26*, 2276–2284. [CrossRef]
69. Kristjansson, S.R.; Nesbakken, A.; Jordhøy, M.S.; Skovlund, E.; Audisio, R.A.; Johannessen, H.O.; Bakka, A.; Wyller, T.B. Comprehensive geriatric assessment can predict complications in elderly patients after elective surgery for colorectal cancer: A prospective observational cohort study. *Crit. Rev. Oncol. Hematol.* **2010**, *76*, 208–217. [CrossRef]
70. Ommundsen, N.; Wyller, T.B.; Nesbakken, A.; Bakka, A.O.; Jordhoy, M.S.; Skovlund, E.; Rostoft, S. Preoperative geriatric assessment and tailored interventions in frail older patients with colorectal cancer: A randomized controlled trial. *Colorectal Dis. Off. J. Assoc. Coloproctol. Great Br. Irel.* **2018**, *20*, 16–25. [CrossRef]
71. Reisinger, K.W.; van Vugt, J.L.; Tegels, J.J.; Snijders, C.; Hulsewé, K.W.; Hoofwijk, A.G.; Stoot, J.H.; Von Meyenfeldt, M.F.; Beets, G.L.; Derikx, J.P.; et al. Functional compromise reflected by sarcopenia, frailty, and nutritional depletion predicts adverse postoperative outcome after colorectal cancer surgery. *Ann. Surg.* **2015**, *261*, 345–352. [CrossRef]
72. Tan, K.Y.; Kawamura, Y.J.; Tokomitsu, A.; Tang, T. Assessment for frailty is useful for predicting morbidity in elderly patients undergoing colorectal cancer resection whose comorbidities are already optimized. *Am. J. Surg.* **2012**, *204*, 139–143. [CrossRef]
73. Kehlet, H. Fast-track colorectal surgery. *Lancet* **2008**, *371*, 791–793. [CrossRef]
74. Vlug, M.S.; Wind, J.; Hollmann, M.W.; Ubbink, D.T.; Cense, H.A.; Engel, A.F.; Gerhards, M.F.; van Wagensveld, B.A.; van der Zaag, E.S.; van Geloven, A.A.; et al. Laparoscopy in combination with fast track multimodal management is the best perioperative strategy in patients undergoing colonic surgery: A randomized clinical trial (LAFA-study). *Ann. Surg.* **2011**, *254*, 868–875. [CrossRef]
75. Varadhan, K.K.; Neal, K.R.; Dejong, C.H.; Fearon, K.C.; Ljungqvist, O.; Lobo, D.N. The enhanced recovery after surgery (ERAS) pathway for patients undergoing major elective open colorectal surgery: A meta-analysis of randomized controlled trials. *Clin. Nutr.* **2010**, *29*, 434–440. [CrossRef]
76. Gonzalez-Ayora, S.; Pastor, C.; Guadalajara, H.; Ramirez, J.M.; Royo, P.; Redondo, E.; Arroyo, A.; Moya, P.; Garcia-Olmo, D. Enhanced recovery care after colorectal surgery in elderly patients. Compliance and outcomes of a multicenter study from the Spanish working group on ERAS. *Int. J. Colorectal Dis.* **2016**, *31*, 1625–1631. [CrossRef]
77. Rubenstein, L.Z.; Stuck, A.E.; Siu, A.L.; Wieland, D. Impacts of geriatric evaluation and management programs on defined outcomes: Overview of the evidence. *J. Am. Geriatr. Soc.* **1991**, *39*, 8S–16S. [CrossRef]
78. Wildiers, H.; Heeren, P.; Puts, M.; Topinkova, E.; Janssen-Heijnen, M.L.; Extermann, M.; Falandry, C.; Artz, A.; Brain, E.; Colloca, G.; et al. International Society of Geriatric Oncology consensus on geriatric assessment in older patients with cancer. *J. Clin. Oncol. Off. J. Am. Soc. Clin. Oncol.* **2014**, *32*, 2595–2603. [CrossRef]
79. Soto-Perez-de-Celis, E.; Aapro, M.; Muss, H. ASCO 2020: The Geriatric Assessment Comes of Age. *Oncologist* **2020**, *25*, 909–912. [CrossRef]
80. Jones, T.S.; Jones, E.L.; Richardson, V.; Finley, J.B.; Franklin, J.L.; Gore, D.L.; Horney, C.P.; Kovar, A.; Morin, T.L.; Robinson, T.N. Preliminary data demonstrate the Geriatric Surgery Verification program reduces postoperative length of stay. *J. Am. Geriatr. Soc.* **2021**. [CrossRef]
81. Shahrokni, A.; Tin, A.L.; Sarraf, S.; Alexander, K.; Sun, S.; Kim, S.J.; McMillan, S.; Yulico, H.; Amirnia, F.; Downey, R.J.; et al. Association of Geriatric Comanagement and 90-Day Postoperative Mortality Among Patients Aged 75 Years and Older With Cancer. *JAMA Netw. Open* **2020**, *3*, e209265. [CrossRef]
82. Ghignone, F.; van Leeuwen, B.L.; Montroni, I.; Huisman, M.G.; Somasundar, P.; Cheung, K.L.; Audisio, R.A.; Ugolini, G.; International Society of Geriatric Oncology Surgical Task Force. The assessment and management of older cancer patients: A SIOG surgical task force survey on surgeons' attitudes. *Eur. J. Surg. Oncol. J. Eur. Soc. Surg. Oncol. Br. Assoc. Surg. Oncol.* **2016**, *42*, 297–302. [CrossRef]

83. Lee, D.Y.; Kwak, J.M. Comprehensive Approach for Older Cancer Patients: New Challenge in an Aging Society. *Ann. Coloproctol.* **2020**, *36*, 289–290. [CrossRef] [PubMed]
84. Shipway, D.; Koizia, L.; Winterkorn, N.; Fertleman, M.; Ziprin, P.; Moorthy, K. Embedded geriatric surgical liaison is associated with reduced inpatient length of stay in older patients admitted for gastrointestinal surgery. *Future Healthc. J.* **2018**, *5*, 108–116. [CrossRef] [PubMed]
85. Ramírez-Martín, R.; JA, G.M.; JL, M.M.; González-Montalvo, J.I. The efficiency of «Cross-speciality Geriatrics» in the co-management of patients older than 80 years admitted to the General Surgery Service. Economic Results. *Rev. Esp. Geriatr. Gerontol.* **2021**, *56*, 87–90. [CrossRef] [PubMed]
86. Tarazona-Santabalbina, F.J.; Llabata-Broseta, J.; Belenguer-Varea, A.; Alvarez-Martinez, D.; Cuesta-Peredo, D.; Avellana-Zaragoza, J.A. A daily multidisciplinary assessment of older adults undergoing elective colorectal cancer surgery is associated with reduced delirium and geriatric syndromes. *J. Geriatr. Oncol.* **2019**, *10*, 298–303. [CrossRef]
87. Indrakusuma, R.; Dunker, M.S.; Peetoom, J.J.; Schreurs, W.H. Evaluation of preoperative geriatric assessment of elderly patients with colorectal carcinoma. A retrospective study. *Eur. J. Surg. Oncol. J. Eur. Soc. Surg. Oncol. Br. Assoc. Surg. Oncol.* **2015**, *41*, 21–27. [CrossRef]
88. Patel, A.V.; Friedenreich, C.M.; Moore, S.C.; Hayes, S.C.; Silver, J.K.; Campbell, K.L.; Winters-Stone, K.; Gerber, L.H.; George, S.M.; Fulton, J.E.; et al. American College of Sports Medicine Roundtable Report on Physical Activity, Sedentary Behavior, and Cancer Prevention and Control. *Med. Sci. Sports Exerc.* **2019**, *51*, 2391–2402. [CrossRef]
89. Schmid, D.; Leitzmann, M.F. Association between physical activity and mortality among breast cancer and colorectal cancer survivors: A systematic review and meta-analysis. *Ann. Oncol.* **2014**, *25*, 1293–1311. [CrossRef]
90. Schmitz, K.H.; Campbell, A.M.; Stuiver, M.M.; Pinto, B.M.; Schwartz, A.L.; Morris, G.S.; Ligibel, J.A.; Cheville, A.; Galvão, D.A.; Alfano, C.M. Exercise is medicine in oncology: Engaging clinicians to help patients move through cancer. *CA Cancer J. Clin.* **2019**, *69*, 468–484. [CrossRef]
91. Schmitz, K.H.; Courneya, K.S.; Matthews, C.; Demark-Wahnefried, W.; Galvao, D.A.; Pinto, B.M.; Irwin, M.L.; Wolin, K.Y.; Segal, R.J.; Lucia, A.; et al. American College of Sports Medicine roundtable on exercise guidelines for cancer survivors. *Med. Sci. Sports Exerc.* **2010**, *42*, 1409–1426. [CrossRef]
92. Lynch, B.M.; van Roekel, E.H.; Vallance, J.K. Physical activity and quality of life after colorectal cancer: Overview of evidence and future directions. *Expert Rev. Qual. Life Cancer Care* **2016**, *1*, 9–23. [CrossRef]
93. McGettigan, M.; Cardwell, C.R.; Cantwell, M.M.; Tully, M.A. Physical activity interventions for disease-related physical and mental health during and following treatment in people with non-advanced colorectal cancer. *Cochrane Database Syst. Rev.* **2020**, *5*, CD012864. [CrossRef]
94. Pollan, M.; Casla-Barrio, S.; Alfaro, J.; Esteban, C.; Segui-Palmer, M.A.; Lucia, A.; Martin, M. Exercise and cancer: A position statement from the Spanish Society of Medical Oncology. *Clin. Transl. Oncol. Off. Publ. Fed. Span. Oncol. Soc. Natl. Cancer Inst. Mex.* **2020**, *22*, 1710–1729. [CrossRef]
95. Berkel, A.E.M.; Bongers, B.C.; Kotte, H.; Weltevreden, P.; de Jongh, F.H.C.; Eijsvogel, M.M.M.; Wymenga, A.N.M.; Bigirwamungu-Bargeman, M.; van der Palen, J.; van Det, M.J.; et al. Effects of Community-based Exercise Prehabilitation for Patients Scheduled for Colorectal Surgery With High Risk for Postoperative Complications: Results of a Randomized Clinical Trial. *Ann. Surg.* **2021**. [CrossRef]
96. Carli, F.; Charlebois, P.; Stein, B.; Feldman, L.; Zavorsky, G.; Kim, D.J.; Scott, S.; Mayo, N.E. Randomized clinical trial of prehabilitation in colorectal surgery. *Br. J. Surg.* **2010**, *97*, 1187–1197. [CrossRef]
97. Dronkers, J.J.; Lamberts, H.; Reutelingsperger, I.M.; Naber, R.H.; Dronkers-Landman, C.M.; Veldman, A.; van Meeteren, N.L. Preoperative therapeutic programme for elderly patients scheduled for elective abdominal oncological surgery: A randomized controlled pilot study. *Clin. Rehabil.* **2010**, *24*, 614–622. [CrossRef]
98. Minnella, E.M.; Ferreira, V.; Awasthi, R.; Charlebois, P.; Stein, B.; Liberman, A.S.; Scheede-Bergdahl, C.; Morais, J.A.; Carli, F. Effect of two different pre-operative exercise training regimens before colorectal surgery on functional capacity: A randomised controlled trial. *Eur. J. Anaesthesiol.* **2020**, *37*, 969–978. [CrossRef]
99. Awasthi, R.; Minnella, E.M.; Ferreira, V.; Ramanakumar, A.V.; Scheede-Bergdahl, C.; Carli, F. Supervised exercise training with multimodal pre-habilitation leads to earlier functional recovery following colorectal cancer resection. *Acta Anaesthesiol. Scand.* **2019**, *63*, 461–467. [CrossRef]
100. Chia, C.L.; Mantoo, S.K.; Tan, K.Y. 'Start to finish trans-institutional transdisciplinary care': A novel approach improves colorectal surgical results in frail elderly patients. *Colorectal Dis. Off. J. Assoc. Coloproctology Great Br. Irel.* **2016**, *18*, O43–O50. [CrossRef]
101. Souwer, E.T.D.; Bastiaannet, E.; de Bruijn, S.; Breugom, A.J.; van den Bos, F.; Portielje, J.E.A.; Dekker, J.W.T. Comprehensive multidisciplinary care program for elderly colorectal cancer patients: "From prehabilitation to independence". *Eur. J. Surg. Oncol. J. Eur. Soc. Surg. Oncol. Br. Assoc. Surg. Oncol.* **2018**, *44*, 1894–1900. [CrossRef]
102. Bousquet-Dion, G.; Awasthi, R.; Loiselle, S.E.; Minnella, E.M.; Agnihotram, R.V.; Bergdahl, A.; Carli, F.; Scheede-Bergdahl, C. Evaluation of supervised multimodal prehabilitation programme in cancer patients undergoing colorectal resection: A randomized control trial. *Acta Oncol.* **2018**, *57*, 849–859. [CrossRef]
103. Carli, F.; Bousquet-Dion, G.; Awasthi, R.; Elsherbini, N.; Liberman, S.; Boutros, M.; Stein, B.; Charlebois, P.; Ghitulescu, G.; Morin, N.; et al. Effect of Multimodal Prehabilitation vs Postoperative Rehabilitation on 30-Day Postoperative Complications for Frail

Patients Undergoing Resection of Colorectal Cancer: A Randomized Clinical Trial. *JAMA Surg.* **2020**, *155*, 233–242. [CrossRef] [PubMed]
104. Gillis, C.; Li, C.; Lee, L.; Awasthi, R.; Augustin, B.; Gamsa, A.; Liberman, A.S.; Stein, B.; Charlebois, P.; Feldman, L.S.; et al. Prehabilitation versus rehabilitation: A randomized control trial in patients undergoing colorectal resection for cancer. *Anesthesiology* **2014**, *121*, 937–947. [CrossRef] [PubMed]
105. Minnella, E.M.; Bousquet-Dion, G.; Awasthi, R.; Scheede-Bergdahl, C.; Carli, F. Multimodal prehabilitation improves functional capacity before and after colorectal surgery for cancer: A five-year research experience. *Acta Oncol.* **2017**, *56*, 295–300. [CrossRef] [PubMed]
106. Campbell, K.L.; Winters-Stone, K.M.; Wiskemann, J.; May, A.M.; Schwartz, A.L.; Courneya, K.S.; Zucker, D.S.; Matthews, C.E.; Ligibel, J.A.; Gerber, L.H.; et al. Exercise Guidelines for Cancer Survivors: Consensus Statement from International Multidisciplinary Roundtable. *Med. Sci. Sports Exerc.* **2019**, *51*, 2375–2390. [CrossRef] [PubMed]
107. Lim, S.H.; Chan, S.W.C.; Chow, A.; Zhu, L.; Lai, J.H.; He, H.G. Pilot trial of a STOMA psychosocial intervention programme for colorectal cancer patients with stomas. *J. Adv. Nurs.* **2019**, *75*, 1338–1346. [CrossRef] [PubMed]
108. Bryan, S.; Dukes, S. The Enhanced Recovery Programme for stoma patients: An audit. *Br. J. Nurs.* **2010**, *19*, 831–834. [CrossRef]
109. Chaudhri, S.; Brown, L.; Hassan, I.; Horgan, A.F. Preoperative intensive, community-based vs. traditional stoma education: A randomized, controlled trial. *Dis. Colon Rectum* **2005**, *48*, 504–509. [CrossRef]
110. Cheung, Y.L.; Molassiotis, A.; Chang, A.M. The effect of progressive muscle relaxation training on anxiety and quality of life after stoma surgery in colorectal cancer patients. *Psycho-Oncology* **2003**, *12*, 254–266. [CrossRef]
111. Danielsen, A.K.; Burcharth, J.; Rosenberg, J. Patient education has a positive effect in patients with a stoma: A systematic review. *Colorectal Dis. Off. J. Assoc. Coloproctology Great Br. Irel.* **2013**, *15*, e276–e283. [CrossRef]
112. Son, H.; Son, Y.J.; Kim, H.; Lee, Y. Effect of psychosocial interventions on the quality of life of patients with colorectal cancer: A systematic review and meta-analysis. *Health Qual. Life Outcomes* **2018**, *16*, 119. [CrossRef]
113. Hoon, L.S.; Chi Sally, C.W.; Hong-Gu, H. Effect of psychosocial interventions on outcomes of patients with colorectal cancer: A review of the literature. *Eur. J. Oncol. Nurs.* **2013**, *17*, 883–891. [CrossRef]
114. Ohlen, J.; Sawatzky, R.; Pettersson, M.; Sarenmalm, E.K.; Larsdotter, C.; Smith, F.; Wallengren, C.; Friberg, F.; Kodeda, K.; Carlsson, E. Preparedness for colorectal cancer surgery and recovery through a person-centred information and communication intervention-A quasi-experimental longitudinal design. *PLoS ONE* **2019**, *14*, e0225816. [CrossRef]
115. Louro, A.C.; Castro, J.F.; Blasco, T. Effects of a positive emotion-based adjuvant psychological therapy in colorectal cancer patients: A pilot study. *Psicooncologia* **2016**, *13*, 113–125.
116. Ellis, J.; Lin, J.; Walsh, A.; Lo, C.; Shepherd, F.A.; Moore, M.; Li, M.; Gagliese, L.; Zimmermann, C.; Rodin, G. Predictors of referral for specialized psychosocial oncology care in patients with metastatic cancer: The contributions of age, distress, and marital status. *J. Clin. Oncol. Off. J. Am. Soc. Clin. Oncol.* **2009**, *27*, 699–705. [CrossRef]
117. Newell, S.A.; Sanson-Fisher, R.W.; Savolainen, N.J. Systematic review of psychological therapies for cancer patients: Overview and recommendations for future research. *J. Natl. Cancer Inst.* **2002**, *94*, 558–584. [CrossRef]

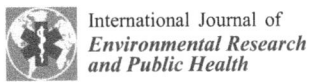

Article

Association between Occupational Dysfunction and Social Isolation in Japanese Older Adults: A Cross-Sectional Study

Keisuke Fujii [1,*], Yuya Fujii [2], Yuta Kubo [3], Korin Tateoka [4], Jue Liu [4], Koki Nagata [5], Shuichi Wakayama [6] and Tomohiro Okura [7,8]

1. Department of Occupational Therapy, Faculty of Health Sciences, Kansai University of Health Sciences, 2-11-1 Wakaba, Kumatori, Sennnan, Osaka 590-0482, Japan
2. Physical Fitness Research Institute, Meiji Yasuda Life Foundation of Health and Welfare, 150 Tobuki, Hachioji, Tokyo 192-0001, Japan; yu3-fujii@my-zaidan.or.jp
3. Division of Occupational Therapy, Faculty of Rehabilitation and Care, Seijoh University, 2-172 Fukinodai, Tokai 476-8588, Japan; kubo-yu@seijoh-u.ac.jp
4. Doctoral Program in Physical Education, Health and Sport Sciences, Degree Programs in Comprehensive Human Sciences, Graduate School of Comprehensive Human Sciences, University of Tsukuba, 1-1-1 Tennodai, Tsukuba 305-8577, Ibaraki, Japan; s2130461@s.tsukuba.ac.jp (K.T.); s1830468@s.tsukuba.ac.jp (J.L.)
5. Doctoral Program in Public Health, Degree Programs in Comprehensive Human Sciences, Graduate School of Comprehensive Human Sciences, University of Tsukuba, 1-1-1 Tennodai, Tsukuba 305-8577, Ibaraki, Japan; s2030441@s.tsukuba.ac.jp
6. Department of Occupational Therapy, Ibaraki Prefectural University of Health Sciences, 4669-2 Ami, Ami, Inashiki 300-0394, Ibaraki, Japan; wakayamas@ipu.ac.jp
7. Faculty of Health and Sport Sciences, University of Tsukuba, 1-1-1 Tennodai, Tsukuba 305-8577, Ibaraki, Japan; okura.tomohiro.gp@u.tsukuba.ac.jp
8. R&D Center for Tailor-Made QOL, University of Tsukuba, 1-1-1 Tennodai, Tsukuba 305-8577, Ibaraki, Japan
* Correspondence: k.fujii@kansai.ac.jp; Tel.: +81-72-453-8251

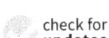

Citation: Fujii, K.; Fujii, Y.; Kubo, Y.; Tateoka, K.; Liu, J.; Nagata, K.; Wakayama, S.; Okura, T. Association between Occupational Dysfunction and Social Isolation in Japanese Older Adults: A Cross-Sectional Study. IJERPH 2021, 18, 6648. https://doi.org/10.3390/ijerph18126648

Academic Editors: Francisco José Tarazona Santabalbina, Sebastià Josep Santaeugènia González, José Augusto García Navarro and José Viña

Received: 15 May 2021
Accepted: 17 June 2021
Published: 21 June 2021

Publisher's Note: MDPI stays neutral with regard to jurisdictional claims in published maps and institutional affiliations.

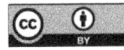

Copyright: © 2021 by the authors. Licensee MDPI, Basel, Switzerland. This article is an open access article distributed under the terms and conditions of the Creative Commons Attribution (CC BY) license (https://creativecommons.org/licenses/by/4.0/).

Abstract: We clarified the relationship between occupational dysfunction and social isolation among community-dwelling adults. We used a self-administered questionnaire with a cross-sectional study for 2879 independently living older adults in Kasama City, Japan. Participants responded to a self-reported questionnaire in November 2019. Occupational dysfunction and social isolation were assessed. The participants were classified into two groups: healthy occupational function group, and occupational dysfunction group. To examine the relationship between occupational dysfunction and social isolation, we performed a logistic regression analysis with social isolation as a dependent variable and occupational dysfunction as an independent variable. In the crude model, the occupational dysfunction group had a higher risk of social isolation than the healthy occupational function group (odds ratio (OR) = 2.04; 95% confidence interval (CI), 1.63–2.55; $p < 0.001$). In the adjusted model, the occupational dysfunction group had a higher risk of social isolation than the healthy occupational function group (OR = 1.51; 95% CI, 1.17–1.94; $p = 0.001$). The results showed that occupational dysfunction was significantly associated with social isolation. These results can be used in constructing a support method for social isolation from a new perspective.

Keywords: occupational therapy; occupational function; social network; social isolation

1. Introduction

The world's population is aging, and Japan has the highest aging rate worldwide. In Japan, as the older adult population has grown in proportion, the composition of households has undergone a change; among older adults, the number of "one-person households" and "households of only a couple" have increased [1]. Therefore, older adults are likely to face increasing social changes, including problems such as social isolation. Social isolation is defined as a state in which an individual lacks a sense of social belongingness, refrains from engaging with others, has a minimal number of social contacts, and displays a deficiency in fulfilling quality relationships [2]. According to a large cohort study of Japanese older adults, the rate of social isolation was reported to be 17.7%, which means that nearly one in five Japanese older adults is experiencing social isolation [3]. Social isolation has been identified as a risk factor for poor health and well-being [4], cognitive decline [5], and mortality [6,7]. Therefore, measures to combat social isolation are important.

Difficulties related to occupational tasks or daily activities are called occupational dysfunction [8]. Occupational dysfunction is recognized worldwide as a major health-related problem in the preventive occupational therapy field [9]. It is a negative experience related to daily life and workplace activities, and it includes occupational marginalization, occupational imbalance, occupational alienation, and occupational deprivation [10]. Occupational dysfunction has been associated with poor mental health [11] and poor health-related quality of life [12]. As mental health and health-related quality of life are associated with social isolation [13–15], occupational dysfunction may also be associated with social isolation. For example, negative subjective daily life performance experiences (occupational dysfunction) may cause people to leave the social community where they participate in occupational activities, which may eventually lead to social isolation. A literature review by Papageorgiou et al. found evidence to support a positive relationship between occupation, participation, and prevention of social isolation among community-dwelling older adults [16]. Therefore, occupational therapists may prevent social isolation by supporting older adults' occupational participation.

However, there are no reports that examined the relationship between occupational dysfunction and social isolation in community-dwelling older adults. The primary purpose of this study is to clarify the relationship between occupational dysfunction and social isolation in older adults living in community-dwellings. The secondary purpose of this study is to determine which occupational dysfunction types are associated with social isolation.

2. Materials and Methods

2.1. Participants and Data Collection

This cross-sectional study was conducted in Kasama City, Ibaraki Prefecture, Japan. Kasama is a rural agricultural area, categorized as a flatland agricultural region and intermediate agricultural region. As of 1 January, 2021, Kasama City's population is 73,589 and the aging rate is 32.4% [17].

Figure 1 shows the participant flowchart. Inclusion criteria were (1) those who are 65–85 years, (2) those without any functional disability. We randomly selected 8000 participants from the basic resident register on 1 October 2019. A self-administered questionnaire was mailed to participants in November 2019. Responses were obtained from 3934 persons (recovery rate: 49.2%). The exclusion criteria were as follows: (1) Those who were in hospital at the time of the response, (2) Those who had a history of cerebrovascular disease, dementia, or psychiatric disorder, and (3) Those who submitted incomplete questionnaires. As a result, 2879 participants were included in the final analysis. All participants were informed of the study details and provided informed consent. This study protocol was approved by the Ethical Committee of the University of Tsukuba (Ref No. Tai 019-101).

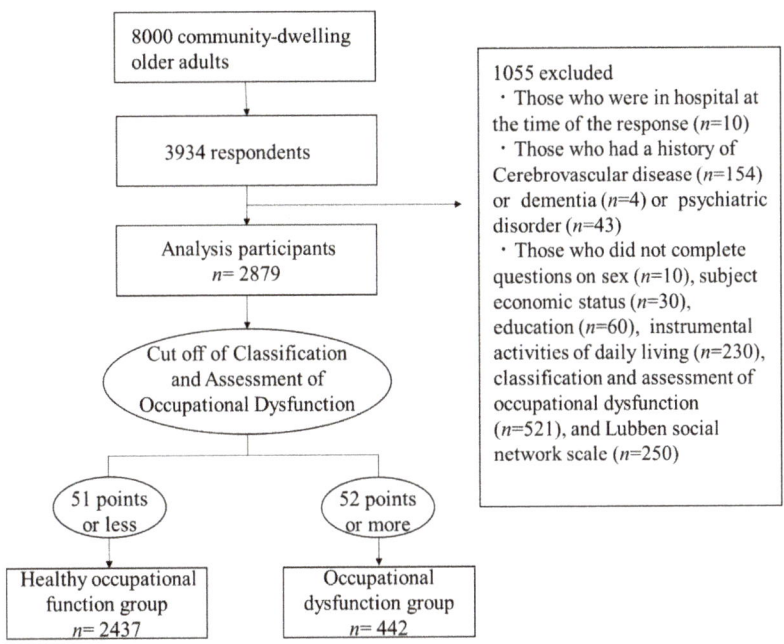

Figure 1. Participant flowchart.

2.2. Measurement Variables

Demographic data including sex, age, household, educational background, subjective economic status, mental health, and instrumental activities of daily living (IADL) were used as covariates. Subjective economic status was assessed by the question, "How do you feel about your current economic situation?" Responses were rated on a scale ranging from "Very difficult," "Slightly difficult," "Normal," "Somewhat rich," "Very rich." The two categories of "Very difficult" and "Slightly difficult" were operationally defined as "Poor." Mental health status was assessed using the Japanese version of the Kessler 6 (K6) scale [18], a screening scale that can effectively measure psychological distress as per the Diagnostic and Statistical Manual of Mental Disorders (DSM-IV) [19]. Respondents answered six items on a 5-point Likert scale and responses on each item were transformed to scores ranging from 0 to 4 points. Total scores range from 0 to 24. A higher total score corresponds to a poorer mental health condition. IADL was evaluated using the five items of the Tokyo Metropolitan Institute of Gerontology Index of Competence (TMIG-IC), based on a subjective evaluation by respondents [20,21]. The TMIG-IC was developed to measure higher-level functional capacity among older adults living in the community and has been commonly used in Japan [22]. These five items of TMIG-IC were used to evaluate IADL ability. Higher values indicate good IADL ability (range: 0–5 points). In this study, IADL disability was defined as an IADL ability score of less than 5 [20,21].

Occupational dysfunction was evaluated using the Classification and Assessment of Occupational Dysfunction (CAOD) [10]. The CAOD measures occupational dysfunction with 16 items. The Cronbach's alpha for this scale was 0.902 [10]. In our study, it was 0.914. Responses are rated on a seven-point Likert-type scale from "strongly agree" = 7 to "strongly disagree" = 1. It has a four-factor structure of occupational imbalance (4–28 points), occupational deprivation (3–21 points), occupational alienation (3–21 points), and occupational marginalization (6–42 points). Occupational marginalization is defined as a person not having the opportunity to engage in desired daily activities, such as when, "I have opinions but nobody hears them," and "It is like being required to talk to a partner who is unpleasant" etc. [23]. Occupational imbalance is a loss of balance in engaging in daily activities, such as feeling, "I am so busy that my life's rhythm is confused," "There is no time to rest, and I am tired," "Daily life is becoming very busy and increasingly exhausting," and "My busy life has led to lack of sleep," etc. [24]. Occupational alienation is defined as a situation when the inner needs of the individual concerning daily activities are not satisfied, such as "I feel my life has no meaning," "There is no sense of accomplishment in daily life," and "Daily life has become tedious," etc. [25]. Occupational deprivation is a lack of opportunity for daily activities beyond the individual's control such as, "There is no place where I can enjoy hobbies," "There is no opportunity to carry out that what I consider important for its own sake," and "I cannot enjoy my favorite activities," etc. [26]. The cutoff value of the CAOD was 52 points, and the higher the score, the more likely it indicated an occupational function impairment. The item characteristics, structural validity, and internal consistency of the CAOD have been confirmed for university students, health care workers, community-dwelling older adults, people with mental disorders, and people with physical disabilities [8,10].

Social isolation was evaluated using the Japanese version of the Abbreviated Lubben Social Network Scale (LSNS) [27]. The LSNS-6 consists of six items, three related to the number of people in the family network and three related to the number of people in the friends and acquaintances network. The Cronbach's alpha for this scale was 0.83 [27]. In our study, it was 0.872. Responses are rated on a six-point scale (range: 0–30 points). Social isolation was defined as an LSNS score of less than 12 points [27].

2.3. Statistical Analysis

According to the cutoff value of CAOD, the participants were divided into the "healthy occupational function group (CAOD score $\leq$ 51 points)" and "occupational dysfunction group (CAOD score $\geq$ 52 points)". We calculated the means and standard deviations for continuous variables and frequencies and percentages for categorical variables. Student's *t*-test and chi-square test were used to compare the characteristics of health occupational function and occupational dysfunction groups. To examine the relationship between occupational dysfunction and social isolation, we performed a logistic regression analysis with social isolation as a dependent variable and occupational dysfunction as an independent variable. We used two models in this study: a crude model and an adjusted model. The latter was adjusted for age, sex, household, educational background, subjective economic status, mental health, and IADL ability. These covariates were selected as potential confounders from previous studies. A logistic regression analysis was conducted to clarify the relationship between occupational dysfunction types and social isolation, and each occupational dysfunction type was entered as a dependent variable.

Analysis was performed using STATA/MP 16.0 (Stata Corp., College Station, TX, USA). In all analyses, a *p*-value of <0.05 was considered to indicate statistical significance.

3. Results

The comparison of characteristics between the healthy occupational function and the occupational dysfunction group is shown in Table 1. The number of people with occupational dysfunction was 442 (15.4%). The occupational dysfunction group was significantly less likely to have an education level beyond high school ($p = 0.001$), have significantly worse subjective economic status ($p < 0.001$), higher mental health scores ($p < 0.001$), higher CAOD scores ($p < 0.001$), and higher scores for the occupational dysfunction types ($p < 0.001$). Social isolation was significantly higher among individuals with evidence of occupational dysfunction ($p < 0.001$).

Table 1. Participants' characteristics.

Characteristic	Healthy Occupational Function Group (n = 2437)	Occupational Dysfunction Group (n = 442)	p-Value
	%(n)	%(n)	
Age (years), Mean ± SD	72.6 ± 5.2	72.7 ± 5.6	0.795
Female, %(n)	49.3 (1202)	46.2 (204)	0.220
Household (living alone), %(n)	12.7 (310)	12.7 (56)	0.976
Educational background (≥high school), %(n)	84.1 (2030)	77.8 (339)	0.001
Subjective economic status (poor), %(n)	17.0 (413)	31.9 (553)	$p < 0.001$
IADL ability (disability), %(n)	7.4 (181)	7.9 (35)	0.718
K6 (score), Mean ± SD	2.8 ± 3.0	6.2 ± 4.0	$p < 0.001$
Social isolation, %(n)	18.4 (448)	31.5 (139)	$p < 0.001$
CAOD (score), Mean ± SD	30.0 ± 10.5	60.6 ± 7.1	$p < 0.001$
Occupational imbalance (score), Mean ± SD	7.5 ± 3.8	14.8 ± 3.8	$p < 0.001$
Occupational deprivation (score), Mean ± SD	6.2 ± 3.2	12.8 ± 2.7	$p < 0.001$
Occupational alienation (score), Mean ± SD	6.4 ± 3.4	12.1 ± 2.8	$p < 0.001$
Occupational marginalization (score), Mean ± SD	9.9 ± 3.8	20.8 ± 3.8	$p < 0.001$

SD: standard deviation; IADL: instrumental activities of daily living; CAOD: classification and assessment of occupational dysfunction.

Table 2 shows the association between occupational dysfunction and social isolation. In the crude model, the occupational dysfunction group had a higher risk of social isolation than those with healthy occupational function group (odds ratio (OR) = 2.04; 95% confidence interval (CI), 1.63–2.55; $p < 0.001$). In the adjusted model, the occupational dysfunction group had a higher risk of social isolation than the healthy occupational function group (OR = 1.51; 95% CI, 1.17–1.94; $p = 0.001$). Table 3 shows the association between the classification of occupational dysfunction and social isolation. In the crude model, occupational imbalance (OR = 1.10; 95% CI, 1.08–1.13; $p < 0.001$), occupational alienation (OR = 1.15; 95% CI, 1.12–1.78; $p < 0.001$), and occupational deprivation (OR = 1.07; 95% CI, 1.05–1.09; $p < 0.001$) were significantly correlated with social isolation. In contrast, in the adjusted model, occupational marginalization (OR = 0.93; 95% CI, 0.90–0.96; $p < 0.001$), occupational alienation (OR = 1.10; 95% CI, 1.06–1.13; $p < 0.001$), and occupational deprivation (OR = 1.04; 95% CI, 1.01–1.07; $p = 0.003$) were significantly correlated with social isolation, but occupational imbalance was not significant (OR = 1.03; 95% CI, 0.99–1.06; $p = 0.134$).

Table 2. Association between occupational dysfunction and social isolation.

	Crude Model			Adjusted Model		
	OR	95%CI	p-Value	OR	95%CI	p-Value
Healthy occupational function group	Ref.			Ref.		
Occupational dysfunction group	2.04	1.63–2.55	$p < 0.001$	1.51	1.17–1.94	0.001

OR: odds ratio, CI: confidence interval, Ref: reference. Adjusted model was adjusted for age, sex, household, educational background, subjective economic status, instrumental activities of daily living, and mental health.

Table 3. Association classification in the relationship between occupational dysfunction and social isolation.

Occupational Dysfunction Type	Crude Model			Adjusted Model		
	OR	95%CI	p-Value	OR	95%CI	p-Value
Occupational imbalance	1.01	0.99–1.03	0.248	0.93	0.90–0.96	$p < 0.001$
Occupational deprivation	1.10	1.08–1.13	$p < 0.001$	1.03	0.99–1.06	0.134
Occupational alienation	1.15	1.12–1.78	$p < 0.001$	1.10	1.06–1.13	$p < 0.001$
Occupational marginalization	1.07	1.05–1.09	$p < 0.001$	1.04	1.01–1.07	0.003

OR: odds ratio, CI: confidence interval. Adjusted model was adjusted for age, sex, household, educational background, subjective economic status, instrumental activities of daily living, mental health, and other types of occupational dysfunction.

4. Discussion

The present study is the first to examine the relationship between occupational dysfunction and social isolation. Social isolation was found to be significantly associated with occupational dysfunction. Those with occupational dysfunction had a significantly higher rate of social isolation (31.5%) compared to those with healthy occupational function (18.4%). Furthermore, compared with those with healthy occupational function, the adjusted odds ratio for social isolation among those with occupational dysfunction was significantly higher at 1.51. The adjusted odds ratio confirmed that the relationship was independent, even after adjusting for the effect of mental health, which was strongly associated with social isolation. A person is expected to relate to society through occupational participation [28]. As a result, occupational dysfunction is associated with social isolation, such as through having fewer relationships with others in the work-place surroundings. This study had a cross-sectional design and therefore, it is difficult to make a strong statement about causality. However, in a previous study reviewing research on social isolation in the field of occupational therapy, the authors identified the paucity of research focusing on social isolation and called for studies on interventions to prevent social isolation in occupational therapy practice [29]; this study meets this need. The findings suggest that occupational dysfunction needs to be considered when occupational therapists think about the problem of social isolation of older adults in the community. The results of this study may provide occupational therapists and other professionals working in the community with a new perspective on social isolation.

Additionally, the present study examined the relationship between occupational dysfunction type and social isolation and revealed that occupational imbalance, occupational alienation, and occupational marginalization, but not occupational deprivation, were associated with social isolation. Occupational alienation and occupational marginalization had significantly higher odds ratios for social isolation. Hence, it is important to pay particularly careful attention to these two occupational dysfunction types. Therefore, when occupational therapists provide support for older adults in the community, they should not only know the occupation of the individual but also understand how they perceive the "internal needs of the individual" and "evaluation by others" regarding the occupation.

In this study, occupational dysfunction was assessed using the CAOD, which detects conditions caused by overwork. Therefore, a state of poor occupational imbalance, as assessed by CAOD, is considered a busy life rhythm in daily activities. People identifying with this condition may maintain social relationships in their busy life. For example, it is believed a person communicates while working. Therefore, the odds ratio of social isolation was lower for those with a poor occupational imbalance status, which was considered an inversion of the odds ratio. However, a state of occupational imbalance has the potential to cause burnout. In a previous study focusing on medical staff, the relationship between occupational dysfunction and occupational stress was examined [11]. High occupational stress has also been reported to be associated with the incidence of cognitive dysfunction [30]. Therefore, it was necessary to keep in mind that, although occupational imbalance was not negatively related to social isolation, it may negatively affect other health conditions.

The present study did not find any relationship between occupational deprivation and social isolation. This result may relate to potential factors not evaluated in this study. For example, if a place to perform an important occupation is not available in the area of residence, occupational deprivation may be attributed to geographical problems and is unlikely to relate to social isolation. In addition, occupational deprivation could also be influenced by issues affecting mobility, accessibility, and availability. It is necessary to further investigate these factors in the future.

The results of this study need to be interpreted with caution. For instance, if the total CAOD score classifies the person into the occupational dysfunction group, but the scores for occupational alienation and work alienation are low, the results may be difficult to interpret. In order to cope with such cases, it is necessary to conduct research to calculate cutoff values for each type of work dysfunction in the future. On the other hand, there are cases in which the total score of CAOD falls into the healthy occupational function group, but the scores of occupational alienation and occupational alienation are high. In such case, these individuals may be considered as those who are in the healthy occupational function group but are at high risk of social isolation.

This study examines the relationship between occupational dysfunction and social isolation, but it has several limitations. First, the cross-sectional research design does not allow inference of causality. In the future, longitudinal studies should be conducted to examine whether occupational dysfunction causes social isolation. Second, although this study had a sufficient sample size, the final study population was approximately 40% of the total. Because there may be a selection bias between those who responded to the questionnaire and those who did not, it is necessary to increase the response rate in the future. In addition, it is necessary to investigate this issue in other countries and various regions in Japan. Third, this study was conducted using a questionnaire survey method, so the results are based on participants' self-reports. Therefore, there is a possibility of overestimation and underestimation. Fourth, in this study, those with a history of cerebrovascular diseases, dementia, and depression were excluded. Additionally, other medical comorbidities, such as arthritis and cardiovascular diseases, were not taken into account. Future studies are advised to consider these medical conditions due to their possible influence on both occupational dysfunction and social isolation. Despite the above limitations, our findings contribute to the development of public health policies and plans that promote the research and practice of new evidence-based occupational therapy approaches that focus on occupational alienation and marginalization to combat social isolation of community-dwelling older adults.

Occupational therapists utilize occupational participation to assist and empower individuals and populations to attain and/or manage their own physical and psychological health, well-being, and participation [31,32]. In addition, occupational therapists facilitate healthy aging in community dwelling older adults by addressing and promoting their occupational needs [32]. Through the results of this study, occupational therapists who provide support for occupational dysfunction may be able to contribute to the social isolation of older people living in the community. In the future, in addition to conducting longitudinal studies, we need to work on (1) practical research on occupational therapy for the prevention of social isolation and (2) practical research on occupational therapy for the improvement of social isolation.

5. Conclusions

In the present study, the relationship between occupational dysfunction and social isolation was examined in a cross-sectional study. The results showed that occupational dysfunction was significantly associated with social isolation. Furthermore, as a result of examining the relationship between the occupational dysfunction type and social isolation, it was found that occupational imbalance, occupational alienation, and occupational marginalization were significantly associated with social isolation. These results can be used in constructing a support method for social isolation from a new perspective. Further research involving longitudinal studies is needed to investigate causality in detail. In addition, there is a need to conduct intervention studies to prevent social isolation. This study adds to the occupational therapy evidence base and supports the important role and future potential of occupation as a form of intervention to facilitate healthy aging. In particular, supporting healthy occupational participation may be a means of addressing social isolation.

Author Contributions: Conceptualization, K.F.; methodology, K.F. and Y.F.; formal analysis, K.F., Y.F., Y.K., S.W. and T.O.; investigation, K.F., Y.F., K.T., J.L. and K.N.; writing—original draft preparation, K.F.; writing—review and editing, Y.F., Y.K., K.T., J.L., K.N., S.W. and T.O. All authors have read and agreed to the published version of the manuscript.

Funding: This study was supported by the Ministry of Education, Culture, Sports, Science and Technology of Japan, Grant-in-Aid for Young Scientist (18K13035).

Institutional Review Board Statement: The study was conducted according to the guidelines of the Declaration of Helsinki, and approved by the by the Ethical Committee of the University of Tsukuba (Ref No. Tai 019-101).

Informed Consent Statement: We used secondary data obtained from the municipal government. Therefore, informed consent was not required, but as an alternative, the following statement was mailed to the participants. "Some of the results obtained from this survey may be published in academic journals or conferences in collaboration with the University of Tsukuba. No personal information will be disclosed. If you wish to refuse participation, please do not return the questionnaire".

Data Availability Statement: The data that support the findings of this study are available on request from the corresponding author. The data are not publicly available due to privacy or ethical restrictions.

Acknowledgments: We are grateful to the participants and Kasama city officials for their cooperation.

Conflicts of Interest: The authors declare no conflict of interest. The funders had no role in the design of the study; in the collection, analyses, or interpretation of data; in the writing of the manuscript, or in the decision to publish the results.

References

1. Ministry of Health, Labour and Welfare. Summary Report of Comprehensive Survey of Living Conditions 2019. 2019. Available online: https://www.mhlw.go.jp/english/database/db-hss/dl/report_gaikyo_2019.pdf (accessed on 5 June 2021).
2. Nicholson, N.R., Jr. Social isolation in older adults: An evolutionary concept Analysis. *J. Adv. Nurs.* **2009**, *65*, 1342–1352. [CrossRef] [PubMed]
3. Saito, M.; Kondo, K.; Ojima, T.; Hirai, H.; The JAGES Group. Criteria for social isolation based on associations with health indicators among older people. A 10-year follow-up of the Aichi Gerontological Evaluation Study. *Jpn. J. Public Health* **2015**, *62*, 95–105. [CrossRef]
4. Courtin, E.; Knapp, M. Social isolation, loneliness and health in old age: A scoping review. *Health Soc. Care Community* **2017**, *25*, 799–812. [CrossRef]
5. Kuiper, J.S.; Zuidersma, M.; Oude Voshaar, R.C.; Zuidema, S.U.; van den Heuvel, E.R.; Stolk, R.P.; Smidt, N. Social relationships and risk of dementia: A systematic review and meta-analysis of longitudinal cohort studies. *Ageing Res. Rev.* **2015**, *22*, 39–57. [CrossRef] [PubMed]
6. Holt-Lunstad, J.; Smith, T.B.; Baker, M.; Harris, T.; Stephenson, D. Loneliness and social isolation as risk factors for mortality: A meta-analytic review. *Perspect. Psychol. Sci.* **2015**, *10*, 227–237. [CrossRef]
7. Steptoe, A.; Shankar, A.; Demakakos, P.; Wardle, J. Social isolation, loneliness, and all-cause mortality in older men and women. *Proc. Natl. Acad. Sci. USA* **2013**, *110*, 5797–5801. [CrossRef]
8. Miyake, Y.; Eguchi, E.; Ito, H.; Nakamura, K.; Ito, T.; Nagaoka, K.; Ogino, N.; Ogino, K. Association between occupational dysfunction and metabolic syndrome in community-dwelling Japanese adults in a cross-sectional study: Ibara Study. *Int. J. Environ. Res. Public Health* **2018**, *15*, 2575. [CrossRef]
9. Kielhofner, G.; Braveman, B.; Baron, K.; Fisher, G.; Hammel, J.; Littleton, M. The model of human occupation: Understanding the worker who is injured or disabled. *Work* **1999**, *12*, 37–45.
10. Teraoka, M.; Kyougoku, M. Development of the final version of the Classification and Assessment of Occupational Dysfunction Scale. *PLoS ONE* **2015**, *10*, e0134695. [CrossRef]
11. Townsend, E.; Wilcock, A.A. Occupational justice and client-centred practice: A dialogue in progress. *Can. J. Occup. Ther.* **2004**, *71*, 75–87. [CrossRef]

12. Anaby, D.; Jarus, T.; Backman, C.L.; Zumbo, B.D. The role of occupational characteristics and occupational imbalance in explaining well-being. *Appl. Res. Qual. Life* **2010**, *5*, 81–104. [CrossRef]
13. Bryant, W.; Craik, C.; McKay, E.A. Living in a glasshouse: Exploring occupational alienation. *Can. J. Occup. Ther.* **2004**, *71*, 282–289. [CrossRef]
14. Whiteford, G. Occupational deprivation: Global challenge in the new millennium. *Br. J. Occup. Ther.* **2000**, *63*, 200–204. [CrossRef]
15. Teraoka, M.; Kyougoku, M. Analysis of structural relationship among the occupational dysfunction on the psychological problem in healthcare workers: A study using structural equation modeling. *PeerJ* **2015**, *19*, e1389. [CrossRef]
16. Morohoshi, N.; Kyougoku, M. Analysis of structural relationships among occupational challenge, occupational participation, occupational dysfunction, depression, and health-related qol in community dwelling elderly with physical disabilities. *Jpn. Occup. Ther. Res.* **2019**, *38*, 294–303.
17. Ge, L.; Yap, C.W.; Ong, R.; Heng, B.H. Social isolation, loneliness and their relationships with depressive symptoms: A population-based study. *PLoS ONE* **2017**, *12*, e0182145. [CrossRef] [PubMed]
18. Hawton, A.; Green, C.; Dickens, A.P.; Richards, S.H.; Taylor, R.S.; Edwards, R.; Greaves, C.J.; Campbell, J.L. The impact of social isolation on the health status and health-related quality of life of older people. *Qual. Life Res.* **2011**, *20*, 57–67. [CrossRef] [PubMed]
19. Matthews, T.; Danese, A.; Wertz, J.; Odgers, C.L.; Ambler, A.; Moffitt, T.E.; Arseneault, L. Social isolation, loneliness and depression in young adulthood: A behavioural genetic analysis. *Soc. Psychiatry Psychiatr. Epidemiol.* **2016**, *51*, 339–348. [CrossRef] [PubMed]
20. Papageorgiou, N.; Marquis, R.; Dare, J.; Batten, R. Occupational Therapy and Occupational Participation in Community Dwelling Older Adults: A Review of the Evidence. *Phys. Occup. Ther. Geriatr.* **2016**, *34*, 21–42. [CrossRef]
21. Government of Kasama City. Statistical Information of Kasama City. 2018. Available online: https://www.city.kasama.lg.jp/data/doc/1547708244_doc_81_0.pdf (accessed on 16 April 2021).
22. Furukawa, T.A.; Kawakami, N.; Saitoh, M.; Ono, Y.; Nakane, Y.; Nakamura, Y.; Tachimori, H.; Iwata, N.; Uda, H.; Nakane, H.; et al. The performance of the Japanese version of the K6 and K10 in the World Mental Health Survey Japan. *Int. J. Methods Psychiatr. Res.* **2008**, *17*, 152–158. [CrossRef]
23. Kessler, R.C.; Andrews, G.; Colpe, L.J.; Hiripi, E.; Mroczek, D.K.; Normand, S.L.; Walters, E.E.; Zaslavsky, A.M. Short screening scales to monitor population prevalences and trends in non-specific psychological distress. *Psychol. Med.* **2002**, *32*, 959–976. [CrossRef]
24. Tomioka, K.; Kurumatani, N.; Hosoi, H. Association between social participation and 3-year change in instrumental activities of daily living in community-dwelling elderly adults. *J. Am. Geriatr. Soc.* **2017**, *65*, 107–113. [CrossRef]
25. Tomioka, K.; Kurumatani, N.; Saeki, K. The differential effects of type and frequency of social participation on IADL declines of older people. *PLoS ONE* **2018**, *13*, e0207426. [CrossRef] [PubMed]
26. Koyano, W.; Shibata, H.; Nakazato, K.; Haga, H.; Suyama, Y. Measurement of competence in the elderly living at home: Development of an index of competence. *Nippon Koshu Eisei Zasshi* **1987**, *34*, 109–114.
27. Lubben, J.; Blozik, E.; Gillmann, G.; Iliffe, S.; von Renteln Kruse, W.; Beck, J.C.; Stuck, A.E. Performance of an abbreviated version of the lubben social network scale among three european community-dwelling older adult populations. *Gerontologist* **2006**, *46*, 503–513. [CrossRef] [PubMed]
28. Larsson-Lund, M.; Nyman, A. Participation and occupation in occupational therapy models of practice: A discussion of possibilities and challenges. *Scand. J. Occup. Ther.* **2017**, *24*, 393–397. [CrossRef] [PubMed]
29. Collins, T.; Davys, D.; Martin, R.; Russell, R.; Kenney, C. Occupational therapy, loneliness and social isolation: A thematic review of the literature. *Int. J. Ther. Rehabil.* **2020**, *27*, 1–23. [CrossRef]
30. Giorgi, G.; Lecca, L.I.; Leon-Perez, J.M.; Pignata, S.; Topa, G.; Mucci, N. Emerging Issues in Occupational Disease: Mental Health in the Aging Working Population and Cognitive Impairment—A Narrative Review. *Biomed. Res. Int.* **2020**, *2020*, 1742123. [CrossRef]
31. American Occupational Therapy Association [AOTA]. Occupational therapy practice framework: Domain and process (3rd ed.). *Am. J. Occup. Ther.* **2014**, *68*, S1–S48. [CrossRef]
32. Stav, W.B.; Hallenen, T.; Lane, J.; Arbesman, M. Systematic review of occupational engagement and health outcomes among community-dwelling older adults. *Am. J. Occup. Ther.* **2012**, *66*, 301–310. [CrossRef]

Article

The Significance of Posterior Occlusal Support of Teeth and Removable Prostheses in Oral Functions and Standing Motion

Kyosuke Oki [1], Yoichiro Ogino [1,*], Yuriko Takamoto [2], Mikio Imai [3], Yoko Takemura [3], Yasunori Ayukawa [1,3] and Kiyoshi Koyano [4]

1. Section of Fixed Prosthodontics, Division of Oral Rehabilitation, Faculty of Dental Science, Kyushu University, Fukuoka 812-8582, Japan; o-ki@dent.kyushu-u.ac.jp (K.O.); ayukawa@dent.kyushu-u.ac.jp (Y.A.)
2. Department of Dentistry, School of Dentistry, Kyushu University, Fukuoka 812-8582, Japan; takamoto.yuriko.997@s.kyushu-u.ac.jp
3. Section of Implant and Rehabilitative Dentistry, Division of Oral Rehabilitation, Faculty of Dental Science, Kyushu University, Fukuoka 812-8582, Japan; mikio@dent.kyushu-u.ac.jp (M.I.); tomitay0804@dent.kyushu-u.ac.jp (Y.T.)
4. Division of Advanced Dental Devices and Therapeutics, Faculty of Dental Science, Kyushu University, Fukuoka 812-8582, Japan; koyano@dent.kyushu-u.ac.jp
* Correspondence: ogino@dent.kyushu-u.ac.jp; Tel.: +81-92-642-6371

Abstract: The purpose of this study was to evaluate the effect of posterior occlusal support of natural teeth and artificial teeth on oral functions and standing motion. Patients who had been treated with removable prostheses were enrolled as the subjects. Their systemic conditions (body mass index (BMI) and skeletal muscle mass index (SMI)) were recorded. The subjects were classified into two groups according to a modified Eichner index: B1–3 (with posterior occlusal support) and B4C (without posterior occlusal support). Maximum occlusal force (MOF), masticatory performance (MP), and standing motion (sway and strength) were evaluated for cases with and without removable prostheses. There were no significant differences in BMI and SMI between the B1–3 group and the B4C group. The subjects with removable prostheses demonstrated significantly higher values in MOF, MP, and sway and strength than the subjects without removable prostheses. The comparison of oral functions between the B1–3 group and the B4C group revealed that the positive effect of posterior occlusal support of natural teeth and removable prostheses and the significant positive effects of posterior occlusal support on standing motion were partly observed in these comparisons. Posterior occlusal support of natural teeth and even of removable prostheses may contribute to the enhancement of oral functions and standing motion.

Keywords: posterior occlusal support; maximum occlusal force; masticatory function; standing motion; removable prostheses; Eichner index

1. Introduction

One of the main causes of disability in the elderly is an accidental fall [1,2]. Falling is a severe problem for the elderly because it results in musculoskeletal injuries, brain injuries, and death in serious circumstances [3,4]. Multiple factors such as aging or aging-related physical dysfunctions, medication, cognitive impairment, and sensory deficits are well known as risk factors contributing to falls in the elderly [2,5–7]. Aging-related physical dysfunctions are inextricably associated with frailty and sarcopenia [8,9]. A decline in muscle mass and function due to the aging-related muscle atrophy is a characteristic feature of sarcopenia and is likely a cause of frailty [8–11]. One's nutritional condition is closely related to muscle and bone aging, and good nutrition and physical exercise may be protective against frailty and sarcopenia [11–14].

Mastication and deglutition play crucial roles in nutritional management [15]. Healthy teeth, oral tissues including the tongue, and well-functioned prostheses are prerequisites for these functions. It has been reported that these functions are also impaired by aging and poor oral management, known as oral frailty, oral sarcopenia, and oral hypofunction [16–20]. The adverse effects of a decline of these functions on systemic and nutritional status have been reported [15–22]. Conversely, occlusal support is also important in oral functions, especially mastication [23–26]. This suggests that rehabilitation of occlusal support contributes to the prevention of frailty and sarcopenia indirectly. This suggestion may imply that rehabilitation of occlusal support has a positive effect on the prevention of accidental falls through the rehabilitation of mastication and nutritional status. Recent observational studies also demonstrated the association between occlusal support and physical function [27–32]. However, comparative studies that evaluate the effect of occlusal support and its rehabilitation on physical functions are still scarce.

The present study aimed to evaluate the effect of posterior occlusal support on standing motion and oral functions in the elderly. The subjects were categorized according to the presence or absence of posterior occlusal support of natural teeth and functional crowns (pontics), and oral functions and standing motion were compared between subjects with and without posterior occlusal support. In addition, the effects of posterior occlusal rehabilitation with removable prostheses on oral functions and standing motion were evaluated. The null hypotheses of this study were that there are no differences in oral functions and standing motion between subjects with and without occlusal support and between subjects with and without removable prostheses.

2. Materials and Methods

2.1. Ethical Approval

The protocol of the present study was developed in accordance with the ethical principles of the Declaration of Helsinki and was approved by our Institutional Review Board for Clinical Research (#2019-167). Patients who participated and provided written informed consent were enrolled as subjects.

2.2. Study Population

The patients who visited the Department of Prosthodontics, Kyushu University Hospital, between April 2019 and February 2020 were considered for enrollment as subjects of this study. The inclusion criteria of the present study were as follows: (1) patients who were more than 65 years old; (2) patients whose activities of daily living (ADL) were almost normal; and (3) patients who were rehabilitated with conventional removable prostheses by the Department of Prosthodontics, Kyushu University Hospital, and who could use their dentures without any specific problems. Thus, subjects were categorized into the groups Eichner B or C according to the original Eichner index. The exclusion criteria were as follows: (1) patients with systemic and/or localized diseases and medications that affect physical functions and with oral diseases that affect masticatory functions; (2) patients who could not understand the aim of this study due to cognitive impairment, etc.; and (3) patients with fixed prostheses supported by implants, implant-assisted partial removable dentures, or implant overdentures. As a result, this study's subjects included 48 patients (21 males and 27 females, median age: 73, and interquartile range (IQR): 70–79).

The subjects were classified into two groups according to the Eichner index with our modifications [23,24,26]. The Eichner index was defined as follows: number of residual teeth was defined as the number of functional tooth crowns. Thus, pontics in fixed partial dentures were counted as residual teeth and remaining roots were excluded. Based on functional teeth and occlusal contacts, the subjects were classified into two groups. The first group included 24 subjects (11 males and 13 females, median age: 73, and IQR: 70–78) who had posterior occlusal support in the molar and/or premolar regions (Eichner B1, B2, and B3: B1–3 group). The second group included 24 subjects (10 males and 14 females, median age: 73, and IQR: 70–79) who had no posterior occlusal support (Eichner B4, C1, C2, and C3: B4C group).

2.3. Patient Profiles

In addition to age, gender, and the Eichner index, body mass index (BMI) for the degree of obesity (a risk factor for falls [33]) and skeletal muscle mass index (SMI) for the prevalence of sarcopenia [34,35] were calculated using the multi-frequency body composition meter (MC–780A, TANITA Corp., Tokyo, Japan) (Figure 1).

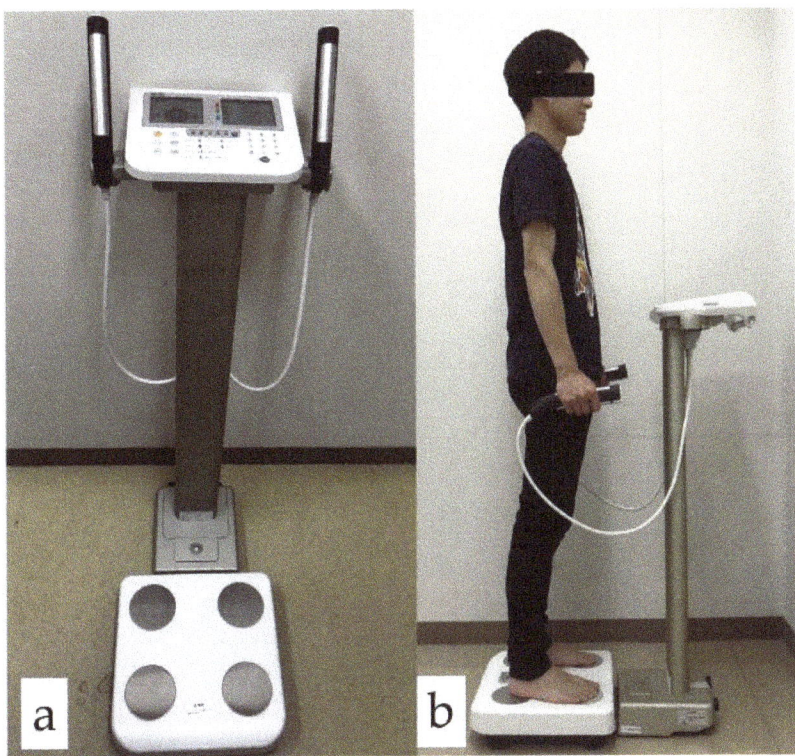

Figure 1. Measurement device (MC–780A) for the skeletal muscle mass index (SMI): (**a**) main unit; (**b**) measurement image.

2.4. Measurements of Oral Function

2.4.1. Maximum Occlusal Force (MOF)

The MOF was measured using a film for the occlusal force measurement system (Dental Prescale II and bite force analyzer, GC Co., Tokyo, Japan) (Figure 2) [18,20,23,24,26]. The subjects were asked to clench the film in the intercuspal position for 3 s. The clenched film was scanned by using the occlusal force analysis software to determine the MOF.

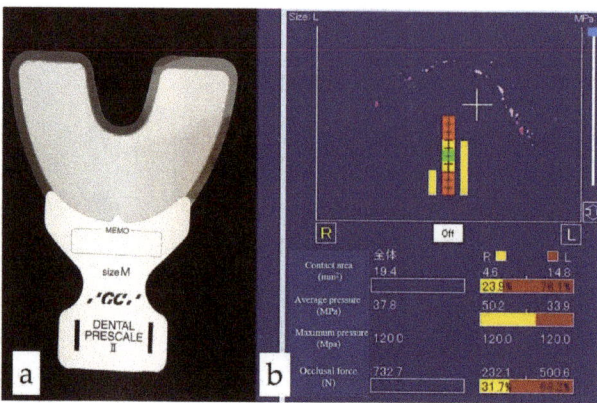

Figure 2. Occlusal force measurement system: (**a**) pressure-sensitive sheet (Dental Prescale II); (**b**) image of occlusal condition using software (bite force analyzer).

2.4.2. Masticatory Performance (MP)

The MP was measured in the manner previous studies utilized to evaluate results [23–26]. In brief, the patients were instructed to voluntarily chew 2 g of gummy jelly for 20 s. The chewed gummy jelly was then moved to a cup with saliva and rinsing water, and the concentration of glucose dissolved in water was measured using a measuring device (Gluco Sensor GS–II, GC Co., Tokyo, Japan) (Figure 3).

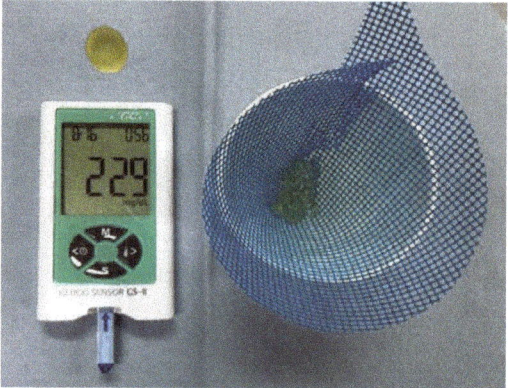

Figure 3. Masticatory performance (MP) measurement system (Gluco Sensor GS–II). The concentration of glucose from the chewed gummy jelly was defined as MP.

2.5. Analyses of Standing Motion

To evaluate physical activity, muscle functions during the action of standing up were analyzed using a motor function analyzer (zaRitz BM–220, TANITA Corp., Tokyo, Japan) according to the manufacturer instructions. In brief, the subjects were asked to sit on a chair with their feet on the analyzer. The subjects stood up quickly, paused for 3 s, and sat down again. The subjects repeated this motion 3 times with and without their removable prostheses. The analyzer could evaluate sway and strength [36]. Sway is an index combining the degree of motion when standing up and the time until the shaking stops, while strength is an index combining leg muscle strength and standing speed (Figure 4).

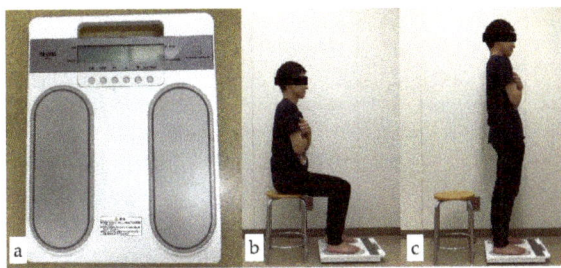

Figure 4. Motor function analyzer (zaRitz BM-220): (**a**) main unit; (**b**) measurement image (the beginning of analysis); (**c**) measurement image (motor function measurement after standing up).

2.6. Statistical Analyses

Numerical data were presented as the median and IQR and demonstrated as a box plot. The statistical analyses were conducted with the statistical package IBM SPSS Statistics 19 software (IBM Corp., Chicago, IL, USA).

The profiles of the subjects (age, BMI, and SMI) were statistically compared between the B1–3 group and the B4C group using the Mann–Whitney U test. To evaluate the effect of removable prostheses on oral functions and standing motion, the measurement items (MOF, MP, and sway and strength) in all subjects and in each group (B1–3 group and B4C group) were statistically compared between the values of those with and without their removable prostheses using the Wilcoxon signed-rank test. To evaluate the effect of posterior occlusal support on oral functions and standing motion, these measurement items were also compared between the B1–3 group and the B4C group using the Mann–Whitney U test. These comparisons were performed in the presence and absence of their removable prostheses. A value of less than 0.05 was considered statistically significant.

3. Results

3.1. Profiles of the Subjects

The profiles of the subjects are shown in Table 1 including the data of age and number of patients. There were no significant differences between the B1–3 group and the B4C group in all items ($p > 0.05$, Mann–Whitney U test). All subjects demonstrated normal ADL, although some patients were defined as underweight (one male and four females) or overweight (six males and nine females) according to the BMI results and the condition of sarcopenia (two males and five females) from the SMI results.

Table 1. Summary of subjects' profiles; IQR: interquartile range; BMI: body mass index; SMI: skeletal muscle mass index. Statistical analyses: B1–3 group vs. B4C group ($p > 0.05$, Mann–Whitney U test in all items).

		All Subjects n = 48	B1–3 Group n = 24	B4C Group n = 24
Age (median and IQR)		73 (70–79)	73 (70–78)	73 (70–79)
Gender (male and female)		21:27	11:13	10:14
BMI (median and IQR)	All	23.1 (20.8–26.4)	22.4 (20.8–25.2)	23.5 (20.6–26.4)
	Male	23.5 (21.5–25.2)	23.2 (21.5–24.7)	24.1 (21.6–25.9)
	Female	22.3 (20.4–26.7)	22.2 (19–26.19)	23.1 (20.6–26.9)
SMI (median and IQR)	All	6.6 (6.1–7.7)	6.5 (6–7.1)	6.6 (6.1–7.7)
	Male	7.8 (7.0–8.5)	7.8 (7.4–8.6)	7.6 (6.6–8.4)
	Female	6.4 (5.9–7.0)	6.5 (5.9–7.2)	6.3 (5.8–6.6)

3.2. Comparisons of Oral Functions and Standing Motion in All Subjects with and without Removable Prostheses

The MOF and MP with and without removable prostheses were compared in all subjects (Figure 5). There were significant differences in both items between subjects with and without their removable prostheses ($p < 0.01$, Wilcoxon signed-rank test), indicating that rehabilitation of posterior occlusal support with removable prostheses could improve MOF and MP.

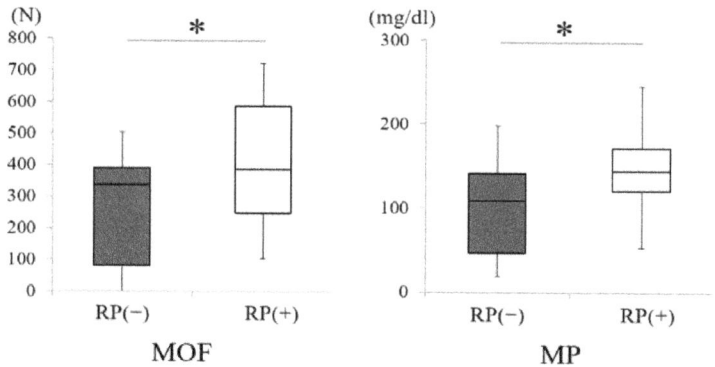

Figure 5. Comparisons of maximum occlusal force and masticatory performance between all subjects with and without removable prostheses. (* $p < 0.01$, Wilcoxon signed-rank test) RP (−)): subjects without removable prostheses; RP (+): subjects with removable prostheses.

The results of standing motion analyses including strength and sway in all subjects with and without their removable prostheses are shown in Figure 6. There were significant differences in strength and sway between those with and without dentures ($p < 0.05$, Wilcoxon signed-rank test).

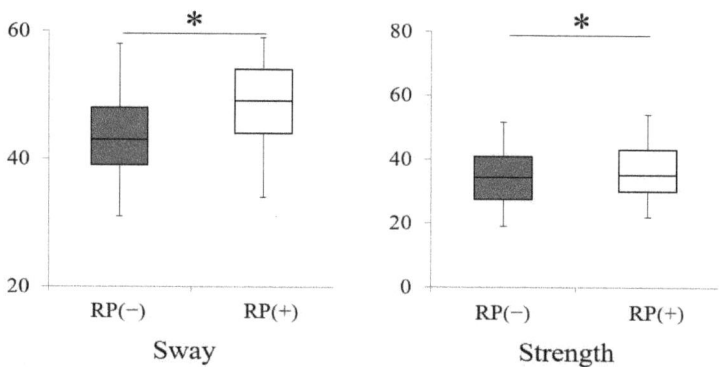

Figure 6. Comparisons of standing motion (sway and strength) between all subjects with and without removable prostheses. (* $p < 0.05$, Wilcoxon signed-rank test) RP (−): subjects without removable prostheses; RP (+): subjects with removable prostheses.

3.3. Comparisons of Oral Functions and Standing Motion between the B1–3 Group and the B4C Group with and without Removable Prostheses

The MOF and MP without removable prostheses were statistically compared between the B1–3 group and the B4C group. Compared with the B4C group, the B1–3 group exhibited significantly higher values in MOF and MP ($p < 0.01$, Mann–Whitney U test) (Figure 7). The MOF and MP with removable prostheses were also compared between the B1–3 group and the B4C group, and the subjects belonging to the B1–3 group exhibited statistically higher values in both functions compared to the subjects in the B4C group ($p < 0.05$, Mann–Whitney U test) (Figure 7). These findings suggest the significance of posterior occlusal support in both oral functions.

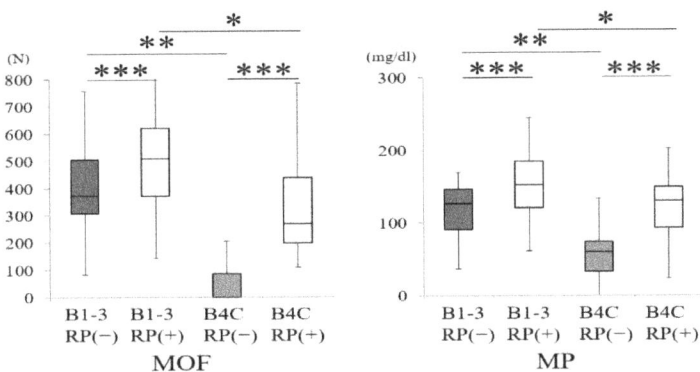

Figure 7. Comparisons of maximum occlusal force and masticatory performance between the B1–3 group and the B4C group with or without removable prostheses in each group (* $p < 0.05$, ** $p < 0.01$, Mann–Whitney U test). Comparisons of maximum occlusal force and masticatory performance between subjects with and without removable prostheses in each group (B1–3 group or B4C group) (*** $p < 0.01$, Wilcoxon signed-rank test). RP (−): subjects without removable prostheses; RP (+): subjects with removable prostheses.

The results of the standing motion analyses with and without removable prostheses are shown in Figure 4. The subjects without removable prostheses in the B1–3 group exhibited significantly higher (better) values in sway than the subjects did without removable prostheses in the B4C group ($p < 0.05$, Mann–Whitney U test), although other comparisons (B1–3 vs. B4C in strength with and without removable prostheses, and B1–3 vs. B4C in sway with removable prostheses) did not detect significant differences ($p > 0.05$, Mann–Whitney U test) (Figure 8).

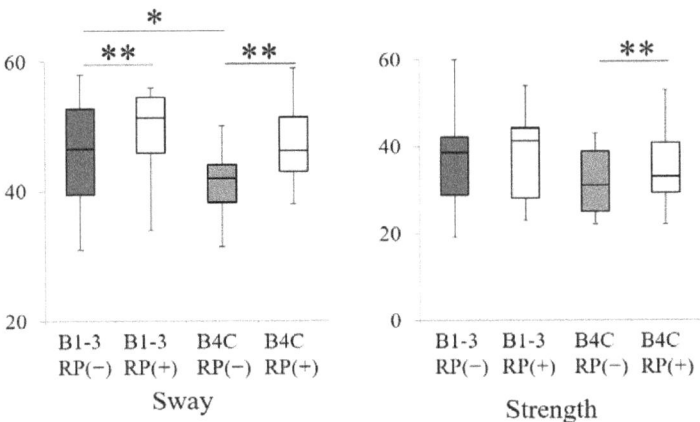

Figure 8. Comparisons of standing motion (sway and strength) between the B1–3 group and the B4C group with or without removable prostheses in each group (* $p < 0.05$, Mann–Whitney U test). Comparisons of standing motion (sway and strength) between subjects with and without removable prostheses in each group (B1–3 group or B4C group) (** $p < 0.05$, Wilcoxon signed-rank test). RP (+): subjects with removable prostheses; RP (−): subjects without removable prostheses.

4. Discussion

It has been reported that poor oral health is closely associated with adverse health outcomes [16,20,21]. Malnutrition is attributed to poor oral status and function [15,22], resulting in sarcopenia and physical frailty [11–14]. Malnutrition has been considered the indirect effect of poor oral health on systemic condition. Several studies demonstrated the direct effect of oral functions on physical condition [37,38]. Above all, the effect of occlusal support on physical condition has been reported [27–32]. However, these studies were conducted as observational studies. The present study evaluated the effect of posterior occlusal support and rehabilitation with removable prostheses on standing motion in the elderly as a comparative study.

The BMI and SMI of the subjects in the present study are shown in Table 1. No significant differences in BMI and SMI between the B1–3 group and the B4C group were observed. All subjects demonstrated normal ADL, although some patients were defined as underweight or overweight and had sarcopenia. These factors might be confounding factors in this study. Comparisons based on the classification by BMI and SMI were not performed because of the limited number of subjects. Future studies that focus on both factors and occlusal support are advised to use more subjects.

Oral functions (MOF and MP) were enhanced in subjects with removable prostheses compared to subjects without removable prostheses (Figures 1 and 3). In addition, the subjects with posterior occlusal support exhibited statistically higher MOF and MP values than the subjects without posterior occlusal support ($p < 0.001$, Mann–Whitney U test) and significant differences were detected when comparing both functions between both subjects with removable prostheses ($p < 0.05$, Mann–Whitney U test) (Figure 3). These findings clearly demonstrate that posterior occlusal support is strongly related to MOF and MP and that rehabilitation with removable prostheses contributes to the recovery or improvement of MOF and MP. The previous studies demonstrated similar results and provided more detailed data [23–26]. It is concluded that posterior occlusal support, even when reconstructed with removable prostheses, can play a crucial role in MOF and MP. Furthermore, based on the findings of the previous studies that demonstrated improvements in MOF and MP with removable prostheses [23–26], it is suggested that removable prostheses in this study works well in oral rehabilitation.

Our results confirmed that rehabilitation of posterior occlusal support with removable prostheses could improve standing motion (sway and strength) (Figure 2). Although the values measured by this device were novel and may lack scientific evidence, the measurement was very simple and an objective assessment considered it possible [36]. While we recognize the weak aspects of the measurements in this study, a significant difference of sway between the B1–3 group and the B4C group without removable prostheses suggests that posterior occlusal support is partly associated with standing motion (Figure 4). Furthermore, sway and strength with removable prostheses were statistically greater that those without removable prostheses, except for strength in the B1–3 group (Figure 4). These results also suggest that the rehabilitation of posterior occlusal support with removable prostheses can contribute to the improvement of standing motion; this effect was more striking in the B4C group in which subjects had no posterior occlusal support. Some discussions regarding the association between physical functions, especially balance (sway in this study), and posterior occlusal support have been reported [39,40]. These suggest plausible evidence for the masticatory and cervical muscles and that afferent signals from dental occlusion may be effective for balance control. These are related to the stability of the jaw position and occlusal support, and the rehabilitation with removable prostheses may also contribute to stability, resulting in improvements in standing motion. A previous study reported the contribution of occlusal support by artificial teeth to improve health and oral function [28]. The present study revealed that standing motion was improved by rehabilitation with removable prostheses and suggests an enhancement of physical functions, although further studies are required to elucidate this hypothesis.

The important issues in the present study are stated as follows. First, the subjects in this study were categorized based on their BMI and SMI, as described above, although they were all healthy and demonstrated normal ADL. It has been reported that these factors may be related to physical functions. Although our statistical analyses illustrated no significant differences between the B1–3 group and the B4C group, future studies will be expected to investigate the effects of occlusal support and these indexes on physical functions with more subjects. Second, there are various methods to assess physical functions [27–31]. The focuses of this study were oral function (MOF and MP) and standing motion (sway and strength), and the results revealed the effect of posterior occlusal support on a portion of physical functions. The background of falls was described previously; however, it is impossible to describe the effect of posterior occlusal support on the prevention of falls.

Lastly, there may be multiple confounding factors that affect the results of this study. The previous study mentioned systemic disease, medicine, and habits as potential confounding factors [31]. more subjects are required to investigate the association of factors such as BMI and SMI with physical function. In addition, the effect of rehabilitation with RPD or the strength of occlusal support with RPD may be different depending on teeth distribution (intermediate or free-end partial edentulism). Furthermore, the number of subjects in this study was limited, as mentioned in the inclusion and exclusion criteria, and it was difficult to calculate the sample size due to the lack of previous studies similar to the present study, unfortunately. However, we believe that this study demonstrated the positive effect of posterior occlusal support of natural teeth and removable prostheses on standing motion and suggests the importance of maintaining healthy teeth and encouraging prosthetic intervention from the viewpoint of physical function.

5. Conclusions

Prosthetic rehabilitation through removable prostheses could improve oral functions (MOF and MP) significantly. Moreover, the results of the present study clearly rejected our null hypotheses that there are no differences in standing motion between subjects with and without occlusal support of natural teeth and between subjects with and without removable denture rehabilitation. However, there are multiple confounding factors including BMI and SMI, and future studies with more subjects are necessary to classify the subjects based on these factors for further evaluations.

Author Contributions: Conceptualization, K.O.; methodology, K.O., M.I. and Y.T. (Yoko Takemura); software, K.O., Y.T. (Yuriko Takamoto), and M.I.; validation, Y.O.; formal analysis, K.O.; investigation, K.O., Y.T. (Yuriko Takamoto), M.I. and Y.T. (Yoko Takemura); resources, K.O. and K.K.; data curation, Y.O.; writing—original draft preparation, K.O. and Y.O.; writing—review and editing, Y.A. and K.K.; visualization, K.O. and Y.O.; supervision, K.K.; project administration, K.O. and Y.A.; funding acquisition, K.K. All authors have read and agreed to the published version of the manuscript.

Funding: This research received no external funding.

Institutional Review Board Statement: The study was conducted according to the guidelines of the Declaration of Helsinki and approved by the Institutional Review Board of the Kyushu University Hospital (#2019-167 and 28 June 2019).

Informed Consent Statement: Informed consent was obtained from all subjects involved in the study.

Data Availability Statement: The datasets used and/or analyzed during the current study are available from the corresponding author upon reasonable request.

Acknowledgments: The authors would like to express our gratitude to Ken Matsunaka, Chiaki Ookawa, and Norifumi Suetsugi for their assistance in data collection.

Conflicts of Interest: The authors declare no conflict of interest.

References

1. Hopewell, S.; Adedire, O.; Copsey, B.J.; Boniface, G.J.; Sherrington, C.; Clemson, L.; Close, J.C.; Lamb, S.E. Multifactorial and multiple component interventions for preventing falls in older people living in the community. *Cochrane Database Syst. Rev.* **2018**, *7*, CD012221. [CrossRef]
2. Gawrońska, K.; Lorkowski, J. Falls, Aging and Public Health-a Literature Review. *J. Ortop. Traumatol. Rehabil.* **2020**, *22*, 397–408. [CrossRef] [PubMed]
3. Ambrose, A.F.; Paul, G.; Hausdorff, J.M. Risk factors for falls among older adults: A review of the literature. *Maturitas* **2013**, *75*, 51–61. [CrossRef] [PubMed]
4. Hill, A.M.; McPhail, S.M.; Waldron, N.; Etherton-Beer, C.; Ingram, K.; Flicker, L.; Bulsara, M.; Haines, T.P. Fall rates in hospital rehabilitation units after individualised patient and staff education programmes: A pragmatic, stepped-wedge, cluster-randomised controlled trial. *Lancet* **2015**, *385*, 2592–2599. [CrossRef]
5. Barker, A.L.; Nitz, J.C.; Choy, N.L.L.; Haines, T.P. Mobility has a non-linear association with falls risk among people in residential aged care: An Fobservational study. *J. Physiother.* **2012**, *58*, 117–125. [CrossRef]
6. Morley, J.E.; Vellas, B.; van Kan, G.A.; Anker, S.D.; Bauer, J.M.; Bernabei, R.; Cesari, M.; Chumlea, W.C.; Doehner, W.; Evans, J.; et al. Frailty consensus: A call to action. *J. Am. Med. Dir. Assoc.* **2013**, *14*, 392–397. [CrossRef]
7. Li, F.; Harmer, P. Prevalence of Falls, Physical Performance, and Dual-Task Cost While Walking in Older Adults at High Risk of Falling with and Without Cognitive Impairment. *Clin. Interv. Aging* **2020**, *15*, 945–952. [CrossRef]
8. Fhon, J.R.; Rodrigues, R.A.; Neira, W.F.; Huayta, V.M.; Robazzi, M.L. Fall and its association with the frailty syndrome in the elderly: Systematic review with meta-analysis. *Rev. Esc. Enferm. USP* **2016**, *50*, 1005–1013. [CrossRef] [PubMed]
9. Larsson, L.; Degens, H.; Li, M.; Salviati, L.; Lee, Y.I.; Thompson, W.; Kirkland, J.L.; Sandri, M. Sarcopenia: Aging-Related Loss of Muscle Mass and Function. *Physiol. Rev.* **2019**, *99*, 427–511. [CrossRef]
10. Cruz-Jentoft, A.J.; Bahat, G.; Bauer, J.; Boirie, Y.; Bruyère, O.; Cederholm, T.; Cooper, C.; Landi, F.; Rolland, Y.; Sayer, A.A.; et al. Sarcopenia: Revised European consensus on definition and diagnosis. *Age Ageing.* **2019**, *48*, 601. [CrossRef]
11. Welch, A.A. Nutritional influences on age-related skeletal muscle loss. *Proc. Nutr. Soc.* **2014**, *73*, 16–33. [CrossRef] [PubMed]
12. Brook, M.S.; Wilkinson, D.J.; Phillips, B.E.; Perez-Schindler, J.; Philp, A.; Smith, K.; Atherton, P.J. Skeletal muscle homeostasis and plasticity in youth and ageing: Impact of nutrition and exercise. *Acta Physiol.* **2016**, *216*, 15–41. [CrossRef]
13. Bloom, I.; Shand, C.; Cooper, C.; Robinson, S.; Baird, J. Diet Quality and Sarcopenia in Older Adults: A Systematic Review. *Nutrients* **2018**, *10*, 308. [CrossRef] [PubMed]
14. Kiuchi, Y.; Makizako, H.; Nakai, Y.; Tomioka, K.; Taniguchi, Y.; Kimura, M.; Kanouchi, H.; Takenaka, T.; Kubozono, T.; Ohishi, M. The Association between Dietary Variety and Physical Frailty in Community-Dwelling Older Adults. *Healthcare* **2021**, *9*, 32. [CrossRef] [PubMed]
15. Mann, T.; Heuberger, R.; Wong, H. The association between chewing and swallowing difficulties and nutritional status in older adults. *Aust. Dent. J.* **2013**, *58*, 200–206. [CrossRef] [PubMed]
16. Tanaka, T.; Takahashi, K.; Hirano, H.; Kikutani, T.; Watanabe, Y.; Ohara, Y.; Furuya, H.; Tetsuo, T.; Akishita, M.; Iijima, K. Oral Frailty as a Risk Factor for Physical Frailty and Mortality in Community-Dwelling Elderly. *J. Gerontol. A Biol. Sci. Med. Sci.* **2018**, *73*, 1661–1667. [CrossRef]
17. Shiraishi, A.; Yoshimura, Y.; Wakabayashi, H.; Tsuji, Y. Prevalence of stroke-related sarcopenia and its association with poor oral status in post-acute stroke patients: Implications for oral sarcopenia. *Clin. Nutr.* **2018**, *37*, 204–207. [CrossRef]
18. Minakuchi, S.; Tsuga, K.; Ikebe, K.; Ueda, T.; Tamura, F.; Nagao, K.; Furuya, J.; Matsuo, K.; Yamamoto, K.; Kanazawa, M.; et al. Oral hypofunction in the older population: Position paper of the Japanese Society of Gerodontology in 2016. *Gerodontology* **2018**, *35*, 317–324. [CrossRef] [PubMed]
19. Shiraishi, A.; Wakabayashi, H.; Yoshimura, Y. Oral Management in Rehabilitation Medicine: Oral Frailty, Oral Sarcopenia, and Hospital-Associated Oral Problems. *J. Nutr. Health Aging* **2020**, *24*, 1094–1099. [CrossRef]
20. Shimazaki, Y.; Nonoyama, T.; Tsushita, K.; Arai, H.; Matsushita, K.; Uchibori, N. Oral hypofunction and its association with frailty in community-dwelling older people. *Geriatr. Gerontol. Int.* **2020**, *20*, 917–926. [CrossRef]
21. Watanabe, D.; Yoshida, T.; Yokoyama, K.; Yoshinaka, Y.; Watanabe, Y.; Kikutani, T.; Yoshida, M.; Yamada, Y.; Kimura, M. Kyoto-Kameoka Study Group. Association between Mixing Ability of Masticatory Functions Measured Using Color-Changing Chewing Gum and Frailty among Japanese Older Adults: The Kyoto-Kameoka Study. *Int. J. Environ. Res. Public Health* **2020**, *17*, 4555. [CrossRef] [PubMed]
22. Iwasaki, M.; Motokawa, K.; Watanabe, Y.; Shirobe, M.; Inagaki, H.; Edahiro, A.; Ohara, Y.; Hirano, H.; Shinkai, S.; Awata, S. A Two-Year Longitudinal Study of the Association between Oral Frailty and Deteriorating Nutritional Status among Community-Dwelling Older Adults. *Int. J. Environ. Res. Public Health* **2020**, *18*, 213. [CrossRef] [PubMed]
23. Ikebe, K.; Matsuda, K.; Murai, S.; Maeda, Y.; Nokubi, T. Validation of the Eichner index in relation to occlusal force and masticatory performance. *Int. J. Prosthodont.* **2010**, *23*, 521–524.
24. Kosaka, T.; Ono, T.; Kida, M.; Kikui, M.; Yamamoto, M.; Yasui, S.; Nokubi, T.; Maeda, Y.; Kokubo, Y.; Watanabe, M.; et al. A multifactorial model of masticatory performance: The Suita study. *J. Oral Rehabil.* **2016**, *43*, 340–347. [CrossRef] [PubMed]
25. Tanaka, Y.; Shiga, H. Masticatory performance of the elderly as seen from differences in occlusal support of residual teeth. *J. Prosthodont. Res.* **2018**, *62*, 375–378. [CrossRef]

26. Kosaka, T.; Kida, M.; Kikui, M.; Hashimoto, S.; Fujii, K.; Yamamoto, M.; Nokubi, T.; Maeda, Y.; Hasegawa, Y.; Kokubo, Y.; et al. Factors Influencing the Changes in Masticatory Performance: The Suita Study. *JDR Clin. Trans. Res.* **2018**, *3*, 405–412. [CrossRef]
27. Okuyama, N.; Yamaga, T.; Yoshihara, A.; Nohno, K.; Yoshitake, Y.; Kimura, Y.; Shimada, M.; Nakagawa, N.; Nishimuta, M.; Ohashi, M.; et al. Influence of dental occlusion on physical fitness decline in a healthy Japanese elderly population. *Arch. Gerontol. Geriatr.* **2011**, *52*, 172–176. [CrossRef]
28. Kimura, M.; Watanabe, M.; Tanimoto, Y.; Kusabiraki, T.; Komiyama, M.; Hayashida, I.; Kono, K. Occlusal support including that from artificial teeth as an indicator for health promotion among community-dwelling elderly in Japan. *Geriatr. Gerontol. Int.* **2013**, *13*, 539–546. [CrossRef]
29. Welmer, A.K.; Rizzuto, D.; Parker, M.G.; Xu, W. Impact of tooth loss on walking speed decline over time in older adults: A population-based cohort study. *Aging Clin. Exp. Res.* **2017**, *29*, 793–800. [CrossRef]
30. Hasegawa, Y.; Horii, N.; Sakuramoto-Sadakane, A.; Nagai, K.; Ono, T.; Sawada, T.; Shinmura, K.; Kishimoto, H. Is a History of Falling Related to Oral Function? A Cross-Sectional Survey of Elderly Subjects in Rural Japan. *Int. J. Environ. Res. Public Health* **2019**, *16*, 3843. [CrossRef]
31. Hatta, K.; Ikebe, K.; Mihara, Y.; Gondo, Y.; Kamide, K.; Masui, Y.; Sugimoto, K.; Matsuda, K.I.; Fukutake, M.; Kabayama, M.; et al. Lack of posterior occlusal support predicts the reduction in walking speed in 80-year-old Japanese adults: A 3-year prospective cohort study with propensity score analysis by the SONIC Study Group. *Gerodontology* **2019**, *36*, 156–162. [CrossRef]
32. Sawa, Y.; Kayashita, J.; Nikawa, H. Occlusal support is associated with nutritional improvement and recovery of physical function in patients recovering from hip fracture. *Gerodontology* **2020**, *37*, 59–65. [CrossRef]
33. Okubo, Y.; Seino, S.; Yabushita, N.; Osuka, Y.; Jung, S.; Nemoto, M.; Figueroa, R.; Tanaka, K. Longitudinal association between habitual walking and fall occurrences among community-dwelling older adults: Analyzing the different risks of falling. *Arch. Gerontol. Geriatr.* **2015**, *60*, 45–51. [CrossRef]
34. Chen, L.K.; Woo, J.; Assantachai, P.; Auyeung, T.W.; Chou, M.Y.; Iijima, K.; Jang, H.C.; Kang, L.; Kim, M.; Kim, S.; et al. Asian Working Group for Sarcopenia: 2019 Consensus Update on Sarcopenia Diagnosis and Treatment. *J. Am. Med. Dir. Assoc.* **2020**, *21*, 300–307. [CrossRef] [PubMed]
35. Sawaya, Y.; Ishizaka, M.; Kubo, A.; Shiba, T.; Hirose, T.; Onoda, K.; Maruyama, H.; Urano, T. The Asian working group for sarcopenia's new criteria updated in 2019 causing a change in sarcopenia prevalence in Japanese older adults requiring long-term care/support. *J. Phys. Ther. Sci.* **2020**, *32*, 742–747. [CrossRef]
36. Tamura, Y.; Ishikawa, J.; Fujiwara, Y.; Tanaka, M.; Kanazawa, N.; Chiba, Y.; Iizuka, A.; Kaito, S.; Tanaka, J.; Sugie, M.; et al. Prevalence of frailty, cognitive impairment, and sarcopenia in outpatients with cardiometabolic disease in a frailty clinic. *BMC Geriatr.* **2018**, *18*, 264. [CrossRef]
37. Izuno, H.; Hori, K.; Sawada, M.; Fukuda, M.; Hatayama, C.; Ito, K.; Nomura, Y.; Inoue, M. Physical fitness and oral function in community-dwelling older people: A pilot study. *Gerodontology* **2016**, *33*, 470–479. [CrossRef] [PubMed]
38. Morita, K.; Tsuka, H.; Kato, K.; Mori, T.; Nishimura, R.; Yoshida, M.; Tsuga, K. Factors related to masticatory performance in healthy elderly individuals. *J. Prosthodont. Res.* **2018**, *62*, 432–435. [CrossRef]
39. Julià-Sánchez, S.; Álvarez-Herms, J.; Burtscher, M. Dental occlusion and body balance: A question of environmental constraints? *J. Oral Rehabil.* **2019**, *46*, 388–397. [CrossRef] [PubMed]
40. Julià-Sánchez, S.; Álvarez-Herms, J.; Cirer-Sastre, R.; Corbi, F.; Burtscher, M. The Influence of Dental Occlusion on Dynamic Balance and Muscular Tone. *Front. Physiol.* **2020**, *10*, 1626. [CrossRef] [PubMed]

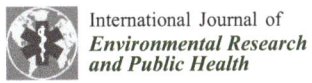

Article

Prognostic Factors of 1-Year Postoperative Functional Outcomes of Older Patients with Intertrochanteric Fractures in Thailand: A Retrospective Cohort Study

Nath Adulkasem [1], Phichayut Phinyo [2,3,4,*], Jiraporn Khorana [2,5], Dumnoensun Pruksakorn [1,4] and Theerachai Apivatthakakul [1]

1. Department of Orthopedics, Faculty of Medicine, Chiang Mai University, Chiang Mai 50200, Thailand; adulkasem.n@gmail.com (N.A.); dumnoensun@hotmail.com (D.P.); tapivath@gmail.com (T.A.)
2. Center for Clinical Epidemiology and Clinical Statistics, Faculty of Medicine, Chiang Mai University, Chiang Mai 50200, Thailand; jiraporn.kho@elearning.cmu.ac.th
3. Department of Family Medicine, Faculty of Medicine, Chiang Mai University, Chiang Mai 50200, Thailand
4. Musculoskeletal Science and Translational Research (MSTR) Cluster, Chiang Mai University, Chiang Mai 50200, Thailand
5. Division of Pediatric Surgery, Department of Surgery, Faculty of Medicine, Chiang Mai University, Chiang Mai 50200, Thailand
* Correspondence: phichayutphinyo@gmail.com; Tel.: +66-89-850-1987

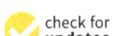

Citation: Adulkasem, N.; Phinyo, P.; Khorana, J.; Pruksakorn, D.; Apivatthakakul, T. Prognostic Factors of 1-Year Postoperative Functional Outcomes of Older Patients with Intertrochanteric Fractures in Thailand: A Retrospective Cohort Study. *IJERPH* **2021**, *18*, 6896. https://doi.org/10.3390/ijerph18136896

Academic Editors: Francisco José Tarazona Santabalbina, Sebastià Josep Santaeugènia Gonzàlez, José Augusto García Navarro and José Viña

Received: 12 May 2021
Accepted: 25 June 2021
Published: 27 June 2021

Publisher's Note: MDPI stays neutral with regard to jurisdictional claims in published maps and institutional affiliations.

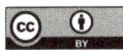

Copyright: © 2021 by the authors. Licensee MDPI, Basel, Switzerland. This article is an open access article distributed under the terms and conditions of the Creative Commons Attribution (CC BY) license (https://creativecommons.org/licenses/by/4.0/).

Abstract: Restoration of ambulatory status is considered a primary treatment goal for older patients with intertrochanteric fractures. Several surgical-related parameters were reported to be associated with mechanical failure without focusing on the functional outcomes. Our study examines the roles of both clinical and surgical parameters as prognostic factors on 1-year postoperative ambulatory outcomes, reaching a good functional outcome (the New Mobility Score: NMS $\geq$ 5) and returning to preinjury functional status at one year, of older patients with intertrochanteric fracture. Intertrochanteric fractures patients age $\geq$65 years who underwent surgical treatment at our institute between January 2017 and February 2020 were included. Of 209 patients included, 149 (71.3%) showed a good functional outcome at one year. The pre-injury ambulatory status (OR 52.72, 95%CI 5.19–535.77, p = 0.001), BMI <23 kg/m^2 (OR 3.14, 95%CI 1.21–8.13, p = 0.018), Hb $\geq$10 g/dL (OR 3.26, 95%CI 1.11–9.57, p = 0.031), and NMS at discharge $\geq$2 (OR 8.50, 95%CI 3.33–21.70, p < 0.001) were identified as independent predictors for reaching a good postoperative functional outcome. Only aged $\leq$80 (OR 2.34, 95%CI 1.11–4.93, p = 0.025) and NMS at discharge $\geq$2 (OR 6.27, 95%CI 2.75–14.32, p < 0.001) were significantly associated with an ability to return to preinjury function. To improve postoperative ambulatory status, orthopedic surgeons should focus more on modifying factors, such as maintaining the preoperative hemoglobin $\geq$10 g/dL and providing adequate postoperative ambulation training to maximize the patients' capability upon discharge. While surgical parameters were not identified as predictors, they can still be used as guidance to optimize the operation quality.

Keywords: fracture fixation; geriatric; intertrochanteric fractures; prognostic factors; Thai

1. Introduction

Intertrochanteric fracture is one of the most common fractures in the geriatric population and is associated with serious consequences [1]. Even though the chance of uneventful bony healing was high, only half of the patients or less could return to their preinjury ambulatory level after operation [2]. The lack of self-ambulatory capability leads to poor quality of life after the injury and subsequently causes significant medical and socioeconomic burdens to both the patients and their families [3]. Therefore, the ultimate treatment goal in treating this fracture type is to enable the patients to return to their previous functional status and social participation [2,4]. As non-operative management was proven to be associated with high morbidity and mortality, operative treatment is currently regarded as the gold standard for the treatment of intertrochanteric fracture [5,6].

Conventionally, the anatomical reduction of the fracture was expected to restore the pre-injury alignment of the patient [7]. Anatomical to slightly valgus femoral neck-shaft angle was generally accepted as an adequate coronal alignment of the proximal femur [8]. Displacement of the femoral cortical support both in the coronal and the sagittal plane should be reduced. Recently, extramedullary reduction was found to have good mechanical properties compared to intramedullary reduction [9]. However, the position of the proximal fixation in three dimensions still greatly affected the fixation stability whether the intramedullary or extramedullary implant was used.

Several parameters were proposed to determine the quality of surgical fixation, such as the tip apex distance (TAD) and its variation calcar reference TAD (CalTAD), which determines the distance of the implant and screw position of proximal fixation in the coronal and axial plane [7,10]. Another important parameter is Parker's ratio, which was used to assess the supero-inferior position of the fixation in the proximal femur [11]. These surgical parameters were widely studied and have proven to be predictive of mechanical failure [7,10], which was the mediator on the causal pathway to the final ambulatory status of the patients [12]. Therefore, it might be reasonable to hypothesize that these surgical-related factors could also have the potential to predict the postoperative functional outcome of the patients.

Several prognostic factors for functional outcomes of patients with intertrochanteric fracture after their surgical treatment were reported in the literature [4,13]. However, most of the evidence tends to focus on clinical parameters and patients' baseline conditions. A previous systematic review of 33 studies identified anemia on admission, comorbidity, pre-fracture function, and cognitive impairment as predictors of postoperative ambulatory status [14]. There was little evidence supporting the association of surgical-related factors with postoperative ambulatory capability. Our study aims to examine the roles of both clinical and surgical parameters as prognostic factors for 1-year postoperative functional outcomes of older patients with intertrochanteric fracture. Two functional outcomes were explored in this study, namely, an ability to reach a good postoperative ambulatory status and an ability to return to preinjury ambulatory status at one year.

2. Materials and Methods

2.1. Design and Setting

Prognostic factor research was conducted with a retrospective observational cohort design. We included patients with intertrochanteric fractures who underwent a surgical operation at Maharaj Nakorn Chiang Mai hospital from January 2017 to February 2020. Our institute is a university-affiliated, tertiary care medical center responsible for the specialized care of patients within the upper Northern region of Thailand. This study was approved by the Research Ethics committee of the Faculty of Medicine, Chiang Mai University (No. 101/2021 Study code ORT-2564-07985).

2.2. Study Patient

We defined the study domain as older patients with an intertrochanteric fracture who underwent surgical management. The medical records of the patients were retrieved and reviewed based on the International Classification of Diseases, 10th revision, Clinical Modification (ICD-10-CM) Diagnosis Code S72.14 Intertrochanteric fracture of the femur. During the study period, all patients aged more than 65 diagnosed with fragility intertrochanteric fracture, which was caused by low energy trauma and treated with internal fixation, were included. Patients whose fractures were caused by a high mechanism of injury, including polytraumatized patients, patients with previously injured ipsilateral hip or major injury affecting lower extremities deformity, or patients diagnosed with a pathological fracture, were excluded. Patients who could not be reached for the telephone interview or who were unable to provide the data (e.g., passed away) were also excluded.

2.3. Treatment Protocol

All patients with intertrochanteric fractures scheduled for operation at our institution are provided with preoperative evaluation by anesthesiologists and medical consultations if required. Closed reduction and internal fixation is generally planned to be performed within the first 72 h after admission. However, if the patients were clinically unstable or deemed unfit for operation, the time to operation would be prolonged. While waiting for the operation, all patients are immobilized with weighted skin traction (2 kg). Board-certified orthopedic trauma surgeons operate using standard surgical techniques [15]. The choice of fixation implants depends on the operating surgeons. For the intramedullary device, Proximal Femoral Nail Antirotation (PFNA) (Synthes, Oberdorf, Switzerland) w used. For extramedullary device, a dynamic hip screw (Synthes, Oberdorf, Switzerland) is used. Postoperative radiography is performed in all cases.

After the operation, all patients are managed according to the standard protocol, including pain management and mechanical venous thromboembolism prophylaxis. Early rehabilitation, including a range of motion and walker-assisted weight-bearing exercises, is performed as tolerated. Patients are evaluated daily by attending orthopedic surgeons. Shared decision making is used to decide appropriate timing for hospital discharge. Patients were scheduled for clinical and radiographic evaluation at two weeks, four weeks, three months, six months, and one year after the operation.

2.4. Data Collection

The data on demographic data (i.e., age at the time of injury and gender) and clinical characteristics (i.e., Charlson's comorbidity index (CCI) [16] and time to surgery) were retrieved from electronic medical records. Body mass index (BMI) was calculated using weight and height, which were preoperatively estimated and recorded by experienced anesthesiologists. Preoperative laboratory investigations, such as hemoglobin level (Hb), and albumin level (Alb), were also collected. Fracture configuration was classified according to AO/OTA classification [17]. The lateral wall thickness was measured according to the methods described in Gotfried's study [18].

Reduction and fixation parameters assessment were measured from the immediate post-operative radiography. Neck shaft angle and Medial and anterior cortical displacement were measured to identify the post-reduction alignment. Fixation parameters, including CalTAD and Parker's ratio, were recorded [10]. Implants were classified into either intramedullary or extramedullary devices.

For avoiding violating the linearity assumption during modeling and interpretability of results, all continuous data were categorized using previously reported cut off points: age less than 80 years [19], preinjury new mobility score (NMS) more than 4 [20], Hb at least 10 g/dL [21], CCI below 5 [16], albumin not lower than 3 mg/L, the lateral wall thickness at least 20.5 mm [18], the neck-shaft angle at least 130° [7], lateral displacement less than 6 mm, posterior displacement less than 7 mm [7,9], CalTAD less than 25 mm [7], Parker's ratio less than 40% [10], time to surgery less than 3 days [22], hospital stay less than 2 weeks [23]. A good ambulatory status at the discharge time was categorized into two groups based on the consensus of two senior authors (TA and DP): those who could walk with or without gait aids (an NMS of at least 2) and those who could not [24].

2.5. Study Endpoint

Postoperative functional outcome at one year was evaluated with the new mobility score (NMS). NMS is comprised of three comprehensive categories describing ambulation ability. The level of dependence was described according to the ability to ambulate with or without aids in the following circumstances: within the house, out of the house, or shopping. The maximum score added up to 9 [20]. This score was widely used and validated with high inter and intra-observer reliability in predicting long-term mortality and rehabilitation outcome in patients with hip fractures [25]. In this study, preinjury NMS, NMS at time of discharge, as well as 1-year postoperative NMS were investigated via structured telephone interviews by investigators who were blinded to the patients' clinical information to avoid interviewer bias [26].

The primary endpoint of this study was the ability to reach a good function outcome at 1-year. According to Parker et al., an acceptable functional outcome was defined as the NMS at least 5 [20]. Other than the ability to reach a good functional outcome at 1-year, another clinically significant endpoint worth exploring was the ability of the patients to return to preinjury functional status at 1-year after the operation, which was set as a secondary endpoint to be explored.

2.6. Statistical Analysis

Based on standard recommendations, a minimum of 10 interested endpoints per predictor is required [27]. Thus, an expected number of 180 patients with an intertrochanteric fracture with good postoperative ambulatory status is required to model 18 predictors. Data distribution was tested using histogram and Shapiro–Wilk test. Normally distributed continuous data were presented with means and standard deviation (SD). In contrast, non-normally distributed data were presented with median and interquartile range (IQR), which were tested using t-test and Mann–Whitney U test, respectively. Categorical data were presented in proportion and compared using Fisher's exact probability test.

Univariable logistic regression analysis was performed to evaluate the individual effect size (univariable odds ratio, uOR) and the statistical significance of each parameter. The dependent variables for the primary and secondary endpoint were NMS $\geq$ 5 and returning to preinjury functional status, respectively. Since this study was an exploratory prognostic factors research, we employed a full model approach where all predictors were entered in multivariable logistic regression modelling without stepwise selection or backward elimination. The mode results were presented with multivariable odds ratios (mOR) and their corresponding 95% confidential intervals (CI). All statistical analysis was computed using Stata 16 (StataCorp LLC, College Station, TX, USA). The level of statistical significance was set at $p < 0.05$.

3. Results

There were 254 patients with an intertrochanteric fracture who underwent surgical treatment during the study period at our institution. Among them, 41 patients who passed away before the interview, three polytraumatized patients, and one patient with pathological fracture were excluded. In summary, a total of 209 patients were included in the analysis (Figure 1).

Of the 209 patients, 149 (71.3%) had good postoperative ambulatory status at one year (i.e., NMS $\geq$ 5). However, only 57 (26.5%) were able to return to preinjury functional status (50 (25%) and 4 (23.5%) in patients with good and poor preinjury ambulatory status respectively). Patients with good postoperative functional outcome had significantly younger age (81 $\pm$ 7 vs. 84 $\pm$ 6 years, $p = 0.008$), better pre-injury NMS (9 (IQR 7, 9) vs. 6 (IQR 4, 9), $p < 0.001$), higher hemoglobin level (10.7 $\pm$ 1.6 vs. 10.2 $\pm$ 1.7 g/dL, $p = 0.022$), lower CCI (4 (IQR 4, 5) vs. 5 (IQR 4, 6), $p < 0.001$), lower length of stay (11 (IQR 8, 14) vs. 14 (IQR 11, 18) days, $p < 0.001$), and better NMS at discharge time (3 (IQR 2, 5) vs. 1 (IQR 0, 2), $p < 0.001$) (Table 1). None of the surgical-related factors showed statistically significant differences between the two groups (Table 2).

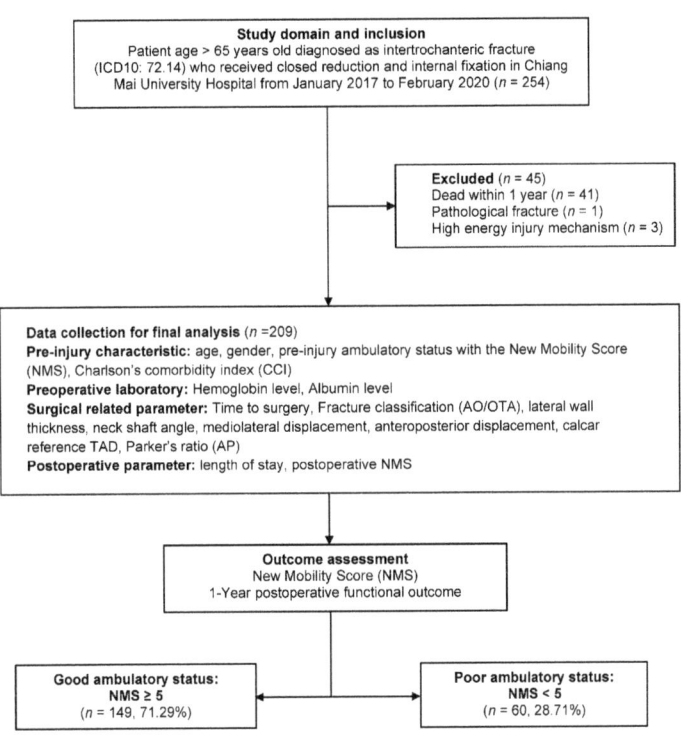

Figure 1. Study flow diagram of eligible patient with fragility intertrochanteric fracture who received reduction and internal fixation. Patient with available 1-year postoperative ambulatory status information were included from January 2017 to February 2020.

Table 1. Demographic data and clinical factors in 209 patients comparing between good and poor functional outcome at one year.

Variable	Total (209)	NMS ≥ 5 (149, 71.3%)	NMS < 5 (60, 28.7%)	p-Value
Age (mean ± SD) years	82 ± 7	81 ± 7	84 ± 6	0.008
Age ≥ 80 years	75 (35.9%)	61 (40.9%)	14 (23.3%)	0.017
Male gender (n.%)	55 (26.3%)	42 (28.2%)	13 (21.7%)	0.388
Pre-fracture NMS [†] (median, IQR)	9 (6, 9)	9 (7, 9)	6 (4, 9)	<0.001
Pre-fracture NMS ≥ 5	192 (91.9%)	148 (99.3%)	44 (73.3%)	<0.001
Hb [‡] (mean ± SD) g/dL	10.6 ± 1.7	10.7 ± 1.6	10.2 ± 1.7	0.022
Hb ≥ 10 g/dL	62 (29.7%)	54 (36.2%)	8 (13.3%)	0.001
CCI [§] (median, IQR)	4 (4, 5)	4 (4, 5)	5 (4, 6)	<0.001
CCI < 5	114 (54.6%)	90 (60.4%)	24 (40.0%)	0.009
BMI [¶] (mean ± SD) kg/m^2	21.7 ± 3.6	21.4 ± 3.6	22.5 ± 3.9	0.062
BMI < 23 kg/m^2	149 (71.3%)	114 (76.5%)	35 (58.3%)	0.011
Albumin (mean ± SD) mg/L	3.6 ± 0.5	3.7 ± 0.5	3.6 ± 0.4	0.117
Albumin ≥ 3 mg/L	183 (87.6%)	129 (86.6%)	54 (90.0%)	0.645
Time to surgery (median, IQR) (d)	5 (3, 8)	4 (2, 7)	5 (3, 8)	0.066
Time to surgery < 3 days	80 (38.3%)	63 (42.3%)	17 (28.3%)	0.083
Length of stay (median, IQR) (d)	12 (9, 15)	11 (8, 14)	14 (11, 18)	<0.001
Length of stay < 14 days	148 (70.8%)	114 (75.5%)	34 (56.7%)	0.007
NMS [†] at discharge (median, IQR)	3 (1, 4)	3 (2, 5)	1 (0, 2)	<0.001
NMS at discharge ≥ 2	109 (52.2%)	96 (64.4%)	13 (21.7%)	<0.001

[†] The New Mobility Scores, [‡] Hemoglobin, [§] Charlson's comorbidity index, [¶] Body Mass Index.

Table 2. Surgical-related factors in 209 patients comparing between good and poor functional outcome at one year.

Variable	Total (209)	NMS ≥ 5 (149, 71.3%)	NMS < 5 (60, 28.7%)	p-Value
Fracture classification (n, %)				
31A1	57 (27.3%)	47 (31.5%)	10 (16.7%)	
31A2	116 (55.5%)	77 (51.7%)	39 (65.0%)	
31A3	36 (17.2%)	25 (16.8%)	11 (18.3%)	0.086
Lateral wall thickness (mean ± SD) mm	21.3 ± 6.6	21.7 ± 6.8	20.5 ± 5.9	0.220
Lateral wall thickness ≥ 20.5 mm	108 (51.7%)	79 (53.0%)	29 (48.3%)	0.545
Neck shaft angle (mean ± SD) °	134.9 ± 8.4	135.3 ± 7.8	133.9 ± 9.8	0.256
Neck shaft angle ≥ 130°	153 (73.2%)	116 (77.9%)	37 (61.7%)	0.024
Medial cortical support (mean ± SD) mm	(+) 0.7 ± 3.7	(+) 0.7 ± 3.5	(+) 0.8 ± 4.2	0.916
Negative medial cortical support < 6 mm	200 (95.7%)	144 (96.6%)	56 (93.3%)	0.282
Anterior cortical support (mean ± SD) mm	(−) 1.2 ± 4.1	(−) 1.1 ± 3.7	(−) 1.4 ± 4.9	0.646
Negative anterior cortical support < 7 mm	193 (92.3%)	140 (94.0%)	53 (88.3)	0.247
CalTAD [†] (mean ± SD) mm	26.6 ± 5.9	26.6 ± 5.9	26.5 ± 6.1	0.957
CalTAD < 25 mm	89 (42.6%)	66 (44.3%)	23 (38.3%)	0.445
Parker's ratio (AP) (mean ± SD) %	47.8 ± 8.2	47.4 ± 8.0	48.8 ± 8.5	0.257
Parker's ratio (AP) < 40%	43 (20.6%)	34 (22.8%)	9 (15.0%)	0.258
Fixation implant				
Extramedullary device	42 (20.1%)	32 (21.5%)	10 (16.7%)	
Intramedullary device	167 (79.9%)	117 (78.5%)	50 (83.3%)	0.567

[†] Calcar reference tip-apex distance.

In univariable logistic regression, the patient's age, pre-injury NMS, preoperative hemoglobin level, CCI, BMI, length of stay, and ambulatory status at discharge time were statistically significant predictors (Table 3). Of the 18 predictors included for the multivariable logistic regression analysis, four were identified as independent predictors of postoperative ambulatory status at one year. Pre-injury NMS ≥ 5 was the predictor with the largest effect size (mOR 52.72, 95%CI 5.19–535.77, p = 0.001). Other influential predictors were preoperative hemoglobin level ≥ 10 g/dL (mOR: 3.26, 95% CI 1.11–9.57, p = 0.031), BMI < 23 kg/m^2 (mOR 3.14, 95% CI 1.21–8.13, p = 0.018), and the ambulatory status of patients at discharge time with NMS at least 2 (mOR 8.50, 95% CI 3.33–21.70, p < 0.001). None of the surgical-related factors have a statistically significant effect on postoperative functional status (Table 3). In multivariable logistic regression analysis for factors associated with the ability to return to preinjury functional status, only patient's age (mOR 2.34, 95% CI 1.11–4.93, p = 0.025) and ambulatory status at discharge time with NMS at least 2 (mOR 6.09, 95% CI 2.75–14.32, p < 0.001) were identified as independent predictors (Table 4). The varying effect of each predictor between two different endpoints was summarized in regression coefficient plots (Figures 2 and 3).

Table 3. Logistic regression analysis of prognostic factors of regaining good 1-year postoperative ambulatory status (NMS ≥ 5).

Variable	Univariable			Multivariable		
	uOR	95% CI	*p*-Value	mOR	95% CI	*p*-Value
Age ≥ 80	2.28	1.15–4.50	0.018	2.50	0.95–6.58	0.064
Male gender	1.42	0.70–2.89	0.334	1.79	0.62–5.14	0.279
Pre-fracture NMS [†] ≥ 5	53.82	6.94–417.27	<0.001	52.72	5.19–535.77	0.001
Hb [‡] ≥ 10 g/dL	3.69	1.63–8.35	0.002	3.26	1.11–9.57	0.031
CCI [§] < 5	2.29	1.24–4.22	0.008	2.02	0.85–4.84	0.113
BMI [¶] < 23 kg/m^2	2.33	1.23–4.40	0.009	3.14	1.21–8.13	0.018
Albumin ≥ 3 mg/L	0.72	0.27–1.88	0.499	0.50	0.14–1.79	0.285
Fracture classification						
31A1	1.00	Reference		1.00	Reference	
31A2	0.42	0.19–0.92	0.030	0.38	0.11–1.26	0.113
31A3	0.48	0.18–1.29	0.148	0.43	0.08–2.28	0.324
Lateral wall thickness ≥ 20.5 mm	1.21	0.66–2.20	0.540	1.19	0.46–3.09	0.722
Neck shaft angle ≥130°	2.19	1.14–4.18	0.018	1.28	0.47–3.48	0.628
Negative medial cortical support < 6 mm	2.06	0.53–7.94	0.295	1.14	0.13–9.85	0.907
Negative anterior cortical support < 7 mm	2.05	0.73–5.80	0.174	2.54	0.56–11.52	0.228
CalTAD [††] < 25 mm	1.28	0.69–2.36	0.431	1.12	0.44–2.83	0.813
Parker's ratio (AP) < 40%	1.68	0.75–3.75	0.209	1.37	0.44–4.22	0.585
Fixation implant						
Extramedullary device	1.00	Reference		1.00	Reference	
Intramedullary device	0.73	0.33–1.60	0.434	1.54	0.42–5.73	0.516
Time to surgery < 3 days	1.85	0.97–3.55	0.062	0.55	0.19–1.55	0.256
Length of stay < 14 days	2.30	1.23–4.30	0.009	2.42	0.91–6.42	0.077
NMS [†] at discharge ≥ 2	6.55	3.25–13.18	<0.001	8.50	3.33–21.70	<0.001

[†] The New Mobility Scores, [‡] Hemoglobin, [§] Charlson's comorbidity index, [¶] Body Mass Index, [††] Calcar reference tip-apex distance.

Table 4. Logistic regression analysis of prognosis factors of returning to preinjury functional status at one year.

Variable	Univariable			Multivariable		
	uOR	95% CI	*p*-Value	mOR	95% CI	*p*-Value
Age ≤ 80	2.23	1.18–4.20	0.013	2.34	1.11–4.93	0.025
Male gender	0.97	0.48–1.97	0.940	0.86	0.37–2.01	0.727
Pre-fracture NMS [†] ≥ 5	1.14	0.36–3.67	0.821	0.51	0.12–2.12	0.356
Hb [‡] ≥ 10 g/dL	0.88	0.44–1.76	0.725	0.66	0.29–1.50	0.320
CCI [§] < 5	1.44	0.76–2.70	0.262	1.17	0.54–2.53	0.689
BMI [¶] < 23 kg/m^2	1.21	0.60–2.43	0.600	1.36	0.57–3.24	0.490
Albumin ≥ 3 mg/L	0.94	0.37–2.37	0.892	0.51	0.16–1.63	0.255
Fracture classification						
31A1	1.00	Reference		1.00	Reference	
31A2	0.82	0.40–1.67	0.577	1.08	0.42–2.73	0.878
31A3	0.99	0.39–2.50	0.976	1.44	0.39–5.30	0.583
Lateral wall thickness ≥ 20.5 mm	1.12	0.60–2.08	0.729	0.95	0.40–2.28	0.911
Neck shaft angle ≥130°	1.60	0.76–3.40	0.218	1.05	0.41–2.66	0.919
Negative medial cortical support < 5 mm	5.26	0.68–41.01	0.113	5.44	0.57–52.35	0.142
Negative anterior cortical support < 7 mm	1.56	0.43–5.69	0.503	1.05	0.21–5.04	0.948
CalTAD [††] < 25 mm	1.36	0.73–2.53	0.338	1.42	0.66–3.06	0.374
Parker's ratio (AP) < 40%	1.14	0.54–2.43	0.728	0.96	0.39–2.37	0.935
Fixation implant						
Extramedullary device	1.00	Reference		1.00	Reference	
Intramedullary device	0.73	0.35–1.53	0.398	0.54	0.19–1.55	0.253
Time to surgery < 3 days	1.28	0.68–2.40	0.449	0.74	0.33–1.69	0.482
Length of stay < 14 days	1.86	0.89–3.91	0.101	2.13	0.90–5.03	0.086
NMS [†] at discharge ≥ 2	6.09	2.86–12.99	<0.001	6.27	2.75–14.32	<0.001

[†] The New Mobility Scores, [‡] Hemoglobin, [§] Charlson's comorbidity index, [¶] Body Mass Index, [††] Calcar reference tip-apex distance.

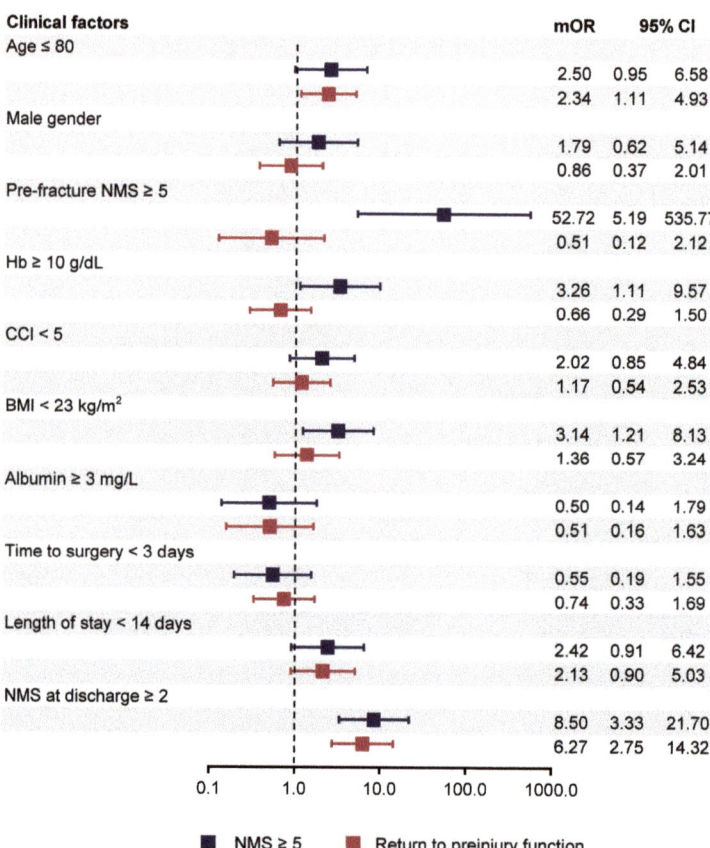

Figure 2. Coefficient plot presenting the odds ratio of each clinical parameter regarding two different endpoints (NMS ≥ 5 and the ability to return to preinjury functional status). Hb: Hemoglobin, CCI: Charlson's Comorbidities index, BMI: Body Mass Index, NMS: The New Mobility Score.

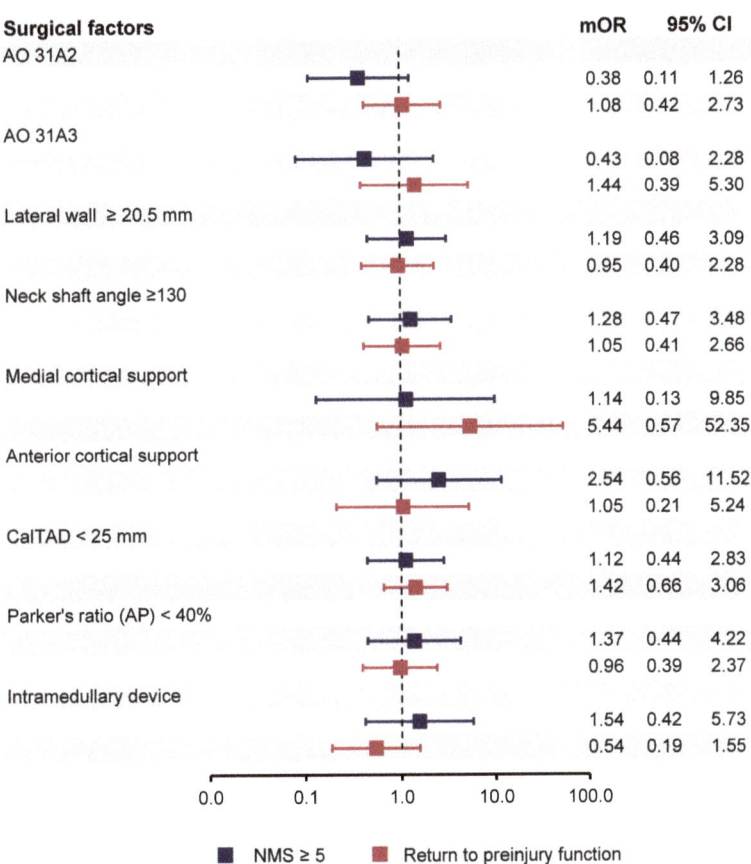

Figure 3. Coefficient plot presenting the odds ratio of each surgical related parameter regarding two different endpoints (NMS ≥ 5 and the ability to return to preinjury functional status). AO: AO/OTA classification, CalTAD: Calcar reference Tip Apex Distance, NMS: The New Mobility Score.

4. Discussion

In this study, it was revealed that the effect of surgical-related factors on the postoperative ambulatory status at one year was outweighed by parameters that reflect the patients' baseline clinical and functional status, such as the pre-injury NMS, which was the strongest predictive factors. The others clinical parameters identified were the NMS at hospital discharge, BMI, and preoperative Hb level. Only patient's age and functional status at hospital discharge were identified as an independent predictor for returning to preinjury functional status.

For patients with an intertrochanteric fracture who underwent surgery, their baseline functional status both before the injury and at discharge were identified as important predictors for their postoperative ambulatory status, which was in consistent with previous evidence. The better the pre-injury ambulatory status, the better the functional outcome would be postoperatively [28]. Patients with lower BMI were more likely to ambulate at one year. We hypothesized that patients with higher BMI might be less physically active and have insufficient caloric expenditure, which leads to the continuous deterioration of their ambulatory status [29]. Therefore, an early rehabilitation intervention to promote sufficient physical activity and nutritional optimization to achieve a balance caloric intake and expenditure should be incorporated into a perioperative protocol for older patients with intertrochanteric fractures.

Admission hemoglobin concentration has been extensively studied and was consistently reported as prognostic factors for functional outcomes and mortality in patients with hip fracture [21]. Based on our results, we recommended that orthopedists should maintain the preoperative Hb level greater than 10 g/dL to improve the postoperative functional recovery [13]. Although an early surgery did not result in a significant improvement of the functional outcome in this study, the surgical operation should still be performed as soon as possible, or within 48 h, in this domain of patients, as it was proven to reduce the length of hospital stay, postoperative complications, and mortality [30]. Ambulatory status at discharge time positively affected the 1-year postoperative outcome of the patients, similar to the previous study [28].

In our study, only less than one-third of the patients could return to their preinjury functional status at one year, similar to the numbers reported by previous studies, from 29% to 39% [2,31]. Interestingly, although a good baseline functional status could strongly predict an acceptable postoperative ambulatory status, it could not predict the ability of the patients to return to their preinjury functional status as the ability to return to preinjury functional status was independent of the patients' baseline functional status. In contrast, only functional status at discharge were significantly associated with both study endpoints. This finding emphasizes the importance of adequate postoperative rehabilitation, which positively influences the patient's long-term functional outcome [28]. Patients aged less than 80 years were more likely to return to their preinjury functional status. Although the statistical significance of this factor was identified only for the secondary endpoint, the direction and magnitude of the association were somewhat similar for the primary endpoint. Thus, it might be reasonable to conclude that age was associated with functional recovery, which was concordance with a previous study [32]. Based on our findings, we suggest that an adequate postoperative rehabilitation to enable the patients to regain at least an NMS of 2, or self-ambulation with a walking aid, is encouraged before hospital discharge.

Contrary to our prior hypothesis, surgical-related parameters were not significantly associated with the postoperative functional outcome at one year, either NMS ≥ 5 or the ability to return to preinjury functional status. However, the absence of statistical evidence should not be construed as the absence of the prognostic ability. Since orthopedic surgeons would attempt to obtain the optimal quality of surgical reduction and fixation in every operation, the effect of these surgical parameters was obscured and might require a larger sample size to identify the statistical significance. Based on the direction and the magnitude of the effect estimates, some surgical-related parameters should not be overlooked, such as the figure configuration. The AO/OTA 31A2 and 31A3 fracture configurations reduced the odds of postoperative ambulation by 0.38 and 0.43, respectively. Intertrochanteric fracture classified as AO/OTA 31A2 creates structural defect at the postero-medial zone, while AO/OTA 31A3 loses the integrity of the supero-lateral zone, which greatly reduces the stability of the intertrochanter area [18,33]. Positive to negative anterior cortical support of less than 7 mm tended to improve the outcome (mOR: 2.54, 95%CI 0.56–11.52), which might be explained according to the previous finite element analysis that shows better reduction stability with positive anterior cortical support by preventing further sliding of proximal fragment [34]. Nevertheless, the standardized surgical techniques that rely on previously reported reduction and fixation parameters should continue to be used regardless of their lack of predictive ability of the postoperative functional outcome as they have been proven to improve the biomechanical properties of the fracture fixation [7,10,18].

Although the effects of baseline clinical factors and pre-injury functional status on postoperative functional status seem to be more pronounced than surgical-related factors, orthopedic surgeons should still optimize the quality of surgery and provide each patient with effective perioperative management to improve functional recovery and promote early ambulation. During the past years, a fast-track perioperative protocol, such as an enhanced recovery after surgery (ERAS), primarily designed to be used in colorectal surgery, has been shown to provide better surgical outcomes if properly implemented. ERAS comprises three main components: preoperative nutritional optimization and education, minimally invasive intraoperative procedure with optimum fluid balance, and adequate postoperative pain control with early rehabilitation [35]. A rehabilitation program in an ERAS protocol promotes pain-free musculoskeletal function and improves overall functional recovery and postoperative ambulation [36]. Several studies had discovered the potential effectiveness of using an ERAS program in the context of orthopedic surgery [37,38]. One propensity score-matched study compared an effect of an ERAS program on patients who underwent hip and knee replacement surgery and found an enhancement in postoperative ambulation and reduction in the length of hospital stay [39]. Our findings could be used to guide the development of an ERAS program specifically designed for older patients with intertrochanteric fractures.

Our study carried some strengths. First, this study was one of few studies to clarify the association between surgical-related and postoperative functional outcomes in patients with an intertrochanteric fracture [40]. Even though statistical significances were not identified among these surgical factors, some have potential predictability of the postoperative ambulation status based on their direction and effect size. Second, our study was able to identify the minimal acceptable NMS score of postoperative ambulation status before hospital discharge, which can be used to guide physicians to consider additional rehabilitation programs.

The results from our study, however, should be considered in light of some limitations. First, the retrospective nature itself is subjected to several biases. Second, the exclusion of patients who passed away before the time of the interview might create an inevitable selection bias. Even though the mortality rate in our study was similar to the previous reports at approximately 15% [41], our samples might not reflect the actual underlying population. Third, using telephone interviews as the data collection method might give rise to both recall and interviewer biases. In our study, these biases were minimized by using valid assessment tools, structured interviews, and blinded interviewers [26]. Fourth, the accuracy of BMI and some other physician-estimated parameters might be questionable. However, clinicians usually perform these estimations in their practice, especially when an actual measurement was not feasible. While using this approach may affect the internal validity of the predictors, it did, however, enhance the generalizability to the real-world practice. Fifth, cognitive status, a potential influencing factor for the functional outcome, was not included in the analysis as it was not routinely evaluated or documented in our practice. Finally, the available sample size was relatively small and was not powered enough to identify the significance of some predictors. The findings of our study regarding the association between surgical-related parameters should be considered preliminary evidence, which still requires further prospective study with a larger sample size to confirm.

5. Conclusions

Our study emphasizes the importance of the patients' preinjury clinical status, which outweighs the surgical-related factors in predicting postoperative functional outcomes of older patients with an intertrochanteric fracture. Pre-injury ambulatory status is the strongest independent predictor, follow by the patient's BMI. Orthopedic surgeons should focus more attention on improving the patient's clinical condition as well as maintaining the optimal quality of surgery. A preoperative hemoglobin level of at least 10 g/dL should be targeted. An adequate rehabilitation program should be included in the postoperative protocol to maximize the ambulatory capability before discharge and ensure a good 1-year postoperative ambulation, allowing patients to return to their previous functional status.

Author Contributions: Conceptualization, N.A., D.P., and P.P.; methodology, N.A., P.P., and J.K.; software, N.A.; validation, D.P. and T.A.; formal analysis, N.A. and P.P.; investigation, N.A.; resources, T.A. and D.P.; data curation, N.A. and P.P.; writing—original draft preparation, N.A.; writing—review

& editing, P.P., J.K., D.P., and T.A.; visualization, P.P.; supervision, T.A.; project administration, N.A. All authors have read and agreed to the published version of the manuscript.

Funding: This research received no external funding.

Institutional Review Board Statement: This study was conducted according to the guidelines of the Declaration of Helsinki and approved by the Research Ethics committee of the Faculty of Medicine, Chiang Mai University (No. 101/2021 Study code ORT-2564-07985).

Informed Consent Statement: Verbal informed consent was obtained from each participant before starting the interview with the approval of the Research Ethics committee of the Faculty of Medicine, Chiang Mai University.

Data Availability Statement: The datasets used and/or analysed during the current study are available from the corresponding author on reasonable request. The data are not publicly available due to their containing information that could compromise the privacy of research participants.

Acknowledgments: The authors acknowledge all relevant medical and nursing staff at Maharaj Nakorn Chiang Mai Hospital (Chiang Mai University Hospital) for their collaboration during the data collection period. This study was partially supported by the Faculty of Medicine, Chiang Mai University.

Conflicts of Interest: The authors declare no conflict of interest.

References

1. Voleti, P.B.; Liu, S.Y.; Baldwin, K.D.; Mehta, S.; Donegan, D.J. Intertrochanteric Femur Fracture Stability: A Surrogate for General Health in Elderly Patients? *Geriatr. Orthop. Surg. Rehabil.* **2015**, *6*, 192–196. [CrossRef] [PubMed]
2. Kulachote, N.; Sa-Ngasoongsong, P.; Sirisreetreerux, N.; Chulsomlee, K.; Thamyongkit, S.; Wongsak, S. Predicting Factors for Return to Prefracture Ambulatory Level in High Surgical Risk Elderly Patients Sustained Intertrochanteric Fracture and Treated with Proximal Femoral Nail Antirotation (PFNA) With and Without Cement Augmentation. *Geriatr. Orthop. Surg. Rehabil.* **2020**, *11*, 2151459320912121. [CrossRef]
3. Adeyemi, A.; Delhougne, G. Incidence and Economic Burden of Intertrochanteric Fracture: A Medicare Claims Database Analysis. *JBJS Open Access* **2019**, *4*, e0045. [CrossRef] [PubMed]
4. Hulsbæk, S.; Larsen, R.F.; Troelsen, A. Predictors of not regaining basic mobility after hip fracture surgery. *Disabil. Rehabil.* **2015**, *37*, 1739–1744. [CrossRef] [PubMed]
5. Vaseenon, T.; Luevitoonvechkij, S.; Wongtriratanachai, P.; Rojanasthien, S. Long-term mortality after osteoporotic hip fracture in Chiang Mai, Thailand. *J. Clin. Densitom.* **2010**, *13*, 63–67. [CrossRef]
6. Chaysri, R.; Leerapun, T.; Klunklin, K.; Chiewchantanakit, S.; Luevitoonvechkij, S.; Rojanasthien, S. Factors related to mortality after osteoporotic hip fracture treatment at Chiang Mai University Hospital, Thailand, during 2006 and 2007. *J. Med. Assoc. Thail.* **2015**, *98*, 59–64.
7. Baumgaertner, M.R.; Curtin, S.L.; Lindskog, D.M.; Keggi, J.M. The value of the tip-apex distance in predicting failure of fixation of peritrochanteric fractures of the hip. *J. Bone Jt. Surg. Am.* **1995**, *77*, 1058–1064. [CrossRef]
8. Pajarinen, J.; Lindahl, J.; Savolainen, V.; Michelsson, O.; Hirvensalo, E. Femoral shaft medialisation and neck-shaft angle in unstable pertrochanteric femoral fractures. *Int. Orthop.* **2004**, *28*, 347–353. [CrossRef]
9. Chang, S.-M.; Zhang, Y.-Q.; Ma, Z.; Li, Q.; Dargel, J.; Eysel, P. Fracture reduction with positive medial cortical support: A key element in stability reconstruction for the unstable pertrochanteric hip fractures. *Arch. Orthop. Trauma Surg.* **2015**, *135*, 811–818. [CrossRef] [PubMed]
10. Kashigar, A.; Vincent, A.; Gunton, M.J.; Backstein, D.; Safir, O.; Kuzyk, P.R. Predictors of failure for cephalomedullary nailing of proximal femoral fractures. *Bone Jt. J.* **2014**, *96*, 1029–1034. [CrossRef]
11. Parker, M.J. Cutting-out of the dynamic hip screw related to its position. *J. Bone Jt. Surg. Br. Vol.* **1992**, *74*, 625. [CrossRef] [PubMed]
12. Broderick, J.M.; Bruce-Brand, R.; Stanley, E.; Mulhall, K.J. Osteoporotic hip fractures: The burden of fixation failure. *Sci. World J.* **2013**, *2013*, 515197. [CrossRef] [PubMed]
13. Buecking, B.; Bohl, K.; Eschbach, D.; Bliemel, C.; Aigner, R.; Balzer-Geldsetzer, M.; Dodel, R.; Ruchholtz, S.; Debus, F. Factors influencing the progress of mobilization in hip fracture patients during the early postsurgical period?—A prospective observational study. *Arch. Gerontol. Geriatr.* **2015**, *60*, 457–463. [CrossRef] [PubMed]
14. Sheehan, K.J.; Williamson, L.; Alexander, J.; Filliter, C.; Sobolev, B.; Guy, P.; Bearne, L.M.; Sackley, C. Prognostic factors of functional outcome after hip fracture surgery: A systematic review. *Age Ageing* **2018**, *47*, 661–670. [CrossRef] [PubMed]
15. Buckley, R.E.; Apivatthakakul, T.; Moran, C.G. *AO Principles of Fracture Management*; Thieme: Stuttgart, Germany, 2017.
16. Charlson, M.E.; Pompei, P.; Ales, K.L.; MacKenzie, C.R. A new method of classifying prognostic comorbidity in longitudinal studies: Development and validation. *J. Chronic Dis.* **1987**, *40*, 373–383. [CrossRef]
17. Müller, M.E. *The Comprehensive Classification of Fractures of Long Bones*; Springer: Berlin, Germany, 1990.

18. Gotfried, Y. The lateral trochanteric wall: A key element in the reconstruction of unstable pertrochanteric hip fractures. *Clin. Orthop. Relat. Res.* **2004**, *425*, 82–86. [CrossRef]
19. Welmer, A.K.; Mörck, A.; Dahlin-Ivanoff, S. Physical activity in people age 80 years and older as a means of counteracting disability, balanced in relation to frailty. *J. Aging Phys. Act.* **2012**, *20*, 317–331. [CrossRef]
20. Parker, M.J.; Palmer, C.R. A new mobility score for predicting mortality after hip fracture. *J. Bone Jt. Surg Br.* **1993**, *75*, 797–798. [CrossRef]
21. Atthakomol, P.; Manosroi, W.; Phinyo, P.; Pipanmekaporn, T.; Vaseenon, T.; Rojanasthien, S. Prognostic Factors for All-Cause Mortality in Thai Patients with Fragility Fracture of Hip: Comorbidities and Laboratory Evaluations. *Medicina* **2020**, *56*, 311. [CrossRef]
22. Kulachote, N.; Sa-Ngasoongsong, P.; Sirisreetreerux, N.; Wongsak, S.; Suphachatwong, C.; Wajanavisit, W.; Kawinwonggowit, V. The Impacts of Early Hip Surgery in High-Risk Elderly Taking Antithrombotic Agents and Afflicted with Intertrochanteric Fracture. *J. Med. Assoc. Thail.* **2015**, *98* (Suppl. 8), S76–S81.
23. Tan, S.T.; Tan, W.P.; Jaipaul, J.; Chan, S.P.; Sathappan, S.S. Clinical outcomes and hospital length of stay in 2,756 elderly patients with hip fractures: A comparison of surgical and non-surgical management. *Singap. Med. J.* **2017**, *58*, 253–257. [CrossRef] [PubMed]
24. Hagino, T.; Sato, E.; Tonotsuka, H.; Ochiai, S.; Tokai, M.; Hamada, Y. Prediction of ambulation prognosis in the elderly after hip fracture. *Int. Orthop.* **2006**, *30*, 315–319. [CrossRef]
25. Kristensen, M.T.; Bandholm, T.; Foss, N.B.; Ekdahl, C.; Kehlet, H. High inter-tester reliability of the new mobility score in patients with hip fracture. *J. Rehabil. Med.* **2008**, *40*, 589–591. [CrossRef]
26. Pannucci, C.J.; Wilkins, E.G. Identifying and avoiding bias in research. *Plast. Reconstr. Surg* **2010**, *126*, 619–625. [CrossRef]
27. Collins, G.S.; Reitsma, J.B.; Altman, D.G.; Moons, K.G. Transparent Reporting of a multivariable prediction model for Individual Prognosis or Diagnosis (TRIPOD): The TRIPOD statement. *Ann. Intern. Med.* **2015**, *162*, 55–63. [CrossRef]
28. Takahashi, A.; Naruse, H.; Kitade, I.; Shimada, S.; Tsubokawa, M.; Kokubo, Y.; Matsumine, A. Functional outcomes after the treatment of hip fracture. *PLoS ONE* **2020**, *15*, e0236652. [CrossRef] [PubMed]
29. Shakouri, S.K.; Eslamian, F.; Azari, B.K.; Sadeghi-Bazargani, H.; Sadeghpour, A.; Salekzamani, Y. Predictors of functional improvement among patients with hip fracture at a rehabilitation ward. *Pak. J. Biol. Sci.* **2009**, *12*, 1516–1520. [CrossRef] [PubMed]
30. Khan, S.K.; Kalra, S.; Khanna, A.; Thiruvengada, M.M.; Parker, M.J. Timing of surgery for hip fractures: A systematic review of 52 published studies involving 291,413 patients. *Injury* **2009**, *40*, 692–697. [CrossRef] [PubMed]
31. Moerman, S.; Mathijssen, N.M.; Tuinebreijer, W.E.; Nelissen, R.G.; Vochteloo, A.J. Less than one-third of hip fracture patients return to their prefracture level of instrumental activities of daily living in a prospective cohort study of 480 patients. *Geriatr. Gerontol. Int.* **2018**, *18*, 1244–1248. [CrossRef] [PubMed]
32. Ortiz-Alonso, F.J.; Vidán-Astiz, M.; Alonso-Armesto, M.; Toledano-Iglesias, M.; Alvarez-Nebreda, L.; Brañas-Baztan, F.; Serra-Rexach, J.A. The pattern of recovery of ambulation after hip fracture differs with age in elderly patients. *J. Gerontol. A Biol. Sci. Med. Sci.* **2012**, *67*, 690–697. [CrossRef]
33. Ye, K.-F.; Xing, Y.; Sun, C.; Cui, Z.-Y.; Zhou, F.; Ji, H.-Q.; Guo, Y.; Lyu, Y.; Yang, Z.-W.; Hou, G.-J.; et al. Loss of the posteromedial support: A risk factor for implant failure after fixation of AO 31-A2 intertrochanteric fractures. *Chin. Med. J.* **2020**, *133*, 41–48. [CrossRef] [PubMed]
34. Shao, Q.; Zhang, Y.; Sun, G.-X.; Yang, C.-S.; Liu, N.; Chen, D.-W.; Cheng, B. Positive or negative anteromedial cortical support of unstable pertrochanteric femoral fractures: A finite element analysis study. *Biomed. Pharmacother.* **2021**, *138*, 111473. [CrossRef] [PubMed]
35. Kaye, A.D.; Urman, R.D.; Cornett, E.M.; Hart, B.M.; Chami, A.; Gayle, J.A.; Fox, C.J. Enhanced recovery pathways in orthopedic surgery. *J. Anaesthesiol. Clin. Pharmacol.* **2019**, *35*, S35–S39. [CrossRef] [PubMed]
36. Kang, Y.; Liu, J.; Chen, H.; Ding, W.; Chen, J.; Zhao, B.; Yin, X. Enhanced recovery after surgery (ERAS) in elective intertrochanteric fracture patients result in reduced length of hospital stay (LOS) without compromising functional outcome. *J. Orthop. Surg. Res.* **2019**, *14*, 209. [CrossRef] [PubMed]
37. Masaracchio, M.; Hanney, W.J.; Liu, X.; Kolber, M.; Kirker, K. Timing of rehabilitation on length of stay and cost in patients with hip or knee joint arthroplasty: A systematic review with meta-analysis. *PLoS ONE* **2017**, *12*, e0178295. [CrossRef] [PubMed]
38. Berg, U.; BüLow, E.; Sundberg, M.; Rolfson, O. No increase in readmissions or adverse events after implementation of fast-track program in total hip and knee replacement at 8 Swedish hospitals: An observational before-and-after study of 14,148 total joint replacements 2011-2015. *Acta Orthop.* **2018**, *89*, 522–527. [CrossRef]
39. Romano, L.U.; Rigoni, M.; Torri, E.; Nella, M.; Morandi, M.; Casetti, P.; Nollo, G. A Propensity Score-Matched Analysis to Assess the Outcomes in Pre- and Post-Fast-Track Hip and Knee Elective Prosthesis Patients. *J. Clin. Med.* **2021**, *10*, 741. [CrossRef]
40. Chopra, M.; Kumar, S.; Mishra, D. Functional and radiological outcomes of intertrochanteric fractures treated with proximal femoral nail. *Int. J. Res. Orthop.* **2020**, *6*, 1001. [CrossRef]
41. Atthakomol, P.; Manosroi, W.; Phinyo, P.; Pipanmekaporn, T.; Vaseenon, T.; Rojanasthien, S. Predicting Survival in Thai Patients After Low Impact Hip Fracture Using Flexible Parametric Modelling: A Retrospective Cohort Study. *J. Clin. Densitom.* **2021**. [CrossRef]

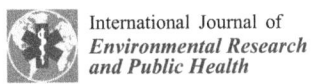

Article

Prescription Habits Related to Chronic Pathologies of Elderly People in Primary Care in the Western Part of Romania: Current Practices, International Recommendations, and Future Perspectives Regarding the Overuse and Misuse of Medicines

Valentina Buda [1,2,*,†], Andreea Prelipcean [1,†], Carmen Cristescu [1,†], Alexandru Roja [3,†], Olivia Dalleur [4,†], Minodora Andor [5,†], Corina Danciu [1,2,†], Adriana Ledeti [1,6,†], Cristina Adriana Dehelean [1,2,†] and Octavian Cretu [5,†]

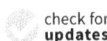

Citation: Buda, V.; Prelipcean, A.; Cristescu, C.; Roja, A.; Dalleur, O.; Andor, M.; Danciu, C.; Ledeti, A.; Dehelean, C.A.; Cretu, O. Prescription Habits Related to Chronic Pathologies of Elderly People in Primary Care in the Western Part of Romania: Current Practices, International Recommendations, and Future Perspectives Regarding the Overuse and Misuse of Medicines. *IJERPH* **2021**, *18*, 7043. https://doi.org/10.3390/ijerph18137043

Academic Editors: Francisco José Tarazona Santabalbina, Sebastià Josep Santaeugènia González, José Augusto García Navarro and José Viña

Received: 13 May 2021
Accepted: 29 June 2021
Published: 1 July 2021

Publisher's Note: MDPI stays neutral with regard to jurisdictional claims in published maps and institutional affiliations.

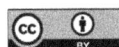

Copyright: © 2021 by the authors. Licensee MDPI, Basel, Switzerland. This article is an open access article distributed under the terms and conditions of the Creative Commons Attribution (CC BY) license (https://creativecommons.org/licenses/by/4.0/).

1. Faculty of Pharmacy, "Victor Babes" University of Medicine and Pharmacy, Eftimie Murgu Square, No. 2, 300041 Timisoara, Romania; andreea.preli@yahoo.com (A.P.); carmencristescu@umft.ro (C.C.); corina.danciu@umft.ro (C.D.); afulias@umft.ro (A.L.); cadehelean@umft.ro (C.A.D.)
2. Research Centre for Pharmaco-Toxicological Evaluation, "Victor Babes" University of Medicine and Pharmacy, Eftimie Murgu Square, No. 2, 300041 Timisoara, Romania
3. Faculty of Economics and Business Administration, West University of Timisoara, Vasile Parvan Boulevard, No.4, 300223 Timisoara, Romania; alexandru.roja@e-uvt.ro
4. Clinical Pharmacy Research Group, Louvain Drug Research Institute, Universite Catholique de Louvain, E. Mounier Street, No. 81, 1200 Woluwe-Saint-Lambert, Belgium; olivia.dalleur@uclouvain.be
5. Faculty of Medicine, "Victor Babes" University of Medicine and Pharmacy Eftimie Murgu Square, No. 2, 300041 Timisoara, Romania; andorminodora@gmail.com (M.A.); cretu.octavian@umft.ro (O.C.)
6. Advanced Instrumental Screening Center, "Victor Babes" University of Medicine and Pharmacy, Eftimie Murgu Square, No. 2, 300041 Timisoara, Romania
* Correspondence: buda.valentina@umft.ro; Tel.: +40-755-100-408
† All authors contributed equally to this work.

Abstract: The European Commission's 2019 report regarding the state of health profiles highlighted the fact that Romania is among the countries with the lowest life expectancy in the European Union. Therefore, the objectives of the present study were to assess the current prescription habits of general physicians in Romania related to medicines taken by the elderly population for chronic conditions in both urban and rural setting and to discuss/compare these practices with the current international recommendations for the elderly (American—Beers 2019 criteria and European—STOPP/START v.2, 2015 criteria). A total of 2790 electronic prescriptions for chronic pathologies collected from 18 community pharmacies in the western part of Romania (urban and rural zones) were included. All medicines had been prescribed by general physicians. We identified the following situations of medicine overuse: 15% of the analyzed prescriptions involved the use of nonsteroidal anti-inflammatory drugs (NSAIDs) for >2 weeks, 12% involved the use of a proton-pump inhibitor (PPI) for >8 weeks, theophylline was the bronchodilator used as a monotherapy in 3.17% of chronic obstructive pulmonary disease cases, and zopiclone was the hypnotic drug of choice for 2.31% of cases. Regarding the misuse of medicines, 2.33% of analyzed prescriptions contained an angiotensin-converting enzyme (ACE) inhibitor and an angiotensin II receptor blocker (ARB) for patients with renal failure in addition to vitamin K antagonists (AVKs) and NSAIDs in 0.43% of cases. Prescriptions for COX2 NSAIDs for periods longer than 2 weeks for patients with cardiovascular disorders accounted for 1.33% of prescriptions, and trihexyphenidyl was used as a monotherapy for patients with Parkinson's disease in 0.18% of cases. From the included medical prescriptions, 32.40% (the major percent of 2383 prescriptions) had two potentially inappropriate medications (PIMs). Rural zones were found to be risk factor for PIMs. Decreasing the chronic prescription of NSAIDs and PPIs, discontinuing the use of hypnotic drugs, and avoiding potentially harmful drug-drug associations will have long term beneficial effects for Romanian elderly patients.

Keywords: aged people; primary health care; STOPP/START; Beers criteria; medical prescriptions for chronic pathologies; inappropriate prescribing

1. Introduction

The European Commission's 2019 report regarding the state of health profiles highlighted the fact that Romania is among the countries with the lowest life expectancy in the European Union (EU) (75.3 years in Romania versus 80.9 years in the EU), with large discrepancies between individuals of different genders and education levels [1]. Women live for an average of 7 years longer than men, and the most educated men (with at least a tertiary education level completed) are expected to live 10 years longer than the least educated (who have not completed secondary education) [2].

Some of the causes of increased mortality involve behavioral risk factors (smoking, obesity, alcohol consumption, low physical activity, and poor nutrition in the form of excessive consumption of salt and sugar and low intake of fruits and vegetables), having a lower number of doctors and nurses per inhabitant, and having much lower health care costs compared with other EU countries (both per patient—1029 versus 2884 EUR/patient in the EU and per percent of gross domestic product (GDP)—5 versus 9.8% in the EU) [1].

It seems that the main causes of death are preventable and treatable pathologies, with diseases of the circulatory system (ischemic heart diseases and stroke) being the primary cause (58.2%), followed by cancer (lung, breast, or colorectal) and respiratory diseases [3].

In light of the current severe acute respiratory syndrome coronavirus (SARS-CoV-2) pandemic, we also have to highlight the susceptibility of elderly people to this virus [4]. Elderly people are more likely to develop a severe and critical form of the disease. Diseases such as cardiovascular diseases, acute respiratory distress syndrome, chronic obstructive pulmonary disease, and diabetes can predict poorer outcomes [5], putting elderly people at risk of faster clinical deterioration [6]. In Romania, The National Institute of Public Health provides a weekly report concerning the COVID-19 situation. Their statistics highlight that the median age of death due to COVID-19 is 71 years and that all people who have died from this disease have had at least one comorbidity. It has also been shown that 59.8% of deaths occurred in males [7]. In a case study, the European Commission's H2020 Expert Group pointed that sex and gender can impact the outcome of contracting COVID-19 and that more men than woman die from acute infection [8]. Regarding the COVID-19 mortality rate in other European countries, data published at the beginning of February 2021 by the WHO Coronavirus Disease Dashboard showed the following: 3.51% in Hungary, 3.46% in Italy, 2.73% in Germany, 2.54% in Romania, 2.41% in France, and 2.09% in Spain (number of deaths/total number of reported cases) [9].

Primary care services in Romania seem to be less often used than hospital emergency services. Emergency services are often used for less urgent cases, thus increasing the inpatient care costs for the Romanian population [1]. Moreover, the vaccination rate is lower than the EU average (8% in Romania versus 44% in the EU among the elderly for influenza in 2017) [1,10].

Several studies have stated that inappropriate prescription is a major health issue among the elderly in all clinical settings [11–13]. The physiological changes that occur during the aging process, result in changes in the pharmacokinetics and pharmacodynamics of administered medicines. Moreover, the presence of comorbidities and polypharmacy, lead to negative outcomes regarding patient safety, such as adverse drug reactions (ADRs). These ADRs will later increase the prevalence and incidence of morbidity and mortality in geriatric patients [14].

In order to counteract this problem, clear rules and recommendations for proper utilization of medicines in the elderly population are required. Explicit criteria have been developed in order to improve the selection, efficiency, and safety of medication as well as the quality of health care services [15]. The first criteria that were developed were the Beers criteria, which were published in 1991 in the USA. They were later adapted and improved for European countries (due to several differences regarding approved medicines in the European market and treatment strategies), giving rise to the Screening Tool of Older Persons' Prescriptions (STOPP) and the Screening Tool to Alert to Right Treatment (START) criteria, which were published in 2008. The American Geriatrics Society updates the Beers criteria every three years (starting from 2012), while the STOPP/START version 1 criteria were updated seven years after first being published, in 2015 [15]. The STOPP/START criteria are now recognized by several institutes and geriatric societies and are used by many European countries in routine clinical practice [16,17].

In 2016, in a population of elderly community members, Wallace et al. showed that when a minimum of two potentially inappropriate medicines were prescribed, the risk of an ADR was increased (according to the STOPP/START criteria). This, in turn, decreased patients' quality of life and increased hospitalization rates over a follow-up period of 2 years [11]. Moreover, in 2016, Wauters et al. concluded that mortality and hospitalization rates are related to inappropriate medication prescription practices, such as overuse (prescribing more medicines than are clinically needed and with potential harmful effects that exceed the potential benefits) and misuse (incorrectly prescribing a medicine) of medicines [13,18–20].

Romania is currently lacking studies that demonstrate the problems in the healthcare system or in real-life situations (lack of current statistical data). Few studies (three in the last 9 years) have assessed the prescription appropriateness in the elderly population [14,21,22]. Moreover, the county and the city hospitals in Romania lack geriatric doctors, and the European guidelines for appropriate prescription in elderly people have not been implemented (and few specialists know about them) [23].

Early detection of frailty and intervention for elderly Romanians living independently (able to take care of themselves without being dependent on another human) must be a priority, as more than 65% of subjects, particularly women (divorced or widowed, with a higher risk, aged >75 years old), were considered frail in a study performed by Pislaru et al. in 2016 [24,25].

Therefore, the objectives of the present study were to assess the current prescription habits of general physicians in Romania regarding medicines taken as chronic treatments by the elderly population (in both rural and urban setting) and to discuss/compare our findings with the current international (USA—Beers 2019 Criteria and European—STOPP/START v.2, 2015) recommendations for the elderly [26,27].

2. Materials and Methods

2.1. Study Design, Setting, and Data Collection

This cross-sectional study included a total of 2790 electronic medical prescriptions for chronic pathologies collected from 18 community pharmacies in the western part of Romania (urban and rural zones) between January 2018 and June 2019, all written by general physicians. Regarding the Romanian classification of urban and rural zone, it is worth mentioning that some of the minimum indicators mentioned by Romanian legislation for urban zones are as follows: 5000 inhabitants/locality, 75% of the total employed population working in non-agricultural activities, 70% of all homes equipped with water supply installations, 55% of all homes equipped with a bathroom and toilet inside the house, seven hospital beds/1000 inhabitants, and 1.8 doctors/1000 inhabitants [28,29]. By chronic pathologies, we understand a human health condition/disease as lasting more than 3 months (long duration and slow progression), that cannot be prevented by vaccines or cured by medication [30].

In Romania, electronic prescriptions for chronic pathologies can be issued over a period of 30, 60, or 90 days and contain a maximum of seven prescribed medicines (usually written using international drug names), which are reimbursed by the national health insurance system (Figure 1) [31].

When medical electronic prescriptions were collected (as the printed version) from community pharmacies (by the "pharmacy group": pharmacist, 2 clinical pharmacist students, and 2 clinical pharmacists), the names and assurance personal identification codes of patients had been already blurred.

Romanian electronic medical prescription
- Example -

Prescription serie .... number ....
1. Prescriber's information
Name of private medical doctor ....
Unique registration code ....
National Assurance contract number ....
Telephone .... E-mail ......

□ General physician
□ Outpatient
□ Hospital
□ Others
....
....

QR code

2. Patient's information Medical record number ....
Name ...... Surname ....
Assurance Personal Identification Code .....
Date of birth day/month/year
Gender .... M .... F, Citizenship ....

Type of Assurance:
□ Employee □ ....
□ Co-insured □ ....
□ Freelance □ ....
□ Child (<18 years) □ ....
□ Student
□ Retired

3. Diagnostic codes ....

4. Prescription date ....

Nr. crt.	Diagnostic code	Type of Diagnostic	International Drug Name / Comercial Name	« Detur Signetur »	Cantity	Number of days of treatment	% Reference price	Assurance list of drug
1.	453 (Essential arterial hypertension)	Cr (chronic)	INDAPAMIDUM prolonged-release tablets 1.5mg	1/day	30 (thirty)	30	90	A
2.	......	......	......	......	.....	.....	.....	....

Doctor's name / stamp ....
Signature ....

Figure 1. Example of a Romanian electronic medical prescription [31].

2.1.1. Inclusion Criteria

Electronic prescriptions were included in this study based on age (≥65 years old), prescriber (general physician), and ambulatory treatment and duration (chronic treatment).

2.1.2. Exclusion Criteria

Prescriptions did not meet the criteria for inclusion in this study if they were duplicates issued for the same patient but in different months (based on the patient's gender, date of birth, prescriber, and medical record number of the patient, using Microsoft Excel). These were excluded by the "pharmacy group" that analyzed the prescriptions. Psychotropic and narcotic medications, such as benzodiazepines, barbiturates, opioids, and zolpidem (and not zopiclone), were also excluded from this study, as Romanian legislation (Law 339/2005) requires different prescription forms that are non-electronic and more secure for these types of medicines [32]. Moreover, over-the-counter (OTC) medicines and food supplements were also excluded, as they are not reimbursed by the national health insurance system and cannot be prescribed via electronic form.

2.2. Data Evaluation

The collected prescriptions were analyzed in face-to-face meetings by an interdisciplinary team of 10 specialists (cardiologist, psychiatrist, gastroenterologist, pulmonologist, generalist, pharmacist, two clinical pharmacists, and two clinical pharmacy students) over a period of 6 months, based on the 2019 Beers criteria and the STOPP/START v.2 criteria [26,27,33]. The meetings were scheduled once per week, and each session lasted for a minimum of 2 h.

First, the collected medical prescriptions were divided in blocks of 250 prescriptions. Each block of medical prescriptions underwent a three-round screening evaluation: first, they were evaluated by the "pharmacy group", then by the general physician and the cardiologist/internist (double specialization), and finally, unanswered questions/problems were managed with the help of other specialists (Figure 2). Final decisions were made based on full agreement by everyone using the Beers 2019 and STOPP/START v.2, 2015 criteria [26,27]. It is worth mentioning that the results of the first review performed by the "pharmacy group" were shared with the first physician reviewers (general physician and the internist).

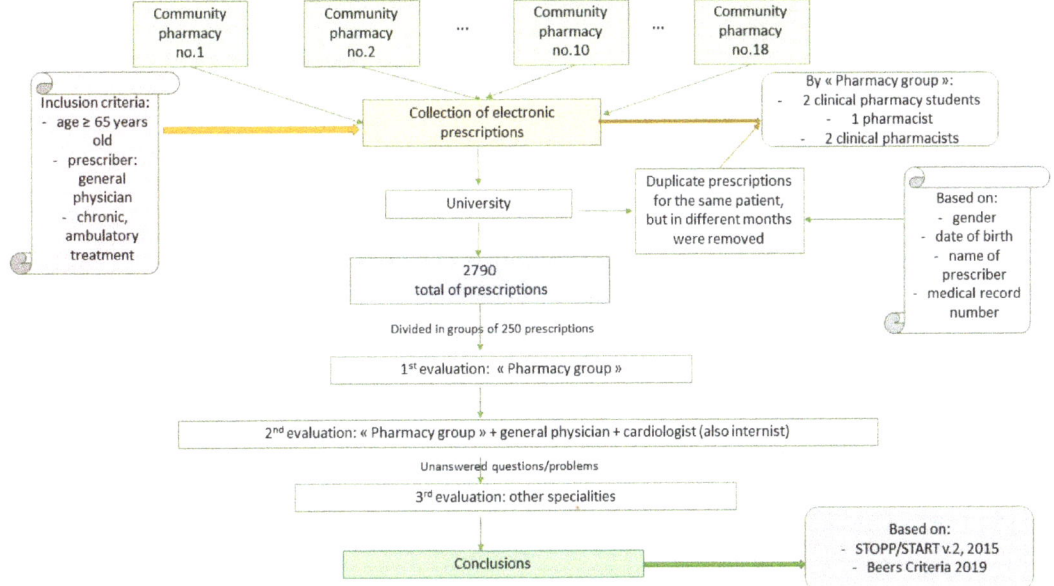

Figure 2. Schematic representation of the study's methodology.

Patients' data were collected using chronic electronic prescriptions, and we did not have access to clinical data. We were able to identify the prescriber (e.g., general physician), the type of treatment (e.g., ambulatory and chronic), and the patients' genders and ages (Figure 1).

Based on the diagnostic codes (attributed by the national health insurance system for each chronic pathology) of each prescription, we identified the main chronic conditions experienced by the patients.

Treatment duration was determined based on the days for which each prescription was issued (number of days of treatment, Figure 1). For the assessment of the duration of use of proton-pump inhibitors (PPIs) and H2 antagonists, only prescriptions issued for 60 or 90 days were counted in the final analysis.

Overall, 26 STOPP v.2, 2015 criteria were applied to the dataset [27]. Regarding the 2019 Beers criteria, only 17 could be applied [26]. All the applied criteria are listed in Appendix A of the present article.

2.3. Statistical Analysis

Data are presented either as the mean ± standard deviation or as percentages. SPSS v.17 statistical software (SPSS Statistics for Windows, version 17.0. Chicago: SPSS Inc.) was used for the analysis. For the sample size calculation, we conducted a power analysis test using G*Power 3.1 software, with 80% power, a significance level of 0.05, and an effect size of 5.31% [34,35]. We determined the descriptive statistics for the numerical variables (means and standard deviations) and for the qualitative variables (absolute and relative frequencies). Logistic regression was applied in order to determine the association between the number of potentially inappropriate medications (PIMs) and zone (rural/urban setting), age, gender, number of chronic conditions and of medicines. Chi-squared test was applied for categorical type variables and Mann–Whitney U test for numerical variables that were not normally distributed [36,37].

All collected electronic prescriptions for chronic conditions are stored under lock and key at the "Victor Babes" University of Medicine and Pharmacy, along with the flash drive containing the electronic data.

3. Results

3.1. Characteristics of the Analyzed Prescriptions and the Studied Population

A total of 2790 electronic prescriptions for chronic conditions (for 2790 patients) were included, of which 53.69% were issued by urban general physicians. Of the total prescriptions, 60.64% were for female patients, and the mean age of patients was 74.54 ± 7.22 years old. The vast majority (78.70%) of included medical prescriptions were written for a period of 30 days, and the mean number of medications per prescription was four (Table 1).

Table 1. Main characteristics of the analyzed prescriptions and patients.

Number of Prescriptions	Zone of Prescriptions		Sex Distribution		Average Age of Patients (years)	Days of Treatment			Average Number of Medicines/ prescriptions
2790	urban	53.69%	female	60.64%	74.54 ± 7.22	30 days 78.70%	60 days 3.66%	90 days 17.64%	4.29 ± 1.60
	rural	46.30%	male	39.36%					

Table 2 presents the average number of medicines per medical prescription based on age category and gender.

Table 2. The average number of medicine/prescriptions based on age.

Age Category	Gender	% of Total Prescriptions	Average Number of Medications/Prescriptions
65–69 years old	female	23.38%	4.14
	male	11.01%	4.72
70–74 years old	female	13.84%	4.36
	male	12.45%	4.53
75–79 years old	female	9.96%	4.40
	male	5.46%	4.77
80–84 years old	female	11.00%	4.51
	male	5.45%	4.51
85–89 years old	female	5.57%	4.32
	male	3.78%	5.27
90–94 years old	female	1.14%	3.11
	male	0.74%	6.63
95–99 years old	female	0.70%	3.00
	male		

From Table 2, it can be observed that for a given age group, men were prescribed more medications than women, suggesting an increased morbidity rate in the male gender.

Figure 3 presents the most common chronic conditions associated with the analyzed prescriptions based on the diagnostic code of each medical prescription. As expected, cardiovascular disorders were the most common chronic conditions encountered (around 79% of cases), followed by metabolic and endocrine disorders (38.7%), gastrointestinal disorders (13.57% of cases), respiratory system disorders, and genitourinary, musculoskeletal, and nervous system disorders (Figure 3).

3.2. Inappropriate Prescription Problems

Table 3 presents the problems associated with the overuse of medicines in elderly Romanian patients.

The prescription of NSAIDs and PPIs was the main problem identified regarding treatment duration. Of the included prescriptions, 15% had an NSAID prescribed for more than 2 weeks, and 12% had an PPI prescribed for more than 8 weeks (Table 3).

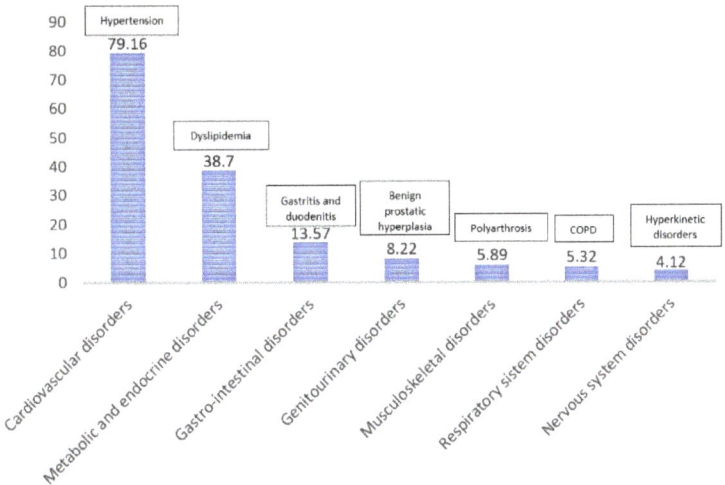

Figure 3. Most common chronic conditions requiring prescriptions.

Table 3. Overuse of medicines according to STOPP/START v.2, 2015 and Beers 2019 Criteria [26,27].

Problem Encountered	Pharmacological Class/Medicine	% of Total Prescriptions	n of Patients	Recommendations for the Elderly
a. Duration of treatment	NSAIDs (>2 weeks) [STOPP/STARRT v.2, 2015; Beers 2019]	15%	418	To be used with caution at the lowest effective dose and for the shortest period of time (acute treatment). Monitoring of side effects.
	PPIs (>8 weeks) [STOPP/STARRT v.2, 2015; Beers 2019]	12%	335	To evaluate the risk/benefit ratio when prescribing for longer periods of time (>8 weeks). Use with caution in patients with polypharmacy (inhibitors of cytochrome P450).
	H_2 antagonist (>8 weeks) [STOPP/STARRT v.2, 2015]	2%	56	To evaluate the risk/benefit ratio when prescribing for longer periods of time (>8 weeks). Potential drug–drug interactions in patients with polypharmacy. [38,39]
b. Treatment indication (i) Bronchodilator used in monotherapy for chronic obstructive pulmonary disease (ii) Hypnotic drugs	Theophylline [STOPP/STARRT v.2, 2015]	3.17%	88	More effective and less toxic agents currently available (beta 2 adrenomimetic or anticholinergic bronchodilators).
	Zopiclone [STOPP/STARRT v.2, 2015; Beers 2019]	2.31%	64	Prefer other treatment options with safer profiles and better tolerance. If used, prescribe in the lowest effective dose (half of the adult dose) and for a maximum period of 4 weeks.
c. Duplication of pharmacological class	Diuretics (loop or thiazide) Beta blockers Dihydropyridines NSAIDs ACE inhibitors H_1 antagonists [STOPP/STARRT v.2, 2015]	2.20%	61	Avoid using two medicines with the same mechanism of action. Minimal clinical benefits when duplicated. Exacerbation of side effects.

Legend: NSAID, nonsteroidal anti-inflammatory drug; PPI, proton-pump inhibitor; ACE, angiotensin-converting enzyme; Screening Tool of Older Persons' Prescriptions (STOPP); Screening Tool to Alert to Right Treatment (START).

Moreover, theophylline was the bronchodilator used as a monotherapy in 3.17% of cases for patients with chronic obstructive pulmonary disease, while zopiclone was the hypnotic medicine used in 2.31% of cases (Table 3).

We also identified duplications of pharmacological class in 2.2% of medical prescriptions (Table 3).

Table 4 presents the identified problems associated with the misuse of medicines in Romanian elderly patients.

Table 4. Misuse of medicines according to STOPP/START v.2, 2015 and Beers 2019 Criteria [26,27].

Problem Encountered	Pharmacological Class/Medicine	% of Total Prescriptions	n of Patients	Recommendations for the Elderly
a. Drug–drug interactions	ACE inhibitors + ARBs [STOPP/STARRT v.2, 2015; Beers 2019]	2.33%	65	Avoid the association. High risk of hyperkalemia, renal injuries.
	α_1 blockers + Furosemide [STOPP/STARRT v.2, 2015; Beers 2019]	1.36%	38	Avoid the association. High risk of urinary incontinence.
	AVK + NSAIDs [STOPP/STARRT v.2, 2015]	0.43%	12	Avoid the association. Major risk of gastro-intestinal bleeding.
	Beta blockers + Verapamil/diltiazem [STOPP/STARRT v.2, 2015]	0.33%	9	Avoid the association. Cardiac depression, heart block.
	Associations of CNS depressants [Beers 2019]	0.18%	5	Avoid the association. Central nervous system depression, with increased risk of falls and fractures.
b. Drug-pathology interactions	Cardiovascular disorders + COX_2 NSAIDs (>2 weeks) [STOPP/STARRT v.2, 2015; Beers 2019]	1.33%	37	Avoid the association. Increased risk of cardiovascular complications (stroke, myocardial infarction).
c. Drug class	Trihexyphenidyl (monotherapy) for Parkinson's disorder in patients $\geq$65 years old [Beers 2019]	0.18%	5	More effective substances currently available. Increased risk of anticolinergic side effects.

Legend: ARB, angiotensin II receptor blocker; AVK, vitamin K antagonist; CNS, central nervous system.

Concerning the misuse of medications, the most commonly encountered problems were drug–drug interactions, the prescription of COX2 NSAIDs for longer than 2 weeks for patients with cardiovascular disorders (1.33% of cases), and the prescription of trihexyphenidyl as a monotherapy for patients with Parkinson's disorder (Table 4).

Regarding drug–drug interactions, 2.33% of analyzed prescriptions contained the association of an ACE inhibitor and an ARB for patients with renal failure (identified based on the diagnostic code), followed by the association of AVK and NSAIDs in 0.43% of cases (Table 4).

The percent of medical prescriptions in function of the number of potentially inappropriate medication (PIM) is presented in Table 5. In addition, 2383 medical prescriptions (85.41%) of total cases had a least one PIM.

Table 5. Percent of medical prescriptions with potentially inappropriate medication (PIM).

n of PIM/Prescription	% of Total Prescriptions with PIM	% of Rural Zones	% of Urban Zones
1	30.96	19.76	11.20
2	32.40	14.69	17.71
3	22.26	17.03	5.22
4	8.48	2.12	5.08
≥5	5.90	1.89	5.30

It can be noticed that the highest percent of potentially inappropriate prescriptions (32.40%) included two potentially inappropriate medications (Table 5), from a total of 2383 prescriptions with PIM.

As presented in Table 6, urban zones were found to be protective factors for PIMs (OR = 0.582, with 95% CI = [0.482, 0.702], as well as a higher duration of treatment (OR = 0.995, with 95% CI = [0.991, 0.999]).

Table 6. Logistic regression considering PIM (Yes/No) as a dependent variable.

Variables in the Equation	B	S.E.	Wald	df	Sig.	Exp(B)	95% CI for EXP(B) Lower	Upper
County	−0.659	0.101	42.125	1	0.000	0.518	0.424	0.631
Zone	−0.541	0.096	32.043	1	0.000	0.582	0.482	0.702
Gender	0.024	0.093	0.068	1	0.794	1.025	0.854	1.229
Age	0.005	0.006	0.732	1	0.392	1.005	0.993	1.017
n of medicines	−0.048	0.041	1.392	1	0.238	0.953	0.880	1.032
n of diagnostics	−0.003	0.053	0.004	1	0.950	0.997	0.899	1.105
Days of treatment	−0.005	0.002	5.878	1	0.015	0.995	0.991	0.999
Constant	1.044	0.513	4.139	1	0.042	2.840		

Rural zones were found to be risk factor for PIMs (Chi-squared test, $p < 0.001$, OR = 2.109, with 95% CI = [1.769, 2.516]) (Tables 5 and 6).

4. Discussion

To the best of our knowledge, this is the first study to assess the prescription habits of general physicians for medications taken as chronic treatments by elderly patients in both urban and rural settings of the western part of Romania and to compare these with the international recommendations for aged people (USA—Beers 2019 criteria and European—STOPP/START v.2, 2015 criteria) [26,27].

This retrospective study, which included a large number of electronic prescriptions for chronic conditions for elderly patients prescribed by Romanian general physicians, showed that more than 85% had medication prescription problems. Below, we discuss some of the most frequent inappropriate prescriptions in light of current recommendations.

4.1. NSAIDs

The most commonly encountered problem in our study was the prescription of NSAIDs and therefore the overuse of this class of medicines by Romanian general physicians for the elderly population. The Beers 2019 criteria state that the administration of NSAIDs increases the risk of gastrointestinal bleeding and peptic ulcer development, especially if they are used as a chronic treatment for more than 1 year. The use of PPIs or misoprostol reduces, but does not eliminate, this risk. Moreover, the use of NSAIDs can increase blood pressure and induce kidney injury, which can aggravate heart failure, as they promote fluid retention and can increase mortality [26]. Therefore, it is recommended to use NSAIDs with caution in the lowest effective dose and for the shortest possible period of treatment (acute treatment), as they can induce several gastrointestinal, renal, and/or cardiovascular side effects, as described in Table 7 [40].

Table 7. Main side effects of NSAIDs [40].

Gastrointestinal	Main Side Effects of NSAIDs Cardiovascular	Renal
• dyspepsia • peptic ulcer • gastrointestinal bleeding • gastrointestinal perforation	• edema • hypertension • myocardial infarction • stroke • congestive heart failure • thrombotic events	• sodium retention • edema • electrolyte imbalance • reduction of glomerular filtration rate • chronic kidney disease
Mechanism: inhibition of prostaglandin synthesis, which decreases the protective action of the gastrointestinal mucosa; fewer side effects with COX2 selective drugs but a higher cardiovascular risk.	Mechanism: inhibition of prostaglandin synthesis and elevation of serum aldosterone, which leads to hypertension and sodium retention.	Mechanism: inhibition of prostaglandin and thromboxane synthesis, which induces renal vasoconstriction, reduced renal perfusion, and impaired renal function.

If these medicines must be used in the elderly, monitoring for common side effects is recommended, especially as several studies have shown that long periods of NSAID exposure increase the risk of acute kidney injury or chronic kidney disease progression, especially if NSAIDs are combined with certain other classes of medicines, such as ACE inhibitors/ARBs and/or diuretics [41–43]. We identified that 2% of cases (56 patients) involved the "triple whammy therapy" (association of RAAS inhibitor + diuretic + NSAID), and 1.15% (32 patients) involved the association of an ACE inhibitor/ARB + NSAID. Several studies have shown that "triple whammy" therapy increases the risk of acute kidney injury, with higher hospitalization rates, especially for men [44,45]. Moreover, the American Geriatric Society noted that NSAID use must be avoided in all patients with end-stage renal failure (CrCl <30 mL/min) [26].

It is important to take the risk of hyponatremia into consideration, as it is the most common electrolyte disorder encountered in clinical practice, especially in the elderly population (due to dehydration, polypharmacy, and comorbidities, which all can induce an electrolyte imbalance) [46]. All NSAIDs can induce hyponatremia, even if they are taken for only a few days, as they inhibit the action of the antidiuretic hormone (due to the reduction of renal prostaglandins), causing also water retention. Thus, physicians must consider this risk, as well as the associations of medicines that can aggravate hyponatremia, as even mild forms of hyponatremia are associated with negative clinical outcomes, such as cognitive impairment, falls, hospitalizations, and mortality [46]. Moreover, a higher mortality rate has been observed in patients with moderate or severe hyponatremia [47,48]. In addition, the STOPP/START v.2 criteria state that the use of selective serotonin reuptake inhibitor (SSRI) antidepressants (the most commonly prescribed medicines nowadays) must be avoided in patients with hyponatremia, as they can exacerbate this condition, while the 2019 Beers criteria also include tramadol in the list of medicines that can aggravate hyponatremia or cause inappropriate antidiuretic hormone secretion (SIADH) [26,27,48]. Thus, it is extremely important to decrease the number of chronic prescriptions of NSAIDs in the Romanian elderly population and to monitor sodium levels in patients undergoing chronic treatment with NSAIDs, as deleterious effects can arise, with extremely dangerous consequences.

In addition to prescriptions, our research group showed (in another study performed) that more than 65% of the Romanian population use NSAIDs for self-medication, especially patients with cardiovascular pathologies, despite the European Medicine Agency recommendations (on safety precautions of particular NSAIDs) and probably because diclofenac formulations are the cheapest medicines on the market [49]. Thus, members of the Romanian population are large consumers of NSAIDs, although Romania is among the EU countries with the highest incidence of acute coronary syndrome [1].

In the elderly, drug-induced nephrotoxicity is a frequent adverse reaction, which can precipitate acute or chronic diseases as well as increase morbidity and mortality. It has been shown to be responsible for 66% cases of renal failure in the elderly population [50]. Moreover, as renal function is affected by senescence, practitioners should avoid prescribing medicines that can increase this risk (for the elderly) when taken in association, as the renal blood flow, number of functional nephrons, and renal filtration rate are already affected by the aging process. Certain prescription associations also increase the risk of community-acquired hyperkalemia in the elderly [44,45].

Furthermore, we also identified associations of NSAIDs and AVKs in chronic electronic prescriptions. It is well known that this kind of association highly increases the hemorrhagic risk. Based on the fact that a very small proportion of the Romanian population has targeted INR (International Normalized Ratio) values under anticoagulant treatment, it is advisable to avoid this association for members of the Romanian elderly population [51].

4.2. PPIs

The second most frequently encountered problem was the prescription of PPIs for a period of more than 2 months. The 2019 Beers criteria mention the risks of bone loss, fracture, and *C. difficile* infection with long-term PPI treatment. Moreover, several publications have shown that long-term use (>2 months) of PPIs is associated with the following side effects, which are particularly harmful in elderly patients: vitamin B_{12} and iron deficiency, hypomagnesaemia, bone demineralization and fragility, intestinal and other infections (bacterial overgrowth, non-typhoidal *Salmonella, Campylobacter, Clostridium difficile*, community-acquired pneumonia), impaired cognition and affect, and increased risk of chronic kidney disease [52–54]. PPI use was recently associated with the onset of dementia and depression in the elderly population, although the exact mechanism by which this occurs is not clear (it might be due to vitamin B_{12} malabsorption). Thus, it is necessary to evaluate the risks and benefits when prescribing PPIs for the elderly for long periods of time and to consider potential drug–drug interactions in patients with polypharmacy, as PPIs are inhibitors of the P450 cytochrome [55,56].

4.3. Theophylline

We also identified the prescription of theophylline as a monotherapy by Romanian general physicians for patients with chronic obstructive pulmonary disease. Theophylline is a narrow therapeutic window bronchodilator. The 2019 Beers criteria and the STOPP/START v2 2015 criteria recommend the use of beta 2 adrenomimetic or anticholinergic bronchodilators, which are more effective and less toxic compared with theophylline, for the treatment of chronic obstructive pulmonary diseases [26,27,57].

Therapy with theophylline requires monitoring of its concentration in the serum, and patients can experience toxicity symptoms like arrhythmia or convulsions before nausea and vomiting occur (Table 8). Moreover, smokers require higher doses of the medication, and smoking cessation increases its toxicity. It is susceptible to drug–drug interactions with the following medicines: phenytoin, ciprofloxacin, co-trimoxazole, levothyroxine, and benzodiazepines [58]. In addition, as cardiovascular diseases are the primary pathologies encountered in the elderly Romanian population (based on our study findings using the percentages of chronic conditions and other European reports) [59], treatment with theophylline can increase the risk of cardiovascular complications with serious side effects, especially in patients with atrial fibrillation and congestive heart failure. Thus, due to the low risk/benefit ratio and despite its low price, it is recommended that theophylline is replaced with other bronchodilator medicines (β_2-agonists or anticholinergics) with safer and more efficient profiles. Further, the 2019 Beers criteria mention an increased risk of theophylline toxicity when the drug is associated with other medicines, especially enzyme inhibitors (e.g., ciprofloxacin), administered for acute treatments [26].

Table 8. The most common side effects of theophylline [60].

Most Common Side Effects of Theophylline			
Neurological	Cardiovascular	Respiratory	Gastrointestinal
• agitation • irritability • tremor • hallucination • insomnia	• tachycardia • atrial fibrillation • hypotension • cardiac arrest	• tachypnea • acute lung injury • respiratory alkalosis	• nausea • vomiting • abdominal pain

4.4. Zopiclone

Regrettably, despite several recommendations not to treat habitual insomnia in the elderly with medications such as benzodiazepines and non-benzodiazepine receptor agonist hypnotics (Z drugs), these medications are still the most commonly prescribed drugs for this age group [61]. The 2019 Beers recommendations state that "Z drugs" produce adverse drug reactions similar to those of benzodiazepines, such as daily sedation, delirium, and increased risk of falls and fractures. Moreover, they induce minimal improvements in sleep latency and duration [26]. Romanian legislation (Law 39/2005) demands that benzodiazepine and zolpidem drugs are prescribed on secure prescription forms and not with the basic electronic formulary; this is why our study did not include these substances [32]. Only zopiclone can be prescribed with the classical electronic prescription form, and as expected, our study shows that it is overprescribed in the elderly population.

It is worth mentioning that older people are the most vulnerable and susceptible to developing side effects of sleep medication, Z drugs, and benzodiazepines, so it is recommended to use them at the lowest effective dose (half the adult dose) and for a short period of time (4 weeks) [61,62]. Moreover, the 2019 Beers criteria mention that they have minimal efficacy in treating insomnia, with a high probability of developing adverse reactions [26]. The current recommendations regarding insomnia treatment focus on cognitive behavioral therapy, as maintaining cognitive functioning is an important aspect that must be taken into account in the elderly [61]. Moreover, sleep-disordered breathing should be diagnosed in a timely manner and treated effectively in elderly patients, as it can be a prime cause of sleep disorders [61,62]. An alternative medicine for the treatment of sleep disorders could be melatonin (as its natural secretion decreases with age), which is better tolerated and has fewer side effects. Moreover, it was recently reported to have renal protective properties, which could be beneficial for elderly patients [50].

4.5. Misuse of Medicines

Regarding the main drug–drug interactions encountered, 2.33% of the prescriptions analyzed in this study involved the association of an ACE inhibitor and an ARB for patients with renal impairment. In 2017, the European Society of Cardiology recommended that this association should be avoided, if possible, because of the unclear results from clinical trials regarding its benefits and the higher risk of acute functional renal failure [63].

It is recommended that COX2 NSAIDs to be avoided as chronic treatments for patients with cardiovascular pathologies due to the high incidence of acute coronary complications (e.g., myocardial infarction) [27]. Moreover, the 2019 Beers recommendations state that COX2 NSAIDs and thiazolidinediones should be used with caution in patients with asymptomatic heart failure and avoided in those with symptomatic heart failure [26]. In the present study, we identified several prescriptions containing COX2 NSAID use for more than 2 weeks.

4.6. Study Limitations

As a study limitation, we must mention the fact that only electronic prescriptions for chronic conditions were included. A clear picture of the entire patient treatment regimen (acute, chronic, OTC drugs, and food supplements) would have provided more information, along with other clinical patient data (e.g., hepatic/renal function, ionogram). Moreover, the assessment of oral anticoagulation therapy in patients with atrial fibrillation/heart failure was not possible, as there is no diagnostic code available from the assurance company for this pathology, and novel oral anticoagulants (NOACs) were not reimbursed by the company when the prescriptions analyzed in this study were written. Due to the limited availability of the included data, only part of the 2019 Beers and STOPP/START v.2, 2015 criteria could be applied [26,27]. Moreover, the present study included prescriptions from only the western part of Romania; thus, the present results cannot be generalized to the entire country. Additionally, patients' frailty was not assessed.

4.7. Correlations with the Scientific Literature

Our study results are in accordance with the studies performed by Primejdie et al. in 2012 and 2016, which highlighted that NSAIDs, benzodiazepines, zopiclone, and zolpidem are the pharmaceutical substances most frequently associated with safety concerns in ambulatory as well as in institutionalized patients [21,22]. In a study performed in Spain in 2019, where the two versions of the Beers criteria (2012 and 2015) and the two versions of the STOPP criteria (v.1, 2008 and v.2, 2015) were applied, benzodiazepines, proton-pump inhibitors, peripheral alpha-1 blockers, and NSAIDs were among the most common potentially inappropriate medications found [64]. Another study performed in Brazil in very old hospitalized patients emphasized (after applying the 2019 Beers criteria) that polypharmacy occurs in approximately 84.6% of cases and that the most commonly encountered PIMs are metoclopramide, omeprazole, regular insulin, and haloperidol [65]. A study performed on South Korean geriatrics and published in 2018 showed that chlorpheniramine and amitriptyline were the most frequently prescribed PIMs (after applying the Beers Criteria) [66].

Other studies on the Romanian elderly population have shown that aged people living in villages have a significantly higher rate of prolonged hospitalization due to the lack of nearby hospitals [67] and the lack of specialists in small cities and rural areas [68]. In addition to this data, in the present study, we found rural zones to be a risk factor for the incidence of PIM which could contribute to the risk of ADR and also to hospitalization rates, as other studies reported [11]. Moreover, a study performed by Simionescu et al. highlighted the fact that in order to reduce the mortality rate due to cardiovascular diseases, the amount of health care spending per person must be increased by the government [68].

Another study that evaluated patients' adherence to antihypertensive therapy in urban family medical practices concluded that Romania needs further strategies and management strategy methods to increase patients' adherence to treatment [69].

4.8. Purpose of Solutions

Regarding health expenditure in Romania compared to other European countries, it can easily be observed that some of the budget allocated to the health sector could be invested more strategically, with higher efficiency, especially for the prevention of diseases that generate high treatment costs (if they are not discovered in time). From the point of view of investing public budgets in health care, there are notable differences between Romania and other EU countries [70]. In the last five years, according to statistics provided by Eurostat and the OECD (Organization for Economic Co-operation and Development), Romania has allocated about 5% of its gross domestic product to health spending [70,71]. When compared to Switzerland, which invests about 12.5% of its GDP in health, or the European average, which is close to 7% of the GDP, it is clear that there is a major difference between Romania and other civilized countries in this regard. Additionally, of interest for our research is that, according to Eurostat statistics, regarding the destination of invested health budgets, in Romania, approximately 54.4% is spent on treating and rehabilitating patients, 27% is spent on equipment and goods needed in the medical process, and only 18% is spent on other expenses, including prevention. We compared this with Switzerland, which ranks first in the allocation of financial resources for other activities, including prevention and found that only half the budget of other countries is allocated for preventive medicine in Romania [70,71]. (The percentage allocated to preventive medicine from the state budget is about 1.8%, far below the European average.)

Another distinctive aspect noted in the OECD statistics is the way in which health budgets are formed at the level of the European Union and the distinct characteristics of Romania. Whereas in states with a high-performing health system, the share of government schemes and private financial instruments prevails, in Romania, the citizens' contributions are the main source of funding for the health system. Almost 70% of Romanian health system costs come from citizen contributions, compared to Switzerland, where citizens contribute 40% and the state identifies other ways, including private ones, to ensure the stability of the national health budget [70,71].

Moreover, the use of technology, digital innovation, and digitalization as part of the national strategy can contribute significantly to making public health spending more efficient [72]. The use of electronic patient medical records is an immediate action that should be implemented in the Romanian health care system. From an economic point of view, the emergence of the eHealthcare field could greatly optimize the spending of budgets and ensure better prevention [73–75].

Teamwork between specialists (doctors, pharmacists, nurses) is also mandatory for a patient-centered approach with a lower incidence of iatrogenic events [76].

4.9. Practical Implications

The present study highlights the urgent need for appropriate pharmacological treatment in order to reduce the iatrogenic risk associated with renal injuries, cardiovascular complications, and electrolyte imbalances. The use of the Beers and STOPP/START criteria could also be beneficial as guides for appropriate treatment, along with clinical judgment and taking into account the specific characteristics of patients [26,27].

Moreover, we emphasize the urgent need to improve and correctly implement prevention strategies and effective treatment programs and to reinforce the proficiency/suitability of primary care, especially for elderly Romanians (who take the largest number of medicines), as the population is aging [77,78].

4.10. Purpose of Further Studies

Larger multi-centric studies are needed in order to get a correct overview of the current Romanian practices of prescribing, based on the entire medical record of the patients.

5. Conclusions

Several prescription problems have been identified in the Romanian primary care setting for patients with chronic pathologies. NSAIDs, PPIs, H2 antagonists, theophylline, and zopiclone were found to be among the medicines prescribed more often than clinically needed and that have potential harmful effects that exceed potential benefits. Additionally, duplication of pharmacological classes was observed. The association of RAAS inhibitors in patients with renal failure in addition to the utilization of COX2 NSAIDs were among the most commonly observed problems involving incorrect prescription.

Thus, decreasing the chronic prescription of NSAIDs and PPIs, discontinuing the use of hypnotic drugs, and avoiding potentially harmful drug–drug associations will have long term beneficial effects for Romanian elderly patients.

Author Contributions: Conceptualization, V.B., C.C., A.P. and O.C.; methodology, V.B., C.C., A.P. and O.D.; software, C.D. and A.L.; writing—original draft preparation, V.B., A.P. and A.R.; writing—review and editing, C.C., C.A.D., M.A., O.C. and O.D. All authors have read and agreed to the published version of the manuscript.

Funding: This research received no external funding.

Institutional Review Board Statement: The study was conducted according to the guidelines of the Declaration of Helsinki.

Informed Consent Statement: Not applicable.

Data Availability Statement: The data presented in this study are available on request from the corresponding author.

Acknowledgments: The authors would like to thank all the healthcare professionals involved in the realization of the present study (data collection and evaluation) for their time and effort.

Conflicts of Interest: The authors declare no conflict of interest.

Appendix A

STOPP/START v.2, 2015 Criteria Used [27]:	2019 Beers Criteria Used [26]:
1. Prescribed medicine with no clinical indication	1. Antiparkinsonian gents (e.g., trihexyphenidyl)—more effective substances are currently available for the treatment of Parkinson disease; not recommended for the prevention/treatment of extrapyramidal symptoms with neuroleptics.
2. Prescribed medicine beyond the recommended period of administration.	
3. The duplication of a drug class e.g., two concurrent NSAIDs, anticoagulants, ACE (angiotensin-converting enzyme) inhibitors, SSRIs (selective serotonin reuptake inhibitors), loop diuretics (before considering a new agent, an optimization of a single drug class should be taken into consideration).	2. Peripheral alpha-1 blockers (e.g., doxazosin, prazosin) for treatment of hypertension—high risk of orthostatic hypotension in the elderly; more effective substances are currently available (superior risk/benefit ratio).
4. The combination of a Beta-blocker with verapamil or diltiazem (risk of heart block).	3. Central alpha-agonists—high risk of central nervous system side effects; risk of bradycardia and orthostatic hypotension if used for chronic treatment of hypertension.
5. The use of centrally-acting antihypertensive (e.g., methyldopa, clonidine, rilmenidine, moxonidine), unless lack of efficacy, or clear intolerance, with other classes of antihypertensive (older people tolerate them less well).	4. Antidepressants (e.g., amitriptyline, doxepin > 6 mg/day, used alone or in combination)—intensive anticholinergic properties, risk of sedation and orthostatic hypotension.
6. The combination of aldosterone antagonists (e.g., spironolactone, eplerenone) with concurrent potassium-conserving drugs (e.g., angiotensin receptor blocker's, ACEI's, amiloride, triamterene) without monitoring of serum potassium (risk of dangerous hyperkalaemia, i.e., >6.0 mmol/l – serum K should be monitored regularly, i.e., at least every 6 months).	5. Neuroleptic drugs used in patients with dementia – higher risk of stroke, cognitive decline, and death.
	6. Benzodiazepine receptor agonist hypnotics (e.g., zopiclone)—side effects comparable to those of benzodiazepines in the elderly population.
7. The use of ACE inhibitors or Angiotensin Receptor Blockers in patients with hyperkalaemia.	7. Metoclopramide—risk of several side effects (e.g., extrapyramidal symptoms), especially with chronic treatment or in frail elderly patients.
8. The use of Loop diuretic as first-line treatment for hypertension (in regard to safety, other effective alternatives should be taken into consideration).	8. Proton-pump inhibitors—risk of *Clostridium difficile* infection and bone loss or fracture.
9. The use of loop diuretic as first line treatment for hypertension in patients associating urinary incontinence (may exacerbate incontinence).	9. Oral NSAIDs—increased risk of gastrointestinal bleeding or peptic ulcer development if administered as a chronic treatment or if associated with other medicines (e.g., corticosteroids, anticoagulants, antiplatelet agents). Higher risk of blood pressure augmentation and renal injuries.
10. Association of antiplatelet agents with direct thrombin inhibitor, vitamin K antagonist or factor Xa inhibitors in patients with cerebrovascular or peripheral arterial disease, stable coronary (the dual therapy did not bring any new benefits).	10. Ketorolac and indomethacin (oral or parenteral use)—higher risk of gastrointestinal and renal problems.
	11. Skeletal muscle relaxants (e.g., chlorzoxazone)—risk of anticholinergic effects, somnolence, fractures.
11. Association of NSAID with direct thrombin inhibitor, vitamin K antagonist or factor Xa inhibitors (risk of major gastrointestinal bleeding).	12. RAAS inhibitors (ACEIs, ARBs) or potassium-sparing diuretics associated with other RAAS inhibitors—risk of hyperkalemia.
12. Association of NSAID with concurrent antiplatelet agent(s) without using the PPI as prophylaxis (increased risk of peptic ulcer disease).	13. Opioids associated with gabapentin/pregabalin—risk of severe sedation, fractures, respiratory depression, and death.
13. The use of tricyclic antidepressants in patients with dementia, prostatism, cardiac conduction abnormalities, narrow angle glaucoma, or prior history of urinary retention (risk of worsening these conditions).	14. Association of two anticholinergic drugs—high risk of cognitive decline.
	15. Association of three or more psychotropic drugs (e.g., antidepressants, antiepileptics, hypnotics, neuroleptics, opioids)—high risk of falls and fractures.

STOPP/START v.2, 2015 Criteria Used [27]:	2019 Beers Criteria Used [26]:
14. Initiation of tricyclic antidepressants as first-line antidepressant treatment (other are available with a lower risk of adverse drug reactions). 15. The use of neuroleptics with moderate-marked antimuscarinic/anticholinergic effects (chlorpromazine, clozapine, promazine flupenthixol, zuclopenthixol) in patients with history of prostatism or previous urinary retention (high risk of urinary retention). 16. The use of antipsychotics (i.e., other than clozapine or quetiapine) in patients with Parkinson disease or Lewy Body Disease (risk of severe extra-pyramidal symptoms). 17. The use of anticholinergics/antimuscarinics in patients with dementia or delirium (risk of exacerbation of cognitive impairment). 18. The use of neuroleptics as hypnotics, unless sleep disorder is due to psychosis or dementia (risk of hypotension, confusion, extra-pyramidal side effects, falls). 19. The use of PPI at full therapeutic dosage for >8 weeks for uncomplicated peptic ulcer disease or erosive peptic oesophagitis (it should be taken into consideration the reduction of dose or earlier discontinuation). 20. The use of theophylline for COPD as monotherapy (there are more effective and safer alternative; due to its narrow therapeutic index the risk of adverse effects is high). 21. The use of NSAID for a long-term (>3 months) for symptom relief of osteoarthritis pain where paracetamol has not been tried (simple analgesics preferable and usually as effective for pain relief). 22. The use of NSAID for a long-term or colchicine (>3 months) for chronic treatment of gout where xanthine-oxidase inhibitor (e.g., febuxostat, allopurinol) are not contraindicated. 23. Prescription of COX-2 selective NSAIDs in patients with concurrent cardiovascular disease (increased risk of stroke and myocardial infarction). 24. Prescription of neuroleptic drugs (may cause gait dyspraxia, Parkinsonism). 25. Prescription of Hypnotic Z-drugs, e.g., zolpidem, zopiclone, zaleplon (risk of fall, protracted day time sedation, ataxia). 26. The association of two or more drugs with antimuscarinic/anticholinergic effects (e.g., tricyclic antidepressants, tricyclic antidepressants, first generation antihistamines) (increased anticholinergic toxicity).	16. Corticosteroids (oral or parenteral)—increased risk of gastrointestinal complications. 17. Peripheral alpha-1 blockers associated with loop diuretics—high risk of urinary incontinence in elderly women.

Legend: NSAID, nonsteroidal anti-inflammatory drug; PPI, proton-pump inhibitor; ACE, angiotensin-converting enzyme; SSRIs, selective serotonin reuptake inhibitors; RAAS inhibitors, renin-angiotensin-aldosterone system inhibitors.

References

1. Eurostat 2019. State of Health in the EU. Romania. Country Health Profiles 2019. Available online: https://www.euro.who.int/__data/assets/pdf_file/0009/419472/Country-Health-Profile-2019-Romania.pdf (accessed on 20 January 2021).
2. Eurostat 2017. State of Health in the Eu. Country Health Profiles 2017. Available online: https://ec.europa.eu/health/sites/health/files/state/docs/chp_romania_english.pdf (accessed on 20 January 2021).
3. European Commission. Country Report 2016. Available online: https://ec.europa.eu/info/sites/info/files/cr_romania_2016_en.pdf (accessed on 20 January 2021).
4. Chen, Y.; Klein, S.L.; Garibaldi, B.T.; Li, H.; Wu, C.; Osevala, N.M.; Li, T.; Margolick, J.B.; Pawelec, G.; Leng, S.X. Aging in COVID-19: Vulnerability, immunity and intervention. *Ageing Res. Rev.* **2021**, *65*, 101205. [CrossRef] [PubMed]

5. Wang, L.; He, W.; Yu, X.; Hu, D.; Bao, M.; Liu, H.; Zhou, J.; Jiang, H. Coronavirus disease 2019 in elderly patients: Characteristics and prognostic factors based on 4-week follow-up. *J. Infect.* **2020**, *80*, 639–645. [CrossRef]
6. Perrotta, F.; Corbi, G.; Mazzeo, G.; Boccia, M.; Aronne, L.; D'Agnano, V.; Komici, K.; Mazzarella, G.; Parrella, R.; Bianco, A. COVID-19 and the elderly: Insights into pathogenesis and clinical decision-making. *Aging Clin. Exp. Res.* **2020**, *32*, 1599–1608. [CrossRef]
7. The National Institute of Public Health (Week 05). Romania. Available online: https://www.cnscbt.ro/index.php/analiza-cazuri-confirmate-covid19 (accessed on 15 February 2021).
8. Oertelt-Prigione, S. The Impact of Sex Gender in the COVID-19 Pandemic. European Commission–Case Study. Research and Innovation. Research and Innovation. 2020. Available online: https://op.europa.eu/en/publication-detail/-/publication/4f419ffb-a0ca-11ea-9d2d-01aa75ed71a1/language-en (accessed on 15 February 2021).
9. World Health Organization. Coronavirus Disease Dashboard. Available online: https://covid19.who.int/table?tableDay=yesterday (accessed on 15 February 2021).
10. Organisation for Economic Co-operation and Development (OECD). Influenza Vaccination Rates. Available online: https://data.oecd.org/healthcare/influenza-vaccination-rates.htm (accessed on 15 February 2021).
11. Wallace, E.; McDowell, R.; Bennett, K.; Fahey, T.; Smith, S.M. Impact of Potentially Inappropriate Prescribing on Adverse Drug Events, Health Related Quality of Life and Emergency Hospital Attendance in Older People Attending General Practice: A Prospective Cohort Study. *J. Gerontol. A Biol. Sci. Med. Sci.* **2017**, *72*, 271–277. [CrossRef]
12. Moriarty, F.; Bennett, K.; Cahir, C.; Kenny, R.A.; Fahey, T. Potentially inappropriate prescribing according to STOPP and START and adverse outcomes in community-dwelling older people: A prospective cohort study. *Br. J. Clin. Pharmacol.* **2016**, *82*, 849–857. [CrossRef]
13. Wauters, M.; Elseviers, M.; Vaes, B.; Degryse, J.; Dalleur, O.; Vander Stichele, R.; Christiaens, T.; Azermai, M. Too many, too few, or too unsafe? Impact of inappropriate prescribing on mortality, and hospitalization in a cohort of community-dwelling oldest old. *Br. J. Clin. Pharmacol.* **2016**, *82*, 1382–1392. [CrossRef] [PubMed]
14. Buda, V.; Prelipcean, A.; Andor, M.; Dehelean, L.; Dalleur, O.; Buda, S.; Spatar, L.; Mabda, M.C.; Suciu, M.; Danciu, C.; et al. Potentially Inappropriate Prescriptions in Ambulatory Elderly Patients Living in Rural Areas of Romania Using STOPP/START (Version 2) Criteria. *Clin. Interv. Aging* **2020**, *15*, 407–417. [CrossRef] [PubMed]
15. O'Mahony, D. STOPP/START criteria for potentially inappropriate medications/potential prescribing omissions in older people: Origin and progress. *Expert Rev. Clin. Pharmacol.* **2020**, *13*, 15–22. [CrossRef] [PubMed]
16. Turner, G.; Clegg, A. Best practice guidelines for the management of frailty: A British Geriatrics Society, Age UK and Royal College of General Practitioners report. *Age Ageing* **2014**, *43*, 744–747. [CrossRef]
17. National Institute for Health and Care Excellence. Medicines Optimization: The Safe and Effective Use of Medicines to Enable the Best Possible Outcomes. Available online: https://www.nice.org.uk/guidance/ng5/chapter/1-Recommendations#medication-review (accessed on 20 January 2021).
18. Cayea, D.; Durso, S.C. Screening and Prevention in the Modern Era. *Clin. Geriatr. Med.* **2018**, *34*, xiii–xvii. [CrossRef]
19. Armstrong, N.; Swinglehurst, D. Understanding medical overuse: The case of problematic polypharmacy and the potential of ethnography. *Fam. Pract.* **2018**, *35*, 526–527. [CrossRef]
20. Spinewine, A.; Schmader, K.E.; Barber, N.; Hughes, C.; Lapane, K.L.; Swine, C.; Hanlon, J.T. Appropriate prescribing in elderly people: How well can it be measured and optimised? *Lancet* **2007**, *370*, 173–184. [CrossRef]
21. Primejdie, D.P.; Bojita, M.T.; Popa, A. Potentially inappropriate medications in elderly ambulatory and institutionalized patients: An observational study. *BMC Pharmacol. Toxicol.* **2016**, *17*, 38. [CrossRef]
22. Primejdie, D.; Bojita, M.; Popa, A. Potential inappropriate medication use in community-dwelling elderly patients: A qualitative study. *Farmacia* **2012**, *60*, 366–378.
23. Ungureanu, M.I.; Brînzac, M.G.; Forray, A.; Paina, L.; Avram, L.; Crișan, D.A.; Donca, V. The geriatric workforce in Romania: The need to improve data and management. *Eur. J. Public Health* **2020**, *30* (Suppl. 4), iv28–iv31. [CrossRef] [PubMed]
24. Pislaru, A.I.; Ilie, A.C.; Pancu, A.G.; Sandu, I.A. Detection and prevention of frailty in independently living pre-elderly and elderly in Northeastern Romania. *Med. Surg. J.* **2016**, *120*, 909–914.
25. Independent Living Institute. Available online: https://www.independentliving.org/toolsforpower/tools11.html (accessed on 15 February 2021).
26. By the 2019 American Geriatrics Society Beers Criteria® Update Expert Panel. American Geriatrics Society 2019 Updated AGS Beers Criteria® for Potentially Inappropriate Medication Use in Older Adults. *J. Am. Geriatr. Soc.* **2019**, *67*, 674–694. [CrossRef]
27. O'Mahony, D.; O'Sullivan, D.; Byrne, S.; O'Connor, M.N.; Ryan, C.; Gallagher, P. STOPP/START criteria for potentially inappropriate prescribing in older people: Version 2. *Age Ageing* **2015**, *44*, 213–218. [CrossRef]
28. Romanian Legislation. Law 351/2001. Available online: http://www.cdep.ro/pls/legis/legis_pck.htp_act_text?idt=28862 (accessed on 20 January 2021).
29. Stanciu, V. Defining the Rural Area in Romania: Legislative Approaches. Econstor. Available online: https://www.econstor.eu/bitstream/10419/163388/1/ICEADR-2016_p293.pdf (accessed on 20 January 2021).
30. Bernell, S.; Howard, S.W. Use Your Words Carefully: What Is a Chronic Disease? *Front. Public Health* **2016**, *4*, 159. [CrossRef]
31. Casa Judetean de Asigurari de Sanatate Dolj. Available online: http://www.cnas.ro/casdj/post/type/local/ordinul-ms-cnas-privind-aprobarea-formularului-de-prescriptie-medicala-electronica.html (accessed on 15 February 2021).

32. Romanian Legislation. Law 339/2005. Available online: https://cmvro.ro/files/download/legislatie/stupefiante-psihotrope/Legea_339_2005_stupefiante_psihotrope-consolidata.pdf (accessed on 15 February 2021).
33. Charles, C.V.; Eaton, A. Highlights from the 2019 AGS Beers Criteria® Updates. *Sr. Care Pharm.* **2020**, *35*, 68–74. [CrossRef]
34. Faul, F.; Erdfelder, E.; Lang, A.-G.; Buchner, A. G*Power 3: A flexible statistical power analysis program for the social, behavioral, and biomedical sciences. *Behav. Res. Methods* **2007**, *39*, 175–191. [CrossRef]
35. Faul, F.; Erdfelder, E.; Buchner, A.; Lang, A.-G. Statistical power analyses using G*Power 3.1: Tests for correlation and regression analyses. *Behav. Res. Methods* **2009**, *41*, 1149–1160. [CrossRef]
36. McHugh, M.L. The chi-square test of independence. *Biochem. Med.* **2013**, *23*, 143–149. [CrossRef] [PubMed]
37. Laerd Statistics. Available online: https://statistics.laerd.com/spss-tutorials/mann-whitney-u-test-using-spss-statistics.php (accessed on 28 June 2021).
38. Miller, J.W. Proton Pump Inhibitors, H2-Receptor Antagonists, Metformin, and Vitamin B-12 Deficiency: Clinical Implications. *Adv. Nutr.* **2018**, *9*, 511S–518S. [CrossRef] [PubMed]
39. *LiverTox: Clinical and Research Information on Drug-Induced Liver Injury*; National Institute of Diabetes and Digestive and Kidney Diseases: Bethesda, MD, USA, 2012.
40. Wongrakpanich, S.; Wongrakpanich, A.; Melhado, K.; Rangaswami, J. A Comprehensive Review of Non-Steroidal Anti-Inflammatory Drug Use in the Elderly. *Aging Dis.* **2018**, *9*, 143–150. [CrossRef] [PubMed]
41. Ungprasert, P.; Cheungpasitporn, W.; Crowson, C.S.; Matteson, E.L. Individual non-steroidal anti-inflammatory drugs and risk of acute kidney injury: A systematic review and meta-analysis of observational studies. *Eur. J. Intern. Med.* **2015**, *26*, 285–291. [CrossRef]
42. Gooch, K.; Culleton, B.F.; Manns, B.J.; Zhang, J.; Alfonso, H.; Tonelli, M.; Frank, C.; Klarenbach, S.; Hemmelgarn, B.R. NSAID use and progression of chronic kidney disease. *Am. J. Med.* **2007**, *120*, 280.e1–280.e7. [CrossRef]
43. Kate, R.J.; Perez, R.M.; Mazumdar, D.; Pasupathy, K.S.; Nilakantan, V. Prediction and detection models for acute kidney injury in hospitalized older adults. *BMC Med. Inform. Decis. Mak.* **2016**, *16*, 39. [CrossRef] [PubMed]
44. Turgutalp, K.; Bardak, S.; Horoz, M.; Helvacı, I.; Demir, S.; Kıykım, A.A. Clinical outcomes of acute kidney injury developing outside the hospital in elderly. *Int. Urol. Nephrol.* **2017**, *49*, 113–121. [CrossRef]
45. Turgutalp, K.; Bardak, S.; Helvacı, I.; İşgüzar, G.; Payas, E.; Demir, S.; Kıykım, A. Community-acquired hyperkalemia in elderly patients: Risk factors and clinical outcomes. *Ren. Fail.* **2016**, *38*, 1405–1412. [CrossRef] [PubMed]
46. Damanti, S.; Pasina, L.; Consonni, D.; Azzolino, D.; Cesari, M. Drug-Induced Hyponatremia: NSAIDs, a Neglected Cause that Should Be Considered. *J. Frailty Aging* **2019**, *8*, 222–223. [CrossRef] [PubMed]
47. Mannesse, C.K.; Vondeling, A.M.; van Marum, R.J.; van Solinge, W.W.; Egberts, T.C.; Jansen, P.A. Prevalence of hyponatremia on geriatric wards compared to other settings over four decades: A systematic review. *Ageing Res. Rev.* **2013**, *12*, 165–173. [CrossRef] [PubMed]
48. Mannesse, C.K.; Jansen, P.A.; Van Marum, R.J.; Sival, R.C.; Kok, R.M.; Haffmans, P.M.; Egberts, T.C. Characteristics, prevalence, risk factors, and underlying mechanism of hyponatremia in elderly patients treated with antidepressants: A cross-sectional study. *Maturitas* **2013**, *76*, 357–363. [CrossRef]
49. Suciu, M.; Suciu, L.; Vlaia, L.; Voicu, M.; Buda, V.; Dragan, L.; Andor, M.; Vlaia, V.; Cristescu, C.; Hirjau, M. The prevalence of inappropriate use of NSAIDs by cardiovascular patients for musculoskeletal disorders. *Farmacia* **2020**, *68*, 628–639. [CrossRef]
50. Raza, Z.; Naureen, Z. Melatonin ameliorates the drug induced nephrotoxicity: Molecular insights. *Nefrologia* **2020**, *40*, 12–25. [CrossRef] [PubMed]
51. Sabau, M. Real life anticoagulant treatment for stroke prevention in patients with nonvalvular atrial fibrillation. *Farmacia* **2020**, *68*, 912–918. [CrossRef]
52. Laine, L.; Nagar, A. Long-Term PPI Use: Balancing Potential Harms and Documented Benefits. *Am. J. Gastroenterol.* **2016**, *111*, 913–915. [CrossRef] [PubMed]
53. Freedberg, D.E.; Kim, L.S.; Yang, Y.X. The Risks and Benefits of Long-term Use of Proton Pump Inhibitors: Expert Review and Best Practice Advice from the American Gastroenterological Association. *Gastroenterology* **2017**, *152*, 706–715. [CrossRef] [PubMed]
54. Sun, J.; Sun, H.; Cui, M.; Sun, Z.; Li, W.; Wei, J.; Zhou, S. The use of anti-ulcer agents and the risk of chronic kidney disease: A meta-analysis. *Int. Urol. Nephrol.* **2018**, *50*, 1835–1843. [CrossRef]
55. Novotny, M.; Klimova, B.; Valis, M. PPI Long Term Use: Risk of Neurological Adverse Events? *Front. Neurol.* **2019**, *9*, 1142. [CrossRef]
56. Cena, C.; Traina, S.; Parola, B.; Bo, M.; Fagiano, R.; Siviero, C. Prescription of proton pump inhibitors in older adults with complex polytherapy. *Eur. J. Hosp. Pharm.* **2020**, *27*, 341–345. [CrossRef]
57. Journey, J.D.; Bentley, T.P. Theophylline Toxicity. In *StatPearls*; StatPearls Publishing: Treasure Island, FL, USA, 2020. Available online: https://www.ncbi.nlm.nih.gov/books/NBK532962/ (accessed on 20 January 2021).
58. Khan, S.; Jones, S. Theophylline interactions. *Respir. Med. J.* **2014**, *293*, 52–54. Available online: https://www.pharmaceutical-journal.com/download?ac=1067077&firstPass=false (accessed on 20 January 2021).
59. Eurostat. Cardiovascular Disease Statistics. Available online: https://ec.europa.eu/eurostat/statistics-explained/index.php/Cardiovascular_diseases_statistics#Self-reporting_of_hypertensive_diseases (accessed on 15 February 2021).
60. Wettengel, R. Theophyllin–Rückblick, Standortbestimmung und Ausblick [Theophylline–past present and future]. *Arzneimittelforschung* **1998**, *48*, 535–539.

61. Abad, V.C.; Guilleminault, C. Insomnia in Elderly Patients: Recommendations for Pharmacological Management. *Drugs Aging* **2018**, *35*, 791–817. [CrossRef] [PubMed]
62. Monti, J.M.; Monti, D. Overview of currently available benzodiazepine and nonbenzodiazepine hypnotics. In *Clinical Pharmacology of Sleep*; Pandi-Perumal, S.R., Monti, J.M., Eds.; Birkhäuser: Basel, Switzerland, 2006. Available online: https://doi.org/10.1007/3-7643-7440-3_14 (accessed on 20 January 2021).
63. Williams, B.; Mancia, G.; Spiering, W.; Agabiti Rosei, E.; Azizi, M.; Burnier, M.; Clement, D.L.; Coca, A.; de Simone, G.; Dominiczak, A.; et al. ESC Scientific Document Group. 2018 ESC/ESH Guidelines for the management of arterial hypertension. *Eur. Heart J.* **2018**, *39*, 3021–3104. [CrossRef] [PubMed]
64. Blanco-Reina, E.; Valdellós, J.; Aguilar-Cano, L.; García-Merino, M.R.; Ocaña-Riola, R.; Ariza-Zafra, G.; Bellido-Estévez, I. 2015 Beers Criteria and STOPP v2 for detecting potentially inappropriate medication in community-dwelling older people: Prevalence, profile, and risk factors. *Eur. J. Clin. Pharmacol.* **2019**, *75*, 1459–1466. [CrossRef]
65. Gorzoni, M.L.; Rosa, R.F. Beers AGS 2019 criteria in very old hospitalized patients. *Rev. Assoc. Med. Bras.* **2020**, *66*, 918–923. [CrossRef] [PubMed]
66. Kim, G.J.; Lee, K.H.; Kim, J.H. South Korean geriatrics on Beers Criteria medications at risk of adverse drug events. *PLoS ONE* **2018**, *13*, e0191376. [CrossRef] [PubMed]
67. Gyalai-Korpos, I.; Ancusa, O.; Dragomir, T.; Tomescu, M.C.; Marincu, I. Factors associated with prolonged hospitalization, readmission, and death in elderly heart failure patients in western Romania. *Clin. Interv. Aging* **2015**, *10*, 561–568. [CrossRef] [PubMed]
68. Simionescu, M.; Bilan, S.; Gavurova, B.; Bordea, E.N. Health Policies in Romania to Reduce the Mortality Caused by Cardiovascular Diseases. *Int. J. Environ. Res. Public Health* **2019**, *16*, 3080. [CrossRef]
69. Tilea, I.; Petra, D.; Voidazan, S.; Ardeleanu, E.; Varga, A. Treatment adherence among adult hypertensive patients: A cross-sectional retrospective study in primary care in Romania. *Patient Prefer. Adherence* **2018**, *12*, 625–635. [CrossRef]
70. Eurostat 2017. Health Expenditure Statistics. Available online: https://ec.europa.eu/eurostat/statistics-explained/index.php?title=Healthcare_expenditure_statistics#Healthcare_expenditure_by_function (accessed on 20 January 2021).
71. OECD. *Health at a Glance 2019: OECD Indicators*; OECD Publishing: Paris, France, 2019. [CrossRef]
72. Bhavnani, S.P.; Narula, J.; Sengupta, P.P. Mobile technology and the digitization of healthcare. *Eur. Heart J.* **2016**, *37*, 1428–1438. [CrossRef]
73. Bucci, S.; Schwannauer, M.; Berry, N. The digital revolution and its impact on mental health care. *Psychol. Psychother.* **2019**, *92*, 277–297. [CrossRef] [PubMed]
74. Agbo, C.C.; Mahmoud, Q.H.; Eklund, J.M. Blockchain Technology in Healthcare: A Systematic Review. *Healthcare* **2019**, *7*, 56. [CrossRef] [PubMed]
75. Abu-Elezz, I.; Hassan, A.; Nazeemudeen, A.; Househ, M.; Abd-Alrazaq, A. The benefits and threats of blockchain technology in healthcare: A scoping review. *Int. J. Med. Inform.* **2020**, *142*, 104246. [CrossRef] [PubMed]
76. Rosen, M.A.; DiazGranados, D.; Dietz, A.S.; Benishek, L.E.; Thompson, D.; Pronovost, P.J.; Weaver, S.J. Teamwork in healthcare: Key discoveries enabling safer, high-quality care. *Am. Psychol.* **2018**, *73*, 433–450. [CrossRef]
77. Charlesworth, C.J.; Smit, E.; Lee, D.S.; Alramadhan, F.; Odden, M.C. Polypharmacy among Adults Aged 65 Years and Older in the United States: 1988-2010. *J. Gerontol. A Biol. Sci. Med. Sci.* **2015**, *70*, 989–995. [CrossRef]
78. United Nations. Aging. Available online: https://www.un.org/en/sections/issues-depth/ageing/ (accessed on 15 February 2021).

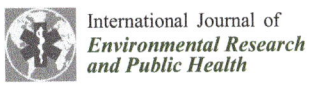

Article

A Machine Learning Approach for Investigating Delirium as a Multifactorial Syndrome

Honoria Ocagli [1], Daniele Bottigliengo [1], Giulia Lorenzoni [1], Danila Azzolina [1,2], Aslihan S. Acar [3], Silvia Sorgato [4], Lucia Stivanello [4], Mario Degan [4] and Dario Gregori [1,*]

[1] Unit of Biostatistics, Epidemiology and Public Health, Department of Cardiac, Thoracic, Vascular Sciences and Public Health, University of Padova, Via Loredan 18, 35121 Padova, Italy; honoria.ocagli@unipd.it (H.O.); daniele.bottigliengo@studenti.unipd.it (D.B.); giulia.lorenzoni@unipd.it (G.L.); danila.azzolina@unife.it (D.A.)
[2] Department of Medical Science, University of Ferrara, Via Fossato di Mortara 64B, 44121 Ferrara, Italy
[3] Department of Actuarial Sciences, Hacettepe University, Ankara 06800, Turkey; aslihans@hacettepe.edu.tr
[4] Health Professional Management Service (DPS) of the University Hospital of Padova, 35128 Padova, Italy; silvia.sorgato@aopd.veneto.it (S.S.); lucia.stivanello@aopd.veneto.it (L.S.); mario.degan@aopd.veneto.it (M.D.)
* Correspondence: dario.gregori@unipd.it; Tel.: +39-049-827-5384

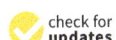

Citation: Ocagli, H.; Bottigliengo, D.; Lorenzoni, G.; Azzolina, D.; Acar, A.S.; Sorgato, S.; Stivanello, L.; Degan, M.; Gregori, D. A Machine Learning Approach for Investigating Delirium as a Multifactorial Syndrome. IJERPH 2021, 18, 7105. https://doi.org/10.3390/ijerph18137105

Academic Editors: Francisco José Tarazona Santabalbina, José Viña, Sebastià Josep Santaeugènia Gonzàlez and José Augusto García Navarro

Received: 26 April 2021
Accepted: 14 June 2021
Published: 2 July 2021

Publisher's Note: MDPI stays neutral with regard to jurisdictional claims in published maps and institutional affiliations.

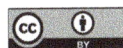

Copyright: © 2021 by the authors. Licensee MDPI, Basel, Switzerland. This article is an open access article distributed under the terms and conditions of the Creative Commons Attribution (CC BY) license (https://creativecommons.org/licenses/by/4.0/).

Abstract: Delirium is a psycho-organic syndrome common in hospitalized patients, especially the elderly, and is associated with poor clinical outcomes. This study aims to identify the predictors that are mostly associated with the risk of delirium episodes using a machine learning technique (MLT). A random forest (RF) algorithm was used to evaluate the association between the subject's characteristics and the 4AT (the 4 A's test) score screening tool for delirium. RF algorithm was implemented using information based on demographic characteristics, comorbidities, drugs and procedures. Of the 78 patients enrolled in the study, 49 (63%) were at risk for delirium, 32 (41%) had at least one episode of delirium during the hospitalization (38% in orthopedics and 31% both in internal medicine and in the geriatric ward). The model explained 75.8% of the variability of the 4AT score with a root mean squared error of 3.29. Higher age, the presence of dementia, physical restraint, diabetes and a lower degree are the variables associated with an increase of the 4AT score. Random forest is a valid method for investigating the patients' characteristics associated with delirium onset also in small case-series. The use of this model may allow for early detection of delirium onset to plan the proper adjustment in healthcare assistance.

Keywords: aging; nursing; delirium; machine learning technique; random forest

1. Introduction

Delirium is a psycho-organic syndrome characterized by an alteration in attention and consciousness, with disorganized psychic activity, fragmentation of psychic processes that appear untied and upset [1]. Delirium has a multifactorial etiology, in which internal predisposing factors (susceptibility) interact with external precipitating ones [2,3]. In contrast to dementia, delirium is often reversible with early detection and treatment of underlying causes [4]. For delirium, there are many risk factors that may change according to the characteristics of the patient. In literature, risk factors for delirium were evaluated in systematic reviews according to the type of patients. Risk of delirium is higher in very old patients [5,6]. Marquetand et al. 2020 [6] in a recent work found that very old patients require only few precipitant factors to develop delirium. Age was a risk factor also for patients after hip fracture surgery [7], vascular surgery [8], in knee and hip replacement patients [9]. Other risk factors are as follows: function dependency [7,10], hypertension [8], hearing or visual impairment [7,8], anesthetic use [11], and cognitive impairment [9,10]. Older adults following elective surgery frailty and psychotropic medication have potentially modifiable prognosis factors [12].

Delirium prevalence in the general population hospitalized is low (1–2%), but increases from 29% to 64% in elderly [13], increasing morbidity, mortality, loss of independence, length of stay, and institutionalization. Delirium prevalence also affects health care costs, which amount to over $164 billion in the United States [14]. In the Italian territory, delirium prevalence is as follows: 11% in medical wards [15], 20% in the general hospital [5], 23% in general wards [16,17] and up to 37% of patients with subsyndromal delirium [18]. Given its pervasive nature and deleterious effects, delirium surveillance is recommended for hospitalized patients [19]. Under-detection or misdiagnosis is estimated in 50–75% of delirium cases [20], and 30–40% of reported delirium episodes are preventable [21]. In addition, delirium detection is complicated by the characteristics of hospitalized patients who are often frail elderly and, therefore, more susceptible to delirium onset, especially during hospitalization where the intensification of treatments and diagnostic interventions become potentially precipitant factors [15].

DSM-V criteria are the standard for the diagnosis of delirium in clinical setting. Recently, time-efficient tools have been developed in the clinical setting for delirium detection and diagnosis [22]. In literature, there are several tools for facilitating delirium detection [22,23], such as the Confusion Assessment Method (CAM) [24], 4AT test [25], and the most recent Nursing DElirium SCreening (Nu-DESC) tool [19]. Both CAM [26–28] and Nu-DESC scales were used to compare the ability of random forest (RF) models in predicting the risk of delirium episodes. The structure of these tools shows similar domains. Nu-DESC has five domains: (1) disorientation, (2) inadequate behavior, (3) inadequate communication, (4) hallucination, and (5) psychomotor delay. CAM consists, instead, of four main themes: (1) acute onset and fluctuating course, (2) inattention, (3) disorganized thinking, and (4) altered level of consciousness. Bellelli [25], for the first time, used the 4AT score to assess patients at risk for delirium. Machine learning techniques (MLTs) have been widely used in data-driven prediction models, for example in dementia [29], or delirium as well with performances comparable with traditional logistic regression [26] and included into clinical workflow [30].

The study has a twofold goal: (1) to identify, using a machine learning approach, which subject's characteristics are mostly associated with 4AT score and how they impact its variability and (2) to evaluate delirium presence/absence in older patients during the first five days of hospitalization using a standardized tool which is the 4AT instrument.

2. Materials and Methods

2.1. Study Design and Inclusion Criteria

This observational study has taken place between August and September 2016 in the Orthopedics, Geriatrics, and General Medicine wards of the University Hospital of Padova. The inclusion criteria for the enrolled patients were as follows; aged above 65 years old, understanding he Italian language and length of stay of at least five days. Patients with a psychiatric illness already diagnosed at admission, with communication problems (such as aphasia, coma status), or with a terminal disease, were excluded from the study.

An experienced nurse explained the purpose of the study and obtained informed consent from the patient or his next of kin when the participant was unable to give his consent. Study participants were evaluated with the 4AT instrument by three trained nursing students. The project was conducted within the framework of thesis preparation of the nursing student and it was approved by the internal offices at the University Hospital of Padova.

2.2. Variables Collected

Each patient was assessed for delirium with the 4AT scale [25] at least 24 h after the admission and each day till the fifth day of hospitalization. For each patient, the following variables were collected in different moments: (i) at hospital admission: socio-demographic characteristics such as ward, age, diagnosis, degree of study, comorbidities potentially affecting the delirium onset (dementia, alcoholism, drugs addiction, depression, other psychiatric diseases, diabetes, cancer, malnutrition); previous admission to hospital, history of delirium, hearing and visual impairment; (ii) daily variables during the hospitalization: sleep deprivation, hours of caregiver assistance, 4AT score; (iii) each shift (three times per day, morning, afternoon and night): mobility (bed transfer-chair, walking, use of stairs); physical restraint; presence/absence of invasive device (urinary catheter, pheripheric venous catheter, central venous catheter, feeding tube, percutaneous endoscopic gastrostomy); pain, fever, surgery; drugs (affecting central nervous system: anticholinergic, dopaminergic, steroid, opioid, antiepileptic, anti-anxiety, neuroleptics, antidepressants); and antibiotics (quinolone, antifungal voriconazole and cephalosporins).

2.3. Instrument

The 4AT [25] is a short and handy instrument for routine detection of delirium and cognitive impairment by unskilled hospital personnel; on average, it takes less than two minutes to fill it. The total score ranges from 0 to 12 and is structured in 4 domains (alertness, orientation, attention and fluctuation). The compilation of items 1–3 is based exclusively on the patient's observation at the time of the evaluation, Item 4 compilation, requires instead the collection of information from multiple sources. A score of 0 suggests that delirium and/or cognitive impairment are unlikely but do not exclude them. A score of 1–3 is suggestive of cognitive impairment and requires a more detailed cognitive examination, whereas a score higher than four suggests for delirium and requires further clinical assessment since the tool is not diagnostic. The instrument has a sensitivity of 89.7% and a specificity of 84.1% with a positive likelihood ratio of 5.62 and a negative likelihood ratio of 0.12 in the validation study [31]. However, it has shown a poor specificity, which ranges from 53.7% (95% CI: 48.1–59.2) [32] to 0.91 (0.88–0.94) [33]. The instrument was validated in the elderly population in several languages [34,35], various contexts such as the emergency department [33], hospice [36], stroke unit [37,38], medical ward [32] and in different cultural backgrounds [39]. The instrument also has some limitations; it is not suitable for patients with impaired communications and the mere presence of changes in alertness or a fluctuating course of the mental status is sufficient to define the patient at risk for delirium [35].

2.4. Statistical Analysis

Categorical variables were summarized according to delirium profile groups, with relative and absolute frequencies. As only categorical variables were considered, the Chi-square test was performed. The *p*-values were also reported for all possible pairwise comparisons between delirium categories. For these comparisons, the Benjamini-Hochberg adjusted *p*-values and the unadjusted *p*-values have been computed [40].

A *p*-value lower than 0.05 is conventionally considered meaningful.

The effective sample size on the observations was computed using Kish [41] formula as follows: (i) the scores of simple standard deviation (SSD) and the robust to heteroskedasticity standard deviation (RSD), were obtained using individuals as clusters; (ii) the ratio between RSD and SSD was computed; (iii) the effective sample size was retrieved as the ratio between the number of observations in the sample and the ratio computed at the previous step. Records with missing assessment of delirium were removed.

A logistic regression model was calculated to assess the time effect on the risk of developing delirium and having delirium during the hospitalization. The variance estimates were calculated by considering the Huber–White [42] estimator to account for the correlation within repeated measurements. Patients with a score higher than one were considered at risk for delirium.

2.5. Machine Learning Approach

An ML approach was used to evaluate the association between the subject's characteristics and the 4AT score. MLTs can easily detect non-linear relationships and interactions and can be used with a low number of subjects, in a case where the standard statistical approaches may have some limitations [43]. The random Forest algorithm, one of the most popular methods in the MLT field [44], was implemented to describe the 4AT score based on the following set of predictors: age, gender, physical restraint, mobility, dementia, diabetes, cancer, ward, degree level, previous episodes of delirium and admission to hospital, and addiction (at least one between alcoholism, drugs addiction, depression, and other psychiatric diseases); at least one antibiotic; at least one drugs affecting the central nervous system, at least one invasive device, at least one among pain and fever, at least one among visual and hearing impairment.

The parameters of the algorithm were chosen such that the root mean squared error (RMSE), i.e., the root of the average squared difference between observed and predicted the 4AT score, was minimized. The RF algorithm was implemented using 10,000 trees.

The database is composed of repeated measurements within-subject; for this reason, the RF algorithm has been forced to use stratified sampling within each subject as indicated in the literature for cluster correlated data [45].

Variable importance using the permutation method [46] was used to assess the predictors that mostly impact the variability of the 4AT score. Partial dependence plots (PDPs) were used to depict how the 4AT score changes given the characteristics of the subjects [47]. Briefly, PDPs represent the score values predicted by the model for predictor's value by marginalizing over the values of the other variables which were observed in the sample. PDPs are often used to aid the interpretation of an ML model by describing the relationship between a predictor and an outcome.

Analyses were performed using R software 3.6.1 (CRAN: Viena, Austria) [48]. The RF algorithm was implemented using the randomForestSRC R package (version 2.9.1) (CRAN: Viena, Austria) [49].

3. Results

In the study, 78 patients were enrolled, for a total of 1149 observations entered in the model and an effective sample size of 95 independent observations computed using the formula from Kish [41]. A total of 49 (63%) patients were at risk for delirium (4AT score higher than 1), 32 (41%) patients experienced delirium at least once (4AT score higher than 4) during their stay. In both cases are prevalently present in geriatrics ward, respectively 23 (96%) and 14 (58%), and in orthopedics ward, 17 (57%) and 12 (40%) respectively. Patients at risk for delirium were mainly females were 52 (64%) of the population, with a medium–low education level and an age between 80 and 90 years. A statistical description of the whole sample according to the 4AT score profile group at baseline assessment is reported in Table 1.

Table 1. Descriptive statistics of the whole sample according to the 4AT score profile group at baseline assessment. Categorical variables were summarized as relative and absolute frequencies. Pearson Chi-square test was used to assess differences across 4AT scale categories.

Variable	Variable Level	n	Delirium or Severe Cognitive Impairment Unlikely (n = 31)	Possible Cognitive Impairment (n = 28)	Possible Delirium +/− Cognitive Impairment (n = 18)	Overall (n = 77) *	p-Value	Unadjusted Pairwise p-Value			Adjusted Pairwise p-Value		
								PCI vs. D/CI	PCI vs. PD	D/CI vs. PD	PCI vs. D/CI	PCI vs. PD	D/CI vs. PD
Ward	Medicine	78	16 (52%)	5 (18%)	3 (17%)	24 (31%)	<0.001	0.235	<0.001	0.004	0.235	0.003	0.006
	Geriatric		1 (3%)	16 (57%)	7 (39%)	24 (31%)							
	Orthopedic		14 (45%)	7 (25%)	8 (44%)	29 (38%)							
Gender	Male	78	12 (39%)	8 (29%)	6 (33%)	26 (34%)	0.71	0.746	0.161	0.305	0.746	0.4575	0.4575
ICD diagnosis	Circulatory system	35	0 (0%)	1 (10%)	0 (0%)	1 (3%)	0.17	0.259	0.135	0.32	0.32	0.32	0.32
	Musculoskeletal system		14 (93%)	7 (70%)	8 (89%)	29 (85%)							
	Digestive system		0 (0%)	0 (0%)	1 (11%)	1 (3%)							
	Respiratory		1 (7%)	0 (0%)	0 (0%)	1 (3%)							
	Undefined		0 (0%)	2 (20%)	0 (0%)	2 (6%)							
Educational level	Bachelor's degree	78	2 (6%)	0 (0%)	1 (6%)	3 (4%)	0.24	0.533	0.044	0.262	0.533	0.132	0.393
	None		0 (0%)	5 (18%)	2 (11%)	7 (9%)							
	Missing		1 (3%)	0 (0%)	0 (0%)	48 (63%)							
	Primary school		23 (74%)	14 (50%)	11 (61%)	13 (17%)							
	Secondary school		4 (13%)	7 (24%)	2 (11%)	5 (7%)							

Table 1. Cont.

Variable	Variable Level	n	Delirium or Severe Cognitive Impairment Unlikely (n = 31)	Possible Cognitive Impairment (n = 28)	Possible Delirium +/− Cognitive Impairment (n = 18)	Overall (n = 77) *	p-Value	Unadjusted Pairwise p-Value			Adjusted Pairwise p-Value		
								PCI vs. D/CI	PCI vs. PD	D/CI vs. PD	PCI vs. D/CI	PCI vs. PD	D/CI vs. PD
Dementia	High school	78	1 (3%) 2 (6%)	2 (11%) 8 (29%)	2 (11%) 8 (44%)	18 (23%) 1 (1%)	0.007	0.181	0.028	0.001	0.181	0.042	0.003
Alcohol use		78	1 (3%)	0 (0%)	0 (0%)	5 (6%)	0.47		0.329	0.454		0.454	0.454
Depression		78	2 (6%)	3 (11%)	0 (0%)	16 (21%)	0.35	0.17	0.586	0.285	0.4275	0.586	0.4275
Diabetes		78	7 (23%)	4 (14%)	5 (28%)	29 (38%)	0.52	0.197	0.379	0.601	0.5685	0.5685	0.601
Cancer		78	10 (32%)	11 (39%)	8 (44%)	71 (92%)	0.68	0.544	0.645	0.311	0.645	0.645	0.645
Previous hospital admission		78	27 (87%)	27 (96%)	17 (94%)	29 (38%)	0.38	0.696	0.185	0.446	0.696	0.555	0.669
Visual impairment		78	13 (42%)	7 (25%)	9 (50%)	29 (38%)	0.19	0.048	0.144	0.464	0.144	0.216	0.464
Hearing impairment		78	8 (26%)	10 (36%)	11 (61%)	14 (18%)	0.047	0.17	0.313	0.024	0.255	0.313	0.072
Antibiotics	>1	78	6 (19%)	8 (28%)	0 (0%)	5 (6%)	0.071	0.02	0.45	0.05	0.05	0.45	0.08
age (classes)	<70	78	4 (13%)	1 (4%)	0 (0%)	3 (4%)	0.035	0.108	0.127	0.039	0.127	0.127	0.117
	>95		1 (3%)	0 (0%)	2 (11%)	5 (6%)							
	71–75		3 (10%)	0 (0%)	2 (11%)	11 (14%)							
	76–80		6 (19%)	4 (14%)	1 (6%)	19 (25%)							
	81–85		8 (26%)	8 (29%)	3 (17%)	21 (27%)							
	86–90		8 (26%)	10 (36%)	3 (17%)	13 (17%)							
	91–95		1 (3%)	5 (18%)	7 (39%)								

n: Reports the number of patients in which calculations were made. * One patient had no assessment in the 4AT score at baseline. Abbreviations: PCI: possible cognitive impairment, D/CI: delirium or severe cognitive impairment unlikely, possible cognitive impairment, PD: possible delirium +/− cognitive impairment.

The logistic regression model shows a *p*-value of 0.09 indicating a non-significant effect of hospitalization time on the risk of developing delirium or cognitive impairment. The same finding has been identified (*p*-value 0.08) by considering the possible time effect on the risk of developing delirium during the hospitalization. The prevalence of patients at risk for delirium for each day varies from 53% to 60% (Figure 1, blue line). Instead, the prevalence of delirium (4AT score higher than 4) for each day varies from 19% to 29% (Figure 1, red line).

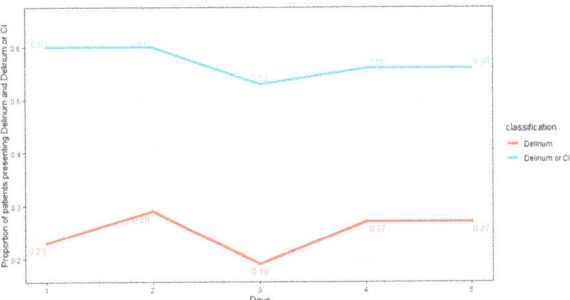

Figure 1. Proportions of patients reporting delirium and risk for delirium during the first five days of hospitalization. The delirium state indicates a 4AT score higher than 4; the delirium or cognitive impairment (CI) state indicates a 4AT score higher than 1.

Patients with a 4AT score that suggest delirium or cognitive impairment were prevalently in geriatrics 7 (39%) and orthopedics 8 (44%) wards (*p*-value < 0.001), had mainly dementia 8 (44%, *p*-value 0.007) and were aged between 91–95 years of age 7 (39%, *p*-value 0.035) (Table 1).

The RF model explained 75.8% of the variability of the 4AT score with an RMSE of 3.29, i.e., the average difference between the observed and predicted 4AT values is 3.29 points. Figure 2 shows the ranking of the predictors according to the importance attributed by the algorithm measured by the associated relative decrease in the model's predictive error.

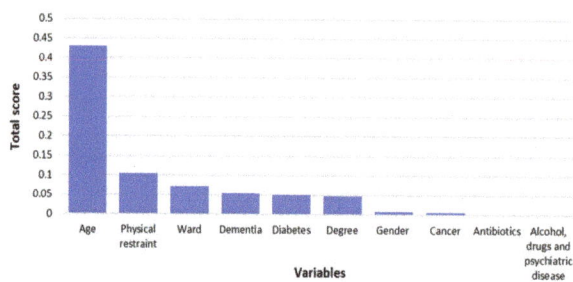

Figure 2. Variables with top importance selected by the RF algorithm according to the permutation approach. The total score measures the predictive impact of the variables, i.e., the relative decrease of the algorithm's predictive error produced by a variable.

For example, when age is considered, the algorithm's predictive error decreases by 43.1%. Age, the presence of physical restraint, dementia, type of ward, educational level, and gender, were the variables most associated with the 4AT score. Table 2 shows the predicted median (I and III quartiles) 4AT score values for each relevant variable marginalized over all the other variables. The 4AT predicted score values were obtained using the PDPs approach.

Table 2. Description of variables' effect on the 4AT delirium score. The "4AT score" column reports the median (I and III quartiles) 4AT delirium score predicted by the model conditional on the variable's values.

Variable		4AT Score
Age	78	2.09 [1.97–2.2]
	84	1.35 [1.25–1.44]
	87	1.58 [1.49–1.68]
	91	2.59 [2.5–2.68]
Dementia	No	2.36 [2.32–2.42]
	Yes	3.72 [3.69–3.79]
Gender	Female	2.69 [2.64–2.77]
	Male	2.97 [2.92–3.07]
Physical restraint	No	1.78 [1.75–1.84]
	Yes	3.2 [3.15–3.28]
Educational level	Bachelor's degree	2.79 [2.74–2.87]
	None	2.69 [2.65–2.75]
	Primary school	2.66 [2.61–2.74]
	Secondary school	2.85 [2.81–2.91]
	High school	3.01 [2.97–3.1]
Diabetes	No	2.51 [2.48–2.6]
	Yes	3.14 [3.07–3.2]
Ward	Medicine	2.77 [2.73–2.85]
	Geriatric	3.57 [3.54–3.62]

Table 2. Cont.

Variable		4AT Score
	Orthopedic	2.32 [2.29–2.4]
Cancer	No	2.78 [2.73–2.86]
	Yes	2.78 [2.73–2.86]
Antibiotics	<1	2.53 [2.49–2.61]
	≥1	2.87 [2.82–2.95]
Previous hospital admission	No	2.73 [2.69–2.82]
	Yes	2.71 [2.67–2.8]
Alcohol, drugs and psychiatric disease	<1	2.72 [2.68–2.82]
	≥1	2.8 [2.76–2.89]

For example, if suffering from dementia, the RF algorithm predicts a median 3.72 4AT score (3.69 as I Quartile and 3.79 as III Quartile), whereas a median 2.36 4AT score (2.32 as I Quartile and 2.42 as III Quartile) is predicted by the model if the subject did not suffer from dementia. The subject's characteristics that increase the 4AT score are higher age (2.59 [2.5–2.68]), the presence of dementia (3.72 [3.69–3.79]), physical restraint (3.2 [3.15–3.28]), diabetes (3.14 [3.07–3.2]), and a lower degree. Moreover, patients in the geriatrics and medicine ward, along with patients that have more than one antibiotic and previous admission to the hospital, are at higher risk of facing delirium onset.

Figures 3 and 4 report the effect of the variables on the 4AT score obtained using the PDPs approach. For example, a patient aged 92 years of age report an estimated 4AT score of 7 (Figure 3).

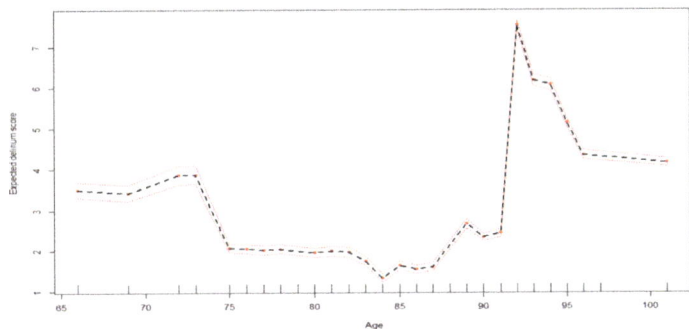

Figure 3. Effect of age on the 4AT delirium score. Expected delirium score estimated with random forest has been reported on the y axis according to ages with 95% confidence bounds.

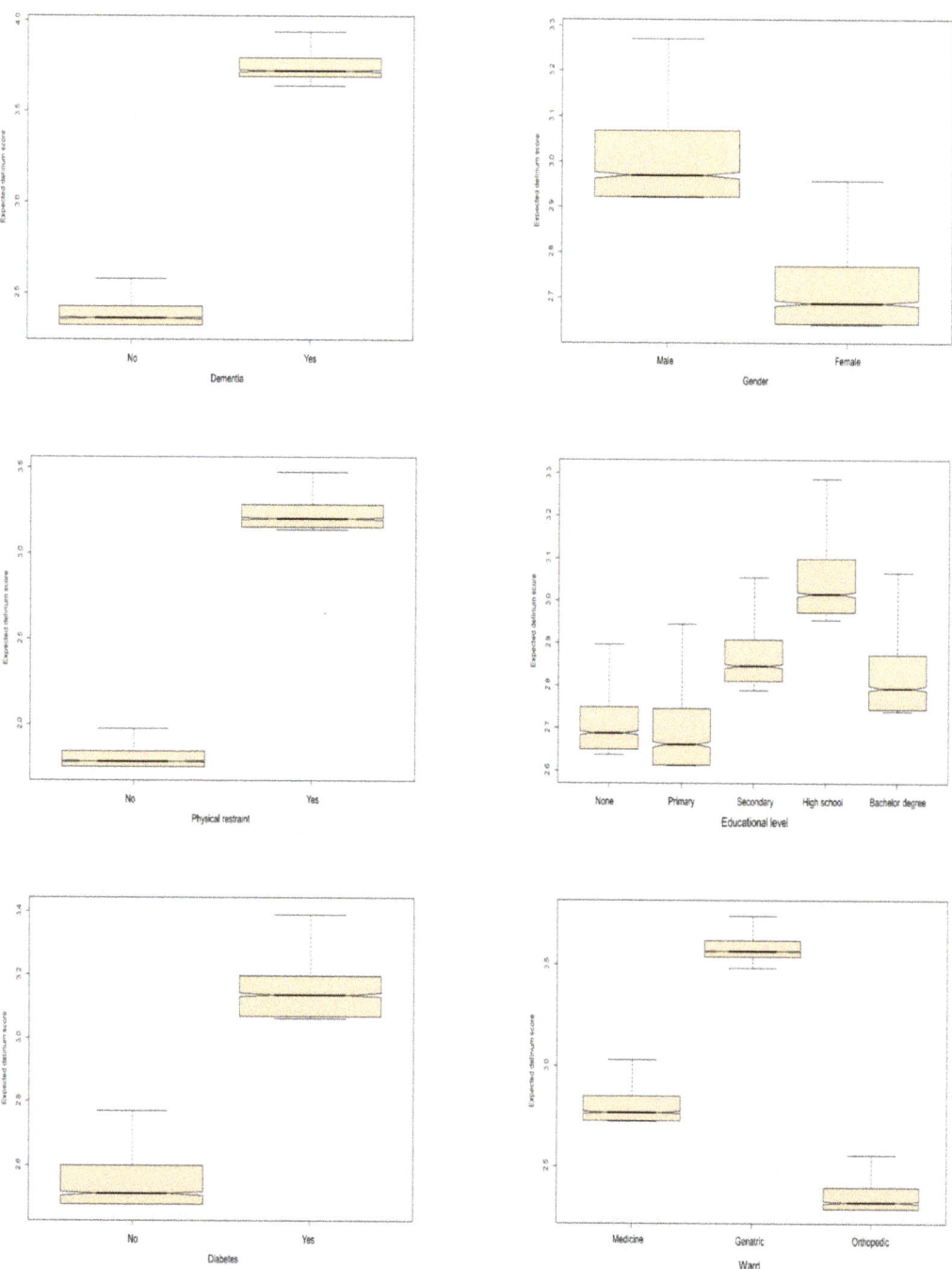

Figure 4. Effect of the presence of dementia, gender, physical restraint, educational level, diabetes, ward, antibiotics, and previous admissions on the 4AT delirium score. The vertical axis displays the ensemble expected predicted delirium score.

4. Discussion

Our findings are consistent with those existing in the literature [24,50], except those related to prevalence. It should be noted that other studies have mainly focused on incidence rather than prevalence [24,51]. Our patients show a higher prevalence of delirium (41%) compared to those of Bellelli [5] (22.9%) and Zuliani [18] (37%), which are studies conducted in similar settings. This difference in the prevalence could be explained by the assessment of delirium in our study in wards such as orthopedics, geriatrics, and general medicine where risk factors for delirium are commonly present [52]. Our results, however, when considering patients at risk for delirium (63%), are similar to those reported in the study of Gehrke in patients older than 90 years in an internal medicine ward (69%) [53] and in a Colombian study in a geriatric unit where the prevalence was 51.03% [54].

As in the study of Belelli, [5], in our RF model, delirium is associated with older age, gender, use of antibiotics, physical restraints, and ward of admission. In this study, the variables that influence the increase of the 4AT score are the ones chosen from the models and already considered as predictors of delirium in other studies [3,5,55]. However, some of the factors such as predisposing ones (e.g., disability) and the precipitating factors (use of drugs active on SNC, peripheral venous and urinary catheters) do not increase the 4AT score in our group.

Several studies have tried to identify risk factors both with traditional statistical methods [55,56] and with MLT [57–60]. The studies on MLT usually use patients' characteristics retrieved in healthcare records only in the first 24/48 h after admission. In our study, we have developed the RF algorithm accounting for all the patient's records observed from the admission to the end of the study. In literature, age is one of the most predictive variables in delirium onset using MLT, regardless of the kind of algorithm [28,57,59,61] as also shown in our results.

Recent applications of the ML technique in predicting the risk factors of delirium onset have shown good results in favor of these techniques. In the study of Wong [59], delirium onset was evaluated using different MLTs, i.e., RF, artificial neural networks, etc., and showed that all ML methods outperform the Nu-Desc clinical tool for delirium risk assessment. The authors observed that gradient boosting machine (GBM) shows the best predictive performances with an AUC of 0.855, suggesting a good predictive ability. Davoudi [62] also, compared different ML approaches in delirium detection risk factors, showing that RF and generalized additive models (GAM) were the ones that best predict it with an AUC of 0.85 (0.83–0.86) and 0.86 (CI: 0.84–0.88) respectively. In the study of Corradi [27] instead, the RF model was the model used for predicting delirium episodes with an AUC of 0.909 (95% CI 0.898 to 0.921). All the models presented in these studies show better performance when compared to a clinical tool. Another recent study have developed a predictive model for post-operative delirium in older surgical patients with better performances than chance, but with similar performances when compared with the traditional stepwise logistic regression [26]. Another recent study has showed the high predictive ability of RF model in detection delirium based on CAM and delirium observation screening scale (DOSS) [28].

Limitations

The present results cannot be generalizable to the whole hospital since the study has taken place in wards, where risk factors for delirium onset are higher compared to the other settings. Furthermore, data are limited thus avoiding the possibility of establishing a setting-specific prevalence of delirium. In this study, the 4AT score was used over several days, although it is suggested to submit it only once for delirium detection. The choice to adopt this tool derives from its simplicity of use and it allows comparison with other studies on the prevalence of delirium in different health contexts. From a statistical point of view, the low number of subjects enrolled in the study and the absence of an external dataset to validate the algorithm performances may limit the generalizability of the findings and the reliability of the model.

The present results show that MLT can identify complex relationship among data, so in the future it would be interesting to use those techniques to define delirium risk factors instead of traditional approaches. Moreover, it would be important to consider delirium as a "dynamic" condition influenced by different factors that are working in different moments as also theorized by Fan et al. [60] and applied in a recent work of our group [61].

5. Conclusions

Early detection of delirium must be a purpose to pursue in wards with a high percentage of risk factors, to adequately treat them and to avoid side effects. The routine uses of a simple instrument, such as the 4AT scale, could help to increase the awareness of delirium among health care workers. Healthcare personnel, especially nurses, thanks to their strictly engagements with patients, must be trained to easily recognize risk factors for delirium. As hypothesized in the recent work of Oberai et al. 2021 [57], nurses require educational intervention that include a variety of teaching style. Moreover, our results, following existing literature, shows that to predict correctly delirium is more useful to use predictive models that consider many factors collected routinely. These methods may also help in small case-series even if they are thought to be useful for large data sets. MLT can identify complex relations between variables and are helpful in structuring predictive models to personalize healthcare assistance.

Author Contributions: Conceptualization, D.G. and M.D.; methodology, D.G.; formal analysis, D.B. and D.A.; resources, M.D. and L.S.; data curation, D.B.; writing—original draft preparation, H.O.; writing—review and editing, S.S., D.A., G.L., A.S.A.; supervision, D.G. and G.L.; project administration, M.D. and L.S. All authors have read and agreed to the published version of the manuscript.

Funding: This research received no external funding.

Institutional Review Board Statement: Ethical review and approval were waived for this study, since the project was conducted within the framework thesis preparation of the nursing student, and it was approved by the internal offices at the University Hospital of Padova. This study is based on data collected in the context of the routine clinical practice. Patients, during hospital admission, provided their consent for the data treatment for scientific purposes. Patients' data of this retrospective study were completely anonymized before analysis. For this reason, it was not necessary to have ethical board approval.

Informed Consent Statement: Informed consent was obtained from all subjects involved in the study.

Data Availability Statement: The data presented in this study are available on request from the corresponding author. The data are not publicly available due to privacy.

Conflicts of Interest: The authors declare no conflict of interest.

References

1. American Psychiatric Association. *Diagnostic and Statistical Manual of Mental Disorders*, 5th ed.; American Psychiatric Association: Washington, DC, USA, 2013; ISBN 978-0-89042-555-8.
2. Bellelli, G.; Brathwaite, J.S.; Mazzola, P. Delirium: A Marker of Vulnerability in Older People. *Front. Aging Neurosci.* **2021**, *13*, 626127. [CrossRef] [PubMed]
3. Inouye, S.K. Predisposing and Precipitating Factors for Delirium in Hospitalized Older Patients. *Dement. Geriatr. Cogn. Disord.* **1999**, *10*, 393–400. [CrossRef] [PubMed]
4. Bull, M.J.; Boaz, L.; Jermé, M. Educating Family Caregivers for Older Adults about Delirium: A Systematic Review. *Worldviews Evid. Based Nurs.* **2016**, *13*, 232–240. [CrossRef] [PubMed]
5. Bellelli, G.; Morandi, A.; Di Santo, S.G.; Mazzone, A.; Cherubini, A.; Mossello, E.; Bo, M.; Bianchetti, A.; Rozzini, R.; Zanetti, E.; et al. "Delirium Day": A Nationwide Point Prevalence Study of Delirium in Older Hospitalized Patients Using an Easy Standardized Diagnostic Tool. *BMC Med.* **2016**, *14*, 106. [CrossRef]
6. Marquetand, J.; Bode, L.; Fuchs, S.; Hildenbrand, F.; Ernst, J.; von Kaenel, R.; Boettger, S. Risk Factors for Delirium Are Different in the Very Old: A Comparative One-Year Prospective Cohort Study of 5831 Patients. *Front. Psychiatry* **2021**, *12*, 655087. [CrossRef]
7. Wu, J.; Yin, Y.; Jin, M.; Li, B. The Risk Factors for Postoperative Delirium in Adult Patients after Hip Fracture Surgery: A Systematic Review and Meta-Analysis. *Int. J. Geriatr. Psychiatry* **2021**, *36*, 3–14. [CrossRef]
8. Visser, L.; Prent, A.; Banning, L.B.D.; van Leeuwen, B.L.; Zeebregts, C.J.; Pol, R.A. Risk Factors for Delirium after Vascular Surgery: A Systematic Review and Meta-Analysis. *Ann. Vasc. Surg.* **2021**. [CrossRef]

9. Rong, X.; Ding, Z.-C.; Yu, H.; Yao, S.-Y.; Zhou, Z.-K. Risk Factors of Postoperative Delirium in the Knee and Hip Replacement Patients: A Systematic Review and Meta-Analysis. *J. Orthop. Surg.* **2021**, *16*, 76. [CrossRef]
10. Tomlinson, E.J.; Phillips, N.M.; Mohebbi, M.; Hutchinson, A.M. Risk Factors for Incident Delirium in an Acute General Medical Setting: A Retrospective Case–Control Study. *J. Clin. Nurs.* **2017**, *26*, 658–667. [CrossRef]
11. Zhou, S.; Deng, F.; Zhang, J.; Chen, G. Incidence and Risk Factors for Postoperative Delirium after Liver Transplantation: A Systematic Review and Meta-Analysis. *Eur. Rev. Med. Pharmacol. Sci.* **2021**, *25*, 3246–3253. [CrossRef]
12. Watt, J.; Tricco, A.C.; Talbot-Hamon, C.; Pham, B.; Rios, P.; Grudniewicz, A.; Wong, C.; Sinclair, D.; Straus, S.E. Identifying Older Adults at Risk of Delirium Following Elective Surgery: A Systematic Review and Meta-Analysis. *J. Gen. Intern. Med.* **2018**, *33*, 500–509. [CrossRef]
13. Maldonado, J.R. Delirium in the Acute Care Setting: Characteristics, Diagnosis and Treatment. *Crit. Care Clin.* **2008**, *24*, 657–722. [CrossRef]
14. Leslie, D.L.; Marcantonio, E.R.; Zhang, Y.; Leo-Summers, L.; Inouye, S.K. One-Year Health Care Costs Associated with Delirium in the Elderly Population. *Arch. Intern. Med.* **2008**, *168*, 27–32. [CrossRef]
15. Fortini, A.; Morettini, A.; Tavernese, G.; Facchini, S.; Tofani, L.; Pazzi, M. Delirium in Elderly Patients Hospitalized in Internal Medicine Wards. *Intern. Emerg. Med.* **2014**, *9*, 435–441. [CrossRef]
16. Morandi, A.; Di Santo, S.G.; Cherubini, A.; Mossello, E.; Meagher, D.; Mazzone, A.; Bianchetti, A.; Ferrara, N.; Ferrari, A.; Musicco, M.; et al. Clinical Features Associated with Delirium Motor Subtypes in Older Inpatients: Results of a Multicenter Study. *Am. J. Geriatr. Psychiatry* **2017**, *25*, 1064–1071. [CrossRef]
17. Mossello, E.; Tesi, F.; Santo, S.G.D.; Mazzone, A.; Torrini, M.; Cherubini, A.; Bo, M.; Musicco, M.; Bianchetti, A.; Ferrari, A.; et al. Recognition of Delirium Features in Clinical Practice: Data from the "Delirium Day 2015" National Survey. *J. Am. Geriatr. Soc.* **2018**, *66*, 302–308. [CrossRef]
18. Zuliani, G.; Bonetti, F.; Magon, S.; Prandini, S.; Sioulis, F.; D'Amato, M.; Zampi, E.; Gasperini, B.; Cherubini, A. Subsyndromal Delirium and Its Determinants in Elderly Patients Hospitalized for Acute Medical Illness. *J. Gerontol.* **2013**, *68*, 1296–1302. [CrossRef]
19. Hargrave, A.; Bastiaens, J.; Bourgeois, J.A.; Neuhaus, J.; Josephson, S.A.; Chinn, J.; Lee, M.; Leung, J.; Douglas, V. Validation of a Nurse-Based Delirium-Screening Tool for Hospitalized Patients. *Psychosomatics* **2017**, *58*, 594–603. [CrossRef]
20. Kean, J.; Ryan, K. Delirium Detection in Clinical Practice and Research: Critique of Current Tools and Suggestions for Future Development. *J. Psychosom. Res.* **2008**, *65*, 255–259. [CrossRef]
21. Hshieh, T.T.; Yue, J.; Oh, E.; Puelle, M.; Dowal, S.; Travison, T.; Inouye, S.K. Effectiveness of Multi-Component Non-Pharmacologic Delirium Interventions: A Meta-Analysis. *JAMA Intern. Med.* **2015**, *175*, 512–520. [CrossRef]
22. Wong, C.L.; Holroyd-Leduc, J.; Simel, D.L.; Straus, S.E. Does This Patient Have Delirium? Value of Bedside Instruments. *JAMA* **2010**, *304*, 779–786. [CrossRef] [PubMed]
23. Van Velthuijsen, E.L.; Zwakhalen, S.M.G.; Warnier, R.M.J.; Mulder, W.J.; Verhey, F.R.J.; Kempen, G.I.J.M. Psychometric Properties and Feasibility of Instruments for the Detection of Delirium in Older Hospitalized Patients: A Systematic Review. *Int. J. Geriatr. Psychiatry* **2016**, *31*, 974–989. [CrossRef] [PubMed]
24. Inouye, S.K.; Westendorp, R.G.J.; Saczynski, J.S. Delirium in Elderly People. *Lancet* **2014**, *383*, 911–922. [CrossRef]
25. Bellelli, G.; Morandi, A.; Davis, D.H.J.; Mazzola, P.; Turco, R.; Gentile, S.; Ryan, T.; Cash, H.; Guerini, F.; Torpilliesi, T.; et al. Validation of the 4AT, a New Instrument for Rapid Delirium Screening: A Study in 234 Hospitalised Older People. *Age Ageing* **2014**, *43*, 496–502. [CrossRef]
26. Racine, A.M.; Tommet, D.; D'Aquila, M.L.; Fong, T.G.; Gou, Y.; Tabloski, P.A.; Metzger, E.D.; Hshieh, T.T.; Schmitt, E.M.; Vasunilashorn, S.M.; et al. Machine Learning to Develop and Internally Validate a Predictive Model for Post-Operative Delirium in a Prospective, Observational Clinical Cohort Study of Older Surgical Patients. *J. Gen. Intern. Med.* **2021**, *36*, 265–273. [CrossRef]
27. Corradi, J.P.; Thompson, S.; Mather, J.F.; Waszynski, C.M.; Dicks, R.S. Prediction of Incident Delirium Using a Random Forest Classifier. *J. Med. Syst.* **2018**, *42*, 261. [CrossRef]
28. Netzer, M.; Hackl, W.O.; Schaller, M.; Alber, L.; Marksteiner, J.; Ammenwerth, E. Evaluating Performance and Interpretability of Machine Learning Methods for Predicting Delirium in Gerontopsychiatric Patients. *Stud. Health Technol. Inform.* **2020**, *271*, 121–128. [CrossRef]
29. Ford, E.; Sheppard, J.; Oliver, S.; Rooney, P.; Banerjee, S.; Cassell, J.A. Automated Detection of Patients with Dementia Whose Symptoms Have Been Identified in Primary Care but Have No Formal Diagnosis: A Retrospective Case–Control Study Using Electronic Primary Care Records. *BMJ Open* **2021**, *11*, e039248. [CrossRef]
30. Jauk, S.; Kramer, D.; Großauer, B.; Rienmüller, S.; Avian, A.; Berghold, A.; Leodolter, W.; Schulz, S. Risk Prediction of Delirium in Hospitalized Patients Using Machine Learning: An Implementation and Prospective Evaluation Study. *J. Am. Med. Inform. Assoc.* **2020**, *27*, 1383–1392. [CrossRef]
31. Hendry, K.; Quinn, T.J.; Evans, J.; Scortichini, V.; Miller, H.; Burns, J.; Cunnington, A.; Stott, D.J. Evaluation of Delirium Screening Tools in Geriatric Medical Inpatients: A Diagnostic Test Accuracy Study. *Age Ageing* **2016**, *45*, 832–837. [CrossRef]
32. O'Sullivan, D.; Brady, N.; Manning, E.; O'Shea, E.; O'Grady, S.; O'Regan, N.; Timmons, S. Validation of the 6-Item Cognitive Impairment Test and the 4AT Test for Combined Delirium and Dementia Screening in Older Emergency Department Attendees. *Age Ageing* **2018**, *47*, 61–68. [CrossRef]

33. Gagné, A.-J.; Voyer, P.; Boucher, V.; Nadeau, A.; Carmichael, P.-H.; Pelletier, M.; Gouin, E.; Berthelot, S.; Daoust, R.; Wilchesky, M.; et al. Performance of the French Version of the 4AT for Screening the Elderly for Delirium in the Emergency Department. *Can. J. Emerg. Med.* **2018**, *20*, 903–910. [CrossRef]
34. Kuladee, S.; Prachason, T. Development and Validation of the Thai Version of the 4 'A's Test for Delirium Screening in Hospitalized Elderly Patients with Acute Medical Illnesses. *Neuropsychiatr. Dis. Treat.* **2016**, *12*, 437–443. [CrossRef]
35. Baird, L.; Spiller, J.A. A Quality Improvement Approach to Cognitive Assessment on Hospice Admission: Could We Use the 4AT or Short CAM? *BMJ Open Qual.* **2017**, *6*, e000153. [CrossRef]
36. Infante, M.T.; Pardini, M.; Balestrino, M.; Finocchi, C.; Malfatto, L.; Bellelli, G.; Mancardi, G.L.; Gandolfo, C.; Serrati, C. Delirium in the Acute Phase after Stroke: Comparison between Methods of Detection. *Neurol. Sci.* **2017**, *38*, 1101–1104. [CrossRef]
37. Lees, R.; Corbet, S.; Johnston, C.; Moffitt, E.; Shaw, G.; Quinn, T.J. Test Accuracy of Short Screening Tests for Diagnosis of Delirium or Cognitive Impairment in an Acute Stroke Unit Setting. *Stroke* **2013**, *44*, 3078–3083. [CrossRef]
38. De, J.; Wand, A.P.F.; Smerdely, P.I.; Hunt, G.E. Validating the 4A's Test in Screening for Delirium in a Culturally Diverse Geriatric Inpatient Population. *Int. J. Geriatr. Psychiatry* **2017**, *32*, 1322–1329. [CrossRef]
39. Benjamini, Y.; Hochberg, Y. Controlling the False Discovery Rate: A Practical and Powerful Approach to Multiple Testing. *J. R. Stat. Soc. Ser. B Methodol.* **1995**, *57*, 289–300. [CrossRef]
40. Kish, L. Survey Sampling. *Am. Polit. Sci. Rev.* **1965**, *59*, 1025. [CrossRef]
41. Long, J.S.; Ervin, L.H. Using Heteroscedasticity Consistent Standard Errors in the Linear Regression Model. *Am. Stat.* **2000**, *54*, 217–224.
42. Friedman, J.; Hastie, T.; Tibshirani, R. *The Elements of Statistical Learning*; Springer Series in Statistics; Springer: New York, NY, USA, 2001; Volume 1.
43. Breiman, L. Random Forests. *Mach. Learn.* **2001**, *45*, 5–32. [CrossRef]
44. Karpievitch, Y.V.; Hill, E.G.; Leclerc, A.P.; Dabney, A.R.; Almeida, J.S. An Introspective Comparison of Random Forest-Based Classifiers for the Analysis of Cluster-Correlated Data by Way of RF++. *PLoS ONE* **2009**, *4*, e7087. [CrossRef]
45. Ishwaran, H. Variable Importance in Binary Regression Trees and Forests. *Electron. J. Stat.* **2007**, *1*, 519–537. [CrossRef]
46. Friedman, J.H. Greedy Function Approximation: A Gradient Boosting Machine. *Ann. Stat.* **2001**, *29*, 1189–1232. [CrossRef]
47. R Core Team. *R: A Language and Environment for Statistical Computing*; R Foundation for Statistical Computing: Vienna, Austria, 2015.
48. Ishwaran, H.; Kogalur, U.B.; Kogalur, M.U.B. *Package 'RandomForestSRC'*, R package version 2; 2019. Available online: http://cran.stat.upd.edu.ph/web/packages/randomForestSRC/randomForestSRC.pdf (accessed on 19 July 2019).
49. Siddiqi, N.; Holt, R.; Britton, A.M.; Holmes, J. Interventions for Preventing Delirium in Hospitalised Patients. *Cochrane Database Syst. Rev.* **2007**. [CrossRef]
50. Landreville, P.; Voyer, P.; Carmichael, P.-H. Relationship between Delirium and Behavioral Symptoms of Dementia. *Int. Psychogeriatr.* **2013**, *25*, 635–643. [CrossRef]
51. Smith, T.O.; Cooper, A.; Peryer, G.; Griffiths, R.; Fox, C.; Cross, J. Factors Predicting Incidence of Post-Operative Delirium in Older People Following Hip Fracture Surgery: A Systematic Review and Meta-Analysis: Predictors of Delirium Post-Hip Fracture Surgery. *Int. J. Geriatr. Psychiatry* **2017**, *32*, 386–396. [CrossRef]
52. Gehrke, S.; Bode, L.; Seiler, A.; Ernst, J.; von Känel, R.; Boettger, S. The Prevalence Rates and Sequelae of Delirium at Age Older than 90 Years. *Palliat. Support. Care* **2020**, 1–6. [CrossRef]
53. Peralta-Cuervo, A.F.; Garcia-Cifuentes, E.; Castellanos-Perilla, N.; Chavarro-Carvajal, D.A.; Venegas-Sanabria, L.C.; Cano-Gutiérrez, C.A. Delirium Prevalence in a Colombian Hospital, Association with Geriatric Syndromes and Complications during Hospitalization. *Rev. Espanola Geriatr. Gerontol.* **2021**, *56*, 69–74. [CrossRef]
54. van Meenen, L.C.C.; van Meenen, D.M.P.; de Rooij, S.E.; ter Riet, G. Risk Prediction Models for Postoperative Delirium: A Systematic Review and Meta-Analysis. *J. Am. Geriatr. Soc.* **2014**, *62*, 2383–2390. [CrossRef]
55. Kim, M.; Park, U.; Kim, H.; Cho, W. DELirium Prediction Based on Hospital Information (Delphi) in General Surgery Patients. *Medicine* **2016**, *95*, e3072. [CrossRef] [PubMed]
56. Davoudi, A.; Ebadi, A.; Rashidi, P.; Ozrazgat-Baslanti, T.; Bihorac, A.; Bursian, A.C. Delirium Prediction Using Machine Learning Models on Preoperative Electronic Health Records Data. In Proceedings of the 2017 IEEE 17th International Conference on Bioinformatics and Bioengineering (BIBE), Washington, DC, USA, 23–25 October 2017; pp. 568–573. [CrossRef]
57. Wong, A.; Young, A.T.; Liang, A.S.; Gonzales, R.; Douglas, V.C.; Hadley, D. Development and Validation of an Electronic Health Record-Based Machine Learning Model to Estimate Delirium Risk in Newly Hospitalized Patients without Known Cognitive Impairment. *JAMA Netw. Open* **2018**, *1*, e181018. [CrossRef] [PubMed]
58. Veeranki, S.; Hayn, D.; Eggerth, A.; Jauk, S.; Kramer, D.; Leodolter, W.; Schreier, G. On the Representation of Machine Learning Results for Delirium Prediction in a Hospital Information System in Routine Care. *Stud. Health Technol. Inform.* **2018**, *251*, 97–100. [PubMed]
59. Veeranki, S.P.K.; Hayn, D.; Kramer, D.; Jauk, S.; Schreier, G. Effect of Nursing Assessment on Predictive Delirium Models in Hospitalised Patients. *Stud. Health Technol. Inform.* **2018**, *248*, 124–131.

60. Fan, H.; Ji, M.; Huang, J.; Yue, P.; Yang, X.; Wang, C.; Ying, W. Development and Validation of a Dynamic Delirium Prediction Rule in Patients Admitted to the Intensive Care Units (DYNAMIC-ICU): A Prospective Cohort Study. *Int. J. Nurs. Stud.* **2019**, *93*, 64–73. [CrossRef]
61. Ocagli, H.; Azzolina, D.; Soltanmohammadi, R.; Aliyari, R.; Bottigliengo, D.; Acar, A.S.; Stivanello, L.; Degan, M.; Baldi, I.; Lorenzoni, G.; et al. Profiling Delirium Progression in Elderly Patients via Continuous-Time Markov Multi-State Transition Models. *J. Pers. Med.* **2021**, *11*, 445. [CrossRef]
62. Oh, J.; Cho, D.; Park, J.; Na, S.H.; Kim, J.; Heo, J.; Shin, C.S.; Kim, J.-J.; Park, J.Y.; Lee, B. Prediction and Early Detection of Delirium in the Intensive Care Unit by Using Heart Rate Variability and Machine Learning. *Physiol. Meas.* **2018**, *39*, 035004. [CrossRef]

MDPI
St. Alban-Anlage 66
4052 Basel
Switzerland
Tel. +41 61 683 77 34
Fax +41 61 302 89 18
www.mdpi.com

International Journal of Environmental Research and Public Health Editorial Office
E-mail: ijerph@mdpi.com
www.mdpi.com/journal/ijerph

www.ingramcontent.com/pod-product-compliance
Lightning Source LLC
LaVergne TN
LVHW070152100526
838202LV00015B/1935

9 7 8 3 0 3 6 5 1 8 2 3 7